MICROBIOLOGY
for the Hospital Environment

MICROBIOLOGY
for the
HOSPITAL ENVIRONMENT

LOIS M. BERGQUIST

Los Angeles Valley College

1817

HARPER & ROW, PUBLISHERS, New York

Cambridge, Hagerstown, Philadelphia, San Francisco,
London, Mexico City, São Paulo, Sydney

Sponsoring Editor: Steven P. Heckel
Project Editor: Holly Detgen
Designer: T. R. Funderburk
Production Manager: Willie Lane
Compositor: Ruttle, Shaw & Wetherill, Inc.
Printer and Binder: Halliday Lithograph Corporation
Art Studio: J & R Technical Services Inc.
Cover Photograph: *Staphylococcus aureus.* Courtesy of Carolyn Luckenbach,
  Los Angeles Valley College, Van Nuys, California.

Microbiology for the Hospital Environment

Library of Congress Cataloging in Publication Data

Bergquist, Lois M
  Microbiology for the hospital environment.

  Includes index.
  1. Medical microbiology. I. Title.
QR46.B44   616'.01   80-19886
ISBN 0-06-040646-1

To T.J., B.J., and the ubiquitous microbe.

Contents

Preface

*There are no such things as pure and applied
science — there are only science and the
applications of science.* — Pasteur

Despite the large number of texts available in introductory microbiology, few are designed to meet the specific needs for training the health-care professional. Changing educational patterns now place students in clinical situations more rapidly than ever before. Many students receive their basic science education and clinical training simultaneously. The mere accumulation of scientific facts is not enough to ensure the effective application of microbiological principles in patient care. The student preparing for a career as a health-care professional needs the guidance provided by the experience of bedside personnel and the microbiology laboratory. Of primary importance are the recognition of the ubiquity of microorganisms and the vulnerability of hospitalized individuals to infectious disease.

Microbiology for the Hospital Environment is designed to provide a foundation in basic microbiology with particular emphasis on the application of its principles in the hospital environment. Two themes are developed in the text. First, pathogenicity is determined by microbial and host factors and their changing interactions. Second, the hospital environment represents a unique ecological niche for microorganisms.

Alterations in the microorganisms, the hosts, and the environment are responsible for changing patterns of infectious disease. Different microorganisms are emerging as pathogens. Today's health-care professional needs a knowledge of the classical pathogens as well as of the opportunistic microorganisms. Hospital-acquired infections were first documented in obstetric wards by Semmelweis and Holmes more than a century ago. Today it is estimated that still from 5 to 16 percent of patients admitted to hospitals in the United States each year develop infections as a result of hospitalization. It is hoped that a synthesis of basic and applied microbiology will lead to a better understanding of the role of all hospital personnel in the diagnosis, treatment, and prevention of infectious disease.

The book is organized into five units: Introduction to Microbiology; Microbial Metabolism and Variation; Host-Parasite Relationships; Microbial and Helminthic Diseases of Humans; and Control of Microorganisms.

Unit One, Introduction to Microbiology, describes a brief history of microbiology with emphasis on the germ theory of disease and the fruitful merger of molecular biology and microbiology. It contains a general survey of the microbial world and separate chapters devoted to a more detailed description of the anatomy of procaryotes and eucaryotes, the acellular viruses, and the multicellular helminths. Techniques for the observation of microorganisms — types of microscopy and preparation of materials for bright-field microscopy — are discussed in a separate chapter.

Unit Two, Microbial Metabolism and Variation, starts with a chapter on basic biochemistry since an understanding of microbial life begins on the molecular level. Emphasis is placed on the functions of major molecules, stressing recognition rather than memorization of structural formulas. One chapter is devoted to metabolism and regulation in microbial cells. Details of aerobic and anaerobic respiration are simplified to clarify understanding of energy turnover in cells. Negative feedback inhibition, repression, and induction are discussed as regulatory mechanisms. Another chapter is devoted to microbial growth and techniques for isolating and enumerating bacteria. A final chapter on microbial genetics includes such topics as phenotypic and genotypic variation, mutation, transformation, conjugation, transduction, and genetic engineering.

Unit Three, Host-Parasite Relationships, introduces the student to the indigenous microorganisms of humans. It contains material on the nature of immunity, with emphasis on the role of the T- and B-cell lymphocytes. The chapter on types of hypersensitivity provides examples of altered states of the immune response. A chapter on *in vitro* antigen-antibody reactions details the basis of those reactions in the diagnosis of infectious diseases. A final chapter is devoted to the nature of pathogenicity as a function of both host and microbial factors. The portal of entry, spread through tissues, effect of toxins, and transmission of infectious disease are presented from the general viewpoint that, regardless of the microbial agent, a variety of both host and microbial factors contribute to the disease process.

Unit Four, Microbial and Helminthic Diseases of Humans, is organized under the major body systems: skin, hair, and nails; respiratory tract; gastrointestinal tract; genitourinary tract; central nervous system; eye and ear; and blood, lymph, and reticuloendothelial system. A brief review of the anatomy of each system is included. The diseases are described in terms of etiological agent, transmission, laboratory diagnosis, immunity, and prevention. An attempt has been made to include laboratory methods that reflect advances in technology during the past several years.

Genus and species names of bacteria are those in the eighth edition of *Bergey's Manual of Determinative Bacteriology*.

Unit Five, Control of Microorganisms, contains a chapter on the principles of disinfection and sterilization with emphasis on the application of chemical, physical, and mechanical agents in the hospital environment. Another chapter discusses the use of antimicrobial and chemotherapeutic agents in the control of infectious agents. An attempt has been made to include drugs of choice for infections caused by fungi, viruses, protozoa, and helminths, as well as for those caused by bacteria. A chapter on the collection and handling of laboratory specimens is included, since an accurate diagnosis depends on adequate sampling, prompt delivery, and proper storage conditions. Finally, a chapter on the control of hospital-acquired infections is designed to help the student apply basic principles of microbiology to the prevention of nosocomial infections.

Each chapter is introduced by a list of student objectives and ends with questions for study. The objectives and questions can both be used by the student as guides for the evaluation of the learning process. Liberal use of diagrams and photographs is designed to clarify the concepts and descriptive material of the book.

The appendixes contain brief classifications of medically important groups or classes of bacteria, fungi, protozoa, viruses, and helminths; a list of proprietary and generic names of selected antimicrobial and chemotherapeutic agents; and descriptions of immunizing agents for some major diseases. The appendixes are intended for reference only, but can be used as a body of teaching material if so desired.

It is hoped that *Microbiology for the Hospital Environment* will help students preparing for the health-care professions to relate basic principles of microbiology to the hospital environment, that it will create an awareness of changing host and microbial factors, that it will focus attention on opportunistic as well as classical pathogens, and that it will stimulate a continuing interest in infection control.

Preparation of the material for any textbook is a shared responsibility. The author is indebted to numerous individuals who reviewed the manuscript, contributed photographs, or supplied art work. Those deserving of special acknowledgment include David Bardell, Kean College of New Jersey; Gertrude Case Buehring, University of California, Berkeley; Joan M. Campbell and Micheline H. Carr of Los Angeles Valley College; Alice C. Helm, University of Illinois, Urbana-Champaign; Mary Jorgenson and Taekyung Kim of Saint Joseph Medical Center, Burbank; Lois H. Lindberg, California State University, San Jose; Leland S. McClung, Indiana University; Eloise A. Nelson, Saint Joseph Medical Center, Burbank; Philip Penner, Borough of Manhattan Community College; Eddie C. Reaux, El Centro College; Angelyn K. Riffenburgh, Los Angeles Valley College; Ruth Russell, California State University, Long Beach; Edward C. Schleg, Mott Community College; Bernice C. Stewart, Prince George's Community College; Muriel H. Svec, Santa Monica City

College; and Priscilla B. Wyrick, University of North Carolina School of Medicine. Special acknowledgment is made to my mother, Teckla J. Bergquist, for her patience and understanding during the preparation of the text; to Ellen M. Swartzenburg, typist extraordináire, who prepared manuscript material; and to staff members of Harper & Row, Publishers, Inc., for their effort and additional expertise.

Lois M. Bergquist

MICROBIOLOGY
for the Hospital Environment

Unit One

INTRODUCTION TO MICROBIOLOGY

Chapter 1

A Brief History of Microbiology

After you read this chapter, you should be able to:

1. Describe the origin of the germ theory of disease.
2. Explain the methods used to disprove the theory of spontaneous generation.
3. Discuss major contributions of nineteenth- and twentieth-century scientists to the developing science of microbiology.
4. Explain the basis of cellular and humoral immunity as purported by Metchnikoff and Ehrlich.
5. Explain the basis of vaccination in prevention of infectious diseases.
6. Explain why chemotherapeutic agents have not eradicated infectious diseases.
7. Identify a role for viruses other than a cause of disease.

Microorganisms have always been a part of the human environment; their actions were observed long before it was possible to see the microorganisms themselves. Antony van Leeuwenhoek (1632–1723) was the first to record microscopic observations of stagnant water, infusions, and scrapings from teeth. His microscope consisted of a primitive biconcave lens mounted between two thin plates of metal (Figure 1-1). The lens had a magnification of approximately 300 so that van Leeuwenhoek was able to discern some differences in size and shape of the protozoa and bacteria which he called "animalcules" (Figure 1-2).

Even before van Leeuwenhoek's observations, Fracastoro of Verona (1483–1553) had suggested that diseases were caused by invisible particles which could be transmitted from person to person. The invisible particles, as well as frogs, mice, and eels, were believed to arise from mud, decaying food, or warm rain. The belief in an inanimate spontaneous origin for living things was known as the *theory of spontaneous generation.* The almost universal acceptance of this theory diverted attention from people as possible sources of infectious agents until the almost simultaneous observations made by two physicians in different parts of the world.

THE GERM THEORY OF DISEASE

In the United States Oliver Wendell Holmes (1809–1894) demonstrated that death following childbirth was often caused by material originating from the

4

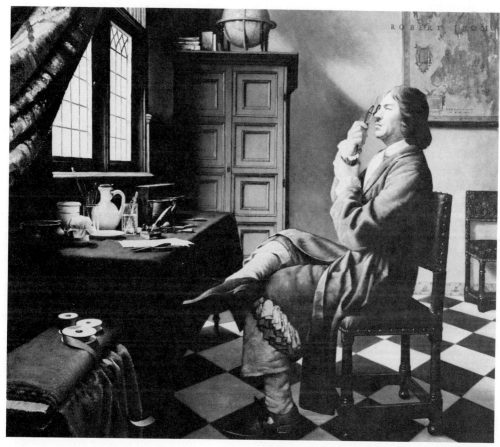

Figure 1-1 Antony van Leeuwenhoek (1632–1723) observing microorganisms he called "animalcules" in his laboratory. (Courtesy, Parke, Davis & Company,© 1959.)

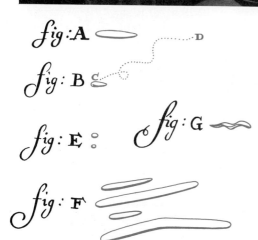

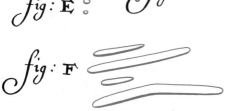

Figure 1-2 Drawings of "animalcules" of the human mouth from van Leeuwenhoek's original engravings showing variation in size and shape as well as the direction of movement for a motile microorganism.

hands of midwives or attending physicians. In a paper published in 1843 he stated:

> The disease known as puerperal fever is so far contagious as to be frequently carried from patient to patient by physicians and nurses. . . .

In Vienna Ignaz Semmelweis (1818–1865), the Hungarian physician, observed that death rates were higher in maternity wards staffed by medical students than in those attended by midwives. Furthermore, he noted that death rates went down in maternity wards during the summer when medical school students were absent. Investigation revealed that medical students were coming immediately from the autopsy room to maternity wards without washing their hands! When the medical students were required to wash their hands in a solution of chlorine before being admitted to the maternity wards, the number of infections and deaths was reduced. Semmelweis's observations were published in 1847, but his recommendations on asepsis were not widely accepted. In the controversy that followed, Semmelweis returned to his native Hungary. He died in 1865 without receiving the recognition he so richly deserved for reducing death rates in maternity wards.

It remained for the French chemist, Louis Pasteur (1822–1895), to disprove the theory of spontaneous generation and to associate living microorganisms with disease (Figure 1-3). The remarkable contributions of Pasteur to the field of microbiology began with his logic, discipline, and ability to ask questions. The questions asked by Pasteur, when studying infectious diseases, are as appropriate today as they were in 1880:

> Where does the disease come from? How is it propagated? Is it not possible that the exact knowledge of its etiology could lead to prophylactic measures?

A consideration of some of Pasteur's contributions is necessary to gain perspective concerning the then emerging science of microbiology.

ORIGIN OF MICROBIAL LIFE

In 1856 Pasteur was commissioned by an industrialist of Lille to investigate a problem which had arisen in the manufacture of alcohol. The beet juice, from which alcohol was derived, was contaminated with a grey material which interfered with alcohol production. Pasteur's decision to accept that challenge was to be the turning point of his career. During the course of the investigation his attention was rather abruptly focused on the role of microorganisms in alcoholic fermentation and spoilage. He was able to demonstrate that particular yeasts were responsible for the fermentation process and that the lack of an alcoholic end product was caused by other acid-producing microscopic rods making up the grey material of the "sick" vats.

In 1863 Napoleon III solicited Pasteur's help on another serious national problem. The usually flavorful wine, for which France had become so famous,

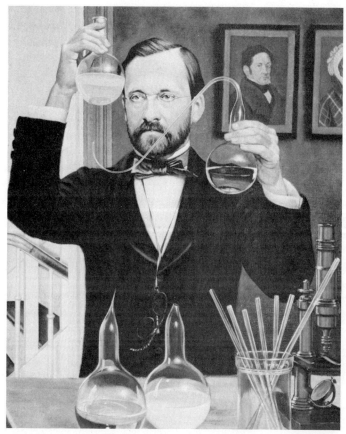

Figure 1-3 Louis Pasteur (1822–1895) at work in his laboratory where he unequivocally disproved the theory of spontaneous generation. (Courtesy, Parke, Davis & Company, © 1962.)

was souring in many parts of the country. The diseased wine was cutting at the heart of both the nation's pride and economy. Pasteur was able to attribute wine spoilage to the presence of contaminating microorganisms. The undesirable forms of life could be destroyed at temperatures of 50° to 60°C in a short period of time. Ultimately, a modified process of heating became known as *pasteurization*.

Pasteur entered the controversy of spontaneous generation with an unparalleled logic and a rigorous experimental approach. In the previous century an English priest, John Needham (1713–1781), and an Italian naturalist, Lazzaro Spallanzani (1729–1799), had experimented with heating infusions and made conflicting observations. Needham had found that living forms developed in both heated closed vessels and unheated open ones. He concluded, therefore, that life arose spontaneously from organic matter in his closed vessels. Spallanzani had shown that prolonged heating prevented microbial growth in closed flasks, but that organic contents of the flasks supported microbial growth when exposed to air. With Antoine Lavoisier's demonstration of the importance of oxygen to life in 1775, some doubted both Needham's and Spallanzani's conclusions and believed it was lack of oxygen which interfered with microbial life.

It was Pasteur who demonstrated the ubiquity of microorganisms in the air. Many of Pasteur's experiments were performed in the now famous swan-necked flasks (Figure 1-4). The tortuous

pathway afforded by the bends in the glass prevented dust particles, laden with microorganisms of the air, from entering heat-sterilized infusions. Instead, dust particles settled by gravity in the bends of the long-necked flasks. No signs of life appeared in sterilized infusions kept in the flasks even over extended periods of time. However, when the top of a flask was removed, the infusion was soon teeming with microbial life. Pasteur summarized the position of the opponents of spontaneous generation by saying:

There is no condition known today in which you can affirm that microscopic beings come into the world without germs, without

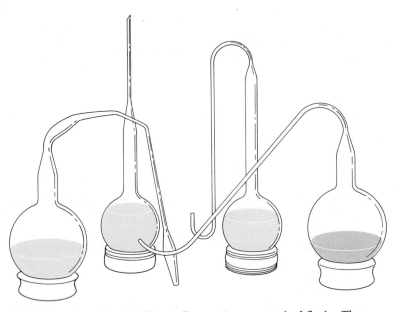

Figure 1-4 A collection of Louis Pasteur's swan-necked flasks. The contours of the flasks prevented the passage of microorganisms from the air to sterilized infusions.

parents, like themselves. They who allege it have been the sport of illusions, of ill-made experiments, vitiated by errors which they have not been able to perceive and have not known how to avoid.

The English physicist John Tyndall (1820–1893), a contemporary of Pasteur's, was able to explain satisfactorily the need for prolonged heating to eliminate microbial life from infusions. By exposing infusions to heat for varying times, Tyndall concluded that bacteria existed in two forms: a heat-stable form and a heat-sensitive form. It took either prolonged or intermittent heating to destroy the heat-stable form. Intermittent heating, now called *tyndallization*, killed both forms since between periods of heat treatment, the heat-stable forms changed to heat-sensitive forms. Almost simultaneously the German botanist, Ferdinand Cohn (1828–1898), described heat-resistant forms as spores. Spores, as well as the heat-sensitive or vegetative forms, were airborne and responsible for the appearance of microbial life in inadequately heated infusions.

Pasteur's latter years were devoted to studying infectious diseases, modes of transmission for causative agents, conditions required for cultivating microorganisms in the laboratory, and means for preventing infectious diseases. Pasteur extended the germ theory of disease from wines to animals and carefully elucidated the characteristics of the microorganisms associated with some diseases causing severe economic losses in France during his time. In 1878

Pasteur, in collaboration with Joubert and Chamberland, described the cause of anthrax, a devastating disease of livestock which sometimes affects humans, and of fowl cholera, a dreaded disease of chickens.

Joseph Lister (1827–1912), an English surgeon and contemporary of Pasteur's, was among the first to appreciate the ramifications of the emerging germ theory of disease. He attributed the frequent disastrous consequences following repair of compound fractures to invasions by airborne microorganisms. To reduce the risk of postsurgical infections, Lister advocated the use of carbolic acid as an aerosol during surgery and for impregnation of dressings. Pasteur was, no doubt, aware of Lister's work when he said:

If I had the honor of being a surgeon, since I am convinced of the dangerous conditions which can be caused by the germs of microbes which are to be found everywhere, especially in hospitals, not only would I use only instruments in a perfect state of cleanliness, but also having cleaned my hands with the greatest of care, I would flame them rapidly. . . .

It is fortunate that it is not necessary in today's hospital routine to flame the hands to prevent contamination!

PREVENTION OF INFECTIOUS DISEASE

There is evidence that both the Chinese and the Turks recognized the value of using material isolated from actual cases of infectious disease to promote a state of resistance. Voltaire described the ancient Chinese custom of placing dried smallpox crusts in the nose to prevent the feared disease. Around 1717 Lady Wortley Montague, the wife of the English ambassador to Turkey, wrote concerning an effective means of preventing smallpox by inoculating material from a smallpox pustule into a vein. Lady Montague permitted her own son to be inoculated in this manner and, although the procedure was not without risk, the child, along with hundreds of Turkish infants, apparently received life-long immunity against the disease.

The English physician, Edward Jenner (1749–1823), is usually credited with introducing the use of cowpox pustules to reduce the risk of the inoculation procedure (Figure 1-5). Jenner acted on the observation that milkmaids did not get smallpox if they had already contracted cowpox. Although some of Jenner's peers doubted the efficacy of using cowpox material for immunization against smallpox, by the time of his death the value of the cowpox inoculum was recognized. Pasteur honored Jenner by calling his own inoculation procedure against fowl cholera and anthrax a *vaccination*, a term derived from vaccinia, the other name for cowpox.

Pasteur decreased the virulence of the microorganisms of anthrax and fowl cholera by repeated culturing in the laboratory. The modification of an infectious agent to a less virulent form is a process referred to as *attenuation*. By 1882 Pasteur had demonstrated the effectiveness of the attenuated agents of anthrax and fowl cholera in the prevention of those diseases.

Perhaps the success which brought Pasteur the greatest satisfaction and

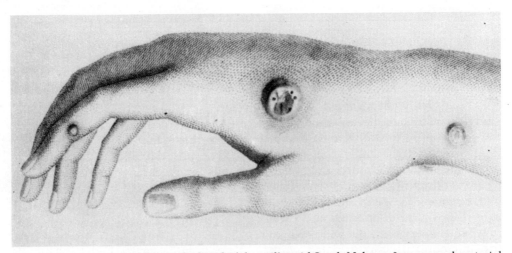

Figure 1-5 Cowpox lesions on the hand of the milkmaid Sarah Nelmes. Jenner used material from the lesions to protect individuals from smallpox in a procedure to become known as vaccination. (Courtesy, National Library of Medicine, Bethesda, Maryland 20014.)

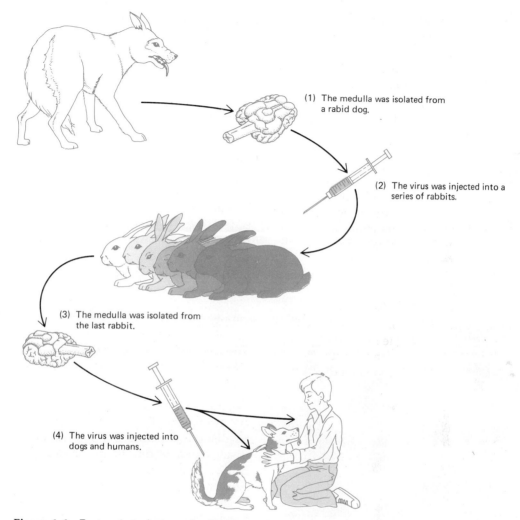

(1) The medulla was isolated from a rabid dog.

(2) The virus was injected into a series of rabbits.

(3) The medulla was isolated from the last rabbit.

(4) The virus was injected into dogs and humans.

Figure 1-6 Pasteur's technique for "taming" the rabies virus.

recognition was the preparation of the first vaccine for rabies, an animal disease that was invariably fatal in humans bitten by a rabid animal. Without ever isolating the causative agent of rabies, he was able to modify the virus by successive inoculations in rabbits. He then used the attenuated virus to immunize dogs against rabies and later to prevent rabies from developing in persons who had been bitten by rabid dogs (Figure 1-6).

In 1888 Pasteur received the honor of having built for him the laboratories of the Pasteur Institute in Paris. The laboratories provided the necessary space for the manufacture of vaccines and for continuing basic research. The Pasteur Institute attracted thousands of talented researchers and remains, to this day, a prestigious institution.

THE DEVELOPING SCIENCE OF MICROBIOLOGY

The work of Robert Koch (1843–1910), a German physician, provided the discipline needed to guide and assure the future of the developing science of microbiology (Figure 1-7). In his study of the anthrax problem in Germany, he was able to isolate the causative organism, to grow it in pure culture in the laboratory, and to show that the disease could be produced in another animal. When the culture was used for inoculation, he was able to recover the same organism in pure culture from the infected animal. The carefully planned experiments were the foundations for Koch's postulates, which consisted of guidelines for the association of particular microorganisms with specific infectious diseases (Figure 1-8). After his studies on anthrax Koch expressed his interest and confidence in the future:

> With a knowledge of comparative etiology of infectious diseases, we can learn to hold at bay the epidemic diseases of man.

In today's modern laboratories the isolation of microorganisms in pure culture is accepted as a necessary prerequisite for identifying specific organisms or for testing them for susceptibilities to antimicrobial agents. It was Koch who tackled the problem of how to grow microbes in pure culture—how to supply the organisms with required nutrients while keeping cultures free from contaminating microorganisms.

Koch first obtained pure cultures using slices of potato, but discovered that all bacteria would not grow on them. The need for a solid medium, as well as for nutrients, became evident. Fanny Hesse, a New Jersey–born wife of one of Koch's colleagues, recommended the use of agar-agar, a product derived

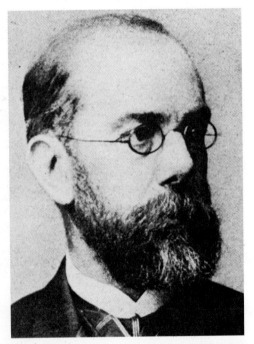

Figure 1-7 Robert Koch (1843–1910), who had a leading role in guiding the future of microbiology. (Courtesy, German Association for the Promotion of International Relations, copyright Presse-und Informationsamt der Bundesregierung.)

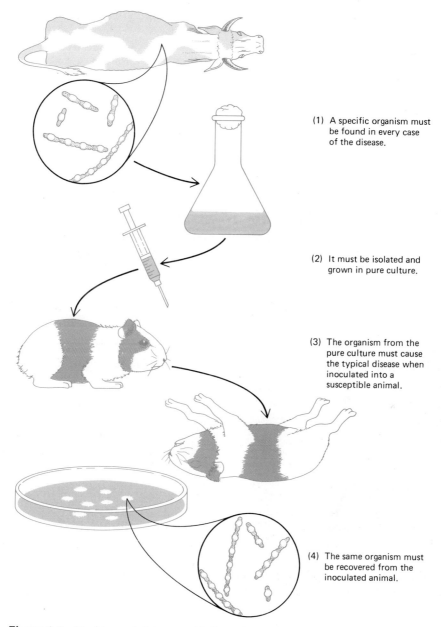

(1) A specific organism must be found in every case of the disease.

(2) It must be isolated and grown in pure culture.

(3) The organism from the pure culture must cause the typical disease when inoculated into a susceptible animal.

(4) The same organism must be recovered from the inoculated animal.

Figure 1-8   Koch's postulates — guidelines for proving that a specific microorganism is the causative agent for a particular disease.

from seaweed, as the solidifying agent. Purified agar is still employed today as the major solidifying agent for many types of media.

The two-part dish for growing bacteria also originated in Koch's laboratory. This dish consists of a round bottom section into which heated agar, enriched with nutrients, can be poured and a slightly larger cover which prevents contamination by airborne bacteria. It is called a *Petri plate* after its inventor, Julius Petri, an assistant of Koch's. Although the first Petri plates were made of glass, many laboratories today prefer to use disposable plastic Petri plates (Figure 1-9). The introduction of agar and Petri plates was a valuable contribution in the development of pure-culture techniques so necessary in studying the causative agents of disease.

Koch's interest in host-parasite relationships led him to undertake a study of tuberculosis. He not only isolated the causative organism in pure culture, but was able to show that it produced a disease characterized by lesions known as tubercles in experimental animals. Koch, furthermore, applied a staining technique, developed by his associate Ehrlich and later referred to as *acid-fast staining*, to differentiate the tubercle bacillus from other microorganisms. He demonstrated modes of transmission for the infecting organisms and then turned his attention to developing a therapeutic agent. Unfortunately, after years of work he had to abandon this pursuit. His proposed therapeutic agent, a material known as *tuberculin*, failed to control the disease, although it was to have value years later as an aid in the diagnosis of tuberculosis by skin testing.

While Koch was occupied with studies on tuberculosis, his students and colleagues were able to describe the infectious agents of erysipelas, tetanus, glanders, acute lobar pneumonia, epidemic cerebrospinal meningitis, typhoid fever, and diphtheria.

In 1881 the Institute of Infectious Diseases, headed by Koch, was established in Berlin. Staff members included Behring, Ehrlich, Pfeiffer, Kitasato, and Wassermann—all of whom turned out to be eminent microbiologists. In 1905 Koch was awarded a Nobel prize for his numerous contributions to medicine. It was, indeed, a golden era for microbiology.

IMMUNITY AND CHEMOTHERAPY

As the germ theory of disease was being so firmly established, associates of Pasteur and Koch turned their attention to an equally provocative subject— how the body resists infectious disease. There was much to be learned concerning the response of a host to the presence of disease-producing microorganisms. Pasteur and others had been able to control some microbial diseases in humans and other animals without understanding the basic mechanisms of infections. Early observations suggested that the concomitant inflammation of infection was caused in some manner by attempts of the body to rid itself of invasive agents.

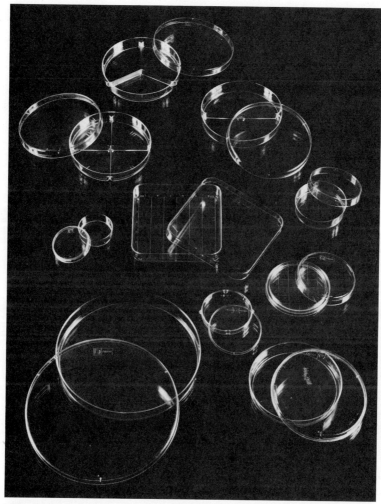

Figure 1-9   An array of plastic Petri plates. Some of the plates are partitioned so more than one type of medium may be used. Other plates contain grid markings for ease of counting colonies. (Courtesy, BBL Microbiological Systems, Division of Becton, Dickinson and Company, Cockeysville, Maryland.)

EMERGING ROLES FOR CELLULAR AND HUMORAL IMMUNITY

Elie Metchnikoff (1845–1916), a Russian working at the Pasteur Institute, formulated the theory of phagocytosis which experimental data later confirmed (Figure 1-10). He maintained that certain white blood cells were able to ingest and destroy invading microorganisms. He called those white blood cells

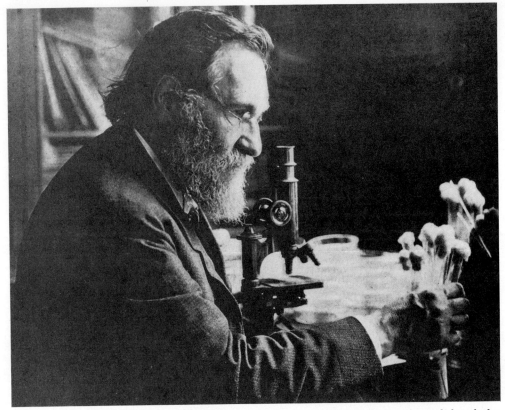

Figure 1-10 Elie Metchnikoff (1845–1916), a pioneer of microbiology who validated the process of phagocytosis. (Courtesy, National Library of Medicine, Bethesda, Maryland 20014.)

phagocytes and the process *phagocytosis*. Metchnikoff's careful observations provided the basis for a type of resistance known as *cellular immunity* (described in Chapter 12).

In Germany Paul Ehrlich (1854–1915), an associate of Koch's, hypothesized that immunity could be explained by the presence of noncellular blood components (Figure 1-11). The theory was later documented by Ehrlich and expanded by Emil von Behring (1854–1917), a Prussian bacteriologist, who, with the Japanese investigator Shibasaburo Kitasato (1856–1931), developed the first immunizing agents for diphtheria and tetanus. Their successful destruction of microorganisms in the absence of white blood cells confirmed the existence of fluid or *humoral immunity* as a major line of defense against disease (described in Chapter 12). A controversy between Metchnikoff and Ehrlich followed as to the importance of cellular and humoral immunity, but in 1908 they shared a Nobel prize for their

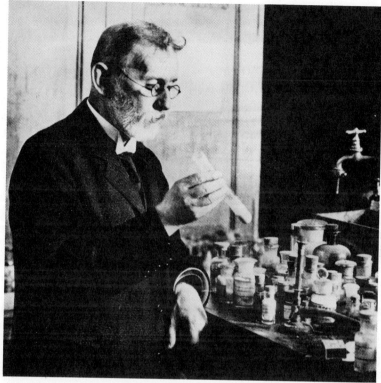

Figure 1-11   Paul Ehrlich (1854–1915) at work in his laboratory where he demonstrated the importance of humoral immunity and developed his "magic bullet" *Salvarsan*. (Courtesy, National Library of Medicine, Bethesda, Maryland 20014.)

contributions to the emerging science of immunology.

THE DISCOVERY OF CHEMOTHERAPEUTIC AGENTS

In 1906 Ehrlich made a discovery that gave him the title Father of Chemotherapy. The discovery was *Salvarsan* or 606, an arsenical compound—sometimes called the "magic bullet," which was capable of destroying the spirochete of syphilis with only moderate toxic side effects. The patience exhibited by this pioneer in investigative research is clearly illustrated by the alternate name of the drug, 606; it was the six hundred and sixth compound tested that finally yielded favorable results. Not satisfied that the drug could not be improved, he continued experimentation until in 1912 he announced the discovery of *Neosalvarsan*—the nine hundred and fourteenth trial drug.

Gerhard Domagk (1895–1964), the German chemist and pathologist, applied Ehrlich's methods to test the action of an azo dye, called *prontosil*, on microorganisms. Prontosil had been derived from para-aminobenzenesulfonamide by the Viennese chemist Gelmo. By careful testing, Domagk found that the agent was active against specific bacteria. The first success in treating streptococcal infections with the sulfonamide drug was reported in 1935. The efficacy of sulfonamides as chemotherapeutic agents received worldwide attention when a sulfa drug was credited with saving the life of Sir Winston Churchill when he contracted pneumonia in Algeria during World War II.

Domagk was to receive the Nobel prize in 1939 for his efforts, but was arrested by the Nazis before he could accept the award. It was not until 1947 that Domagk was able to go to Stockholm for the delayed presentation of his gold medal and diploma. The prize money had reverted back to the Nobel Foundation after the long delay. According to the rules of the foundation, money must be claimed within one year of the announcement of the award.

The testing of another antimicrobial agent that was to have an unmatched impact was proceeding in a laboratory in England. In 1928 Sir Alexander Fleming (1881–1955) accidentally discovered that a substance produced by the mold *Penicillium notatum* inhibited the growth of bacteria (Figures 1-12, 1-13). During experimentation on bacteria known as staphylococci, Fleming had neglected to discard inoculated Petri plates promptly. The additional time of incubation afforded by the delay had permitted a contaminating mold to grow and to elaborate a material that had destroyed colonies of the staphylococci.

Subsequent testing showed that this mold inhibited a number of disease-producing organisms. Furthermore, *penicillin*, an extract of the mold prepared by Fleming, appeared to be only slightly toxic to animals. Investigations on the chemotherapeutic agent continued until 1941 with the aid of Sir Howard Florey and Sir Ernst Chain. With the help of the United States, wide-scale production of penicillin began during World War II. The "miracle drug" was used successfully to treat Allied troops wounded in action and was effective against the causative organisms of both syphilis and gonorrhea. Fleming, Florey, and Chain shared the Nobel prize in 1945 for their work on penicillin.

The discovery that one microbe could produce an agent so potent against other microorganisms, but at the same time could be used without harm to patients, opened a new avenue of investigation — the search for additional substances with similar qualities derived from other molds or bacteria. There followed the isolation of antibiotics, such as streptomycin, the tetracyclines, and chloramphenicol.

The large-scale use of such drugs has not eradicated infectious diseases because many microorganisms demonstrate remarkable powers of survival. Some strains of bacteria, for example, are capable of producing an enzyme which destroys the antimicrobial activity of penicillin. Other microorganisms

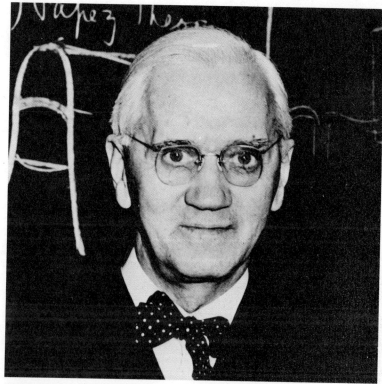

Figure 1-12 Sir Alexander Fleming (1881–1955), whose discovery of penicillin initiated the era of antibiotics. (Courtesy, National Library of Medicine, Bethesda, Maryland 20014.)

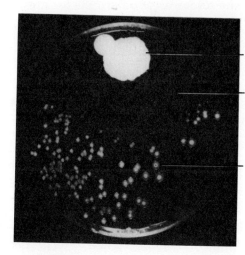

Penicillium colony

Staphylococci undergoing lysis

Normal staphylococcal colony

Figure 1-13 The original plate showing dissolution of staphylococcal colonies by a colony of the mold *Penicillium notatum,* as observed by Fleming in 1929. (From A. Fleming, *Brit. J. Exper. Path.* 10:228, 1929. Courtesy, National Library of Medicine, Bethesda, Maryland 20014.)

achieve a state of "antimicrobial indifference" and subsist at low levels of metabolic activities. The reason for this type of resistance to antibiotics is not well understood. There is evidence that genetic material, responsible for some types of resistance, is transferable from one bacterium to another.

Antimicrobial activity of naturally occurring products and resistance to their action represent powerful forces and complex processes in all natural microbial habitats. Medicine, and this textbook, focus on those processes involved when the human is the host to disease-producing organisms.

THE BEGINNINGS OF VIROLOGY

For many years the term *virus* was used to describe any poison or microbial agent capable of causing an infection. Unique characteristics of the particles now known as viruses permitted them to escape discovery for years. Not only are viruses ultramicroscopic, but they require living cells for replication. Viruses can pass through filters which retain larger microorganisms. Sophisticated laboratory techniques have shown that some particles, once thought to be viruses, actually are very small bacteria, some of which also need the resources of other cells for growth and multiplication.

DISCOVERY OF FILTERABLE AGENTS

The first man to describe a filtered extract capable of causing disease in plants was Dmitri Ivanovski (1864–1920), a Russian scientist, who started his studies on diseases of tobacco while he was still a student (Figure 1-14). In 1892 he found that the sap of leaves infected with mosaic disease retained its infectious properties even after passage through a filter designed to retain bacteria. He was unsure if he had discov-

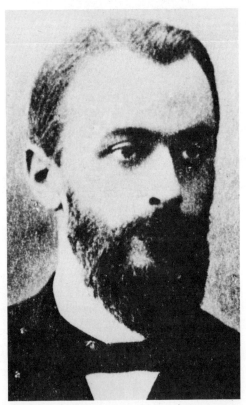

Figure 1-14 Dimitri Ivanovski (1864–1920), an early investigator of filterable agents. (Courtesy, National Library of Medicine, Bethesda, Maryland 20014.)

ered a small microorganism or a product of bacterial metabolism which had the ability to cause tobacco-mosaic disease. Mosaic or leaf spot disease is characterized by spotty blanching of leaves and localized death of tissue (Figure 1-15).

In 1898 Friedrich Loeffler (1852–1915) and Paul Frosch (1860–1928) reported from Germany that the causative organism of foot-and-mouth disease in cattle, likewise, could pass through a bacteriological filter. The same year Martinus Beijerinck (1851–1931), a Dutch botanist, unaware of Ivanovski's observations, attributed the cause of tobacco-mosaic disease to *contagium vivum fluidum*. In describing his conclusions he stated,

> The infection is not caused by microbes, but by a living liquid virus.

Many investigators still referred to the small particles as "filterable viruses," but in time the term filterable was dropped and the tiny infectious agents were merely called viruses. Thus, Ivanovski and Beijerinck became the pioneers of yet another branch of microbiology to be known as *virology*.

VIRUSES AS PREDATORS OF BACTERIA

After the turn of the century not only were viruses that caused diseases of other plants and animals described, but viruses which specifically attacked bacteria were discovered. In 1915 Frederick Twort (1877–1950) found that filter-passing particles could destroy bacteria

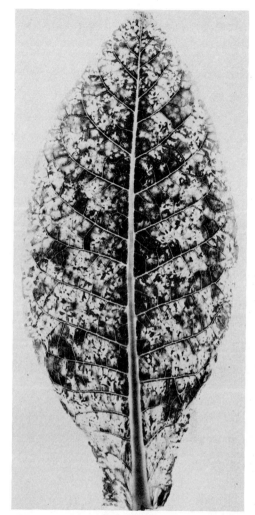

Figure 1-15 Tobacco leaf showing characteristic appearance of mosaic disease. (USDA photo.)

(Figure 1-16). In 1917 the same finding was made independently by Felix d'Hérelle (1873–1949) when he discovered a "transmissible" disease of bacteria while studying diarrhea of locusts (Figure 1-17). The excitement that the

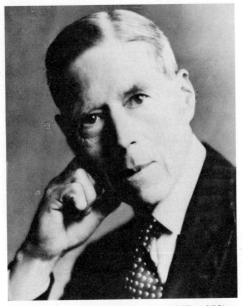

Figure 1-16 Frederick Twort (1877–1950), a bacteriologist who demonstrated the existence of bacteriophages, filter-passing agents that destroy bacteria. (Courtesy, The Wellcome Trustees, The Wellcome Institute for the History of Medicine, London.)

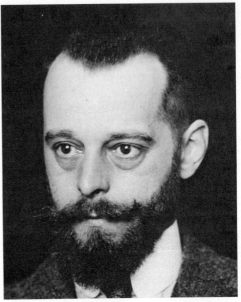

Figure 1-17 Félix d'Hérelle (1873–1949), who discovered a filterable virus which was parasitic on bacteria. (Courtesy, Archives photographiques du Musée Pasteur, Institut Pasteur, Paris.)

discovery of this event generated can be felt in d'Hérelle's own words.

> The next morning, on opening the incubator, I experienced one of those rare moments of intense emotion. . . . at first glance I saw the broth culture, which the night before had been very turbid, was perfectly clear; all the bacteria had vanished, they had dissolved away like sugar in water. As for the agar spread, it was devoid of all growth. . . . what caused my clear spots was in fact an invisible microbe, a filterable virus, but a virus parasitic on bacteria.

The newly discovered agents were called *bacteriophages*, meaning "bacteria eaters" (now frequently called simply *phages*). The use of phages and their specific bacterial hosts has made invaluable contributions to our understanding of host-parasite relationships because both host bacterial cells and their viral predators may be grown successfully in large quantities under laboratory conditions.

THE MOLECULAR BASIS OF LIFE

While progress was being made identifying the agents of infectious disease, elucidating the host's response to infection, and combating microbial diseases through immunization or chemotherapy, another challenging frontier of inquiry emerged—the discipline of molecular biology. The developing science, which attempted to explain life processes in molecular terms, occupied many eminent scientists.

Microorganisms proved to be invaluable models for studying the metabolism and genetics of cells. The rapidity with which bacteria grow permits investigators to study energy production and utilization under a variety of environmental conditions. Furthermore, the short generation times of microorganisms make it possible to observe inheritance in a large number of succeeding generations.

In 1944 the discovery of the chemical nature of hereditary material by Oswald Avery, Colin MacLeod, and Maclyn McCarty heralded the beginning of the merger between microbiology and molecular biology (Figure 1-18). The

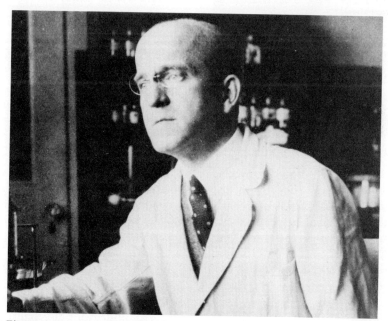

Figure 1-18 Oswald Avery (1877–1955), who with Colin MacLeod and Maclyn McCarty, showed that deoxyribonucleic acid (DNA) transformed nonvirulent pneumococci to virulent organisms. (Courtesy, National Library of Medicine, Bethesda, Maryland 20014.)

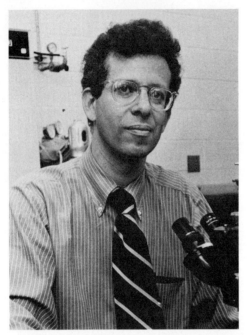

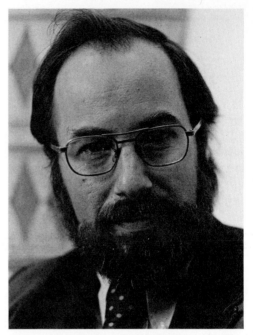

Figure 1-19 Howard Temin (born 1934), who was one of the first to demonstrate the process of reverse transcription and continues to study host cell-virus interactions. (Courtesy, University of Wisconsin, Madison.)

Figure 1-20 David Baltimore (born 1938), who independently demonstrated the presence of an RNA-directed enzyme in tumor viruses and shared the Nobel Prize in Physiology and Medicine in 1975 with Howard Temin and Renato Dulbecco. (Courtesy, Massachusetts Institute of Technology, Cambridge.)

role of that material, now known as deoxyribonucleic acid (DNA), as the sole agent of heredity was not challenged until 1970, when cumulative evidence from the research of Renato Dulbecco, Howard Temin, and David Baltimore demonstrated the presence of an RNA-directed enzyme in tumor viruses (Figures 1-19, 1-20).

The pertinence of the discovery of the RNA-dependent DNA polymerase to cell biology was summed up by Baltimore when he said:

It is important that investigation of such systems continue because the results have implications if for no other reason than to illustrate how virology can illuminate cell biology. . . . It is possible to imagine such systems having a role in the processes of differentiation, the workings of the immunological system and in the mechanisms of memory storage.

The fruits of the merger between microbiology and molecular biology continue to emerge as we enter a new century of microbiology.

SUMMARY

More than 100 years has passed since the early microbiologists began their studies on the cause and prevention of infectious diseases. More than 30 years has elapsed since DNA was discovered to be the major carrier of genetic material. As a result of the diligent efforts of microbiologists and molecular biologists, revolutionary changes in health, longevity, and economic productivity have occurred. Never before has this statement of Pasteur's had more meaning:

> There are no such things as pure and applied science—there are only science and the applications of science. . . .

The exploration of the nature and prevention of infectious disease continues in the laboratories of twentieth-century microbiologists and molecular biologists. When the emerging principles of microbiology are applied in everyday life, the fruits of their labor will be realized.

QUESTIONS FOR STUDY

1. List one contribution of each of the following men to microbiology.

van Leeuwenhoek	Ehrlich
Pasteur	Fleming
Koch	Ivanovski
Metchnikoff	Avery

2. How was the theory of spontaneous generation disproved?
3. Differentiate between cellular and humoral immunity as described by Metchnikoff and Ehrlich.
4. How can vaccinations and chemotherapy be used to combat infectious diseases?
5. Why did bacteria prove to be valuable in defining the roles of DNA and RNA in cells?

SELECTED REFERENCES

Brock, T. D. *Milestones in Microbiology.* Englewood Cliffs, N.J.: Prentice-Hall, 1961.

Bulloch, W. *The History of Bacteriology.* New York: Oxford University Press, 1938.

Dobell, C. *Antony van Leeuwenhoek and His "Little Animals."* New York: Dover, 1960.

Dubos, R. *The Unseen World.* New York: Rockefeller Institute Press, 1962.

Hayes, W. *The Genetics of Bacteria and Their Viruses.* 2d ed. New York: Wiley, 1968.

Lapage, G. *Man Against Disease.* New York: Abelard-Schuman, 1964.

Lechevalier, H. Dmitri Iosifovich Ivanovski (1864–1920). *Bacteriol. Rev.* 36:135, 1972.

Reid, R. *Microbes and Men.* New York: Saturday Review Press, 1975.

Roller, A. *Discovering the Basis of Life.* New York: McGraw-Hill, 1965.

Shaffer, M. F. A sesquicentennial reappraisal. *Amer. Soc. Microbiol. News* 38:280, 1972.

Stent, G. S. *Molecular Biology of Bacterial Viruses.* San Francisco: Freeman, 1963.

Chapter 2

A Survey of the Microbial World

After you read this chapter, you should be able to:

1. Describe two general patterns of cellular organization found in microorganisms.
2. Identify the metric units used in measuring microorganisms.
3. Differentiate between cyanobacteria and bacteria.
4. Describe three groups of nonphotosynthetic bacteria.
5. Explain the dependence of rickettsiae and chlamydiae on host cells.
6. Compare the morphology and structure of algae, protozoa, and fungi.
7. Differentiate between yeasts and molds.
8. Explain why viruses cannot be classified as procaryotes or eucaryotes.
9. Classify the particular groups of procaryotes and eucaryotes as photosynthetic or nonphotosynthetic organisms.
10. Describe several benefits derived from microbial populations on earth.
11. Explain the basis of the binomial system of nomenclature.
12. Differentiate between a scientific and a vernacular name.

The microbial world is made up of a diverse population of organisms usually visible only with the aid of a microscope. Many microorganisms consist of single cells; some are multicellular; still others, like the viruses, lack cellular organization and replicate only within the cytoplasm or nucleus of living cells.

Microorganisms are divided into two major groups on the basis of cell structure. Organisms with cells lacking internal membrane systems are called *procaryotes*. In procaryotic cells the nuclear region, though distinct from the cytoplasm, is not bounded by a membrane. Those organisms with cells having internal membrane systems enclosing specialized units of structure, including the nucleus, comprise the more complex group known as *eucaryotes*.

Because viruses do not exhibit cytological characteristics of either group, the ultramicroscopic forms must be considered apart from procaryotes or eucaryotes.

Microorganisms are measured in units known as *micrometers* (μm) or *nanometers* (nm). One micrometer is 0.0001 (10^{-4}) of a centimeter (cm) or about 0.00025 of an inch. One nanometer is 0.0000001 (10^{-7}) of a centimeter or 0.001 (10^{-3}) of a micrometer (Figure 2-1).

Some organisms which are macroscopic in size are included in the study of microbiology because of their role in the cause or transmission of disease. Some of the parasitic helminths or worms cause disease in vertebrate hosts. Their size, structure, and metabolic characteristics are so different from typical eucaryotic microorganisms that they, too, like the viruses, are studied as a separate category.

27

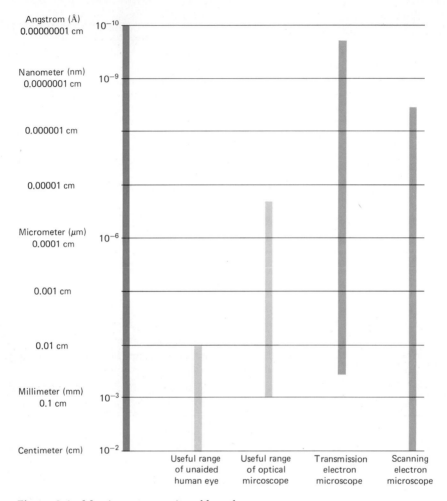

Figure 2-1   Metric system units of length.

Arthropods, such as fleas, flies, mosquitoes, true bugs, lice, ticks, and mites, transmit infectious diseases to humans; a few actually parasitize humans. Some knowledge of their role as vectors is required in studying particular microbial diseases.

THE PROCARYOTES

A procaryote may consist of a single cell or an association of simple cells having morphological, physiological, and biochemical similarities. The procaryotes have many characteristics in common, but the most important structural property they share is lack of internal membrane systems. Classification of the diverse forms in this group is summarized in Table 2-1.

PHOTOSYNTHETIC PROCARYOTES

Cyanobacteria. The cyanobacteria constitute a major group of structurally diverse microorganisms distinguished by the presence of chlorophyll a and one or more accessory pigments known as phycobiliproteins. The popular use of the term blue-green algae to describe the cyanobacteria is misleading and probably should be abandoned since the microorganisms resemble bacteria more than algae. Phycocyanin, a blue pigment, and chlorophyll a are responsible for the blue-green appearance. Some species contain phycoerythrin, a red pigment. (Their presence in large numbers in the Red Sea accounts in part for its name.) Cyanobacteria may be unicellular forms, ranging from 0.5 μm in diameter to cells as large as 60 μm in diameter. The cells, frequently, aggregate into colonies surrounded by sheaths or form filaments (Figure 2-2).

Cyanobacteria live in fresh water, salt water, or the soil. They may sometimes be found floating on the surface of lakes and ponds. A prominent feature of the cytoplasm is the accumulation of gas in clear spaces called *vacuoles*, that provide the buoyancy necessary for flota-

Table 2-1 AN ABBREVIATED CLASSIFICATION OF THE PROCARYOTES

I. Photosynthetic procaryotes
  A. Cyanobacteria
  B. Photopigmented bacteria
II. Nonphotosynthetic procaryotes
  A. Free-living forms and extracellular parasites
    1. Bacteria with cell walls
      a. with monolayered cell walls
      b. with double-layered cell walls
    2. Cell-wall deficient bacteria (mycoplasmas)
  B. Obligate intracellular parasites
    1. Rickettsiae
    2. Chlamydiae

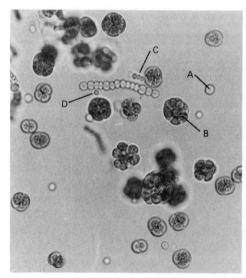

Figure 2-2 Cells of *Chlorogloea fritschii* illustrating major morphological types of cyanobacteria. *A,* single granulated cells; *B,* colonial aggregates surrounded by a sheath; *C,* small cells in short filaments; *D,* larger cells in long filaments. (From E. H. Evans, I. Foulds, and N. G. Carr, *J. Gen. Microbiol.* 92:149, 1976, Cambridge University Press.)

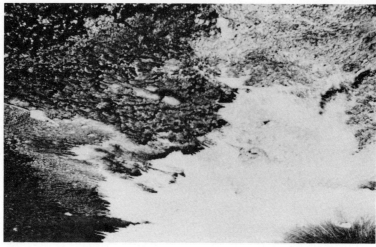

Figure 2-3 Cyanobacteria in hot springs where temperatures may reach 85°C. The photosynthetic procaryotes are more tolerant to extremes in temperature than the photosynthetic eucaryotes. (Courtesy, Carolina Biological Supply Company, Burlington, North Carolina.)

tion. The buoyancy also exposes the primitive forms to the sunlight required for the process of photosynthesis. Cyanobacteria are more tolerant to environmental extremes than photosynthetic eucaryotes. Some species are found, for example, in the hot springs of Yellowstone National Park where temperatures may reach 85°C (Figure 2-3).

Photopigmented Bacteria. The photopigmented bacteria are primarily aquatic forms containing pigments known as bacteriochlorophylls and carotenoids. They include the purple and green bacteria. Individual cells may be spherical (cocci), rod-shaped (bacilli), spiral-shaped (spirilla), or comma-shaped (vibrios). Some spheri-

cal forms measure only 0.3 μm in diameter, while some rod- or spiral-shaped organisms attain lengths of over 15μm (Figure 2-4). In photopigmented bacteria photosynthesis occurs under anaerobic conditions, differing from that process in cyanobacteria and green plants which requires atmospheric oxygen.

Mud, stagnant water, lakes, sewage lagoons, and ponds, which are rich in hydrogen sulfide, are popular habitats of the photosynthetic bacteria. Many exhibit motility in aquatic environments. Others are nonmotile under all conditions. Some photosynthetic bacteria contain gas vacuoles which resemble those found in cyanobacteria. A few species form aggregates with other bacteria or protozoa.

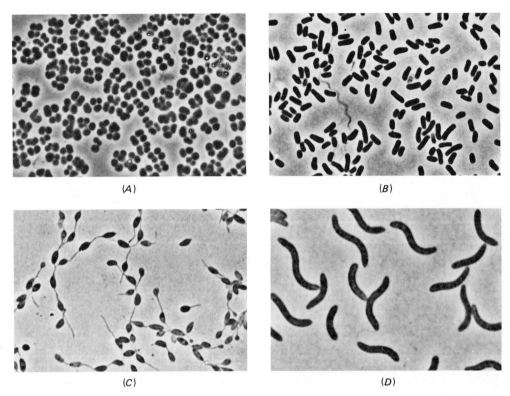

Figure 2-4   Four types of photosynthetic bacteria. (*A*) Aggregates of cocci. (*B*) Bacilli. (C) Ovoid cells originating from filaments. (*D*) Spirilla. (Courtesy, N. Pfenning, Gottingen, West Germany.)

NONPHOTOSYNTHETIC BACTERIA

The nonphotosynthetic bacteria are a heterogeneous group of microorganisms that do not contain photopigments. Most depend on organic compounds as sources of energy; a few obtain energy from inorganic sources. The nonphotosynthetic bacteria are ubiquitous in nature and are predominantly unicellular; some form simple associations of cells. The bacteria which

cause disease include (1) the free-living organisms with cell walls, (2) the free-living cell-wall deficient mycoplasmas, and (3) the obligate intracellular parasites with cells walls (the rickettsiae and the chlamydiae). Free-living organisms are able to live independently in nature without the cooperation of a host. The bacteria that produce cell walls can be classified according to shape as bacilli, cocci, or spirilla (Figure 2-5). Some of the organisms with cell walls synthesize monolayered cell walls; others

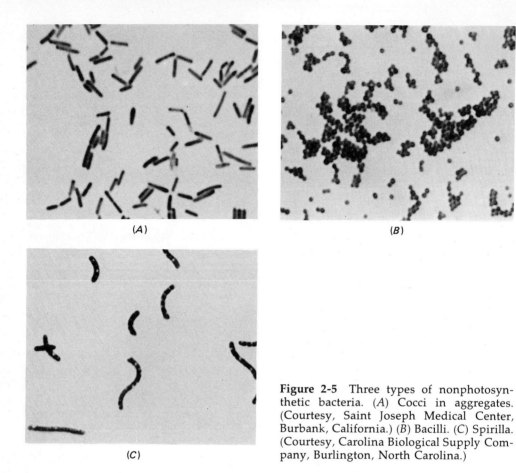

(A)

(B)

(C)

Figure 2-5 Three types of nonphotosynthetic bacteria. (A) Cocci in aggregates. (Courtesy, Saint Joseph Medical Center, Burbank, California.) (B) Bacilli. (C) Spirilla. (Courtesy, Carolina Biological Supply Company, Burlington, North Carolina.)

produce cell walls having at least two layers.

Mycoplasmas, another free-living form, are the smallest of the cellular organisms. The absence of protective cell walls makes them exceedingly vulnerable to environmental influences. The mycoplasmas are, therefore, often quite bizarre in shape.

The obligate intracellular parasites (the rickettsiae and chlamydiae) are dis-

tinguished by their limited metabolic capacity and requirement for host cells for multiplication.

Bacteria with Cell Walls. Although other characteristics of nonphotosynthetic bacteria with cell walls differ markedly, the basic shapes are usually constant for each species. *Bacilli* are rod-shaped and vary from 0.5 to 1.0 μm in width and from 1.0 to 3.0 μm in length. *Cocci* are spherical and usually measure 0.5 to 1.0 μm in diameter. *Vibrios* are short, slightly curved rods measuring 0.5 by 1.5 to 3.0 μm. *Spirilla* are curved rods which may attain lengths up to 60 μm, but more often are shorter. *Spirochetes* are flexuous, helical cells about 0.2 μm in width and up to 500 μm in length. Elongated coccal forms are sometimes called *coccobacilli.* Bacilli which occur as long threads are designated as *filamentous* bacilli; those with tapered ends are referred to as *fusiform* bacilli. Most bacteria exhibit some variation in size and shape depending on environmental conditions. The variation in morphology is called *pleomorphism.*

When viewed microscopically, some bacteria tend to appear in groups, rather than singly. Since fission may occur along more than one plane in cocci, those organisms are frequently observed in pairs, chains, tetrads, or clusters (Figure 2-6). Bacilli divide only across their short axes. Most often they occur singly, but may be seen in pairs, chains, or a steplike arrangement called a palisade.

Many bacteria exhibiting motility propel themselves by means of long, thin appendages called *flagella* arising from the ends of cells or from multiple sites on the surfaces of cells (Figure 2-7).

A majority of the nonphotosynthetic bacteria are beneficial to man, but those that cause disease have had the greatest notoriety. Many species are able to fix atmospheric nitrogen; some do so independently and others symbiotically, that is, with the aid of a leguminous plant such as alfalfa, clover, or soybean (Figure 2-8). Large numbers of bacteria are able to degrade carbon-containing compounds in nature and return carbon dioxide to the atmosphere. Certain other bacteria are involved in the recycling of sulfur and phosphorus. Still others produce valuable food products or antimicrobial substances as a result of their fermentative or synthetic abilities. The extraordinary variety of metabolic characteristics found among the bacteria is responsible for the benefits derived from that sector of the microbial population.

Mycoplasmas. Mycoplasmas appear microscopically as long branched or unbranched filaments or as coccoidal forms (Figure 2-9). Coccoidal structures usually range from 0.3 to 0.9 μm in diameter. Many species require cholesterol or other sterols and long-chain fatty acids for growth.

As early as 1898 mycoplasmas were implicated in a disease of cattle called contagious bovine pleuropneumonia and subsequently became known as PPLO's (pleuropneumonialike organisms). At one time they were believed to be derived from a bacterial parent possessing a cell wall. The designation of the wall-less microorganisms as PPLO's is not common today, but, for historical reasons, it is important to know the earlier name given to them.

L-Phase Variants. Although the L-phase variants are not separate biological entities, their superficial resemblance to mycoplasmas caused confu-

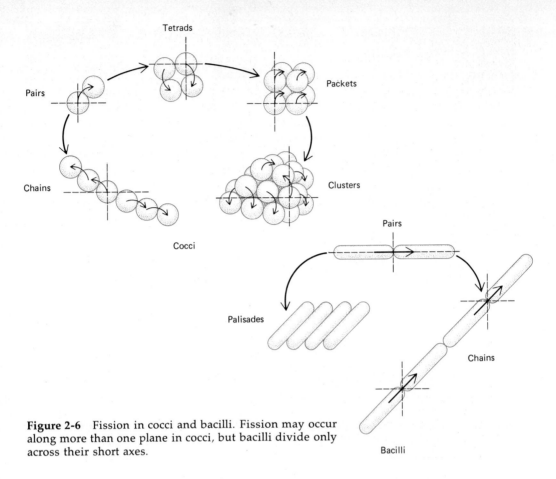

Tetrads

Pairs

Packets

Chains

Clusters

Cocci

Pairs

Palisades

Chains

Bacilli

Figure 2-6 Fission in cocci and bacilli. Fission may occur along more than one plane in cocci, but bacilli divide only across their short axes.

Figure 2-7 Types of flagella in bacteria.

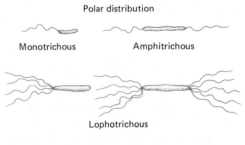

Polar distribution

Monotrichous

Amphitrichous

Lophotrichous

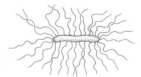

Peritrichous distribution

34

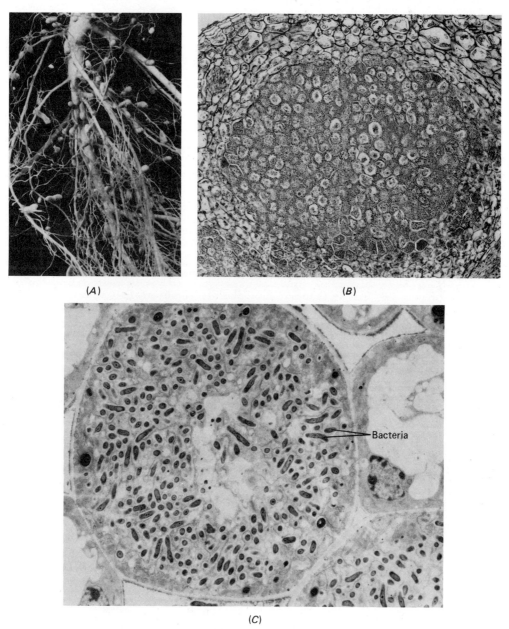

(A)

(B)

Bacteria

(C)

Figure 2-8 Symbiotic nitrogen-fixation. (A) Nodules on a crimson clover plant. (USDA photo.) (B) Appearance of a cross-section of a nodule under the bright-field microscope. (Courtesy, Carolina Biological Supply Company, Burlington, North Carolina.) (C) Appearance of an individual nodule cell under the electron microscope. (Courtesy, L. Nesbitt, National Research Council of Canada, Saskatoon, Saskatchewan.)

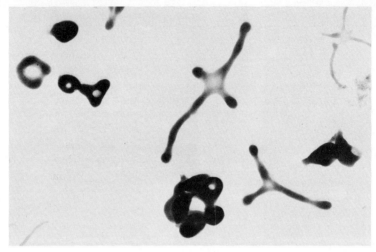

Figure 2-9   Bizarre shapes of mycoplasmas. (Courtesy, E. S. Boatman, University of Washington, Seattle.)

sion for many years (Figure 2-10). L-forms are pleomorphic variants of bacteria differing from typical bacteria in that they, like mycoplasmas, lack cell walls. The wall-less variants were called L-forms because they were first discovered at the Lister Institute in London in 1935 during the investigations of Emmy

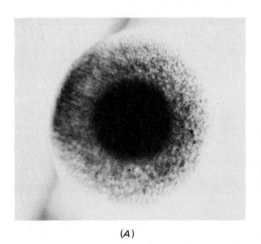

(A)

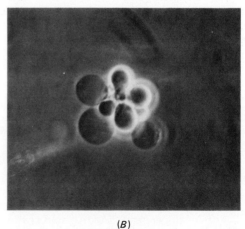

(B)

Figure 2-10   L-phase variants of *Staphylococcus aureus*. (A) L-colony with typical "fried-egg" appearance. (B) Wall-defective cells (spheroplasts) of the same organism. (From C. Watanakunakorn, *J. Infect. Dis.* 119:67, 1969.)

Klieneberger-Nobel. The wall-defective L-phase variants, unlike mycoplasmas, can revert to the parent wall-containing bacterial strains.

L-forms can be induced artificially in a large number of bacterial species by inhibiting the synthesis of cell wall components. The significance of L-phase variants in humans is not well understood. Unfortunately, specific information on the incidence of L-phase variants in a majority of infections is not available. It is likely, however, that the induction of L-forms is a relatively common phenomenon, occurring under the type of environmental stress caused by some kinds of antimicrobial therapy.

Rickettsiae. Rickettsiae are rod-shaped organisms with cell walls; they vary in size from 0.3 to 0.7 μm in width and 1.5 to 2.0 μm in length (Figure 2-11). It appears that rickettsiae may have descended from other bacteria, but in

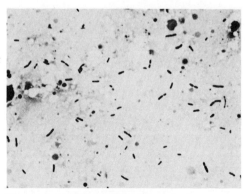

Figure 2-11 *Rickettsia rickettsii*, the causative agent of Rocky Mountain spotted fever, growing in an egg yolk sac. (Courtesy, Rocky Mountain Laboratory, U.S. Public Health Service, Hamilton, Montana.)

the process lost the ability to synthesize some essential metabolites. Arthropods, such as fleas, lice, and ticks, host rickettsiae without apparent disease. If transmitted to humans, the intracellular parasites produce severe and sometimes fatal infections.

Chlamydiae. Chlamydiae are coccoidal forms measuring approximately 0.2 to 0.7 μm in diameter. Like rickettsiae, the chlamydiae possess limited synthetic abilities. Chlamydiae were probably also derived from other bacteria, but are transmitted to humans or animals in the absence of an arthropod vector.

THE EUCARYOTES

The eucaryotes consist of a heterogeneous group of unicellular or multicellular organisms having a structural complexity which permits specialization of function not found among the procaryotes. Microbial eucaryotes include the photosynthetic *algae* and the nonphotosynthetic *protozoa* and *fungi* (Table 2-2).

Table 2-2 AN ABBREVIATED CLASSIFICATION OF EUCARYOTES

I. Photosynthetic eucaryotes
   Unicellular and multicellular algae
II. Nonphotosynthetic eucaryotes
   A. Unicellular organisms
      1. Protozoa
      2. Yeast phases of fungi
   B. Coenocytic organisms
      Mold phases of fungi

The algae comprise a diverse group of morphological types, most of which have cell walls and all of which are photosynthetic. The protozoa occur as unicellular or colonial forms and are devoid of cell walls. Most are motile during at least one stage of their development. Most fungi are *coenocytic* organisms, that is, they are characterized by continuous cytoplasm, uninterrupted by cell walls, and many nuclei. Most have distinct cell walls and produce a filamentous vegetative structure known as a *mycelium*. None are motile.

One or more nuclei can usually be observed with a light microscope in all eucaryotic cells at some stage of their development. Nuclei appear as dense areas bounded by membranes. Within the nuclei an even more dense area, known as a *nucleolus*, is often identifiable as a rough spherical structure. Sometimes more than one nucleolus is discernible. Membrane-bound structures of the cytoplasm are sometimes beyond the limit of visibility of a light microscope and require electron microscopy for definition and substructure analysis.

ALGAE

The algae include microscopic forms as well as some plantlike organisms such as the seaweed kelp (Figure 2-12). Motile cells usually have one or two flagella. All algae contain chlorophyll a and either chlorophyll b or c. Some produce phycobiliproteins which cause them to appear yellow-green, brown, or red. Algae may be classified by the types of photopigments found in the chloroplasts, by the chemical nature of cell walls, by numbers and positions of flagella, and by the type of material in storage depots of the cells.

Most algae live in the oceans of the world although some are found in fresh water and soil. Most of us are more familiar with the green foliage of plants than with algae, but it is the microscopic algae which represent the principal site of photosynthesis on earth. The algae are far more similar both in structure and chemical complexity to plants than are cyanobacteria.

It is their morphological and chemical relationships to the protozoa and fungi, however, that provide the basis for our

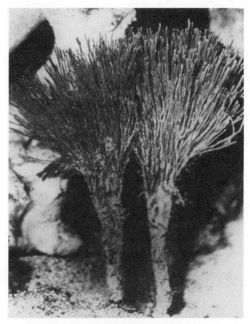

Figure 2-12   A macroscopic green alga. The marine alga with a brushlike appearance occurs in a colonial form. (From A. O. Wasserman, *Biology*, 1973.)

interest in algae since, for the most part, algae do not cause disease. An exception is a marine dinoflagellate, ingested with shellfish muscle or viscera, which is capable of causing a paralytic type of poisoning.

PROTOZOA

The protozoa include a group of unicellular organisms as diverse in morphology as unicellular algae. They vary a good deal in both size and shape and were probably derived from unicellular algae. Some spherical forms may be only 1.0 μm in diameter whereas elongated cells may be 60 μm or more in length. The protozoa do not typically possess photopigments or cell walls, but a few exceptions exist. For example, members of the genus *Euglena* contain distinct chloroplasts and carry on photosynthesis, but have no cell walls (Figure 2-13).

Although biology has long been divided into the classical disciplines of zoology and botany, the microbiologist no longer feels obligated to classify microorganisms as animals or plants. On the basis of nuclear and cytoplasmic structures, it is possible to classify *Euglena* species as eucaryotes, but difficult to identify these microorganisms as typical protozoa or algae. The lack of cell walls is usually associated with animal cells, whereas chloroplasts are typically found in plant cells. These organisms serve to point out an important lesson. Because of the dynamic continuum of life forms, it is not always possible, or indeed practical, to place living things into distinct groups.

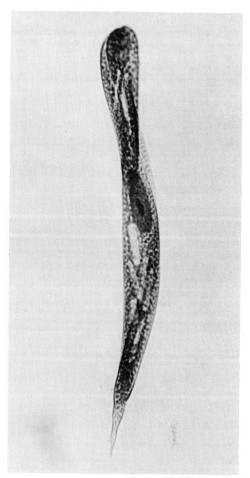

Figure 2-13 *Euglena oxyuris.* The organism has distinct chloroplasts and lacks a cell wall. (Courtesy, Carolina Biological Supply Company, Burlington, North Carolina.)

Protozoa live in oceans, lakes, ponds, streams, and moist soil. Many protozoa have specialized appendages such as flagella or *cilia*, small filamentous processes, for locomotion. Others project portions of cytoplasm from the cell as *pseudopodia* or false feet in the process

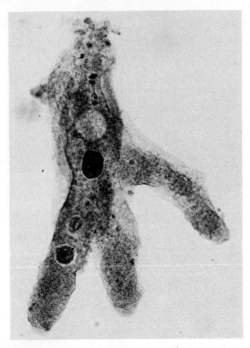

Figure 2-14 *Amoeba proteus.* The organism moves by means of extensions of cytoplasm called pseudopodia. (Courtesy, Carolina Biological Supply Company, Burlington, North Carolina.)

of moving (Figure 2-14). Amebas demonstrate this method of movement and for that reason cells with pseudopodia are said to show ameboid movement. Some protozoa have complex life cycles and are nonmotile during part of their lives. Other free-living ameboid protozoa, the foraminifera, produce white shells containing pores through which pseudopodia pass to obtain nutrients. The famous White Cliffs of Dover are actual deposits of residual white shells of calcium carbonate derived from foraminifera which at one time inhabited the coastal water.

The majority of protozoa are, like the algae, free-living forms which do not cause disease in animals. Many are beneficial to humans. Some protozoa play a role in degradative processes that return CO_2 to the atmosphere. An interesting partnership exists between termites and the flagellate *Trichonympha.* The protozoa live in the gut of the wood-eating insects and digest the cellulose of the wood ingested by the termites. A few protozoa inhabit the intestinal track of animals, including humans, and do produce disease; others have a predilection for the blood, lungs, liver, or brain and may cause serious damage.

FUNGI

The fungi include both microscopic organisms and larger plantlike organisms, like mushrooms or toadstools, which are substantial in size. The microscopic forms include a homogeneous group of unicellular organisms known as *yeasts* and a heterogeneous group of coenocytic organisms known as *molds.* Some fungi are *dimorphic,* that is, capable of growth as a yeast or as a mold depending on environmental conditions. All fungi lack chlorophyll; most have rigid cell walls.

The basic structural unit of molds is a tubular filament called a *hypha.* A mass of hyphae constitutes a vegetative structure, such as that often seen on moldy bread or cheese. The vegetative structure, consisting of the intertwined hyphae, is known as a *mycelium* (Figures 2-15, 2-16). Hyphae may have no cross walls (*septae*) or may be divided at

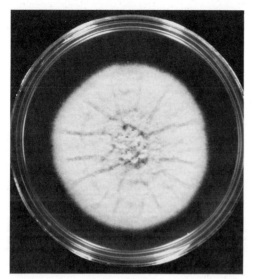

Figure 2-15 Macroscopic appearance of a mold. Typical vegetative structure, or mycelium, seen growing on agar in a Petri plate. (Courtesy, E. W. Koneman, Denver, Colorado.)

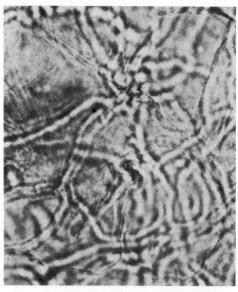

Figure 2-16 Microscopic appearance of a mold showing a mass of intertwined hyphae. (Courtesy, E. W. Koneman, Denver, Colorado.)

irregular intervals into individual compartments. Nonseptate hyphae are multinuclear; septate hyphae may be uninuclear, binuclear, or multinuclear. The mycelium continues to grow as long as nutrients and moisture are available.

Yeasts are spherical, oval, or elongated and may be as large as 3.0 to 5.0 μm long and 2.5 μm wide (Figure 2-17). Elongated yeast cells sometimes appear so similar to hyphae that the chains of cells are called *pseudohyphae* (Figure 2-18).

Fungi are found in both moist and arid soils and can withstand very warm temperatures. They have been isolated from the sands of Death Valley, California, where summer temperatures may reach 50°C. Other fungi can survive in the temperatures of the polar regions. A few molds are aquatic and grow submerged in salt or fresh water. It is estimated that approximately one hundred species of fungi can adapt to parasitism of humans, although not all of them are commonly associated with human infections. Either the yeastlike or filamentous forms of pathogenic fungi can invade susceptible tissues.

NOMENCLATURE AND CLASSIFICATION OF MICROORGANISMS

It became evident to early microbiologists that the tiny organisms observ-

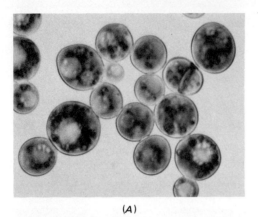

(A)

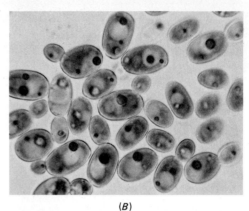

(B)

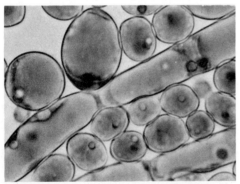

(C)

Figure 2-17 Three types of yeast cells. (A) Spherical cells. (B) Oval cells. (C) Elongated forms. (Courtesy, G. Svihla, Portage, Indiana.)

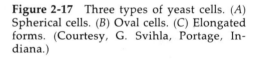

Figure 2-18 Morphological variation of cells of *Candida albicans*. Pseudohyphae appear as elongated cells. (Courtesy, G. Svihla, Portage, Indiana.)

able only under the microscope were not typical plants or animals. In 1866 Ernest Haeckel (1834–1919), a German biologist, proposed that a separate category, the kingdom *Protista*, be established for microscopic forms of life. Yet for many years plant and animal taxonomists continued to place algae, bacteria, fungi, and protozoa in their schemes of classification. As more was learned about the true nature of the protists, however, the justification for separating the protists from plants and animals seemed more and more apparent. Demonstration of the lack of internal membrane systems in cyanobacteria and bacteria was the primary basis for recognizing the two patterns of cellular organization—the procaryotes and eucaryotes. The cyanobacteria and bacteria are classified as members of the kingdom of procaryotes (*Procaryotae*). The eucaryotic algae, protozoa, and fungi constitute the groups now comprising the kingdom of protists (*Protista*).

The eighth edition of *Bergey's Manual of Determinative Bacteriology* (1974) is recognized as the authoritative source for the classification and nomenclature of bacteria. In the manual the kingdom of procaryotes (*Procaryotae*) is divided into two divisions, the *Cyanobacteria* and the *Bacteria*. The bacteria are subdivided into nineteen groups with vernacular descriptions (see Appendix A). The groups are divided again into orders (*-ales*), families (*-aceae*), and tribes (*-ieae*). Order, family, or tribe names are used very little in the hospital laboratory. One exception, however, is the use of the family designation *Enterobacteriaceae* to describe certain enteric bacteria. The *Enterobacteriaceae* consist of a large and diverse group of bacilli. More will be learned about the characteristics of members of the *Enterobacteriaceae* in subsequent chapters.

Sometimes a vernacular name is used in referring to particular groups of bacteria. For example, bacteria belonging to the genus *Mycoplasma, Salmonella,* or *Yersinia* may be called mycoplasmas, salmonellae, or yersiniae. Vernacular designations are not italicized or capitalized. Occasionally, other simplified terms are employed for particular bacteria. The terms meningococcus and pneumococcus are descriptive for *Neisseria meningitidis* and *Streptococcus pneumoniae*, respectively.

The nomenclature used in this textbook is that recognized in *Bergey's Manual* with the exception of a few changes in taxonomy and nomenclature of the *Enterobacteriaceae* recommended in 1977 by the Enteric Section of the Center for Disease Control in Atlanta, Georgia.

The binomial system of naming organisms, first proposed by Carolus Linnaeus (1707–1778), a Swedish botanist, provided an orderly approach for dividing living things into groups (taxons) and for naming specific organisms. According to the Linnaean system of binomial nomenclature, each organism is given two names: a generic name (*genus*), usually of Latin or Greek derivation, and a specific name (*species*), consisting of a descriptive adjective pertaining to a source, characteristic, or even discoverer of the organism. All microorganisms belonging to a particular genus share many characteristics with each other; each species is different in some characteristics from other members of a genus. Bacteria belonging to a genus are frequently compared with a so-called type species for that genus. Names of genera are always capitalized; names of species begin with lowercase letters. Genus and species names are italicized in print or underlined in handwriting.

SUMMARY

The microbial world consists of a diverse population of unicellular and multicellular organisms and the acellular viruses, all of which are ubiquitous in nature. Two patterns of cellular organization are recognized among the organisms with cellular structure—the procaryotes and eucaryotes. The procaryotes consist of the cyanobacteria and the bacteria. Cyanobacteria and bacteria belong to the kingdom *Procaryotae*. The eucaryotes consist of the algae, protozoa, and fungi and make up the kingdom *Protista*. The ability of some microorganisms to carry on photosynthesis, recycle nitrogen, carbon, sulfur, and phosphorus, or synthesize antimicrobial substances makes it possible for people to survive on earth. Some bacteria, protozoa, and fungi, however, possess predatory characteristics which cause disease in other living forms, including humans.

QUESTIONS FOR STUDY

1. Classify the following groups of microorganisms as procaryotes or eucaryotes.

   cyanobacteria   mycoplasmas
   molds   protozoa
   L-phase variants chlamydiae
   rickettsiae   yeasts
   red algae   green algae

2. Which of the above groups of microorganisms are able to carry on photosynthesis?
3. List the three basic shapes of bacteria according to size in decreasing order.
4. Differentiate between mycoplasmas and L-phase variants.
5. How do yeasts differ from molds?
6. Why are species of *Euglena* not typical protozoa or algae?
7. Name the major groups of the protists and procaryotes which cause disease in humans.
8. Define the following terms and name the groups of microorganisms with which each is identified.

   cilia   mycelium
   chloroplasts   hyphae
   pseudohyphae   pseudopodia
   flagella   nuclear membrane
   nucleolus

SELECTED REFERENCES

Brock, T. D. *Biology of Microorganisms.* 2d ed. Englewood Cliffs, N.J.: Prentice-Hall, 1970.

Buchanan, R. E., and Gibbons, N. E. *Bergey's Manual of Determinative Bacteriology.* 8th ed. Baltimore: Williams & Wilkins, 1974.

Evans, E. H.; Foulds, I.; and Carr, N. G. Environmental conditions and morphological variation in the blue-green alga *Chlorogloea fritschii. J. Gen. Microbiol.* 92:147, 1976.

Hayflick, L. *The Mycoplasmatales and the L-Phase of Bacteria.* Englewood Cliffs, N.J.: Prentice-Hall, 1969.

Palmer, C. W. *Algae in Water Supplies.* Washington, D.C.: U.S. Department of Health, Education and Welfare, 1962.

Stanier, R. Y.; Adelberg, E. A.; and Ingraham, J. L. *The Microbial World.* 4th ed. Englewood Cliffs, N.J.: Prentice-Hall, 1976.

Chapter 3

Observation of Microorganisms

After you read this chapter, you should be able to:

1. Describe five types of microscopes and one purpose for which each is used.
2. Differentiate between the magnifying and resolving power of a microscope.
3. Compare advantages of wet mounts, hanging-drop wet mounts, and stained smears in making microscopic observations of microorganisms.
4. Explain the significance of gram reactivity and acid-fastness.
5. Describe the major uses for polychromatic stains.
6. Differentiate between negative and fluorescent stains.

Microbial anatomy has been revealed by the application of principles of optics and the development of special techniques for preparing specimens of microorganisms. One can envision the progress made in *microscopy,* the use of the microscope to examine objects, when one realizes that the magnification possible with van Leeuwenhoek's microscope in the seventeenth century was only 300 times. With today's electron microscope magnification of 1 million times or more makes it possible to see minute details of cellular and viral structure.

TYPES OF MICROSCOPES

THE BRIGHT-FIELD MICROSCOPE

Various types of microscopy are available to today's microbiologist, but the bright-field microscope remains the most widely used optical instrument. The bright-field microscope is an optical instrument which uses ordinary light to magnify images of objects. Most bright-field microscopes made today contain two sets of lenses for magnification and are therefore called compound microscopes (Figure 3-1). The lens closer to the eye when viewing an object is called the *ocular lens;* the lens closer to the object being viewed is called the *objective lens.*

Magnification refers to the increase in diameter of the microscopic field. It depends on the focal length and the magnifying power of the lens system. The focal length is the distance between the center of a lens and the point required for focus (Figure 3.2). The ocular lens commonly has a magnifying power of 10, although lenses with a power of 5 or 15 are also used. The usual laboratory microscope has at least three

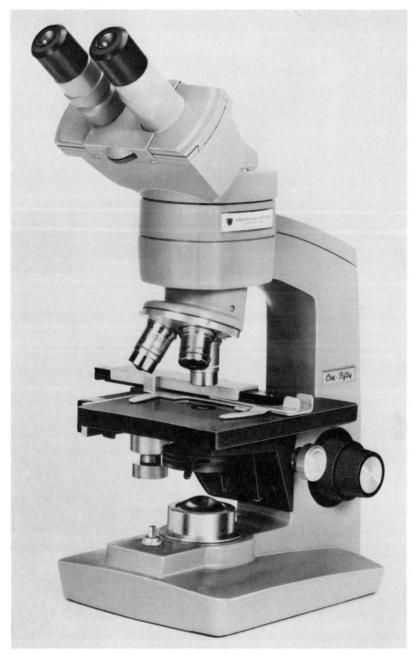

Figure 3-1 A binocular compound bright-field microscope. (Courtesy, American Optical Corporation, Buffalo, New York.)

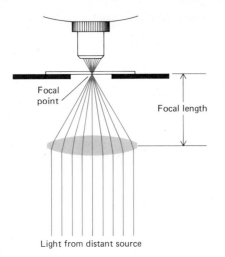

Focal point

Focal length

Light from distant source

Figure 3-2   A beam of light is converged to a focal point from the center of a lens. The distance between the two is the focal length of an objective.

objective lenses mounted on a revolving nosepiece so that they can be rotated according to need. The low-power objective contains a lens with a magnifying power of 10. The total magnification possible with an ocular lens with a magnifying power of 10 and an objective lens with a magnifying power of 10 would be 10 × 10 or 100. The high-power objective frequently contains a lens with a magnifying power of 40, 43, 45, or 47, making a total magnification of over 400 possible when the 10× ocu-

lar lens is used. The lens of a third or oil-immersion objective may magnify 95, 97, or 100 times; it requires a drop of immersion oil to be placed between the specimen and the objective lens. A single bacterium appears approximately 1000 times its actual size when viewed under oil.

The resolving power of a microscope is the minimum distance between two points permitting two objects to be seen as separate entities. It is quantitatively related to the amount of observable detail: the more resolving power, the greater the degree of detail observable. The factors limiting resolution are the wavelength of visible light and the aperture of the lens system. The wavelength of visible light is 4000 to 7000 Å and is a constant when using a bright-field microscope. The numerical aperture (NA) is a mathematical expression of the light-gathering ability of a lens. It is derived from the refractive index of the lens and the angle of the cone of light entering the lens (Figure 3-3).

The magnification, numerical aperture, and equivalent focal length of objective lenses are usually engraved on the sides of objectives (Table 3-1). The equivalent focal lengths are the distances required between the objectives and the object for focusing. Thus, an object should be in focus using the oil-

Table 3-1   OPTICAL PARAMETERS FOR COMMON OBJECTIVES

OBJECTIVE	NUMERICAL APERTURE	EQUIVALENT FOCAL LENGTH	DEPTH OF FIELD	RESOLVING POWER
10×	0.25	16.0 mm	7.0 μm	2.00 μm
40×	0.65	4.0 mm	1.3 μm	0.45 μm
100×	1.25	1.8 mm	0.5 μm	0.20 μm

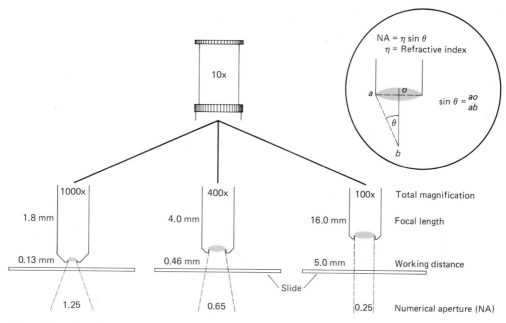

Figure 3-3 A comparison of the light-gathering ability of three objective lenses. The lens with the largest numerical aperture has the greatest ability to gather light.

immersion lens (100× lens) when there is approximately 1.8 mm between the lens and the object. Objectives containing lenses with numerical apertures of 0.5 or more, generally, need a condenser for regulation of light. The depth of field or thickness of a specimen observable at one time decreases as the numerical aperture and magnification increase. The depth of field diminishes somewhat with lesser ability of an observer's eye to accommodate, that is, to adjust for distance. With age the lens of the human eye gradually loses elasticity required for accommodation.

The actual size of a field observable with the three objectives is often difficult to conceive. A comparison of the sizes of observable fields is given in Figure 3-4.

In general, the greater the power of the lens, the more light is required for

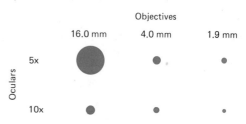

Figure 3-4 Approximate diameters of fields seen through a microscope with three objectives. (Adapted from I. Davidsohn and J. B. Henry, *Todd-Sanford Clinical Diagnosis by Laboratory Methods*, 14th ed., Philadelphia, Saunders, 1969.)

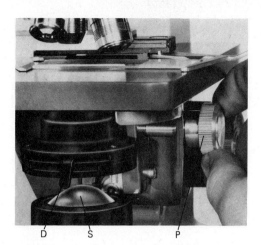

Figure 3-5 Mechanism for adjusting condenser and diaphragm to obtain proper illumination. *S*, substage lamp; *D*, diaphragm; *P*, pinion knob to raise and lower condenser. (Courtesy, American Optical Corporation, Buffalo, New York.)

detailed observations of an object under the microscope. Proper illumination is best obtained by a substage lamp and adjustment of the condenser and diaphragm to regulate the amount of light (Figure 3-5). If daylight or light from an unattached lamp is not emitted directly into the condenser lens, an adjustable concave mirror is used to obtain the correct light reflection for best observation. Frequent adjustments may be necessary to observe appropriate detail during a single microscopic examination.

For best visualization an object should be placed in the center of the field. The coarse and fine adjustment knobs are used to obtain a sharp image. A good microscopist constantly adjusts both light and focal distance for optimal viewing. Careful interpretations based on bright-field microscopy take both time and patience as well as familiarity with a particular microscope.

THE DARK-FIELD MICROSCOPE

A dark-field microscope has one or more special condensers which block out the central rays of light and cause the peripheral rays to hit the object from the side (Figure 3-6). Under dark-field illumination microorganisms appear light against a black background. Some bright-field microscopes are constructed in such a way that the light condenser can easily be replaced by a dark-field condenser. Bacteria which are difficult to stain, such as spirochetes, are best seen with a dark-field microscope. The dark-field technique is frequently used to observe living spiro-

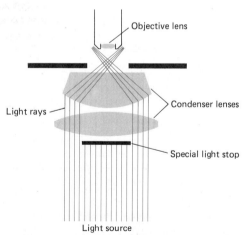

Figure 3-6 The dark-field microscope. A special condenser blocks central rays of light and directs peripheral rays to a focal point. The small portion of light reflected into the objective lens causes objects to appear light against a black background.

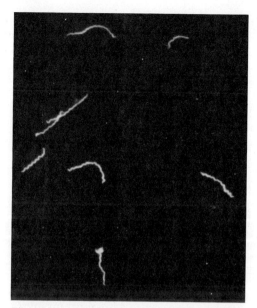

Figure 3-7 Dark-field preparation showing spirochetes of *Treponema pallidum* in scrapings from a chancre of a patient with syphilis. (Courtesy, Beckman Diagnostics, Fullerton, California.)

chetes that cause syphilis, in lesion scrapings, or to visualize capsules of yeast cells (Figure 3-7). Since no special staining is necessary, there is little or no distortion in shape or size of microorganisms observed with a dark-field microscope.

THE FLUORESCENCE MICROSCOPE

Another type of microscope which is gaining in importance as a tool in the diagnosis of infectious diseases is the fluorescence microscope. The use of fluorescence to accentuate objects is based on the principle that objects emit a light of one color when a light of another color is the source of illumination. Ultraviolet is employed to visualize objects stained with fluorescent dyes such as fluorescein, auramine, or rhodamine B. Special filters limit the wavelength to that required for fluorescence.

There are many applications of fluorescent techniques in microbiology, including those employed for the identification of bacteria, viruses, rickettsiae, and protozoa and, perhaps more importantly, those used for the identification of specific antibodies produced in response to the invasion of a host by microorganisms. Fluorescein-tagged antibodies react with particular antigens of microorganisms causing observable fluorescence at the site of antigen-antibody combinations.

THE PHASE-CONTRAST MICROSCOPE

More detailed observation of living cells is possible with a phase-contrast microscope. Organelles of varying density retard transmitted light, resulting in phase differences perceptible when accentuated by special filters and diaphragms. The phase change is proportional to the difference in density between an organelle and the surrounding medium. Phase differences appear as variations in brightness through a phase-contrast microscope (Figure 3-8). The addition or subtraction of wavelengths, by use of a special condenser, produces contrasts which reveal detailed structures. No greater magnification or resolution is obtainable with phase-contrast microscopy,

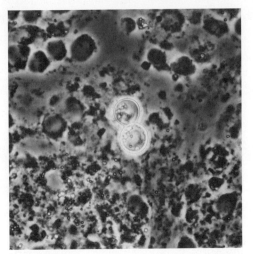

Figure 3-8 A phase-contrast micrograph of a budding cell of the yeast *Blastomyces dermatitidis*. The contrast between the background and the yeast cell is accomplished with special filters and diaphragms. (Courtesy, G. D. Roberts, Rochester, Minnesota.)

but the greater clarification of detail makes it an especially useful tool in studying microbial anatomy.

Phase-contrast microscopy is also valuable in demonstrating motility, cytoplasmic streaming, and the dynamic states of organelles. The application of cinemamicrography to phase-contrast microscopic studies has recorded vividly such processes as mitosis, binary fission, budding, fragmentation, and phagocytosis.

THE ELECTRON MICROSCOPE

In recent years the most valuable tool of microbial cytologists and virologists has been the electron microscope (Figure 3-9). Electron microscopy employs a stream of fast-moving electrons which

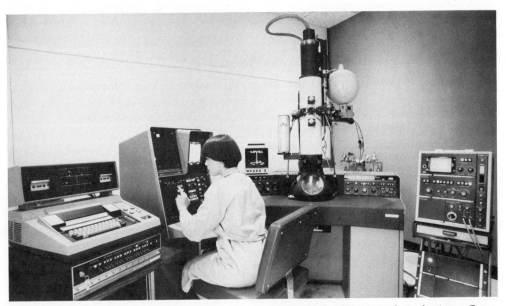

Figure 3-9 One of many electron microscopes available to cytologists and virologists. (Courtesy, Philips Electronic Instruments, Inc., Mahwah, New Jersey.)

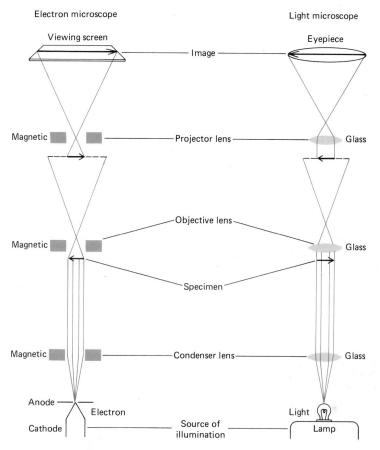

Figure 3-10 Comparison of the structure of a light and an electron microscope.

behave like light with a very short wavelength. Magnetic fields rather than optical lenses are used to focus electron beams and project an image on a fluorescent screen (Figure 3-10). Magnifications 100 times greater than can be obtained with the bright-field microscope are possible. If photographs are taken and enlarged, magnifications of 1 million or more can be obtained.

Furthermore, a resolving power of 0.0003 μm or about 600 times greater than that of the bright-field microscope can be achieved. Drawbacks of the electron microscope are the expense of the equipment, elaborate and time-consuming procedures necessary to prepare specimens, and requirement of specially-trained personnel for its operation.

Despite cumbersome procedures and the inability to examine living material, the electron microscope has no counterpart for ultrastructural analysis of structures which are beyond the resolving power of light microscopes. Virologists are completely dependent on electron microscopy for elucidation of the anatomy of viruses. Observation of structural characteristics of viruses on electron micrographs has enabled virologists to classify the tiny particles according to size, shape, and symmetry (Figure 3-11).

The freeze-etching technique is often used to prepare material for electron microscopy. Specimens are frozen and then thin sections are chipped off and coated with a thin layer of carbon. This technique has two major advantages over chemical fixation. First, it eliminates *artifacts*, that is, aberrations produced by the fixation process. Second, it gives the images a new dimension; electron photomicrographs can reveal the topography or surface appearance of specimens (Figure 3-12).

A recent modification of electron microscopy is the scanning electron microscope which provides three-dimensional images with concurrent magnification. The images show realistic contours of specimens rather than the two-dimensional representations of the conventional electron microscope (Figure 3-13). The scanning electron microscope has a resolving power of 100 to 200 Å and a magnification of up to 100,000 diameters.

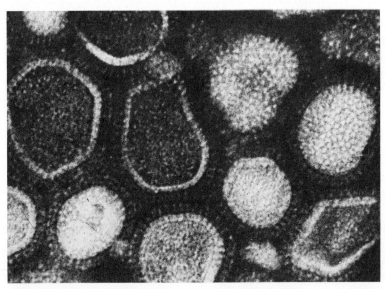

Figure 3-11   An electron photomicrograph of the influenza virus. The viral particles vary in size from 80 to 120 nm. (From R. W. Horne, A. P. Waterson, A. Farnham, and P. Wildy, *Virology* 11:79, 1960.)

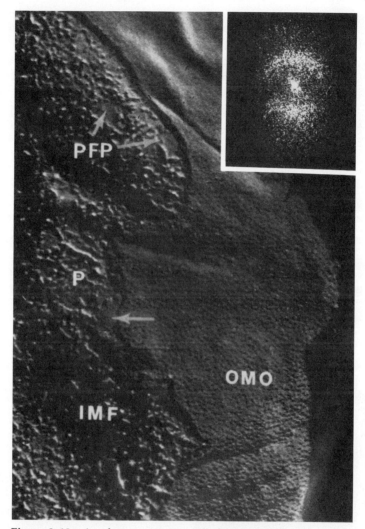

Figure 3-12 An electron micrograph showing the surface of the bacterium *Escherichia coli,* taken by freeze-etching. A concave and a convex surface can be discerned. *IMF,* inner membrane's fracture plane; *OMO,* outer face of outer membrane; *P,* particle within fracture plane; *PFP,* particle-free patches. The insert is a diffractogram of central pitted area showing a random arrangement of pits. (From M. E. Bayer and L. Leive, Effect of ethylenediaminetetracetate upon the surface of *Escherichia coli, J. Bacteriol.* 130:1367, 1977.)

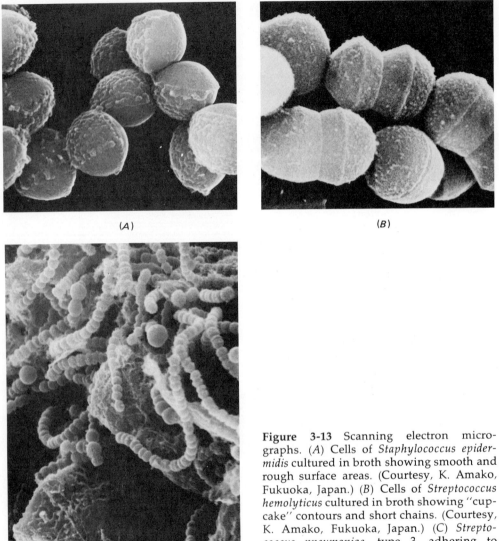

(A)

(B)

(C)

Figure 3-13 Scanning electron micrographs. (*A*) Cells of *Staphylococcus epidermidis* cultured in broth showing smooth and rough surface areas. (Courtesy, K. Amako, Fukuoka, Japan.) (*B*) Cells of *Streptococcus hemolyticus* cultured in broth showing "cupcake" contours and short chains. (Courtesy, K. Amako, Fukuoka, Japan.) (*C*) *Streptococcus pneumoniae*, type 3, adhering to human conjunctival epithelial cells. (Courtesy, W. P. Reed, Albuquerque, New Mexico.)

PREPARATION OF MATERIALS FOR BRIGHT-FIELD MICROSCOPIC EXAMINATION

The preparation of materials for microscopic examination varies with the type of microscope and the type of specimen. Specimens to be examined may be living microorganisms suspended in a liquid medium, but more often are dead microorganisms to which chemical fixatives and stains have been applied. Only fixed and dried specimens can be examined with an electron microscope since life is not compatible with the vacuum required to prevent scattering of the electron beam. Since the bright-field microscope remains the basic tool of most microbiology laboratories, only methods used to prepare materials for examination with that microscope are presented.

WET AND HANGING-DROP WET MOUNTS

A simple wet mount of a specimen, such as urine, cerebrospinal fluid (CSF), or stool, can reveal the presence of microorganisms. It is made by putting a drop of the specimen or sediment, obtained by centrifugation, on a clean glass slide and placing a cover slip over the material (Figure 3-14). Low power is frequently adequate to observe the gross morphology of larger organisms and ova of helminths. High power will reveal additional details. Small bacteria are often difficult to see and reduced illumination may be required.

Although motility may be discernible on a simple wet mount, a hanging-drop wet mount is often more reliable. A small quantity of petrolatum is applied to the corners of one surface of a cover slip. A drop of liquid is placed on the cover slip and a special slide, with a depression, is inverted and positioned

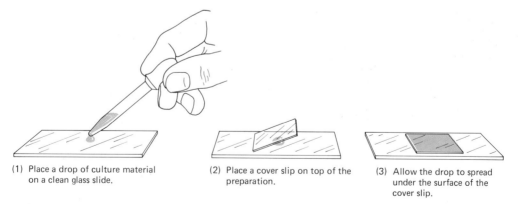

(1) Place a drop of culture material on a clean glass slide.

(2) Place a cover slip on top of the preparation.

(3) Allow the drop to spread under the surface of the cover slip.

Figure 3-14 Steps in the preparation of a wet mount.

so that the petrolatum touches and adheres to the slide. The slide is carefully turned right side up so that the drop of liquid is suspended from the cover slip into the depression (Figure 3-15). The specimen is viewed under the high-power or oil-immersion objective.

True motility must be differentiated from *Brownian movement,* a type of movement exhibited by both living and nonliving small particles in an aqueous suspension. Brownian movement is caused by forces created by movement of water molecules. A particle exhibiting Brownian movement moves in a haphazard fashion. A motile bacterium progresses in a definite direction and

may often be observed turning end-to-end as well.

Microscopic examination is not a practical method for detecting motility of bacteria on a wide scale. A cultural method, which employs a semisolid medium, is reliable for demonstrating motility.

FIXED STAINED SMEARS

Materials which have been dried on glass slides are most useful for detecting the presence of microorganisms or their morphological characteristics. The preparations are called *smears.* The dried smears are first fixed, that is, fastened to the slide, by treatment with

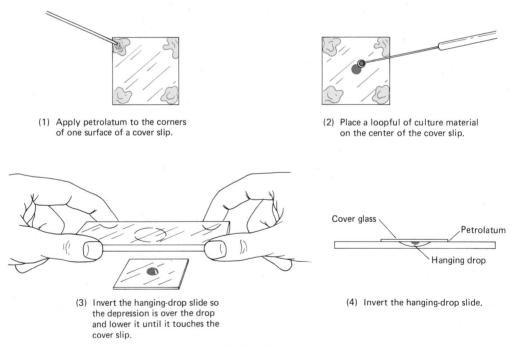

(1) Apply petrolatum to the corners of one surface of a cover slip.

(2) Place a loopful of culture material on the center of the cover slip.

(3) Invert the hanging-drop slide so the depression is over the drop and lower it until it touches the cover slip.

(4) Invert the hanging-drop slide.

Cover glass
Petrolatum
Hanging drop

Figure 3-15 Steps in the preparation of a hanging-drop wet mount.

chemicals or heat and then stained. Unstained bacteria are difficult to distinguish from their surroundings. Staining provides the means for obtaining contrast between bacteria and background material.

Solutions of a number of organic dyes may be applied for staining smears. An organic dye is classified chemically as a salt because it contains positively and negatively charged ions. A basic dye contains the staining component in the positive (cationic) portion of the molecule; an acid dye has the staining component associated with the negative (anionic) portion of the molecule. Some stains are called polychromatic because they produce a variety of colors.

Bacteria have an affinity for basic aniline dyes, such as crystal violet, safranin, and methylene blue, a property attributed to the nucleic acid content of bacterial protoplasm. Acid dyes, such as acid fuchsin, eosin, and Congo red, are repelled by the negative charge of bacteria. Polychromatic stains are valuable for staining blood, tissue, and fecal smears or any materials suspected of containing eucaryotic cells. Negative charges of nucleic acid are confined to nuclei which take up basic components of dyes. The basic charges of the eucaryotic cytoplasm have an affinity for acid stains. The contrast, provided by mixtures of dyes in polychromatic stains, makes it possible to differentiate the types of eucaryotic cells from one another. Such differentiation can be very important in mixed infections and for observing white blood cells in peripheral blood.

Smears may be prepared from bacteria suspended in a liquid or from actual clinical specimens, such as pus, skin scrapings, sputum, stool, CSF, or blood. Rarely can bacteria be identified by microscopic examination alone for there are too many "look-alikes." However, careful examination of stained smears can provide information on staining and morphological characteristics such as shape, size, and groupings of bacteria. Microorganisms must be differentiated from other cells and debris on smears prepared from clinical specimens.

The fact that microorganisms cannot be seen upon microscopic examination of a clinical specimen does not necessarily mean that no organisms are present. The organisms may not be present in sufficient numbers to be observable in the limited sampling of the specimen placed on the slide. For this reason cultures are more reliable for detecting the presence of infectious agents. In those instances when culturing is not feasible, repeated samplings of clinical specimens and multiple smears should be prepared.

SIMPLE STAINS

Simple staining is the application of a single stain to a fixed smear. Methylene blue, crystal violet, safranin, or another stain is allowed to react with bacteria on a heat-fixed smear for several seconds. The smear is then washed with water and blotted dry.

The simple-stain technique will allow the shape, size, and groupings of bacteria to be discerned using the oil-immersion objective. Sometimes the presence of inclusions or spores can also be detected. Most inclusions have a greater affinity for basic dyes than the surrounding protoplasm and stain darker than the rest of the cell. Spores do not take up dyes readily and appear colorless unless special procedures are used for staining.

DIFFERENTIAL STAINS

Differential staining is the application of more than one stain to a fixed smear. The procedure is used to demonstrate different staining characteristics of cells. A number of differential staining techniques are used in microbiology, but the most widely used is the Gram stain (Table 3-2).

Gram Stain. Crystal violet is allowed to react with bacteria on a heat-fixed smear for one minute and the smear is rinsed in tap water. Gram's iodine, a mordant, is applied and allowed to react for an additional minute before the smear is rinsed in tap water. Gram's iodine reacts specifically with the crystal violet to form intracellular complexes. At this point in the procedure all bacteria are stained purple. The smear is next subjected to decolorization by applying a mixture of acetone and alcohol or 95 percent alcohol drop by drop until the primary stain of crystal violet fails to wash from the smear. The smear is rinsed once again in tap water. In the final step the smear is flooded with a counterstain of safranin for 30 seconds before rinsing in tap water for the last time. The most critical step in successful Gram staining is the decolorizing procedure. Bacteria retaining the primary stain of crystal violet are designated as *gram-positive;* bacteria taking on the color of the counterstain safranin are described as *gram-negative.*

The gram reaction is not an all-or-none phenomenon. The crystal violet–iodine precipitate forms in both types of cells, but the cells must be heavily charged with precipitate for good gram differentiation. Differences in retention of the dye-iodine complex have been attributed to the amount of unbound crystal violet present in cells and the selective extractability of the Gram stain reagents or the dye-iodine complex by the decolorizer. Intact cell envelopes do not appear to be necessary, since ruptured cells can be differentiated. The thickness of the cell wall, "pore" size available for molecular diffusion, and the amount of water in cell-wall material may be additional significant factors in gram reactivity. Typically, gram-negative cells do have thinner cell walls and more interstitial cell space than gram-positive cells.

The Gram-stain technique is useful

Table 3-2   THE GRAM-STAIN
            PROCEDURE

1. Cover the smear with crystal violet for 1 minute and rinse in tap water.
2. Cover the smear with Gram's iodine for 1 minute and rinse in tap water.
3. Decolorize by adding 95 percent alcohol drop by drop to the slide in a tilted position until the primary stain fails to wash from the smear, but *no longer*. Rinse in tap water.
4. Cover the smear with safranin for 30 seconds. Wash in tap water and blot dry.

for dividing bacteria into two major groups. The implications of differences in staining go beyond mere differences in physical and chemical characteristics of cell walls, however. The gram reactivity is of significance in the choice of other procedures needed for identification of bacterial species. Furthermore, a physician can sometimes make a presumptive etiological diagnosis on the basis of a Gram stain and thus begin appropriate antimicrobial therapy.

Acid-Fast Stain. Another differential staining technique is the *acid-fast stain* which is employed on centrifuged sediments in the diagnosis of diseases caused by bacteria belonging to the genus *Mycobacterium* or *Nocardia*. In the Ziehl-Neelsen acid-fast procedure carbolfuchsin is used as the primary stain; a stain of contrasting color, such as methylene blue, is employed for counterstaining (Table 3-3). Acid alcohol is used as a decolorizer. It contains 3 percent hydrochloric acid (HCL) in 95 percent ethanol and is a much more potent decolorizer than the 95 percent

Table 3-3 THE ZIEHL-NEELSEN ACID-FAST STAIN PROCEDURE

1. Cover the smear with carbolfuchsin and heat slowly to the steaming point.
2. Steam gently for 5 to 10 minutes replacing stain as necessary.
3. Allow slide to cool and wash in tap water.
4. Decolorize by adding acid alcohol drop by drop to the slide in a tilted position until the primary stain fails to wash from the smear. Wash in tap water.
5. Cover the smear with methylene blue for 30 seconds. Wash in tap water and blot dry.

alcohol used in the Gram-stain technique. Acid-fast bacteria appear red against a blue (or other contrasting color) background. The organisms are called acid fast because they retain the primary stain despite decolorization with acid alcohol. Other bacteria or background material take up the counterstain.

The Ziehl-Neelsen acid-fast procedure requires heat to permit carbolfuchsin to permeate the resistant wax-containing walls of mycobacteria. The lipid-rich walls of these bacteria make them resistant not only to dyes, but also to the action of some antimicrobial agents and disinfectants. A modification of the Ziehl-Neelsen procedure permits visualization of *Nocardia* or *Mycobacterium* species in tissue.

Special Stains. Differential staining techniques are also used to demonstrate flagella, capsules, nuclei, endospores, and inclusions of bacteria. A number of differential staining techniques are also used for the demonstration of protozoa and fungi in tissue.

Many protozoan-staining procedures employ hematoxylin as a dye because it has remarkable polychromic properties. It is possible to obtain several shades intermediate between blue and red for differentiation of cell types and structures. An iron-hematoxylin or a trichrome stain is particularly valuable for making permanent mounts of fecal specimens. The iron-hematoxylin staining procedure permits good differentiation of nuclei and chromatin material, but it is time consuming. The trichrome staining technique is a rapid procedure

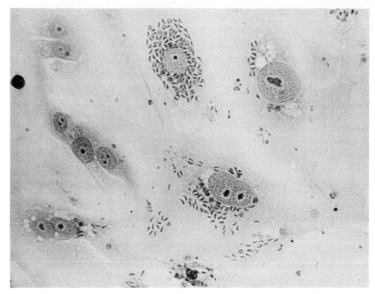

Figure 3-16 Appearance of a Giemsa-stained culture of the protozoan *Toxoplasma gondii,* strain C-56, in primary cat kidney cells after four days. (Courtesy, H. G. Sheffield, Bethesda, Maryland.)

and convenient for identification of some protozoa and ova of helminths. The cytoplasm of cysts and trophozoites appears blue-green with tinges of purple, whereas nuclei stain red. Ova usually also appear red.

Wright's stain and Giemsa's stain are used to examine some spirochetes, rickettsiae, chlamydiae, microfilariae, and protozoa and to differentiate white cell types (Figure 3-16). Mycoplasmas are not usually recognizable by direct examination using the ordinary light microscope. Both stains are compound stains containing eosin and methylene blue. The most important systemic parasites detected by these stains are the species of protozoa causing malaria. A more frequent use of Wright's stain in

the hospital laboratory, however, is the routine staining of blood smears.

Special stains containing silver nitrate may be necessary to demonstrate fungi in tissue. Fungi impregnated with silver nitrate appear dark brown against a yellow background.

NEGATIVE STAINS

The application of acid stains, such as India ink or nigrosin, to microorganisms produces a dark background against which unstained bacteria or fungi can be observed. The appearance of the organisms is somewhat analogous to their appearance in dark-field microscopy. Little distortion of microorganisms occurs with negative stains since no fixing is required. Furthermore, only a bright-field microscope is necessary. Negative-staining techniques are particularly valuable for demonstrating capsules of yeasts and some spirochetes that are resistant to staining with aniline dyes.

SUMMARY

Advances in microbiology have closely paralleled the development of microscopic techniques and equipment. Although the bright-field microscope is the most frequently used instrument, dark-field, phase-contrast, fluorescence, and electron microscopy have revealed anatomic details of cellular and viral structure.

The most widely used technique for staining bacteria, the Gram stain, divides the bacteria into two major groups. Organisms retaining the primary stain of crystal violet are designated as gram-positive, whereas those taking on the color of the counterstain safranin are called gram-negative. A variety of staining techniques may be applied in the laboratory to demonstrate acid-fast bacteria, fungi, protozoa, or helminths.

QUESTIONS FOR STUDY

1. How is the magnification of a microscope determined?
2. Name the microscope which is commonly used to observe each of the following:
   causative agent of syphilis
   cytoplasmic streaming
   topography of a bacterium
   site of antigen-antibody combinations
   dynamic state of organelles
   phagocytosis
   structure of viruses
   sediments of urine
   ameba in three dimensions
3. What factors account for gram reactivity of bacteria?
4. List two stains which can be used for staining protozoa.
5. Name two advantages associated with use of negative stains.

SELECTED REFERENCES

Barer, R. *Lecture Notes on the Use of the Microscope.* 3rd ed. Oxford: Blackwell, 1968.

Bartholomew, J. W.; Cromwell, T.; and Gan, R. Analysis of the mechanism of gram differentiation by use of a filter-paper chromatographic technique. *J. of Bact.* 89:766, 1965.

Beishir, L. *Microbiology in Practice.* San Francisco: Harper & Row (Canfield Press), 1974.

Blazevic, D. J., and Ederer, G. M. *Principles of Biochemical Tests in Diagnostic Microbiology.* New York: Wiley, 1975.

Davidsohn, I., and Henry, J. B. *Todd-Sanford Clinical Diagnosis by Laboratory Methods.* 14th ed. Philadelphia: Saunders, 1969.

Difco Manual. 9th ed. Detroit: Difco Laboratories, Inc., 1974.

Everhart, T. E., and Hayes, T. L. The scanning electron microscope. *Sci. Am.* 226:55, 1972.

Goldman, M. *Fluorescent Antibody*

Methods. New York: Academic Press, 1968.

Isenberg, H. D., and Berkman, J. I. Microbial diagnosis in a general hospital. *Ann. N.Y. Acad. Sci.* 98:647, 1962.

Lennette, E. H.; Spaulding, E. H.; and Truant, J. P. *Manual of Clinical Microbiology.* 2d ed. Washington, D.C.: American Society for Microbiology, 1974.

Lillie, R. D. *H. J. Conn's Biological Stains.* 8th ed. Baltimore: Williams & Wilkins, 1969.

Chapter 4

Anatomy of Procaryotes and Eucaryotes

After you read this chapter, you should be able to:

1. Define organelle, cytoplasm, cell boundary, colloid, protoplasm, and fluidity.
2. Describe the structure and function of the cell wall and cell membrane.
3. Explain the role of passive and active transport in permitting molecules to enter or leave cells.
4. Compare the internal membrane systems of eucaryotic and procaryotic cells.
5. Describe the major differences between procaryotic and eucaryotic cells.
6. Describe the major similarities between procaryotic and eucaryotic cells.
7. Name the DNA-containing structures within cells.
8. Describe a function for each type of microbial appendages.
9. Differentiate between a gene and a chromosome.
10. Explain the roles of microtubules in procaryotic and eucaryotic cells.
11. Describe the importance of reproductive and resting structures in microorganisms.

One can study microbial anatomy, or substructure of procaryotic and eucaryotic microorganisms, in much the same manner as one studies the anatomy of the human body. There is, of course, much less detail and specialization of function. Cellular structures with particular functions are called *organelles*. Unfortunately, some organelles are visible only with the aid of an electron microscope, but analytical physiochemical methods have provided detailed information about their properties.

Most procaryotic cells have a cell envelope which includes cell walls and cytoplasmic membranes; some have an additional external surface enclosure. Eucaryotic cells may be bounded only by cytoplasmic membranes or have both cell membranes and walls. The cytoplasmic membrane of both eucaryotes and procaryotes surrounds a colloidal mixture of compounds known as the *cytoplasm*. The particles of a colloid—in this case, molecules of organic substances and inorganic salts—vary between 1 and 100 nm in size and remain suspended, but dispersed in an aqueous environment. The entire living material is frequently called *protoplasm*.

Eucaryotic cells are structurally more diverse and complex than procaryotic cells. The diversity is exemplified by observable differences in the internal structure of algae, protozoa, and fungi. The complexity of structure, however, is not necessarily associated with any increase in chemical complexity. As a matter of fact, it is somewhat paradoxical that the cell envelopes of eucaryotes are less complex chemically than the cell envelopes of procaryotes. Some major organelles are found in both types of cells, but eucaryotic cells have some very distinct organelles which show varying degrees of functional specialization. Among those with specialized functions are the mitochondria and chloroplasts, which are membrane-enclosed and capable of independent replication. Electron microphotographs demonstrate details of the differences in structure and organization between procaryotic and eucaryotic cells of microorganisms (Figures 4-1, 4-2).

CELL ENVELOPE

The cell envelope consists of the integuments surrounding a cell. It is made up of a cell wall and a cytoplasmic membrane in cyanobacteria, bacteria, algae, and fungi, but only of a cytoplasmic membrane in protozoa. In addition, some cyanobacteria and bacteria produce a layer of slime which surrounds the cell wall. Cell envelopes generally range from 0.150 μm to 0.500 μm in thickness.

The visible slime layer of bacteria is called a *capsule;* an analogous layer in cyanobacteria is called a *sheath.* Some capsules or sheaths are refractile, that is, they can be seen as clear areas surrounding organisms because of the way light is refracted by them, but others may require special staining techniques to be observed (Figures 4-3, 4-4). With ordinary light microscopy capsular surfaces of bacteria appear to be smooth and continuous, but electron microscopy has revealed that capsules sometimes consist of localized patches of discontinuous components (Figure 4-5). Encapsulated bacteria are often highly

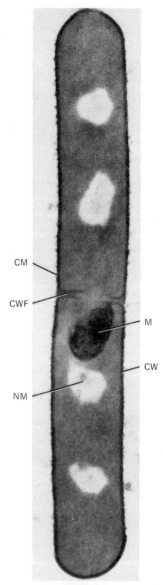

Figure 4-1 Morphology of procaryotic microbial cells. The electron micrograph of *Bacillus subtilis* shows *CW,* cell wall; *CM,* cytoplasmic membrane; *NM,* nuclear material; *M,* mesosome; *CWF,* initial stage of crosswall formation. (Courtesy, S. F. Zane and G. B. Chapman, Washington, D.C.)

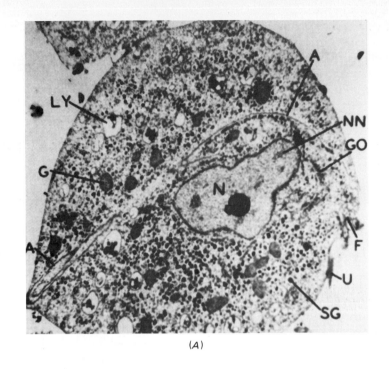

(A)

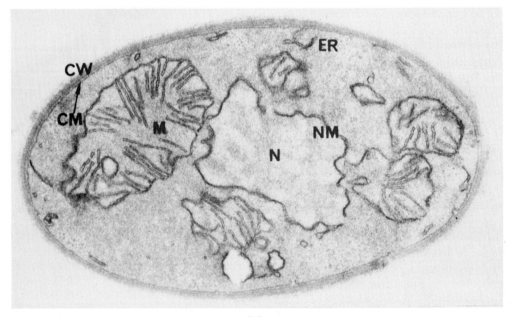

(B)

◄ **Figure 4-2** Morphology of eucaryotic microbial cells. (*A*) Electron micrograph of a longitudinal section of the eucaryotic protozoan *Trichomonas vaginalis*. *N*, nucleus; *NN*, nucleolus; *GO*, Golgi complex; *A*, axostyle; *F*, flagella; *U*, undulating membrane; *G*, large granule; *SG*, small granule; *LY*, lysosome-like vesicles. (From M. H. Nielsen and J. Ludvik, *Electron Microscopy*, vol. B., Prague, Academia, Publishing House of the Czechoslovak Academy of Sciences, 1964.)

(*B*) Electron micrograph of a thin section of *Rhodotorula mucilaginosa*. *ER*, endoplasmic reticulum; *M*, mitochondria; *N*, nucleus; *CW*, cell wall; *CM*, cell membrane; *NM*, nuclear membrane. (From M. Osumi and S. Kitsutani, *Journal of Electron Microscopy* 20:27, 1971, Japanese Society of Electron Microscopy, Tokyo.)

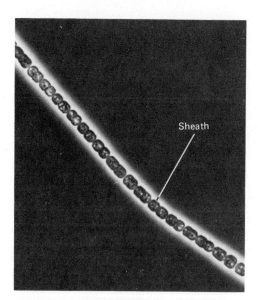

Figure 4-3 Refractile sheath surrounding a filament of vegetative cells of the cyanobacterium *Anabaena cylindrica*. (Courtesy, I. J. Foulds, Liverpool, England.)

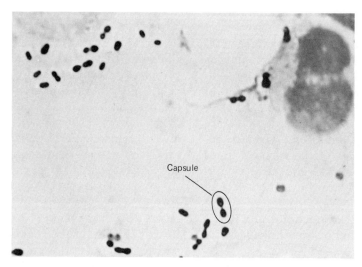

Figure 4-4 Refractile capsules surrounding cells of *Streptococcus pneumoniae* in sputum. (Courtesy, Abbott Laboratories, *Atlas of Diagnostic Microbiology*, p. 9-1, July, 1974.)

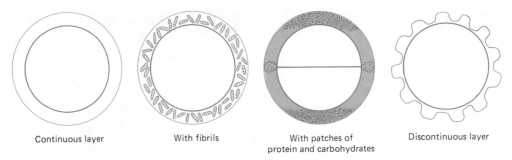

Continuous layer   With fibrils   With patches of protein and carbohydrates   Discontinuous layer

Figure 4-5 Types of capsular structure. (From J. Salton, *Bact. Rev.* 25:77, 1961.)

virulent because the protection afforded by the extra layer allows organisms to resist phagocytosis.

CELL WALL

The cell wall enables cyanobacteria, bacteria, algae, and fungi to maintain rather rigid shapes despite environmental stress because of its unique physicochemical structure. In typical bacteria the cell wall is composed of large molecules derived from glucose and amino acids. Diaminopimelic acid, an amino acid found in cell walls of procaryotes, is not known to exist elsewhere in nature. The amino acids are arranged in a cross-link fashion between molecules of the carbohydrates n-acetylglucosamine and n-acetylmuramic acid (Figure 4-6). The walls of typical bacteria vary in thickness, in the amount of carbohydrate, and in the type and number of cross linkages with amino acids.

Many fungi and algae have cell walls composed of cellulose. The glucose molecules, which make up the subunits of cellulose, form a cross network of microfibrils which impart strength and durability to the walls of fungi and algae. The walls of other fungi contain chitin, a hard substance also present in the external coverings of arthropods. Some algae, such as diatoms and chrysophytes, have walls of silica which form interesting geometric patterns (Figure 4-7).

CYTOPLASMIC MEMBRANE

The space between the cell wall and the cytoplasm contains a continuous layer of a lipid-protein "mosaic" called the cell or cytoplasmic membrane. The enclosure consists of six layers of lipids and proteins, some of which are intermingled in spatial arrangements that provide integrity to the membrane (Figure 4-8). Two layers of lipids, situated back to back, are surrounded by two layers of lipid-bound proteins interspaced with lipids. Two layers of adsorbed proteins enclose the inner lipid-protein portions. The adsorbed proteins are only loosely attached to the outside surface of the membrane. It has been estimated that there are approxi-

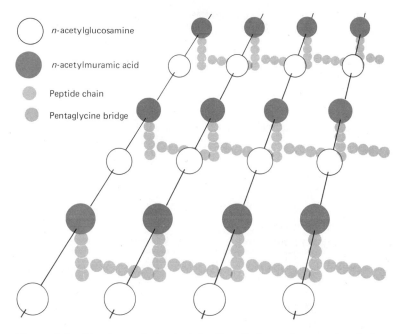

n-acetylglucosamine

n-acetylmuramic acid

Peptide chain

Pentaglycine bridge

Figure 4-6 Structure of a bacterial cell wall. A continuum of carbohydrates (n-acetylglucosamine and n-acetylmuramic acid) is wound around the cell. Reinforcement is supplied by cross-linkages with chains of amino acids. (Modified from *Sci. Am.* 220, No. 5:92, 1969.)

mately a hundred different membrane proteins. There are probably even greater differences in the lipid content of membranes. The membranes of all eucaryotic cells contain lipids known as sterols. Membranes of procaryotes, with the exception of some mycoplasmas, contain no sterols.

TRANSPORT ACROSS MEMBRANES

Water is the chief component of all cells, including those of microorganisms. Water passes freely across the cytoplasmic membrane by the process of *osmosis*. Water molecules move from an area of greater concentration to an area of lesser concentration across membranes. The water content of the cell exerts a pressure within the cell. Cells having no walls may exhibit significant changes in size or form or even burst as osmotic pressure increases within the cells. Microorganisms with rigid cell walls are less subject to alterations in morphology unless large inequities exist between the concentration of water molecules inside and outside of the cells.

The liquid lipid bilayer is responsible for a characteristic of membranes

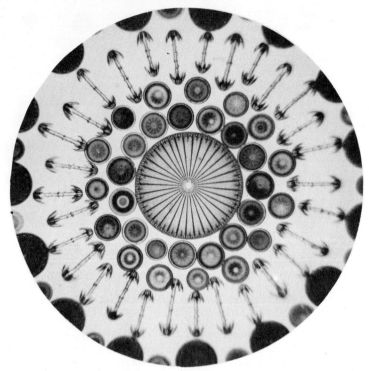

Figure 4-7   A photomicrograph of a diatom with radial symmetry. The cell wall is covered with markings which form an interesting geometric pattern. (Courtesy, Bausch and Lomb Optical Company, Rochester, New York.)

known as *fluidity*—a characteristic which permits passage of molecules by a solvent action. Soluble molecules can gain access to cells or leave cells as particles dissolved in the liquid lipid bilayer. The specific membrane lipids of a number of microorganisms can vary considerably without affecting the integrity of the membrane. The proteins reinforce the lipid layers and promote the selective exchange of materials with the environment. The mechanisms of selectivity are not well understood because it is difficult to extract intact proteins from membranes.

The selective permeability of the cytoplasmic membrane acts as an effective barrier in preventing large molecules from entering or leaving the cell. Small fragments of deoxyribonucleic acid (DNA) represent the only exception and the circumstances for the uptake of those fragments are very special. There is a continuous exchange of small molecules between cells and the environment.

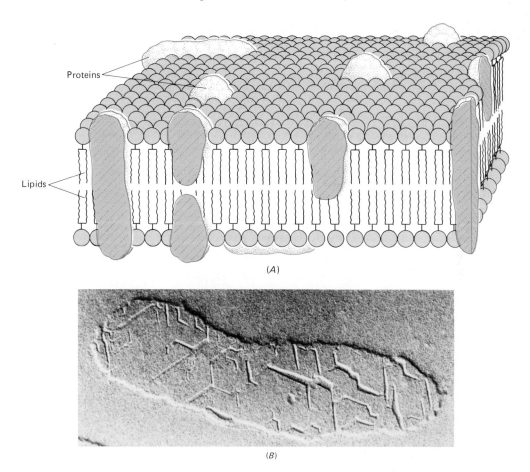

(A)

(B)

Figure 4-8 Cytoplasmic membrane. (A) Diagram of the lipid-protein "mosaic" making up the cytoplasmic membrane. Layers of protein surround or are interspaced with two inner layers of lipid. (B) Electron micrograph of an isolated membrane from a purple bacterium. Upon drying, the membrane surface develops cracks consistent with the presence of protein molecules. (Courtesy, National Aeronautics and Space Administration, Washington, D.C.)

Passive Transport. The random movement of molecules is called *Brownian movement*. Particles can be observed under the microscope to dart here and there in a haphazard manner. However, the direction of molecular movement is not always random. Movement of molecules and random collisions of molecules supply the energy for transporting molecules from an area of greater concentration to an area of lesser concentration. This type of movement is called

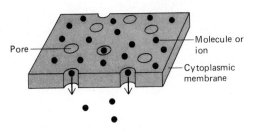

Figure 4-9 Passive transport of molecules or ions. Forces from movement and random collisions of molecules supply energy for transporting molecules from an area of greater concentration to an area of lesser concentration.

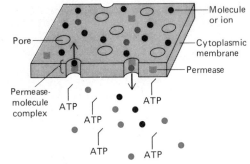

Figure 4-10 Active transport of molecules or ions across the cytoplasmic membrane of a bacterial cell. Cellular energy, supplied by adenosine triphosphate (ATP), and permeases permit molecules to move against a concentration gradient.

passive transport or *diffusion*. It occurs only in the presence of a differential in concentration gradient (Figure 4-9).

Molecules move freely across a membrane by diffusion if they are small enough to permeate the cytoplasmic membrane. The rate of diffusion is dependent on concentration gradients and the temperature of the environment. The greater the difference in concentration of molecules separated by the membrane, the greater is the rate of diffusion from the area of greater concentration to the area of lesser concentration. A rise in temperature increases the rapidity with which molecules move and, therefore, speeds up the rate of diffusion in the direction of the lower concentrations. The higher the temperature, the greater is the rate of diffusion within limits compatible with life of the microorganism. When equilibrium is reached, the rates of diffusion are the same in both directions across the membrane.

Active Transport. Molecules can also be transported against concentration gradients, that is, from areas of lesser concentration to areas of greater concentration, by an expenditure of cellular energy. If energy from a cell provides the momentum for movement of molecules, the process is called *active transport* (Figure 4-10). Active transport of molecules through the cytoplasmic membrane is facilitated in bacteria by enzymes known as *permeases*. Permeases are sensitive to the temperature of the environment; in general, they are less active at low temperatures.

The cytoplasmic membranes of bacteria vary extensively in permeability characteristics. The differences can be explained by variation in pore size and by the presence or absence of an outer lipopolysaccharide layer, but can also be attributed to the diversity of microbial permeases. Some permeases facilitate the transport of a wide variety of substances; others are highly specific in their facilitating ability and act as carriers for single substances only. Most molecules move across cytoplasmic membranes of both procaryotic and eucaryotic cells as a result of an active transport mechanism.

INTERNAL MEMBRANES

Electron microscopy reveals the presence of internal membranes in most procaryotes and eucaryotes. The internal membranes are diverse in structure and function, but have the same chemical composition as the layered cytoplasmic membrane. Sometimes groups of internal membranes lie on a parallel plane; other membranes remain isolated as separate units.

MESOSOMES

Some internal membranes of procaryotic cells appear to be undifferentiated extensions of the cytoplasmic membrane; others are highly organized lamellar, tubular, or vesicular structures called *mesosomes* (Figure 4-11). The formation of mesosomes occurs in a series of events beginning with the infolding of the membrane to form a sac. Subsequent invaginations produce an internal membrane system which varies in conformation among the bacteria.

Mesosomes provide substantial increases in surface area of membranes and are rich in respiratory enzymes. *Septal* mesosomes, located at the point of cross-wall formation following binary fission, are involved in cell division. *Lateral* mesosomes, found in other regions of the cell, have a secretory function. During the induced formation of penicillinase in at least one species of *Bacillus,* the mesosomes excrete penicillinase.

ENDOPLASMIC RETICULUM

The cytoplasm of eucaryotic cells contains a system of internal membranes known as the *endoplasmic reticulum* (ER) (Figure 4-12). The endoplasmic reticulum may appear continuous with the cytoplasmic membrane. It may have a simple structure, but often appears in

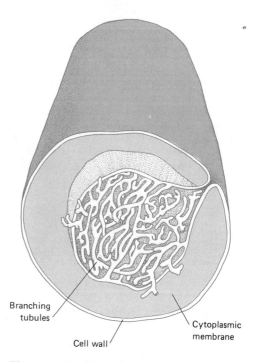

Branching tubules

Cell wall

Cytoplasmic membrane

Figure 4-11 Diagram of a mesosome of *Chromobacterium violaceum* as branching tubules of an invagination of the cytoplasmic membrane. (From T. E. Rucinsky and E. H. Cota-Robles, *J. of Bacteriol.* 118:717, 1974.)

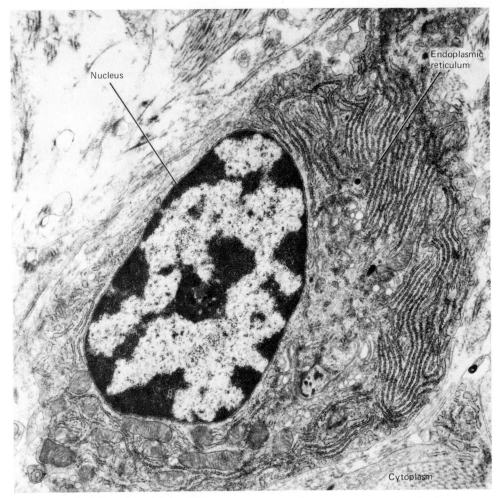

Figure 4-12   A typical eucaryotic cell showing membranous channels of endoplasmic reticulum. (Courtesy, G. D. Rose, Houston, Texas.)

the form of elaborate convolutions and infoldings. The membrane system provides for a primitive type of communication within cells and represents an accumulative site for enzymes. The association of ribosomes with the endoplasmic reticulum gives it a rough appearance. Endoplasmic reticulum which lacks ribosomal attachments appears smooth.

THE GOLGI COMPLEX

The Golgi complex consists of prominent membranous structures found in some aquatic fungi and algae. The

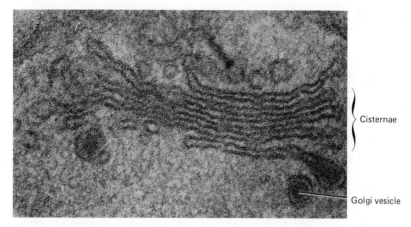

Cisternae

Golgi vesicle

Figure 4-13 A Golgi complex in the aquatic fungus *Chytridiomyces*. (Courtesy, R. T. Moore, The New University of Ulster, Coleraine, Northern Ireland.)

membranous organelles are connected to the ER and are usually located near the nucleus (Figure 4-13). The parallel, narrowly stacked membranes are known as *cisternae*. Vesicles, which are isolated from the cisternae and expanded into a closed membrane system, make up the *Golgi bodies*. The Golgi complex appears to have a role in cell-wall synthesis and may be somewhat analogous to the mesosomes of procaryotic cells.

CYTOPLASM

The cytoplasm of both procaryotic and eucaryotic cells consists of a heterogeneous colloidal mixture of water, carbohydrates, proteins, lipids, and inorganic salts. The cytoplasm of microorganisms contains accumula-tions of nonliving material in the form of *granules* or *vacuoles*. A few species of bacteria and cyanobacteria have granules or vacuoles throughout their lives (Figure 4-14). Granules and vacuoles appear particularly conspicuous in some eucaryotic cells.

In some cells granules are composed of stored insoluble nutrients; vacuoles contain soluble nutrients or gases or, as is the case in some protozoa, have a digestive or a contractile function. Digestive vacuoles contain hydrolytic enzymes which degrade ingested food particles. Contractile vacuoles aid in regulation of osmotic pressure within the cell by excreting water and other materials.

The streaming (flowing movement) of cytoplasm, readily visible in eucaryotic cells of protozoa, algae, and fungi, but not observable in procaryotes, provides the basis for the dynamic interaction of organelles.

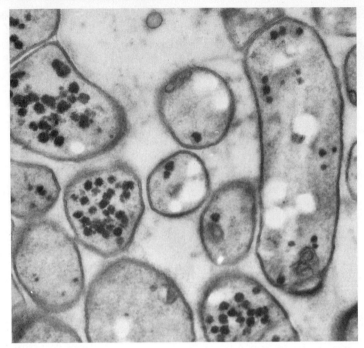

Figure 4-14 A thin section of a young culture of *Nocardia asteroides* showing dark staining glycogen granules and clear lipid-containing vacuoles. (From J. R. DiPersio, *J. of Gen. Microbiol.* 83:355, 1974, Cambridge University Press.)

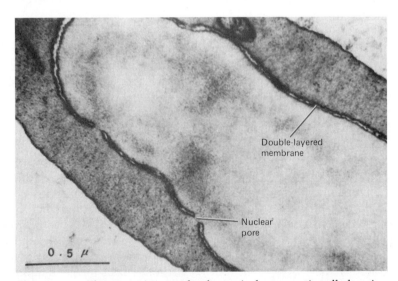

Double-layered membrane

Nuclear pore

0.5 μ

Figure 4-15 Electron micrograph of a typical eucaryotic cell showing the double-layered nuclear membrane and nuclear pores. (From R. Sugihara et al., in *Electron Microscopy*, vol. 2, Tokyo, Maruzen, 1966.)

NUCLEUS

The nuclear material of procaryotes is found in distinct regions, but is not separated from the cytoplasm by a membrane. In eucaryotes the nuclear material is contained within a membrane consisting of two layers with numerous pores through which large molecules may pass (Figure 4-15). The structure bounded by the membrane is often referred to as a *true nucleus*. True nuclei are found in algae, fungi, and protozoa as well as all plant and animal cells at some stage of their development. DNA is the major nuclear substance in both procaryotic and eucaryotic cells; in eucaryotes the DNA is complexed with specific proteins known as *histones*. A more dense area within the nucleus, called a *nucleolus*, is visible in some eucaryotic cells. The nucleolus is very rich in ribonucleic acid (RNA).

CHROMOSOMAL UNITS OF HEREDITY

The DNA of both procaryotes and eucaryotes contains the units of heredity known as *genes*. These units of genetic information make up distinct entities known as *chromosomes*. The number of chromosomes of particular species of eucaryotes is usually fixed. The DNA of a procaryote can be called a chromosome even though it differs vastly in physical appearance from chromosomes of eucaryotic cells (Figure 4-16). Every procaryotic cell has but a single chromosome except under unusual circumstances. The DNA of some bacteria has been demonstrated to be tightly coiled into a circle, but if stretched end to end, it would be 1000 or more times longer than a single bacterial cell.

EXTRACHROMOSOMAL UNITS OF HEREDITY

In some species of bacteria extrachromosomal DNA appears in the form of *plasmids* in the cytoplasm. The genes of plasmids are classified as nonessential since loss of them does not interfere with cell life. Plasmids are capable of independent replication and under special conditions can be transferred from one bacterium to another. Among the plasmids of special interest are those which are responsible for resistance to antimicrobial agents.

RIBOSOMES

The organelles responsible for protein synthesis in both procaryotic and eucaryotic cells are called *ribosomes* (Figure 4-17). There are probably 10,000 or more ribosomes in a metabolically active cell, each containing two subunits made up of approximately 65 percent RNA and 35 percent protein by weight and measuring approximately 15 nm. Since the subunits are different sizes and move under centrifugal force at different rates, the ribosomal subunits can be obtained by subjecting ribosomes to a high velocity ultracentrifuge. The rate of sedimentation is expressed as a sedi-

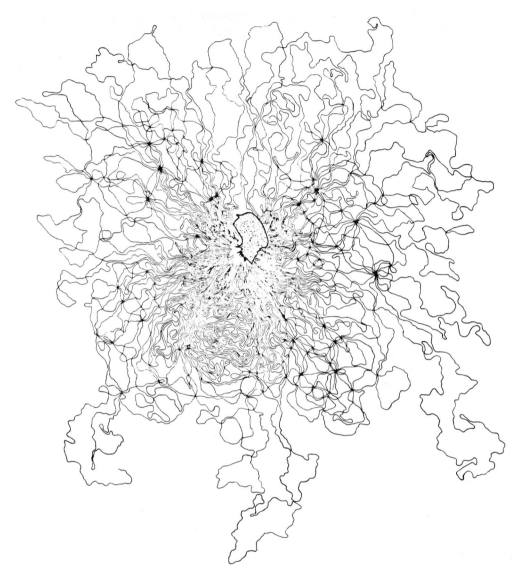

Figure 4-16 Tracing of an electron microphotograph of DNA released from *Haemophilus influenzae* and spread into a monolayer. (From B. D. Davis et al., *Microbiology*, 2d ed., New York, Harper & Row, 1973.)

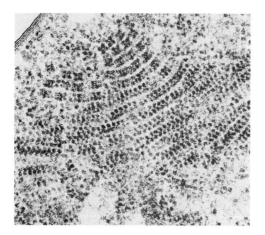

Figure 4-17 Ribosomes as helices in the bacterium *Escherichia coli*. (From E. W. Kingsbury and H. Voelz, *Science* 166:768. Copyright 1969 by the American Association for the Advancement of Science.)

mentation constant or Svedberg (S) unit. A 30S and a 50S particle are obtained from ribosomes of procaryotic cells; a 40S and a 60S particle are isolated from ribosomes of eucaryotic cells.

MITOCHONDRIA

In eucaryotic cells mitochondria are the sites of respiration and fatty acid synthesis. The oval or rod-shaped structures are often called "power houses of energy." Mitochondria are enclosed by a two-layered membrane and contain a system of inner membranes or *cristae* (Figure 4-18). The numbers of mito-

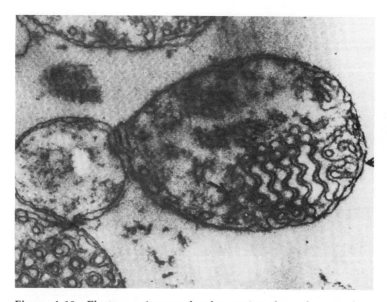

Figure 4-18 Electron micrograph of a section through part of an ameba (*Pelomyxa carolinensis*) showing a mitochondrion formed by infoldings of the inner membrane. Arrow indicates fibrous inclusions in the matrix space. (From G. D. Pappas and P. W. Brandt, *J. Biophys. Biochem. Cytol.* 6:85, 1959.)

chondria in a eucaryotic cell may vary from a very few to over 500,000, depending on the amount of cellular activity. The size of mitochondria varies somewhat with species. However, most mitochondria are 1 to 2 μm long and 0.3 to 0.7 μm wide.

CHLOROPLASTS

The photosynthetic pigments and enzymes of procaryotes are associated with the cytoplasmic membrane or platelike membranes known as *thylacoids*. However, in algae photosynthesis occurs in distinct chlorophyll-containing organelles called *chloroplasts*. Chloroplasts may be highly pleomorphic and consist of both motile and nonmotile portions. Like mitochondria, chloroplasts have both a double-layered outer membrane and inner membranes called *stroma lamellae* with which the chlorophyll is associated (Figure 4-19). Sometimes the membranes are stacked in a parallel arrangement forming *grana lamellae*.

Chloroplasts also contain DNA and ribosomes. The presence of nuclear ma-

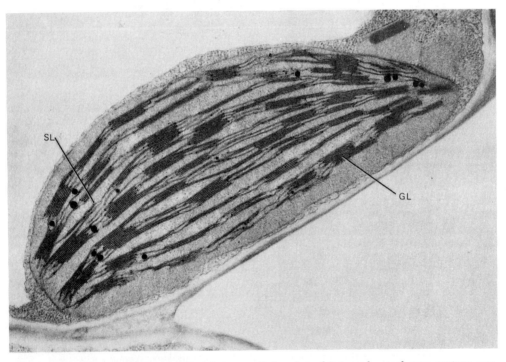

Figure 4-19   Mature chloroplast containing well-developed internal membrane system consisting of grana lamellae (*GL*) and stroma lamellae (*SL*) (From W. P. Wergin, *Sci. Am.* 223:24, 1970.)

terial and ribosomes within these organelles provides the chloroplasts with a degree of independence within host cells. It is tempting to speculate that chloroplasts also were derived from a form of chlorophyll-containing procaryotic life that colonized larger non-photosynthetic cells.

LYSOSOMES

The *lysosomes* are membrane-bound organelles of eucaryotic cells containing large quantities of hydrolytic enzymes (Figure 4-20). These small particles, often below the lower limit of visibility of the light microscope, act as the digestive tract of cells.

The confinement of hydrolytic enzymes to particular sites in the cell is advantageous to the cell since the enzymes can dissolve (or *lyse*) the cell itself if they escape into the surrounding cytoplasm. Rupture of lysosomal membranes and subsequent digestion of cell constituents does occur when a cell dies. Sometimes lysosomes of seemingly normal cells release their enzymes and cause cell death by dissolution; for this reason lysosomes are referred to as "suicide bags." The granules of some white blood cells are believed to be lysosomes which release enzymes capable of destroying invading microorganisms phagocytized by the cells.

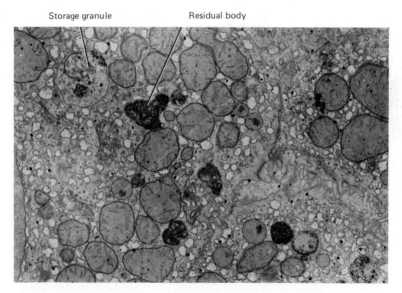

Figure 4-20 An electron micrograph showing two physical states of lysosomes in a rat kidney cell. The dark irregularly shaped structures are storage granules. The rounded structure is a residual body. (Courtesy, H. Beaufay, Brussels, Belgium.)

The digestive enzymes of procaryotes are associated with the cytoplasmic membrane or are stored temporarily in an area between the cytoplasmic membrane and the cell wall known as the *periplasmic space*. Most bacteria release hydrolytic enzymes into the environment, but the mechanism is unknown. Specific permeases transport extracellular products of digestion across the membrane.

MICROTUBULES

Eucaryotic cells contain filamentous cytoplasmic organelles known as *micro-tubules* which are composed of a protein called *tubulin*. Microtubules are particularly prominent in eucaryotes as spindle fibers during the process of mitosis, but they also are involved in locomotion and determination of cell shape. The spindle fibers appear to be assembled just prior to mitosis and disassembled after the process of cell division. A unique feature of tubulin is its apparent ability to alternate between insoluble and soluble states. Despite the instability of state, the intact microtubule is uniform in various types of cells. Each microtubule has thirteen protofilaments arranged in a precise pattern with cross bridges linking not more than four protofilaments (Figure 4-21). The imperfect symmetry is be-

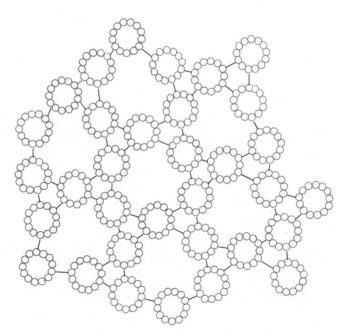

Figure 4-21 Diagrammatic representation of a group of microtubules. Each tubule has 13 protofilaments and 4 asymmetric attachments. (From L. B. Tilney, *J. Cell Biol.* 51:837, 1971.)

lieved to be a major reason for the insta-bility of microtubules.

APPENDAGES

Some microorganisms have distinct ap-pendages which can be seen with an or-dinary light microscope. Other micro-organisms have appendages which can be viewed only by electron microscopy. The primary functions of appendages are locomotion and adherence. The mo-tility of cells is not completely random, but may be oriented in a direction to-ward specific nutrients or away from harmful substances. When this orienta-tion or movement is initiated by chemi-cals in the environment, the phenome-non is called *chemotaxis.*

Appendages other than those in-volved in motility appear to be respon-sible for adherence, the ability of cer-tain bacteria to stick to one another or to surfaces of other cells or body sur-faces. The presence of either or both types of appendages probably provides microorganisms with a selective advan-tage over those without the specialized structures.

FLAGELLA

The presence of long, thin filamentous appendages known as *flagella* permits some bacteria and cyanobacteria to move about freely in aqueous environ-ments. Flagella cannot be observed with an ordinary light miscroscope unless special stains are employed, but they are frequently longer than the or-ganism from which they emanate (Fig-ure 4-22). Flagellar protein is called *flagellin,* and the fibrous and contractile

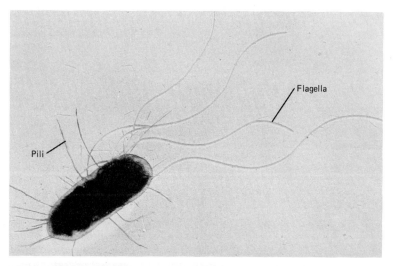

Figure 4-22 Appendages of a typical bacterium, *Escherichia coli.* (Courtesy, G. Fonte, Boulder, Colorado. From H. C. Berg, *Sci. Am.* 233:36, 1975.)

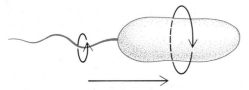

Figure 4-23 Diagrammatic representation of a bacterium showing clockwise rotary movement of the body as a flagellar filament completes one counterclockwise rotation.

nature of that material is not unlike that of muscle fibers.

A procaryotic flagellum consists of a single fiber anchored in a minute basal organelle in the cytoplasm. Energy expended by the cell produces a rotary type of motion. A complete counterclockwise rotation of a flagellar filament is necessary to propel a bacterium

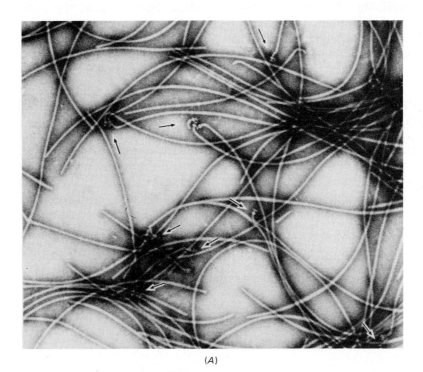

(A)

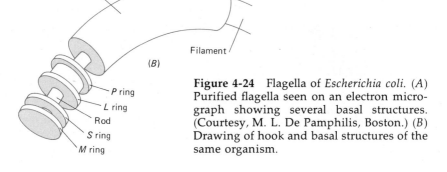

Hook

Filament

(B)

P ring
L ring
Rod
S ring
M ring

Figure 4-24 Flagella of *Escherichia coli*. (A) Purified flagella seen on an electron micrograph showing several basal structures. (Courtesy, M. L. De Pamphilis, Boston.) (B) Drawing of hook and basal structures of the same organism.

a small fraction of its length in a clockwise rotary movement (Figure 4-23). One model of a flagellum suggests that torque is generated by a rotary motor consisting of a hook and basal structures (Figure 4-24). *Escherichia coli* has been shown to move at speeds of approximately 20 μm per second. The organism has special surface proteins that act as chemoreceptors permitting it to modify movements in response to changes in the environment.

Some algae and protozoa have flagella, but the eucaryotic flagella vary considerably in structure from procaryotic flagella. Eucaryotic flagella are large enough to be seen readily with a light microscope. Each flagellum contains a ring of nine double fibrils surrounding two central fibrils; a membrane encloses the fibrils (Figure 4-25). The flagella are anchored in a basal body which converges in a bundle near the nucleus.

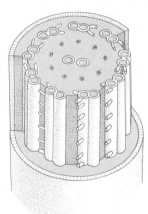

Figure 4-25 Diagrammatic representation of a eucaryotic flagellum containing a ring of nine double fibrils surrounding two central fibrils. The fibrils are enclosed by a plasma membrane.

CILIA

One group of protozoa moves by means of shorter, more numerous, hairlike appendages known as *cilia*. Each cilium arises from a basal body which is analogous in its anchoring function to the basal body of a flagellum. A cilium differs from a flagellum in that the ciliary basal body is structurally more complex. Also, cilia tend to beat in a coordinated manner which causes ciliates to be propelled more rapidly than flagellates with the whiplike type of motility.

Tubulin has been isolated from both flagella and cilia, indicating a relationship between the unstable microtubules and the stable appendages arising from the cytoplasm. Microtubules, flagella, and cilia do not always appear to form at specific sites, but the control mechanisms for differentiation into particular appendages and dissolution of microtubules remain unknown.

PILI

A number of bacteria have shorter, finer appendages known as *pili* or fimbriae surrounding the cells (Figure 4-22). The pili apparently have no role in motility, but allow some organisms to adhere to inert surfaces. Particular pili, designated as sex pili, have a role in the transfer of DNA from one bacterium to another during conjugation.

AXIAL FIBRILS

Spirochetes differ morphologically from other procaryotic bacteria by having *axial fibrils*, internal structures that lie

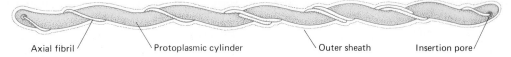

Axial fibril   Protoplasmic cylinder   Outer sheath   Insertion pore

Figure 4-26   Axial fibril and related structures of a typical spirochete.

between an outer sheath of the organism and the outermost layer of the
protoplasmic cylinder (Figure 4-26).
Axial fibrils wind around organisms
with some overlapping. The internal
structure of axial fibrils is similar to that
of bacterial flagella. The axial fibrils are
believed to rotate in a manner analogous to flagella. Rotation of axial fibrils
promotes movement of the protoplasmic cylinder in the opposite direction.
Spirochetes demonstrate motility of

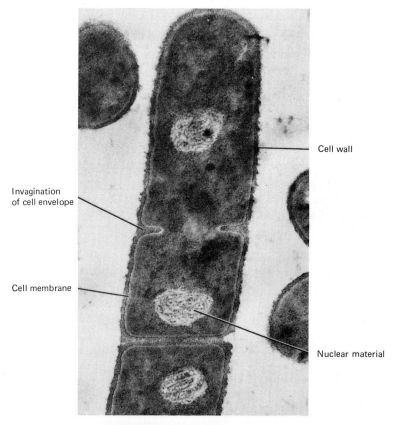

Cell wall

Invagination
of cell envelope

Cell membrane

Nuclear material

Figure 4-27   Ultrathin section of a bacterium, *Bacillus subtilis,* showing
elongation and invagination of cell envelope. (Courtesy L. Archer and
G. B. Chapman, Washington, D.C.)

three types: flexion of the cells, rotation along the long axis of the helix, and a corkscrew type of movement. Structures other than axial fibrils, such as the microtubulelike cytoplasmic or perimural fibrils or the sheath itself, may contribute in some manner to the motility of spirochetes.

REPRODUCTIVE STRUCTURES

The apparent simplicity of asexual reproduction is misleading because the processes of nuclear replication and organization which precede actual division must be among the most orderly processes in nature. Most procaryotic and many eucaryotic microorganisms reproduce by means of *binary fission*, a type of asexual reproduction in which one cell splits into two daughter cells. Bacilli may be observed to elongate before invagination of cell walls (Figure 4-27). A few bacteria, protozoa, and some fungi reproduce by *budding*, a process whereby small extensions of cell substances pinch off from the parent cell and start an independent existence (Figure 4-28). *Fragmentation*, another form of asexual reproduction, occurs in filamentous procaryotes, fungi,

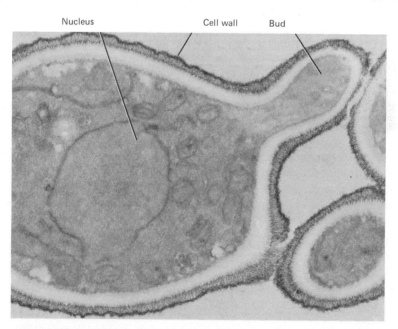

Nucleus   Cell wall   Bud

Figure 4-28 An electron microphotograph showing a bud, nucleus, and cell wall in a three-day culture of yeast (*Sporothrix schenckii*). (From R. G. Garrison et al., *J. Bact.* 124:955, 1975.)

Table 4-1   DESCRIPTIONS OF FUNGAL SPORES

TYPE OF SPORE	DESCRIPTION	EXAMPLE
Asexual spores		
arthrospores	cylindrical or cask-shaped cells arising from fragmentation of hyphae	*Geotrichum*
blastospores	cells occurring as buds pinched off from parent cells	*Saccharomyces*
chlamydospores	thick-walled cells occurring as intercalary or terminal cells of hyphae	*Candida*
conidiospores	spherical, elliptical, or pear-shaped cells (microconidia) or frequently septate, club-, or spindle-shaped cells (macroconidia)	*Penicillium*
sporangiospores	cells formed within a sac (sporangium) at ends of hyphae	*Mucor*
Sexual spores		
ascospores	cells contained in a sac (ascus) and formed by modified hyphal branches	*Neurospora*
basidiospores	cells borne on club-shaped structure (basidium)	*Cryptococcus*
oospores	thick-walled cells formed by fusion of large female and small male gametes	*Saprolegnia*
zygospores	thick-walled cells formed by fusion of similar gametes	*Rhizopus*

and some protozoa. Small portions of filaments break off and develop into independent organisms. Some cyanobacteria and fungi reproduce by terminal release of cells called *exospores* or short motile chains of cells called *hormogonia.*

The life cycles of most eucaryotic microorganisms tend to be relatively complex. In many organisms the equivalent of egg and sperm cells are produced. Very often protozoa, algae, and fungi are able to reproduce both asexually and sexually.

As molds mature, specialized reproductive cells known as *spores* are borne on tips of hyphae. The spores can be divided into sexual and asexual spores (Table 4-1). Typically, cellular and nuclear fusion occurs in the sexual reproductive process. Fungi in which sexual reproduction has not been observed are placed in the class *Fungi Imperfecti.* Most of the pathogens of humans belong to that group of fungi. Sexual reproduction does not usually occur under the conditions employed to grow fungi in the laboratory. Asexual spores tend to occur in abundance on the hyphae or modified hyphae of actively growing molds (Figure 4-29).

Some protozoa divide by *binary* or *multiple fission;* other protozoa, like the

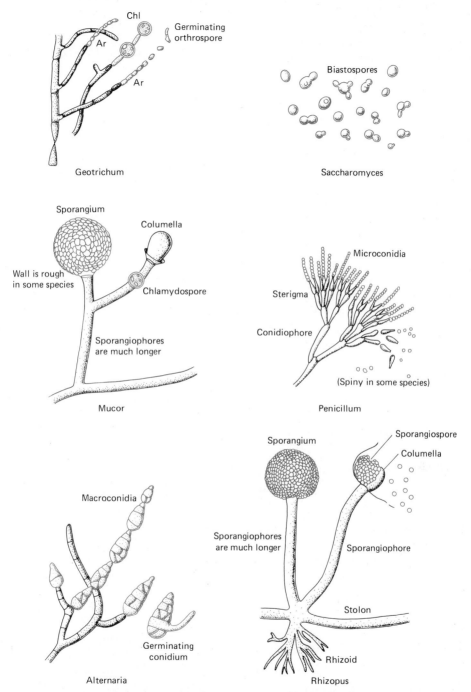

Figure 4-29 Asexual spores of common molds.

malarial parasite, reproduce asexually in humans by fragmentation and sexually in mosquitoes by the union of male and female sex cells.

Many algae, as well as a few protozoa, reproduce sexually by a mating process known as *conjugation* (Figure 4-30). During conjugation contact between cells is established and genetic material is exchanged. The products of conjugation are known as *zygotes*. Some zygotes develop immediately; others remain dormant and begin independent existences only when liberated upon death of the parent colony. The details of such complex forms of sexual reproduction are outside the scope of this textbook. However, it is important to realize that the varied forms of reproduction contribute to the diversity of the microbial world.

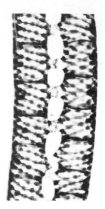

Figure 4-30 *Spirogyra* filaments in conjugation. Tubular outgrowths develop and fuse to form zygotes. (Courtesy, Fisher Scientific Company, Chicago.)

RESTING STRUCTURES

Certain procaryotes and eucaryotes form resting structures during the course of their life cycles. The resting structures permit the organisms to remain dormant for many years in soil or dust. Metabolically active stages of cells are called *vegetative cells* to differentiate them from the dormant forms. The vegetative cells of some protozoa are sometimes called *trophozoites.*

Resting structures are especially adapted to withstand environmental pressures resulting from lack of moisture and nutrients. The ability to form such specialized resistant cells provides microorganisms with a distinct survival advantage.

HETEROCYSTS, AKINETES, AND ENDOSPORES

Some cyanobacteria and bacteria form dormant cells which can be readily recognized under the bright-field microscope. Rounded empty-appearing cells known as *heterocysts* form along filaments of certain cyanobacteria, although they rarely germinate. In other species of cyanobacteria resting cells called *akinetes* are formed when the organisms are subjected to extremes of temperature. Certain bacteria, most usually bacilli and only rarely cocci and vibrios, form specialized resting structures known as *endospores*. Although the term *endospores* is frequently shortened to the word "spores" in describing the structures formed as a part of the natural life cycle of those organisms,

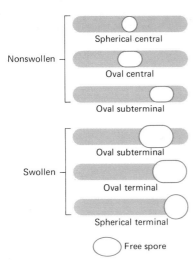

Nonswollen

Spherical central

Oval central

Oval subterminal

Swollen

Oval subterminal

Oval terminal

Spherical terminal

Free spore

Figure 4-31 Types of spores formed by bacilli. Spores may occupy three regions of a bacillus and be nonswollen or swollen. (Adapted from R. Cruickshank et al., *Medical Microbiology*, 12th ed., London, Churchill Livingston, 1973.)

it should not be confused with the asexual or sexual spores of fungi.

Endospores may occupy space within the confines of the cell (called nonswollen spores) or be greater in diameter than the parent cell (swollen spores). Furthermore, the spores can form in a central, subterminal, or terminal position of the cell. Typically, spores are spherical or oval (Figure 4-31). Alterations in chemical contents of the cell occurring during sporulation give rise to a refractile quality which is observable with an ordinary bright-field microscope; the spores are seen as dense-walled intracytoplasmic structures by electron microscopy (Figure 4-32). A more detailed discussion of endospore

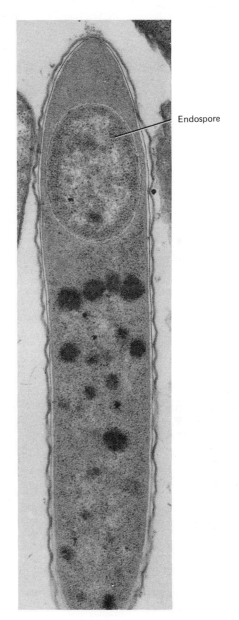

Endospore

Figure 4-32 Developing endospore in a thin section of *Bacillus brevis*. (Courtesy, S. G. Lee, New York.)

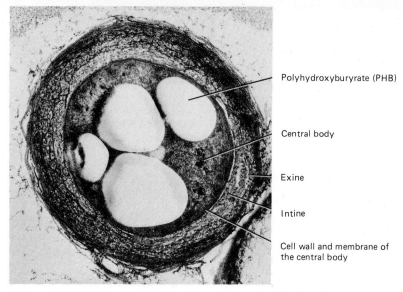

Polyhydroxyburyrate (PHB)

Central body

Exine

Intine

Cell wall and membrane of
the central body

Figure 4-33   Mature cyst of the soil bacterium *Azotobacter,* showing internal morphology. (Courtesy, H. L. Sadoff, East Lansing, Michigan.)

formation and germination is presented in Chapter 9.

CYSTS

Some soil organisms, such as bacilli belonging to the genus *Azotobacter* and many protozoa, can be induced to form thick-walled structures known as cysts in the presence of adverse environmental conditions (Figure 4-33). Cysts are quite resistant to drying, but, unlike endospores, are not particularly resistant to heat. Cysts, like endospores, may remain dormant for long periods of time.

Table 4-2   COMPARISON OF PROCARYOTIC AND EUCARYOTIC CELLS

CHARACTERISTIC	PROCARYOTES	EUCARYOTES
Size	0.2–60.0 μm	5–>100 μm
Nuclear membrane	none	present
Chromosome	one	multiple
Cytoplasmic streaming	not visible	visible
Sterols in cytoplasmic membrane	usually absent	present
Internal membranes	simple	complex
Membranous organelles	few	abundant
Photosynthetic apparatus	membrane-associated	chloroplast function
Mode of reproduction	asexual	asexual and sexual
Mitotic apparatus	none	microtubular spindles
Resting structures	endospores and cysts	cysts
Appendages	flagella and pili	flagella and cilia

SUMMARY

Microscopic studies reveal morphological variation not only between procaryotic and eucaryotic microorganisms, but also among major groups of procaryotes and eucaryotes. Eucaryotes are structurally more diverse and complex than procaryotic cells. Many of the differences in microbial anatomy become apparent only when microbial cells are studied by electron microphotography. Major differences between procaryotic and eucaryotic microorganisms are summarized in Table 4-2.

QUESTIONS FOR STUDY

1. How does the chemical composition of cell walls differ from cell membranes?
2. Explain how molecules can move against a concentration gradient.
3. Compare the chemical and structural complexity of eucaryotic and procaryotic cells.
4. Identify the following organelles as structures of eucaryotic or procaryotic cells or both:

   nucleus   Golgi complex
   ribosome   lysosome
   mitochondrion   nucleolus
   chloroplast   microtubule
   endospore   capsule
   heterocyst
5. What characteristic of tubulin accounts for the appearance and disappearance of spindle fibers during mitosis?

SELECTED REFERENCES

Berg, H. C. How bacteria swim. *Sci. Am.* 233:36, 1975.

Brock, T. D. *Biology of Microorganisms.* 2d ed. Englewood Cliffs, N.J.: Prentice-Hall, 1970.

Buchanan, R. E., and Gibbons, N. E. *Bergey's Manual of Determinative Bacteriology.* 8th ed. Baltimore: Williams & Wilkins, 1974.

Danielli, J. F. The bilayer hypothesis of membrane structure. *Hosp. Pract.* 8:63, 1973.

de Duve, C. The lysosome. *Sci. Am.* 208:64, 1963.

Delwiche, C. C. The nitrogen cycle. *Sci. Am.* 223:137, 1970.

Emmons, C. W.; Binford, C. H.; and Utz, J. P. *Medical Mycology.* 2d ed. Philadelphia: Lea & Febiger, 1970.

Goodenough, U. W., and Levine, R. P. The genetic activity of mitochondria and chloroplasts. *Sci. Am.* 223:22, 1970.

Nomura, M. Ribosomes. *Sci. Am.* 221:28, 1969.

Palmer, C. M. *Algae in Water Supplies.* Washington, D.C.: U. S. Department of Health, Education and Welfare, 1962.

Stanier, R. Y.; Adelberg, E. A.; and Ingraham, J. L. *The Microbial World.* 4th ed. Englewood Cliffs, N.J.: Prentice-Hall, 1976.

Chapter 5

The Viruses

After you read this chapter, you should be able to:

1. Define capsid, capsomer, virion, nucleocapsid, and peplos.
2. Explain the basis for classification of viruses into two major groups.
3. Describe three major morphological types of viruses.
4. Describe the sequence of events occurring in the replicative cycle of viruses.
5. Describe two *in vitro* methods of cultivating viruses.
6. Describe two techniques used for enumerating virus particles.
7. Explain the significance of the 50 percent infectious dose (ID_{50}).
8. Describe five groups of DNA and ten groups of RNA viruses affecting vertebrates.
9. Explain the role of unclassified and subviral entities in disease.

Immunization for the viral diseases smallpox and rabies was practical long before the viruses were identified. Beijerinck, in 1899, was the first to propose the concept of *contagium vivum fluidum* or contagious living fluid. More than 35 years later, after exhaustive experimentation, W. M. Stanley (1904–1971) concluded that the tobacco mosaic virus was a protein with properties of an infectious agent. Scientists were undecided whether the virus was an "organule" or a "molechism." The physical and chemical characterization of viruses was possible only when cell culture techniques, analytical centrifugation, X-ray diffraction, radioactive tracers, and electron microscopy were developed. Information accumulated during the past 40 years has revealed that viruses are ultramicroscopic biological entities containing either DNA or RNA surrounded by a protein coat.

The particles exhibit properties of life only within host cells so may be considered obligate parasites.

Viruses that affect vertebrates are divided into two major groups on the basis of the type of nucleic acid contained within the particles. A virus may contain either DNA or RNA, but not both. Additional characteristics, such as molecular weight of nucleic acids, number of nucleic acid strands (either single or double strand), and particle structure permit the two major groups to be divided into even smaller groups (Tables 5-1, 5-2).

MORPHOLOGY OF VIRUSES

Electron microphotographs reveal that viruses are not merely particles of ill-

Table 5-1   PROPERTIES OF DNA VIRUSES OF VERTEBRATES

Group	Number of Strands	Size of Virion (nm)	Shape of Virion	Nucleocapsid Symmetry	Envelope
Parvovirus	1	18–24	cubical	isosahedral	−
Papovavirus	2	40–55	cubical	icosahedral	−
Adenovirus	2	70–80	cubical	icosahedral	−
Herpesvirus	2	180–200	pleomorphic	icosahedral	+
Poxvirus	2	230–300	brick shaped	complex	+

SOURCE: Adapted from J. D. Acton et al., *Fundamentals of Medical Virology* (Philadelphia: Lea & Febiger, 1974).

Table 5-2   PROPERTIES OF RNA VIRUSES OF VERTEBRATES

Group	Number of Strands	Size of Virion (nm)	Shape of Virion	Nucleocapsid Symmetry	Envelope
Reovirus	2	54–75	cubical	icosahedral	−
Picornavirus	1	18–30	cubical	icosahedral	−
Togavirus	1	35–40	cubical	icosahedral	+
Orthomyxovirus	1	80–120	roughly spherical	helical	+
Paramyxovirus	1	100–300	pleomorphic	helical	+
Rhabdovirus	1	60–225	bullet shaped	helical	+
Retrovirus	1	100	roughly spherical	icosahedral	+
Arenavirus	1	110–130	oval or pleomorphic	unknown	+
Coronavirus	1	80–160	roughly spherical	unknown	+
Bunyavirus	1	90–100	oval	helical	+

SOURCE: Adapted from J. D. Acton et al., *Fundamentals of Medical Virology* (Philadelphia: Lea & Febiger, 1974).

defined shape or detail, but actually consist of almost geometrically perfect architectural designs. Although viruses show more morphological diversity than bacteria, they do share many structural components. Clarification of morphological details has paralleled the development of purification techniques for virus-laden suspensions.

The life cycle of viruses consists of an extracellular phase and an intracellular parasitic phase. In the extracellular phase viruses exist as inert infectious particles known as *virions*. In the intracellular parasitic phase the particles exist as *replicating forms*.

Virions are composed of an inner core of nucleic acid surrounded by a protein coat or *capsid*. Aggregates of the structural units of the protein, which can be seen by electron microscopy, are called *capsomers*. The nucleic acid and the capsid make up the *nucleocapsid*.

SIZE AND SHAPE

Groups of viruses have virions which vary in size and symmetry of nucleocapsids, but individual viruses of the same type show little pleomorphism. Most nucleocapsids demonstrate helical or polyhedral symmetry (Figure 5-1). The tobacco mosaic virus is a good example of a helical virus. The inner core

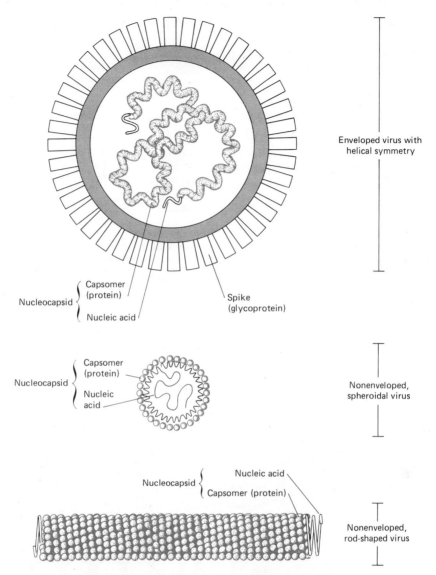

Figure 5-1 Morphology of viruses. The drawings are representations of three forms of viruses: enveloped with helical symmetry; nonenveloped, spheroidal; and nonenveloped, rod-shaped. (From C. A. Knight, *Chemistry of Viruses,* 2d ed., New York, Springer-Verlag, 1975.)

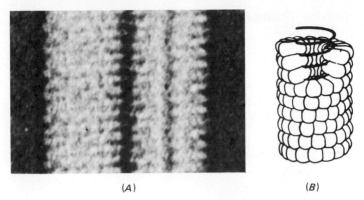

Figure 5-2 Tobacco mosaic virus. (*A*) Actual appearance of rigid rods. (*B*) Drawing of the virus showing helical symmetry. The RNA is embedded in the protein. (From A. W. Horne, J. M. Harnden, and R. Markham, *J. Gen. Virol.* 31:265, 1976, Cambridge University Press, New York.)

of RNA is surrounded by a capsid made up of about 2000 capsomers (Figure 5-2). Many of the polyhedral nucleocapsids are icosahedrons—geometric figures with 12 corners, 20 triangular faces, and 30 edges. The herpes simplex virus is an example of a virus with icosahedral symmetry (Figure 5-3). It contains

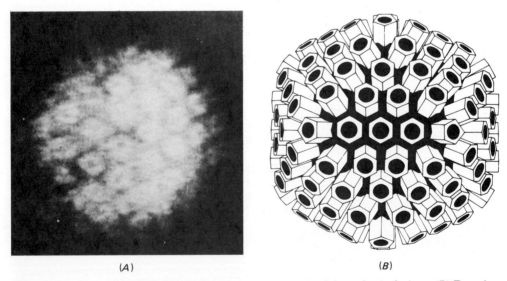

Figure 5-3 Herpes simplex virus. (*A*) Actual appearance of the spherical virus. (*B*) Drawing of the virus showing icosahedral symmetry with five- and six-sided capsomers. (From R. W. Horne, *Virus Structure*, New York, Academic Press, 1974.)

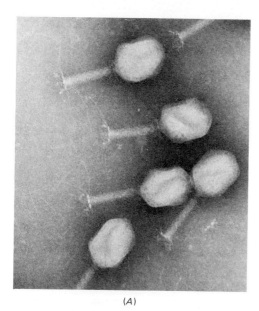

(A)

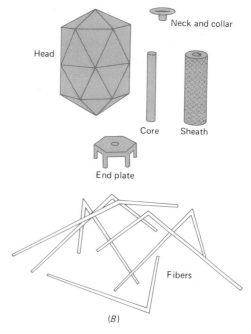

Head

Neck and collar

Core Sheath

End plate

Fibers

(B)

Figure 5-4 T4 phage. (A) Actual appearance with extended tail. (Courtesy, V. Chapman and S. Delong, Denver, Colorado.) (B) Drawing of component parts and assembled phage.

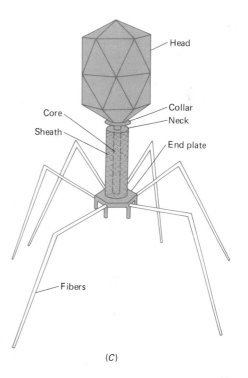

Head

Core

Collar

Neck

Sheath

End plate

Fibers

(C)

12 five-sided capsomers and 150 six-sided capsomers.

Some nucleocapsids are enclosed in an envelope or *peplos* of host-cell membrane or viral origin; others are nonenveloped. Electron microphotographs reveal that some envelopes have surface projections called *spikes* which are made up of glycoproteins. Most virions range in size from 20 nm to 300 nm.

Some viruses cannot be classified as helical or polyhedral because of more complex morphology or inadequate data. Most bacteriophages, for example, have *heads* with icosahedral symmetry and distinct appendages known as *tails* with helical symmetry. The T-even phages of *Escherichia coli* are typical of the tailed bacterial viruses (Figure 5-4).

The heads of bacteriophages contain DNA or RNA surrounded by protein; the tail contains several proteins. An inner core of protein is surrounded by a contractile sheath and is attached to an end plate and tail fibers. The tail is the attachment organ and structure through which nucleic acid makes its way to the surface of the host bacterium.

The poxviruses are examples of morphologically complex viruses. Many of the virions are brick-shaped with the DNA arranged as a tubular structure in a crisscross pattern. The Orf virus, which causes infectious pustular dermatitis, mainly in sheep and rarely in humans, is a virus with this complex morphology (Figure 5-5).

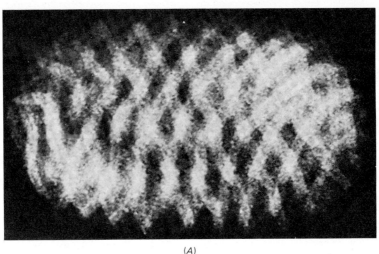

(A)

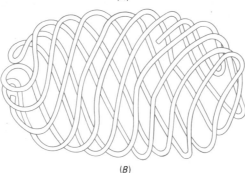

(B)

Figure 5-5 Orf virus. (A) A highly magnified view of the virus with crisscross effect. (B) Drawing of the virus showing origin of crisscross pattern. (From R. W. Horne, *Virus Structure*, New York, Academic Press, 1974.)

REPLICATION OF VIRUSES

The host-parasite relationship between cells and viruses is unique in that energy and synthetic resources of the cells are used for viral replication. Cells of algae, bacteria, fungi, plants, vertebrates, or invertebrates can supply the support necessary for replication of particular viruses. The replicative cycle, or series of events occurring during reproduction, constitutes the infectious process. The sequence of events includes attachment, penetration, multiplication, assembly, and release.

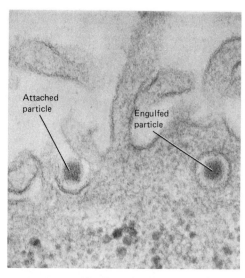

Figure 5-6 Attachment and engulfment of adenovirus. One particle is attached to the surface of a cell; the second has been engulfed by the process of viropexis. (From Y. Chardonnet and S. Dales, *Virology* 40:462, 1970.)

ATTACHMENT

The initial contact between viruses and susceptible cells is a random event. After collision, the virus particles may attach to receptor sites if a type of structural or electrostatic complementarity exists; if it does not, attachment is blocked. The tail fibers of bacteriophages and the spikes of enveloped viruses are well adapted for attachment; other viruses have no discernible morphological characteristic which has a role in this initial event. Picornaviruses, retroviruses, and orthomyxoviruses attach to specific receptor sites on the surface of host-cell membranes. The receptor sites may, in addition to attracting viruses, have a role in capsid disruption.

PENETRATION

Viruses may play an active or a passive role in the penetration process whereby they enter cells following attachment. The T2 bacteriophage of *Escherichia coli* injects only the nucleic acid portion of the virus particle through the bacterial cell wall; it is distinctly an active process. Transfer of animal viruses across cell membranes requires no activity by viruses. Some viruses appear to be engulfed by cells in a process called *viropexis* (Figure 5-6). Sometimes a fusion of cell and virus seems to occur, thereby facilitating entry of the virus. Degradation of capsids at attachment sites may also facilitate penetration of particular viruses.

MULTIPLICATION

Before replication of viral nucleic acid can occur within cells, viruses must be denuded of all capsid material. The penetration process of bacteriophages leaves the capsid behind, but capsids of other viruses are apparently destroyed by proteolytic enzymes of host cells. The genomes of a few viruses retain small amounts of protein.

In some cells multiplication of viruses occurs only in the cytoplasm or nucleus, while in others both the cytoplasm and nucleus support replication (Figure 5-7). The synthetic processes involved in the production of more infective particles are the same as for normal cell synthesis except that the viral nucleic acid supplies the genetic information. Transcription of RNA from host chromosomes ceases almost immediately after penetration. An infecting virus containing single-stranded RNA can code for its own replication. In some RNA virus–host cell systems the RNA is transcribed into DNA by a viral reverse transcriptase. Some viruses may supply more than one enzyme needed for replication. The host cell supplies the ribosomes, tRNA, amino acids, nucleotides, most of the enzymes, and all of the energy for synthesis of new viruses.

ASSEMBLY

The assembly of newly synthesized nucleic acids and proteins may require special enzymes made by virus-directed synthetic processes. Assembly of the components of a few viruses has been accomplished *in vitro*. Within cells transfer of capsid proteins from the cy-

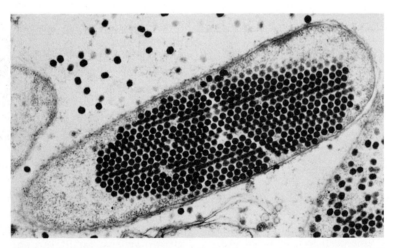

Figure 5-7   Electron micrograph of ultrathin section of T-2–infected *Escherichia coli*. The polyhedral bodies represent condensates and intact phage particles. (Courtesy, G. B. Chapman and J. Pisani, Washington, D.C.)

toplasm to the viral nucleic acid in the nucleus may be necessary. If both proteins and nucleic acids are synthesized in the cytoplasm, the assembly process is less complex. The period from the entry of a virus particle to the time of the appearance of progeny with infectious capabilities is called the *eclipse phase*.

RELEASE

Mature progeny are liberated from bacterial cells when a viral enzyme, lysozyme, promotes cell lysis by destroying cell walls. Infective particles of animal cells are extruded by a budding process on the cell membrane or by the formation of specialized tubular structures (Figure 5-8). The yield of viruses from infected cells varies with the host-virus system. A bacterium may produce 100 to 1000 new infective particles; a human cell frequently produces as many as 10^5 to 10^6 particles.

CULTIVATION OF VIRUSES

Since viruses need the resources of living cells for replication, the techniques for cultivating viruses are more complex than those required for growing bacteria. Most bacteria and some other microorganisms can serve as hosts to viruses. The propagation of type-specific bacteriophages can be accomplished by adding infectious phage particles to a culture of susceptible bacteria. Within a few hours, lysis of cells

occurs and phage particles can be harvested. Animals or plants were employed in the earliest attempts to propagate viruses affecting those organisms, but only limited information on host cell–virus relationships could be obtained. It became feasible to cultivate cells *in vitro* when plant or animal cells could be freed from tissue by the en-

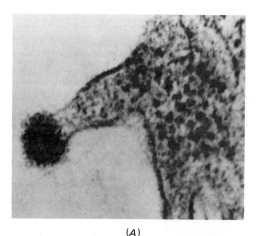

(A)

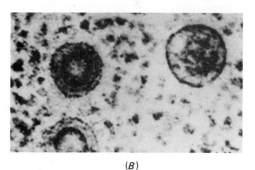

(B)

Figure 5-8 A virus bud and particles from a Friend ascites tumor of a mouse. (A) Bud is on the membrane of a tumor cell. (B) Particles are in supernatant of ascites fluid. (From K. Maruyama and S. Oboshi, in *Electron Microscopy*, vol. 2, Tokyo, Japan, 1966.)

zyme trypsin and when antibiotics became available for preventing contamination of cultures with fungi and bacteria. The three most common methods for culturing animal viruses employ embryonated eggs, cells, and animals.

EMBRYONATED EGGS

The developing chicken embryo is a suitable medium for growing a variety of viruses including those of influenza, vaccinia, rabies, canine distemper, measles, and mumps. It takes 21 days for a fertilized ovum to develop into a chick. During the first week after fertilization the extraembryonic membranes and cavities are formed. Viruses show

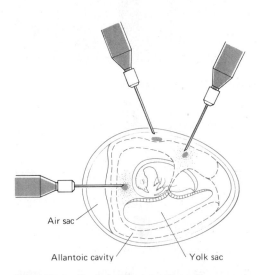

Air sac

Allantoic cavity   Yolk sac

Figure 5-9 Inoculation into the yolk sac, on the chorioallantoic membrane, and into the allantoic cavity of embryonated eggs. (Adapted from R. H. A. Swain and T. C. Dodds, *Clinical Virology*, Edinburgh, Churchill Livingstone, 1967.)

some selectivity for particular embryonic structures. The age of the embryo required and route of inoculation depend on the virus to be grown (Figure 5-9). Some grow best in the allantoic or amniotic cavities; others multiply more readily on the chorioallantoic membrane, in the yolk sac, or, less frequently, in the developing embryo.

Prior to inoculation a candling device, which exposes embryonated eggs to a concentrated beam of light, identifies the vascular structure of the chorioallantois. Eggs are marked on the shell at a point for inoculation that avoids large blood vessels. Shells are disinfected, punctured, and viruses are injected into the appropriate structure of the eggs. Eggs are examined for evidence of virus infection after a week or more of incubation at 35° to 37°C. With some viruses distinct lesions known as pocks occur on the chorioallantoic membrane (Figure 5-10). Sometimes growth of the embryo is only stunted; other times the embryo dies. The presence of viruses in embryonic fluids is detected by animal inoculation or hemagglutination activity. Viruses, such as vaccinia, mumps, and influenza, bind to receptor sites of some red blood cells producing visible agglutination.

CELLS

Cell cultures are the most desirable method for studying host cell–virus relationships. Viruses may be grown in *primary* cell cultures, that is, those with limited capacities for subculture, or in *continuous* cell lines, that is, those capable of indefinite numbers of transfers in media containing essential nutrients. Primary cells can usually be successfully propagated for only one to three months. The term *cell strain* is sometimes used to refer to cells capable of limited serial culturing.

Cell strains, like primary cells, retain the diploid number of chromosomes of the parent tissue, but may undergo other alterations with serial culturing.

Cell strains can usually be subcultured approximately 50 times.

Continuous cell lines have adapted to an *in vitro* environment, but no longer resemble the original host cells. The chromosome number usually increases —a condition called *polyploidy*. Other changes may occur so that continuous cell lines actually consist of *transformed* cells. The continuous cell lines in use

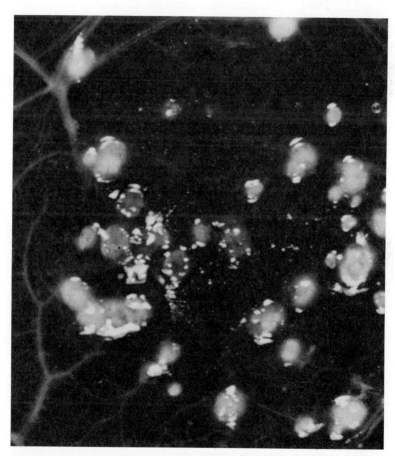

Figure 5-10 Pocks on a chorioallantoic membrane of a chicken embryo infected with vaccinia virus. (Armed Forces Institute of Pathology Photograph, Neg. No. 58-13966-4.)

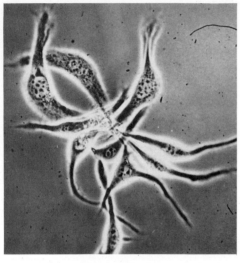

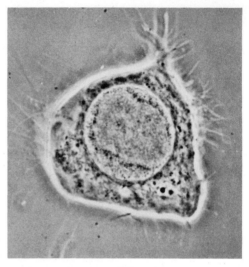

(A)   (B)

Figure 5-11 Effect of virus infection on cells. (*A*) Uninfected ovarian cells. (*B*) Early stage of a viral infection characterized by rounding up of a cell and formation of viral particle in center of cell. (From L. E. Volkman and M. D. Summers, *J. of Virol.* 16:1632, 1975.)

today, such as monkey kidney cells, human fibroblasts, and human neoplastic cells, emerged from successful repeated culturing of cell strains.

Viruses may destroy host cells or have no apparent effect on them. Infected cells often become round and more refractile than uninfected cells (Figure 5-11). A distinct morphological change, known as a *cytopathic effect* (CPE), may occur. The CPE is generally characteristic of a particular host cell–virus system. For example, multinucleated giant cells can be observed in tissue cultures infected with measles virus (Figure 5-12). The CPE produced by some other viruses takes the form of

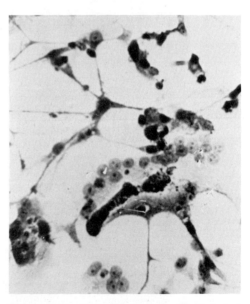

Figure 5-12 Human amnion cells infected with measles virus. Changes include formation of stellate-shaped and multinuclear giant cells. Cells lyse in three or four weeks, releasing infective particles. (From J. W. Frankel and M. K. West, *Proc. Soc. Exp. Biol. and Med.* 97:741, 1958.)

cytoplasmic or nuclear inclusion bodies in infected cells. The inclusion bodies appear at the site of viral replication and may consist of actual viral particles, components, or remnants.

Virus-infected cells may show no apparent cytological aberration, but have alterations in cell membrane or metabolic activities. For example, the membranes of some myxovirus-infected cells have an affinity for red blood cells and will adsorb them (Figure 5-13). Cells infected with adenoviruses sometimes clump because of a cell-membrane–associated affinity for one another. Infected cells may bring about a change in the pH of the surrounding medium. With some viruses host cell injury is associated with an increase in pH; other viruses cause cells to produce acidic end products.

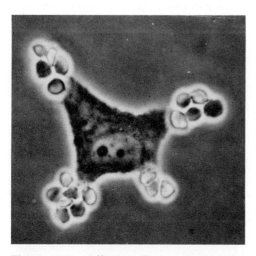

Figure 5-13 Affinity of a myxovirus-infected cell for red blood cells. Bovine red blood cells are adsorbed to the cell membrane of an infected cell. (Courtesy, P. I. Marcus, Storrs, Connecticut.)

ANIMALS

Animals are still used for the isolation and identification of some viruses. For example, mice are employed for demonstration of the causative agents of encephalitis and rabies. In addition, chickens, mice, hamsters, guinea pigs, and rats are valuable in studying the oncogenic (tumor-inducing) viruses. Animals may be inoculated intracerebrally, intraperitoneally, intravenously, intranasally, intratracheally, or intradermally with nasal or throat washings, urine, or body fluids. When mice are inoculated with rabies virus, the animals exhibit muscle incoordination and paralysis a week or more after injection. Sections of nerve tissue may demonstrate cytoplasmic inclusions (Negri bodies) as a CPE or rabies viruses may react with fluorescein-tagged antibodies for definitive diagnosis. With other viruses it is necessary to mince tissue to free viruses for serological testing.

ENUMERATION OF VIRUSES

The small size of viruses and complex cultural methods required for their propagation preclude the use of bacteriological assay techniques for enumeration of virus particles. A count of physical particles provides limited information because the ability of the particles to infect cells remains unmeasured. Both counts and infectivity assays may require equipment available only in research laboratories.

PARTICLE COUNTS

Highly purified preparations of the larger viruses can be counted with an electron microscope. In one method, a known concentration of latex particles of approximately the same size as the viruses to be counted is mixed with the virus preparation. The ratio of latex to virus particles multiplied by the concentration of latex particles equals the concentration of virus particles (Figure 5-14).

An alternate method for estimating virus particles employs the property of

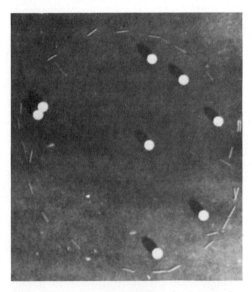

Figure 5-14 Enumeration of viruses by particle count. Suspensions of tobacco mosaic virus and latex particles in dried droplets under the electron microscope. The ratio of latex to virus particles multiplied by the concentration of latex particles equals the concentration of virus particles. (From M. Yamada, B. Commoner, and J. Symington, *Proc. Nat'l. Acad. Sci.* 48:1675, 1962.)

viruses to agglutinate red blood cells. If twofold dilutions of virus preparation are incubated with red cell suspensions, the hemagglutination titer, that is, the highest dilution of virus causing hemagglutination, can be determined.

INFECTIVITY ASSAYS

A measure of the infectivity of virus particles can be obtained by inoculating embryonated eggs, cell cultures, or animals with dilutions of virus suspensions. After appropriate incubation, effects attributable to virus infection are analyzed. The highest dilution of virus causing a noticeable effect contains at least one infective particle. The titer is expressed as the 50 percent infectious dose (ID_{50}), that is, the reciprocal of the highest dilution that causes an effect attributable to a virus in one-half of the embryonated eggs, cell cultures, or animals. For example, if 0.1 ml of a dilution of a virus suspension infected 50 percent of the test animals, the titer would be expressed as

$$\frac{1}{0.1 \times 10^{-6}} = 10^7 ID_{50}/ml$$

Large numbers of tests are frequently necessary to obtain valid results.

A more precise and less costly estimation of viral infectivity is obtained by the plaque method. Dilutions of virus are added to monolayers of susceptible cells or, in the case of phage counting, to agar seeded with susceptible bacteria. Agar is sometimes added to monolayers of animal host cells. The growing host cells produce a so-called "lawn" of growth interrupted by clear

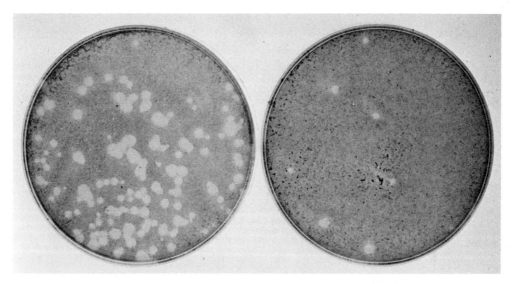

Figure 5-15 Typical plaque formation in a monolayer of human kidney cells infected with adenovirus 12. Each plaque represents a plaque forming unit (PFU) where cells have been destroyed by the progeny of an infective particle. (Courtesy, B. C. Casto, BioLabs, Inc., Northbrook, Illinois.)

areas called plaques (Figure 5-15). Each plaque is produced by the progeny of a single infectious particle called a *plaque-forming unit* (PFU). When compared with physical counts, the number of PFU is greater for phage particles than for animal viruses. The *efficiency of plating* (EOP) is obtained by comparing the infectious titer with the electron microscope count.

THE DNA VIRUSES OF VERTEBRATES

All the vertebrate deoxyribonucleic acid viruses (DNA viruses) contain double-stranded DNA in the virion with the exception of the parvoviruses, which have single-stranded DNA. All except the poxviruses have icosahedral nucleocapsid symmetry. All except the poxviruses replicate in the nucleus. Human disease is caused by viruses belonging to all of the DNA viral groups except the parvoviruses.

PARVOVIRUS

The parvovirus group contains the smallest viruses of the DNA viruses. The single-stranded DNA of the virion serves as a template for a complementary form of DNA in host-mammalian cells. The double-stranded DNA is known as the replicative form (RF). From it, additional molecules of DNA, only one of which contains a DNA

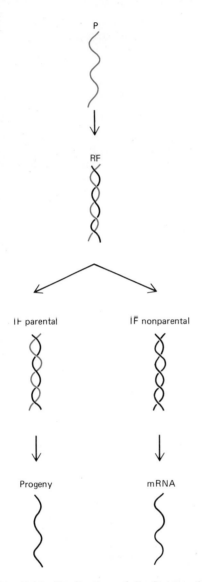

Figure 5-16 Replication of single-stranded DNA viruses. Parental DNA (P) serves as a template for the complementary strand of a replicative form of DNA (RF). Intermediate forms of DNA (IF) serve as templates for mRNA and progeny. (Adapted from J. D. Acton et al., *Fundamentals of Medical Virology*, Philadelphia, Lea & Febiger, 1974.)

strand of parental origin, are synthesized. The double-stranded DNA molecules of nonparental origin serve as templates for mRNA to code for virus proteins. DNA of the progeny is transcribed from the intermediate DNA which has one strand of parental DNA (Figure 5-16).

The parvoviruses contain no viruses producing disease in humans, but include the Kilham rat virus and some adeno-associated viruses which replicate only in the presence of an adenovirus as a "helper."

PAPOVAVIRUS

The papovavirus group, like other DNA viruses except the parvoviruses, contain double-stranded DNA. However, unlike other DNA viruses, the nucleic acid of papovaviruses is cyclic rather than linear in structure. The double-stranded DNA serves as a template for mRNA and progeny (Figure 5-17).

The papovaviruses produce tumors or tumorlike lesions in the rabbit, human, dog, cattle, hamster, horse, and monkey. One group of papovaviruses, known as papilloma viruses, causes warts in a number of species, including humans. Another member of the papovaviruses, the SV40 virus, was originally isolated from the rhesus monkey. In its natural host the SV40 virus has no effect, but it produces malignant tumors in hamsters. Some of the first oral poliovirus vaccines used were contaminated with SV40 viruses because monkey kidney cell cultures employed to grow the polio viruses contained SV40 viruses. However, there have been no

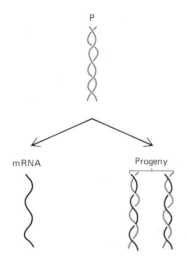

Figure 5-17 Replication of double-stranded DNA viruses. Parental DNA (P) serves as a template for mRNA and progeny. (Adapted from J. D. Acton et al., *Fundamentals of Medical Virology*, Philadelphia, Lea & Febiger, 1974.)

cases of tumor induction reported in individuals who received the contaminated vaccines.

ADENOVIRUS

The adenovirus group is a large group of viruses, all of which contain double-stranded DNA in linear form. Replication is similar to that of other double-stranded DNA viruses.

Adenoviruses infect many species of animals, including humans. There are at least 33 serotypes of human adenoviruses, some of which are oncogenic in animals (Figure 5-18).

HERPESVIRUS

The viruses of the herpesvirus group are unique among the DNA viruses in

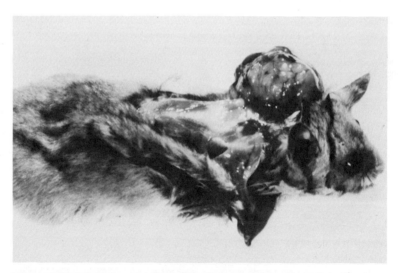

Figure 5-18 A tumor produced by human adenovirus 12 in hamster 34 days after injection. (Courtesy B. C. Casto, BioLabs, Inc., Northbrook, Illinois.)

that they possess an envelope acquired by budding from the nucleus or cytoplasm of host cells during maturation. Some herpesviruses appear to have "empty" centers in electron micrographs, but the significance of these barren cores is not clear (Figure 5-19).

The viruses of fever blisters, chickenpox, shingles, cytomegalic inclusion disease, and infectious mononucleosis belong to the herpesvirus group. In addition, the causative agent of infectious mononucleosis, known as the Epstein-Barr (EB) virus, is frequently found in association with Burkitt's lymphoma. The etiological role of the EB virus in the lymphoma, which is endemic in some parts of Africa, remains uncertain.

POXVIRUS

The viruses of the poxvirus group are not only the largest of all DNA viruses,

but they exhibit the most complex nucleocapsid symmetry. All poxviruses contain lipid in addition to nucleic acid and protein. Both a DNA-dependent RNA polymerase and a DNA-dependent DNA polymerase are associated with the virion.

Viruses of the poxvirus group cause variola (smallpox), vaccinia (cowpox), and a benign tumor known as molluscum contagiosum in humans.

THE RNA VIRUSES OF VERTEBRATES

The vertebrate ribonucleic acid viruses (RNA viruses), with the exception of the reovirus group, contain single-stranded RNA. Some are without an envelope, while others have a distinct

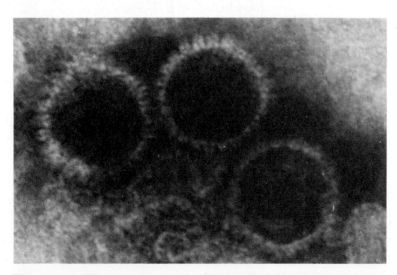

Figure 5-19 Electron micrograph of herpes simplex viruses showing barren cores. (Courtesy, R. W. Horne, P. Wildy, and the John Innes Institute, Norwich, England.)

envelope. The group contains examples of both helical and icosahedral nucleocapsid symmetry. The mechanisms of replication are more complex than for DNA viruses, often involving replicative intermediates and RNA-DNA hybrids, that is, molecules with one strand of each nucleic acid. Most replicate in the cytoplasm, but a few multiply in the cytoplasm or nucleus. There are viruses in each RNA-virus group that can cause human disease. The retroviruses are oncogenic in animals.

REOVIRUS

The viruses belonging to the reovirus group are nonenveloped, contain icosahedral nucleocapsids, and are double stranded. They contain RNA polymerase which transcribes mRNA from the genome (Figure 5-20). Newly synthesized RNA also serves as a template for progeny.

Members of the reoviruses may cause mild fever, diarrhea, or upper respiratory infections in humans.

PICORNAVIRUS

The viruses of the picornavirus group are the smallest of the RNA viruses. They are nonenveloped with icosahedral nucleocapsids. The single strand of RNA acts directly as mRNA or as a template for a replicative form (RF) from which a replicative intermediate (RI) is transcribed (Figure 5-21). Single-stranded RNA progeny, identical to parental RNA, are formed from the RI in some manner. Progeny RNA can function, in turn, as mRNA, as a template for more RF, or associate with pro-

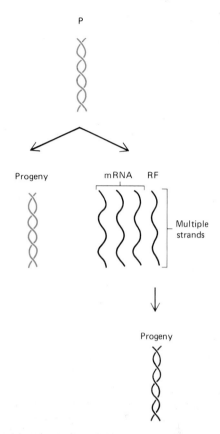

Figure 5-20 Replication of double-stranded RNA viruses. Parental RNA (P) serves as a template for multiple strands of RNA which serve as mRNA or as templates for progeny. (Adapted from J. D. Acton et al., *Fundamentals of Medical Virology*, Philadelphia, Lea & Febiger, 1974.)

teins for capsid production. Synthesis of an RNA-dependent RNA polymerase is not viral-coded, but rather a cellular function.

The viruses causing polio, coxsackie disease, and some enteric infections belong to the picornavirus group. The group also includes a large number of viruses associated with common colds.

TOGAVIRUS

The togavirus group consists of heterogeneous enveloped particles with icosahedral nucleocapsid symmetry. Many are not only transmitted by arthropod vectors, but can replicate both in insect vectors and animal hosts. The difference in size of togaviruses may be a reflection of variability in the deposition of lipoprotein in the envelope during budding. Details of the mode of replication of the togaviruses have not been studied as thoroughly as some other viruses. The biological cycle for the arthropod-borne viruses belonging to this group is complex since both vertebrate and nonvertebrate hosts are required.

The viruses causing yellow fever, rubella, and encephalitis belong to this group.

ORTHOMYXOVIRUS

Viruses of the orthomyxovirus group are roughly spherical, have envelopes, and demonstrate helical nucleocapsid symmetry. Spikes can usually be observed radiating from the surface of virions. Replicative phases occur in both the nucleus and the cytoplasm of host cells. RNA complementary to virion RNA, catalyzed by virion RNA-dependent RNA polymerase, serves as mRNA, as a template for progeny, and for a replicative intermediate (RI) (Figure 5-22). Virus replication of the orthomyxovirus group appears to require cell-coded proteins.

Types A, B, and C of the influenza virus are orthomyxoviruses. Their role

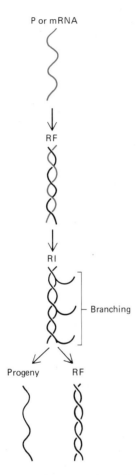

Figure 5-21 Replication of single-stranded RNA viruses involving a replicative form (RF) and a replicative intermediate (RI). Initial viral RNA can act as mRNA or as a template for RF. Progeny RNA which function as mRNA or a template for additional RF or which associate with protein for capsid production are formed from RI. (Adapted from J. D. Acton et al., *Fundamentals of Medical Virology*, Philadelphia, Lea & Febiger, 1974.)

in respiratory infections of humans is well documented.

PARAMYXOVIRUS

The paramyxoviruses are highly pleomorphic, enveloped viruses with helical nucleocapsid symmetry (Figure 5-23). Replication usually occurs in the cytoplasm in a manner similar to that of the orthomyxovirus group. Viral antigens are frequently found on cell membranes of infected cells. Virus particles are released by budding.

The viruses of mumps, measles (rubeola), and some respiratory infections belong to this group.

RHABDOVIRUS

Viruses of the rhabdovirus group are unique in that they have bullet-shaped virions (Figure 5-24). They are enveloped and have helical nucleocapsid symmetry. Their replication cycle is similar to that of the orthomyxovirus and paramyxovirus groups. Infected cells characteristically produce cytoplasmic inclusions.

The viruses of vesicular stomatitis and rabies are the most studied members of the group.

RETROVIRUS

The retroviruses consist of roughly spherical, enveloped virions in icosahedral nucleocapsids. They replicate in the nucleus forming both RNA-DNA hybrids and DNA intermediates. The DNA intermediates can be incorporated into the host-cell genome (Figure

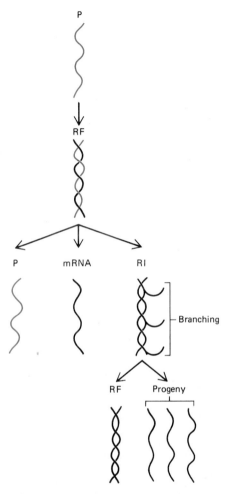

Figure 5-22 Replication of single-stranded RNA viruses in which mRNA is complementary to virion RNA. The replicative form (RF) can act as a template for the mRNA, progeny, or a replicative intermediate (RI). The RI can serve as a template for RF or progeny. (Adapted from J. D. Acton et al., *Fundamentals of Medical Virology*, Philadelphia, Lea & Febiger, 1974.)

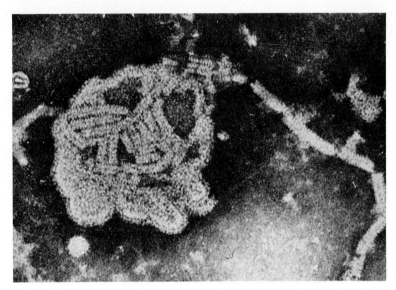

Figure 5-23   A paramyxovirus. The enveloped Newcastle virus with its helical symmetry is typical of the group. (From R. W. Horne and A. P. Waterson, *J. Mol. Biol.* 2:75, 1960.)

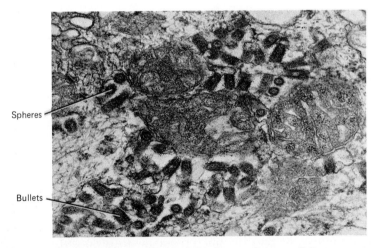

Figure 5-24   An electron micrograph of a cow brain cell line containing dark "bullets" and spheres of rabies viruses, strain CVS, seen longitudinally and in cross-section. (Courtesy, P. D. Lunger, Newark, Delaware.)

5-25). The virion contains both an RNA-directed DNA polymerase and a DNA-dependent DNA polymerase.

The discovery that DNA synthesis can be directed by reverse transcription in cells infected with RNA oncogenic viruses has challenged the central dogma of DNA. More than that, it has provided a possible explanation for RNA virus–host cell interactions. Viral coded DNA, once incorporated into a host-cell genome, may be expressed only under appropriate environmental circumstances.

The retroviruses produce tumors in chickens, mice, rats, cats, and guinea pigs. The Rous sarcoma virus of chickens, the murine leukemia viruses, and the mouse mammary tumor viruses have been studied extensively and remain model systems for studying oncogenic properties of viruses. Although RNA-containing particles have been found in human cancers, no proof exists to show that the particles are either infectious or oncogenic.

ARENAVIRUS

Little is known about arenaviruses except that they are pleomorphic, enveloped, and often have dense granules in the core. Lymphocytic choriomeningitis (LCM) virus, which infects a variety of mammals including humans, belongs to this group.

CORONAVIRUS

The coronaviruses are similar to the influenza viruses, but infected cells are surrounded with petal-like structures.

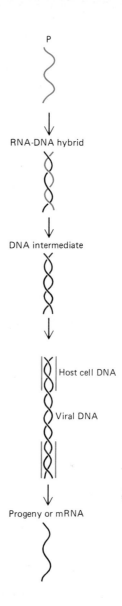

Figure 5-25 Replication of single-stranded RNA viruses having RNA-DNA hybrids and double-stranded DNA intermediates. The DNA intermediate is integrated into the host cell genome. Progeny or mRNA can be transcribed from integrated viral DNA. (Adapted from J. D. Acton et al., *Fundamentals of Medical Virology*, Philadelphia, Lea & Febiger, 1974.)

They are one cause of upper respiratory infections.

BUNYAVIRUS

The bunyaviruses make up the largest group of arthropod-borne viruses, but little is known about their structure or method of replication. These single-stranded RNA viruses have a helical nucleocapsid. They are named after the African locality of Bunyamwera, but are not limited to Africa. At least 10 serotypes are found as a cause of encephalitis in California. All bunyaviruses are carried by mosquitoes, but, fortunately, most do not cause disease in humans.

UNCLASSIFIED VIRUSES

The viruses of hepatitis (type A), hepatitis (type B), and non-A, non-B (NANB) viruslike particles have not yet been studied sufficiently to classify them as members of one of the DNA or RNA virus groups. An antigen (HB$_s$Ag) is found on the surface of the type B hepatitis virus; a second antigen (HB$_c$Ag) is associated with the core of the virion. Numerous attempts to grow the hepatitis viruses have produced a variety of possible etiological agents, but more study is needed to characterize the isolates.

SUBVIRAL ENTITIES

A number of incomplete viruses, designated as subviral entities or *viroids*, have been isolated from diseased plants and chronic diseases associated with cell dysfunction of vertebrates. The term slow viruses was used to describe the subviral entities of vertebrates until it was discovered that the particles can grow quite rapidly under appropriate circumstances.

The viroids range in size from 15 to 100 nm. Some consist of nucleic acid alone; others have an envelope surrounding the genome. Those that have been characterized appear to contain single-stranded RNA.

A number of subviral particles appear to be the possible agents of chronic neurologic disease, such as Guillain-Barré syndrome, kuru, Creutzfeldt-Jakob disease, multiple sclerosis, and Parkinson's disease. Much remains to be learned of subviral entities and their interactions with host cells.

SUMMARY

Viruses are submicroscopic biological entities exhibiting the characteristics of life only in host cells. They can be classified according to the type of nucleic acid in the virion and further grouped by shape and size of virions, presence or absence of an envelope, number of nucleic acid strands, and type of nucleocapsid symmetry. Replication can occur in the nucleus or cytoplasm and sometimes involves replicative intermediates of DNA, RNA, or RNA-DNA hybrids.

Cells of bacteria, plants, animals, and humans can host specific viruses. Both DNA and RNA viruses of vertebrates can transform host cells. The oncogenic RNA viruses provide the most striking examples of transformation leading to tumor production in animals. The possible roles of viruses in human cancer and of subviral entities in neurological diseases need further clarification.

QUESTIONS FOR STUDY

1. How does a virion differ from a replicating form of a virus?
2. By what means do viruses enter cells?
3. Name three continuous cell lines in use today.
4. Name three retroviruses which are oncogenic in animals.
5. Define the following terms and indicate how each is related to the study of viruses:
   primary cells
   continuous cell lines
   plaque
   cytopathic effect (CPE)
   50 percent infectious dose (ID_{50})
   hybrid

SELECTED REFERENCES

Acton, J. D.; Kucera, L. S.; Myrvik, Q. N.; and Weiser, R. S. *Fundamentals of Medical Virology for Students of Medicine and Related Sciences.* Philadelphia: Lea & Febiger, 1974.

Fenner, F.; McAuslan, B. R.; Mims, C. A.; Sambrook, J.; and White, D. O. *The Biology of Animal Viruses.* New York: Academic Press, 1974.

Goodheart, C. R. *An Introduction to Virology.* Philadelphia: Saunders, 1969.

Horne, R. W. *Virus Structure.* New York: Academic Press, 1974.

Knight, C. A. *Chemistry of Viruses.* 2d ed. New York: Springer-Verlag, 1975.

Lennette, E. H.; Spaulding, E. H.; and Truant, J. P. *Manual of Clinical Microbiology.* 2d ed. Washington, D.C.: American Society for Microbiology, 1974.

Maramorosch, K., and Kurstak, E. *Comparative Virology.* New York: Academic Press, 1971.

Chapter 6

The Helminths

After you read this chapter, you should be able to:

1. Differentiate between an obligate and a facultative parasite.
2. Differentiate between a definitive and an intermediate host.
3. Describe morphological differences among three groups of parasitic helminths.
4. Explain how the helminths are adapted for parasitism.
5. Describe the infective stages of nematodes, cestodes, and trematodes.
6. Describe the relationship between filarial worms and particular arthropods.

The helminths make up a heterogeneous group of worms, which, unlike the procaryotes, simple eucaryotes, and viruses, are macroscopic in size. They include both free-living and parasitic forms and belong to the animal kingdom. There are diverse morphological and metabolic types of helminths, many of which require more than one host to complete their life cycles.

Helminths unable to exist without resources supplied by one or more hosts are *obligate parasites;* those able to live either independently or by means of resources provided by a host, when extended the opportunity, are *facultative parasites. Ectoparasites* live on the external surfaces of a host. *Endoparasites* live within the body of a host. The requirements of some helminths are so special that they survive only in a single species of an animal host or in particular types of tissue.

Helminths, despite their macroscopic size, are included in the study of microbiology. As we have said, the reason for this anomaly is that in the course of their life cycle many species of helminths cause disease in their animal hosts. The helminths exhibit direct life cycles in which there is a single *definitive host* or indirect life cycles with one or more *intermediate hosts.* Definitive hosts harbor adult parasites, whereas intermediate hosts support the *larvae,* the immature parasites. There may also be *alternate hosts,* that is, animals other than natural hosts capable of supporting an immature or mature helminth. Frequently, humans become *accidental hosts* when they ingest microscopic ova (eggs) of worms or are bitten by an arthropod carrying disease-producing organisms.

Some parasitic helminths may exhibit free-living larval stages. Only the primitive roundworm *Strongyloides* can

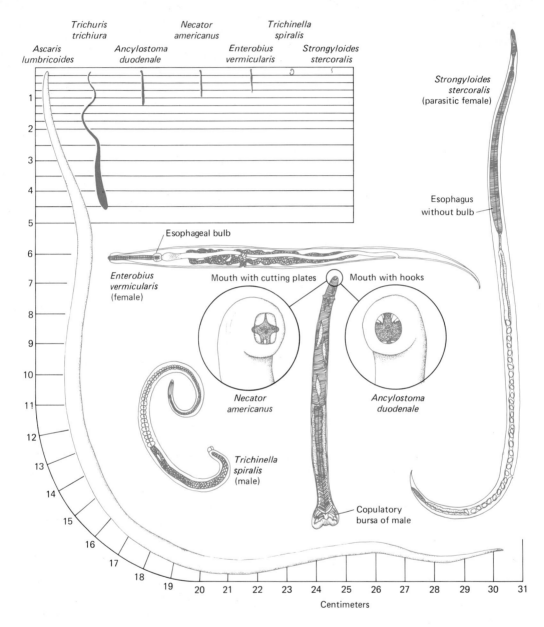

Figure 6-1 Actual size of medically important female roundworms. (Adapted from U.S. Naval Medical School, *Medical Protozoology and Helminthology,* Washington, D.C., U.S. Government Printing Office, 1965.)

exist as a free-living adult. Helminths with direct life cycles tend to be widespread in distribution; parasites with indirect life cycles are more restricted geographically.

Some stages of helminths develop only in aquatic environments; some infective stages require particular physiological environments or specific sites for development. Helminths may have complex metamorphoses before attaining sexual maturity. The continuing survival of helminth species is made possible by the production of tremendous quantities of ova and availability of appropriate hosts.

THE NEMATODES

The nematodes or roundworms include numerous aquatic and terrestrial free-living forms as well as more than 80,000 parasites of vertebrates. The adult worms are cylindrical and vary in size from 2.0 mm to over 1 m in length. They are nonsegmented and have rounded anterior ends and somewhat pointed posterior ends. They are usually *dioecious* (the sexes are separate) and the male is smaller than the female (Figure 6-1). The anterior end sometimes contains special organs of attachment such as hooklets, suckers, setae, or papillae. The body wall consists of a noncellular cuticle, epithelium, and muscle fibers. Nematodes can find refuge in a wide variety of locations within the human host (Figure 6-2).

ANATOMY OF NEMATODES

The nematodes have an alimentary tract with two openings, a mouth and an anus. The tubular digestive system is divided into a buccal cavity, esophagus, intestine, and rectum (Figure 6-3). In the male the rectum and genital duct are joined forming a common passage, the cloaca, which opens into the anus. In the female a short rectum extends directly from the intestine. Some adult worms have two lateral excretory canals or tubules which empty into a ventral excretory pore. The metabolic processes of the parasitic nematodes, as well as other parasitic worms, are anaerobic since there is little, if any, free oxygen available to them in their vertebrate hosts.

Nematodes have no circulatory system. Instead, a fluid containing hemoglobin and nutrients circulates within the body cavity meeting metabolic needs of cells.

The nervous system is rudimentary, consisting only of six longitudinal nerves, an anal ganglion, and two connecting bands of nerve tissue, the circumesophageal ring and the circumcloacal commissure.

The reproductive system of nematodes is exceptionally well developed and adapted for production of 20 to 200,000 fertilized ova daily. Parts of the male reproductive system are differentiated into a testis, vas deferens, seminal vesicle, and ejaculatory duct. Some species have accessory organs, such as spicules, which function as copulatory organs. Parts of the female re-

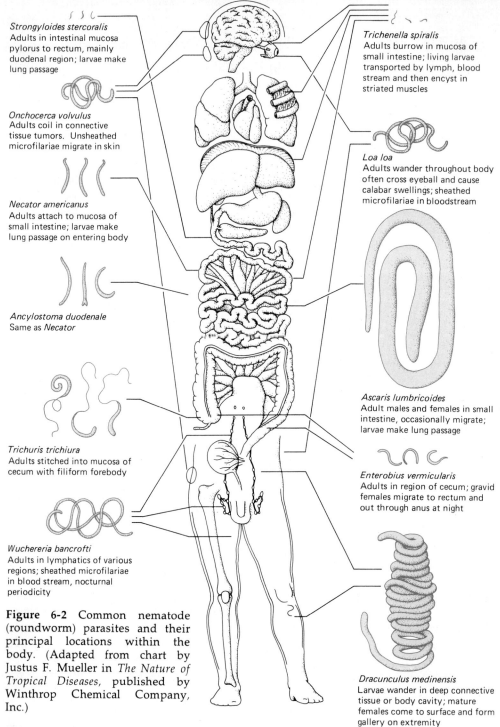

Strongyloides stercoralis
Adults in intestinal mucosa
pylorus to rectum, mainly
duodenal region; larvae make
lung passage

Onchocerca volvulus
Adults coil in connective
tissue tumors. Unsheathed
microfilariae migrate in skin

Necator americanus
Adults attach to mucosa of
small intestine; larvae make
lung passage on entering body

Ancylostoma duodenale
Same as *Necator*

Trichuris trichiura
Adults stitched into mucosa of
cecum with filiform forebody

Wuchereria bancrofti
Adults in lymphatics of various
regions; sheathed microfilariae
in blood stream, nocturnal
periodicity

Trichenella spiralis
Adults burrow in mucosa of
small intestine; living larvae
transported by lymph, blood
stream and then encyst in
striated muscles

Loa loa
Adults wander throughout body
often cross eyeball and cause
calabar swellings; sheathed
microfilariae in bloodstream

Ascaris lumbricoides
Adult males and females in small
intestine, occasionally migrate;
larvae make lung passage

Enterobius vermicularis
Adults in region of cecum; gravid
females migrate to rectum and
out through anus at night

Dracunculus medinensis
Larvae wander in deep connective
tissue or body cavity; mature
females come to surface and form
gallery on extremity

Figure 6-2 Common nematode
(roundworm) parasites and their
principal locations within the
body. (Adapted from chart by
Justus F. Mueller in *The Nature of
Tropical Diseases,* published by
Winthrop Chemical Company,
Inc.)

126

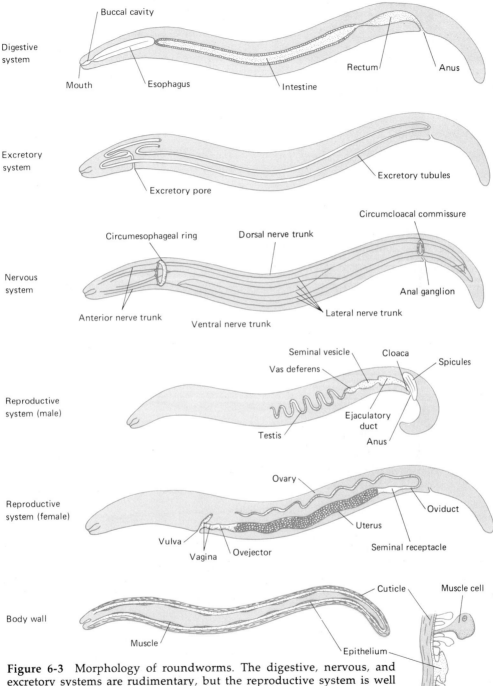

Figure 6-3 Morphology of roundworms. The digestive, nervous, and excretory systems are rudimentary, but the reproductive system is well developed. (From U.S. Naval Medical School, *Medical Protozoology and Helminthology*, Washington, D.C., U.S. Government Printing Office, 1965.)

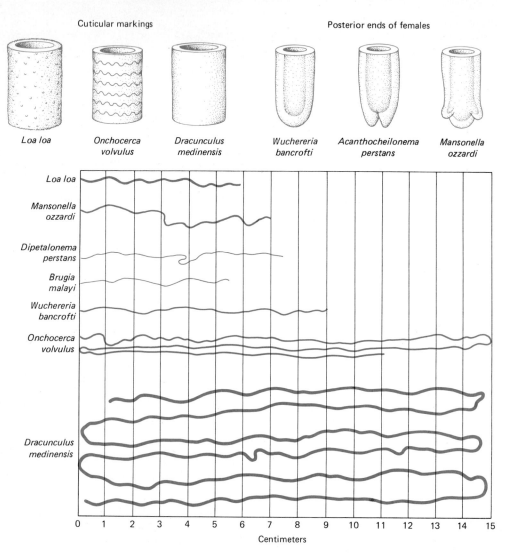

Figure 6-4 Characteristics of female filarial worms. Females may be distinguished from one another by size, cuticular markings, and posterior ends. (From U.S. Naval Medical School, *Medical Protozoology and Helminthology*, Washington, D.C., U.S. Government Printing Office, 1965.)

productive system are differentiated into the ovary, oviduct, seminal receptacle, uterus, ovejector, vagina, and vulva. Unlike the male systems, the female's genital and digestive tracts have separate openings.

One group of slender, threadlike roundworms, the filarial worms, do not attain lengths greater than 50 cm. Female filarial worms are always twice the size of their male counterparts. The different species can be distinguished in the females by characteristic size, well-defined transverse striations on the cuticle, and characteristics of the tail (Figure 6-4).

A unique feature of filarial worms is the production of a prelarval stage known as a *microfilaria*. Two characteristics by which species can be identified are the presence or absence of a sheath surrounding the microfilaria and the presence or absence of cells with outstanding nuclei at the tips of tails (Figure 6-5).

INFECTIVE STAGES

Favorable environmental circumstances enable some nematodes to develop into first and second stages of larvae. The first larval stage or *rhabditiform larva* is a noninfective feeding form, whereas the second larval stage or *filariform larva* is an infective nonfeeding form (Figure 6-6).

A single definitive host is required for completion of the life cycles of ne-

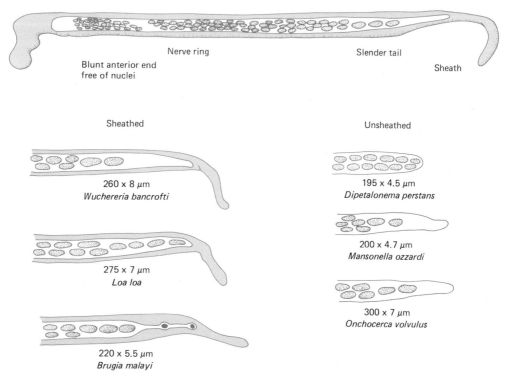

Figure 6-5 Diagnostic characteristics of microfilariae of man. (From H. W. Brown, *Basic Clinical Parasitology*, 4th ed., Englewood Cliffs, N.J., Prentice-Hall, 1975.)

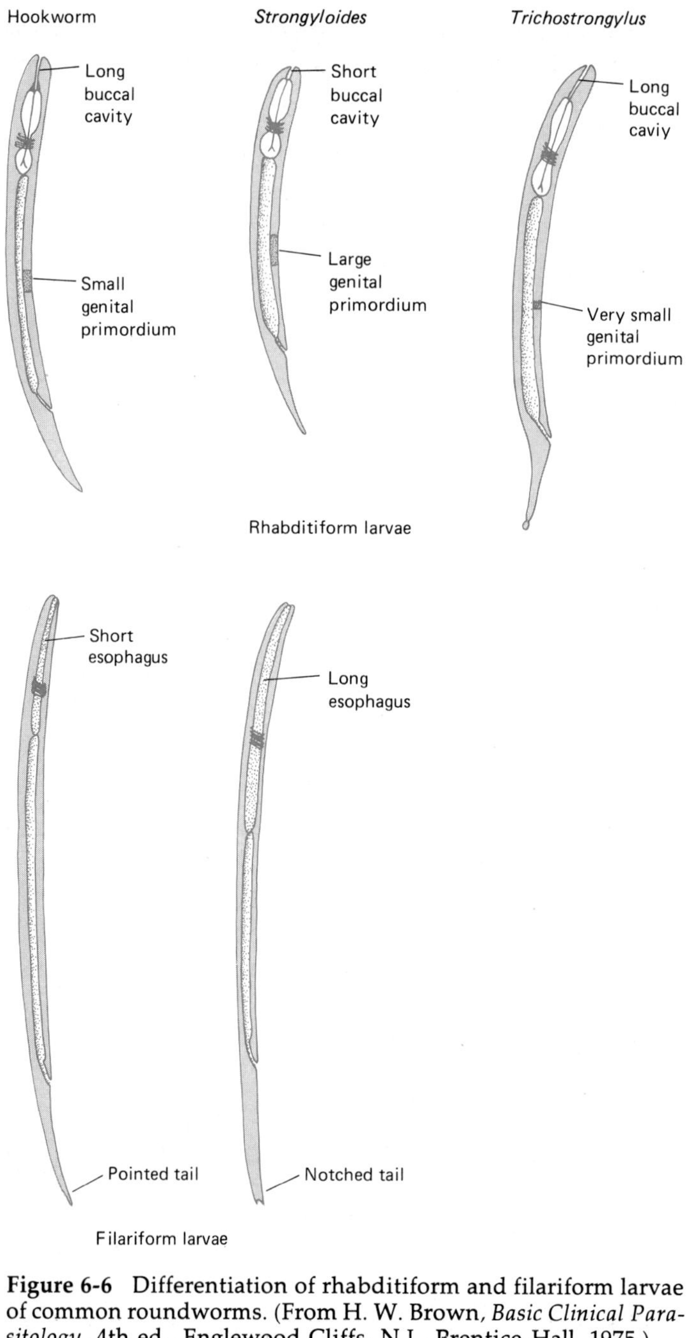

Hookworm

Long
buccal
cavity

Small
genital
primordium

Strongyloides

Short
buccal
cavity

Large
genital
primordium

Trichostrongylus

Long
buccal
caviy

Very small
genital
primordium

Rhabditiform larvae

Short
esophagus

Long
esophagus

Pointed tail

Notched tail

Filariform larvae

Figure 6-6   Differentiation of rhabditiform and filariform larvae
of common roundworms. (From H. W. Brown, *Basic Clinical Parasitology*, 4th ed., Englewood Cliffs, N.J., Prentice-Hall, 1975.)

matodes other than filarial worms. Larval forms may be ingested or may penetrate the skin, travel by way of the blood to the lungs, pass into the pharynx, and ultimately, be swallowed to reach the intestines. If larvae are unable to develop within a host, an infection called larva migrans results. Larva migrans may be cutaneous, subcutaneous, or visceral. The disease is self-limiting because larvae eventually die within the host, but the larvae may persist long enough to cause serious symptoms and predispose the host to secondary bacterial infections.

The life cycle of filarial worms requires an arthropod as an intermediate host. Microfilariae are ingested from the blood or tissue of a definitive host by a blood-sucking insect. Metamorphosis into a rhabditiform larva and then into a filariform larva occurs in the insect. The filariform larva penetrates the skin of a new host with the help of a biting fly or mosquito. Microfilariae do not appear in the blood of the host for months. The microfilariae of some species of filarial worms are present in the blood only at night: that phenomenon is called *nocturnal periodicity.*

Life spans of nematodes vary from one or two months to several years. Most nematodes can withstand extreme environmental conditions, including exposure to human digestive enzymes.

Life cycles of specific nematodes that parasitize humans will be considered in Chapters 21 and 25. In humans they may be associated with intestinal or extraintestinal sites (Table 6-1). Diagnosis of infections caused by roundworms is usually made microscopically by finding ova or larval forms in stool or tissue specimens.

THE CESTODES

The cestodes consist of a group of parasitic worms that live, for the most part, as adults in intestinal tracts of vertebrates, including humans (Figure 6-7). The cestodes are more commonly called tapeworms because of their elongated ribbonlike appearance. The tissues of vertebrates and some invertebrates support larval stages of tapeworms. Their presence in the tissue interferes with normal organ function.

The length of adult worms varies from 3 mm to 10 m. The cestodes are covered with a continuous layer of cellular cuticle which can absorb materials from the environment. The body of a tapeworm consists of a head or *scolex* and a series of segments known as *proglottids* (Figure 6-8). The scolex bears attachment organs such as suckers, bothria, and hooks. The groove-shaped

Table 6-1 GENERA OF COMMON ROUNDWORMS

INTESTINAL	EXTRAINTESTINAL
Ancylostoma	Brugia
Ascaris	Dipetalonema
Enterobius	Dracunculus
Necator	Loa
Strongyloides	Mansonella
Trichuris	Onchocerca
	Toxocara
	Trichinella
	Wuchereria

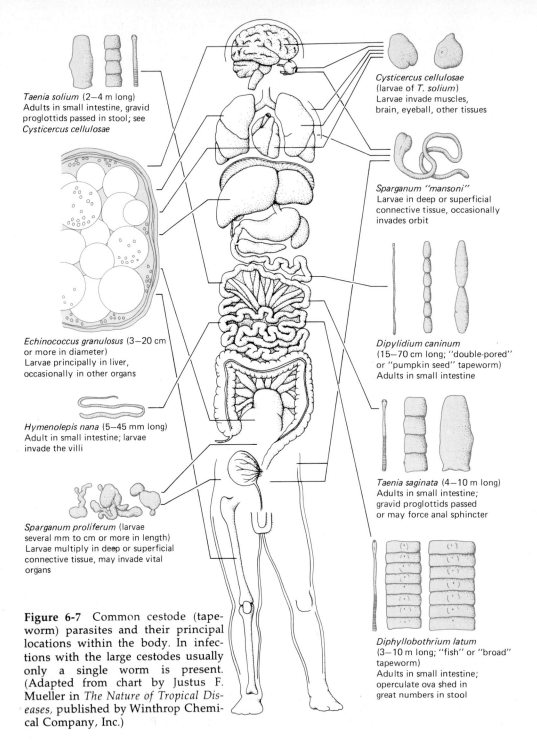

Taenia solium (2–4 m long)
Adults in small intestine, gravid
proglottids passed in stool; see
Cysticercus cellulosae

Cysticercus cellulosae
(larvae of *T. solium*)
Larvae invade muscles,
brain, eyeball, other tissues

Sparganum "mansoni"
Larvae in deep or superficial
connective tissue, occasionally
invades orbit

Echinococcus granulosus (3–20 cm
or more in diameter)
Larvae principally in liver,
occasionally in other organs

Dipylidium caninum
(15–70 cm long; "double-pored"
or "pumpkin seed" tapeworm)
Adults in small intestine

Hymenolepis nana (5–45 mm long)
Adult in small intestine; larvae
invade the villi

Taenia saginata (4–10 m long)
Adults in small intestine;
gravid proglottids passed
or may force anal sphincter

Sparganum proliferum (larvae
several mm to cm or more in length)
Larvae multiply in deep or superficial
connective tissue, may invade vital
organs

Figure 6-7 Common cestode (tape-worm) parasites and their principal locations within the body. In infections with the large cestodes usually only a single worm is present. (Adapted from chart by Justus F. Mueller in *The Nature of Tropical Diseases,* published by Winthrop Chemical Company, Inc.)

Diphyllobothrium latum
(3–10 m long; "fish" or "broad"
tapeworm)
Adults in small intestine;
operculate ova shed in
great numbers in stool

132

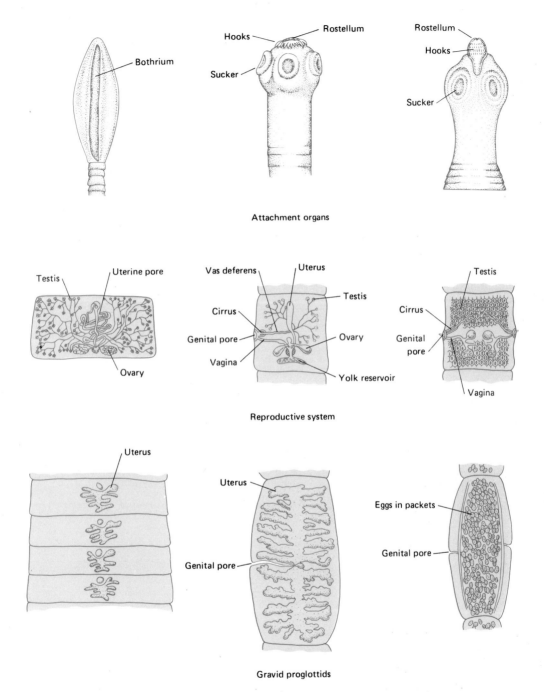

Figure 6-8 Morphology of an adult tapeworm. The worm has specialized attachment organs and a well-developed reproductive system. (From U.S. Naval Medical School, *Medical Protozoology and Helminthology*, Washington, D.C., U.S. Government Printing Office, 1965.)

bothria or the spherical suckers permit the scolex to attach firmly to cells which line the intestinal tract. In some species of tapeworms hooks, mounted on the rostellum (crown) of the scolex, penetrate the intestinal mucosa. The proglottids develop from the scolex and differentiate first into segments called *mature proglottids,* having both male and female sex organs, and later into *gravid proglottids,* each of which contains a uterus distended with ova. Organisms possessing reproductive organs of both sexes are called *hermaphroditic* or *monoecious.* A single gravid proglottid may contain more than 100,000 ova.

ANATOMY OF CESTODES

The cestodes have a well-developed muscular system consisting of circular, transverse, longitudinal, and dorsoventral muscle fibers.

The worms have a rudimentary nervous system with ganglia in the scolex and both sensory and motor peripheral nerve fibers.

Digestive and circulatory systems are absent. Nutrients are absorbed through the cuticle and are transported by the fluid of the body cavity.

Most tapeworms have highly developed male and female reproductive systems (Figure 6-8). The vas deferens of the male and vagina of the female share a genital pore on each mature proglottid. The vas deferens, testis, and the muscular cirrus, making up the male reproductive system, are in the dorsal part of each mature proglottid. The uterus, ovary, vagina, and yolk reservoir, making up the female reproductive system, are located near the ventral surface of each mature proglottid. Self-fertilization is the usual process, but cross fertilization can occur.

The excretory system consists of dorsal and ventral longitudinal tubules extending from the scolex to openings in

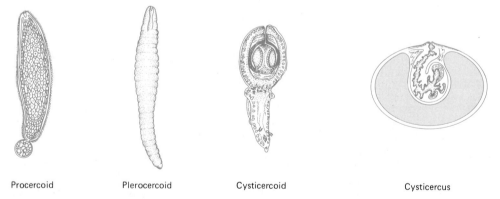

Procercoid   Plerocercoid   Cysticercoid   Cysticercus

Figure 6-9   Solid and vesicular larvae of tapeworms. Procercoid and plerocercoid are examples of solid forms. Cysticercoid and cysticercus are vesicular forms. (From H. W. Brown, *Basic Clinical Parasitology,* 4th ed., Englewood Cliffs, N.J., Prentice-Hall, 1975.)

the terminal proglottid, transverse tubules from the posterior portion of each proglottid, and deep-seated ciliated cells. The ciliated cells aid in the collection of fluid wastes from the parenchyma and their transport to the tubules. The flickering motion exhibited by the ciliated cells has earned them the title of *flame cells*.

INFECTIVE STAGES

Most tapeworms require one or more intermediate hosts and demonstrate a good deal of species selectivity for both definitive and intermediate hosts. In the most common type of tapeworm infection the definitive hosts ingest larvae in meat or fish. Larvae are described as solid or vesicular (bladder) forms (Figure 6-9). The term bladder is used because the immature forms are contained within cysts (sacs) which appear bladderlike in shape. Usually larvae develop into adults in the intestine of the vertebrate host. The ova of a few species of cestodes, such as the echinococcal tapeworm, if swallowed accidentally by man, may develop into an extraintestinal cyst (Figure 6-10). The hydatid cyst, or fluid sac, constitutes a larval form of the parasite in which daughter cysts and scolices are formed. Striated muscle and brain tissue are common sites for cysts to occur, but they may also develop in the eye, heart, or lungs

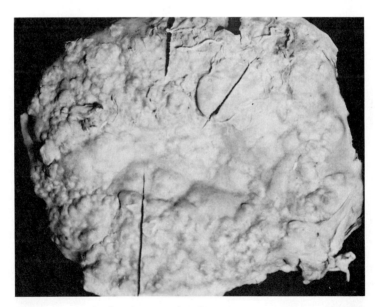

Figure 6-10 Hydatid cyst of *Echinococcus granulosus*. Human echinococcosis depends on the intimate association of human hosts with infected dogs. (Armed Forces Institute of Pathology Photograph, Neg. No. N-81062.)

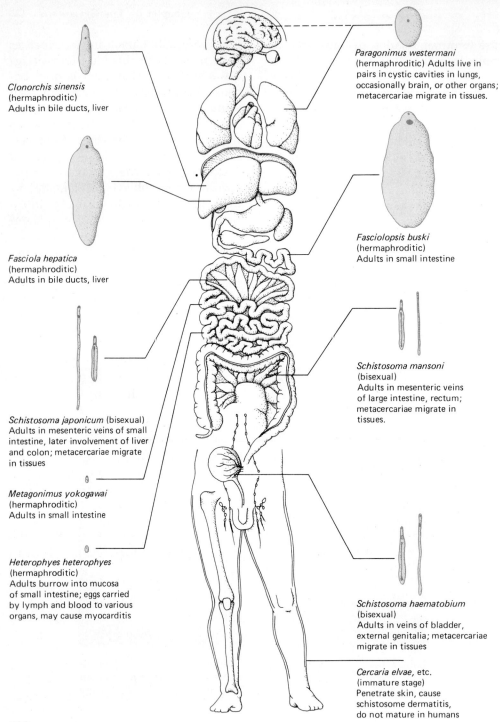

Clonorchis sinensis
(hermaphroditic)
Adults in bile ducts, liver

Paragonimus westermani
(hermaphroditic) Adults live in
pairs in cystic cavities in lungs,
occasionally brain, or other organs;
metacercariae migrate in tissues.

Fasciola hepatica
(hermaphroditic)
Adults in bile ducts, liver

Fasciolopsis buski
(hermaphroditic)
Adults in small intestine

Schistosoma japonicum (bisexual)
Adults in mesenteric veins of small
intestine, later involvement of liver
and colon; metacercariae migrate
in tissues

Schistosoma mansoni
(bisexual)
Adults in mesenteric veins
of large intestine, rectum;
metacercariae migrate in
tissues.

Metagonimus yokogawai
(hermaphroditic)
Adults in small intestine

Heterophyes heterophyes
(hermaphroditic)
Adults burrow into mucosa
of small intestine; eggs carried
by lymph and blood to various
organs, may cause myocarditis

Schistosoma haematobium
(bisexual)
Adults in veins of bladder,
external genitalia; metacercariae
migrate in tissues

Cercaria elvae, etc.
(immature stage)
Penetrate skin, cause
schistosome dermatitis,
do not mature in humans

136

Table 6-2 GENERA OF COMMON
TAPEWORMS

INTESTINAL	EXTRAINTESTINAL
Diphyllobothrium	Cysticercus
Dipylidium	Echinococcus
Hymenolepsis	Sparganum
Taenia	Spirometra

(Table 6-2). Life cycles of specific intestinal and extraintestinal tapeworms will be studied in Chapter 21. Diagnosis of intestinal infections is made by finding ova, proglottids, or scolices in stool specimens. Diagnosis of extraintestinal cestodal infections is more difficult and often can be made only upon surgical excision of cysts.

THE TREMATODES

The trematodes include ecto- and endoparasites having complex life cycles involving both aquatic and terrestrial hosts. Adult trematodes, called *flukes*, are generally flat, unsegmented, and oval or leaf-shaped. They range in size from a millimeter to several centimeters. Most flukes are hermaphroditic and are parasitic to humans only in the adult stage (Figure 6-11). Almost all species have two suckers: an oral sucker

◄ **Figure 6-11** Common trematode (fluke) parasites and their principal locations within the body. (Adapted from a chart by Justus F. Mueller in *The Nature of Tropical Diseases*, published by Winthrop Chemical Company, Inc.)

surrounding the mouth and a larger ventral sucker or *acetabulum*. Flukes are covered by a noncellular cuticle which, as in the cestodes, plays a role in absorption of nutrients.

ANATOMY OF TREMATODES

Three distinct layers of muscles consisting of circular, oblique, and longitudinal fibers lie beneath the cuticle of trematodes. Additional bands of muscle fibers occur with a dorsoventral orientation. The well-developed muscles enable the fluke to undergo multiple changes in size and shape.

There is no body cavity. The digestive system is composed of a mouth, pharynx, esophagus, and cecum (Figure 6-12).

Two lateral ganglia, near the region of the pharynx, and anterior and posterior nerve fibers constitute the nervous system.

The excretory system consists of tubules, the ciliated cells known as flame cells, a bladder, and an excretory pore.

The male and female reproductive systems are exceedingly well developed. All except the blood flukes are monoecious. Most of the ova have a conventional egg shape. In addition, the ova are characterized by a polar cap known as an *operculum* which pops open like a lid to release larvae; the ova of some species contain spines (Figure 6-13).

INFECTIVE STAGES

Most flukes are *digenetic*, that is, they demonstrate an alternation of genera-

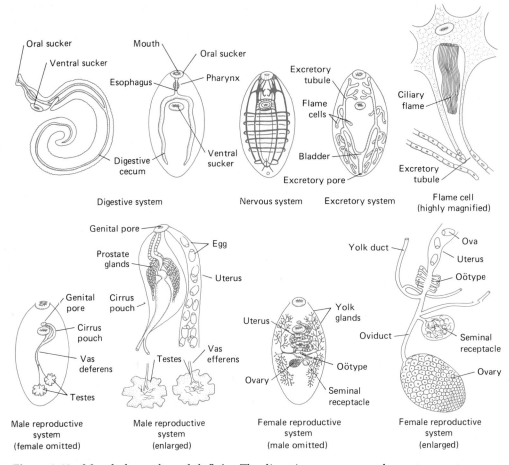

Figure 6-12   Morphology of an adult fluke. The digestive, nervous, and excretory systems are rudimentary. The reproductive system is exceedingly well-developed. (From U.S. Naval Medical School, *Medical Protozoology and Helminthology*, Washington, D.C., U.S. Government Printing Office, 1965.)

tions in which sexual reproduction of adult forms in vertebrate hosts is followed by asexual reproduction of larval forms in snails. Some flukes have an aquatic animal as a second intermediate host. For others an aquatic or terrestrial plant may serve as a vehicle of transfer. The lifespan of flukes ranges from sev-eral years to as long as 30 years for some of the blood flukes.

There are several immature stages of flukes. A ciliated larva known as a *miracidium* hatches from an ovum (Figure 6-14). The miracidium develops into the nonciliated saclike *sporocyst* within a snail. An intermediate larva

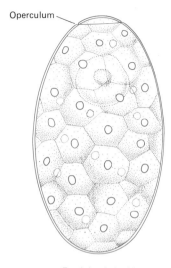

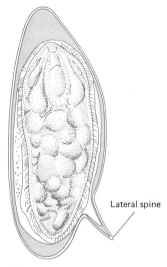

Fasciolopsis buski   *Schistosoma mansoni*

Figure 6-13 Characteristics of fluke ova. (From U.S. Naval Medical School, *Medical Protozoology and Helminthology*, Washington, D.C., U.S. Government Printing Office, 1965.)

called a *redia* may arise from a sporocyst or miracidium. Germ balls bud from the redia to produce a *cercaria*, a free-swimming stage, containing two suckers, a rudimentary alimentary canal, and a tail. A cercaria can penetrate the skin of a definitive host, enter the tissue of an intermediate host, or attach itself to a leafy vegetable where it loses its tail and becomes encysted as a *metacercaria*

Table 6-3 SITE OF ENCYSTMENT FOR COMMON FLUKES

SITE	TYPE OF FLUKE
Aquatic plants	liver, intestinal
Crayfish, crabs	lung
Fish	liver, intestinal
Snails, fresh- water clams	intestinal fluke (one species)

(Table 6-3). One miracidium can produce thousands of cercariae.

Once ingested, flukes may undergo complex migrations before reaching sexual maturity. Particular species of trematodes have predilections for specific organs or tissues (Table 6-4). Diag-

Table 6-4 HABITAT OF ADULT FLUKES IN MAN

FLUKE	HABITAT
Clonorchis	bile ducts, liver
Fasciola	bile ducts, liver
Fasciolopsis	small intestine
Heterophyes	small intestine, heart
Metagonimus	small intestine
Opisthorchis	bile ducts, liver
Paragonimus	lungs, brain
Schistosoma	blood

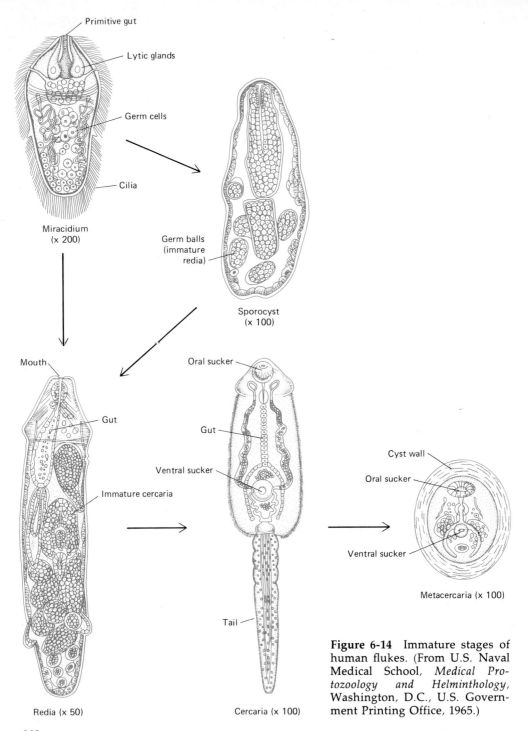

Miracidium
(x 200)

Primitive gut

Lytic glands

Germ cells

Cilia

Sporocyst
(x 100)

Germ balls
(immature
redia)

Mouth

Gut

Immature cercaria

Redia (x 50)

Oral sucker

Gut

Ventral sucker

Tail

Cercaria (x 100)

Cyst wall

Oral sucker

Ventral sucker

Metacercaria (x 100)

Figure 6-14 Immature stages of human flukes. (From U.S. Naval Medical School, *Medical Protozoology and Helminthology*, Washington, D.C., U.S. Government Printing Office, 1965.)

nosis of trematode disease is made by finding typical ova in stool, blood, urine, or sputum specimens.

SUMMARY

The helminths causing disease in man are nematodes (roundworms), cestodes (tapeworms), and trematodes (flukes). Helminths exhibit direct life cycles having a single definitive host and indirect life cycles having one or more intermediate hosts. Those requiring particular species of intermediate hosts to complete their life cycles tend to be restricted in nature. Both adult worms and developmental stages can parasitize humans. Identification of helminths in the laboratory depends on a knowledge of the morphological characteristics of adults, developmental forms, or ova of the parasites.

QUESTIONS FOR STUDY

1. Identify each structure as a part of nematodes, cestodes, or trematodes.

   microfilaria   rhabditiform larva
   proglottid   flame cell
   redia   scolex
   cercaria   metacercaria
   miracidium   filariform larva
2. What is the source of most helminthic infections in humans?
3. Since most helminths are not microscopic in size, why are they included in the study of microbiology?

SELECTED REFERENCES

Brown, H. W. *Basic Clinical Parasitology.* 4th ed. Englewood Cliffs, N.J.: Prentice-Hall, 1975.

Koneman, E. W.; Richie, L. E.; and Tiemann, C. *Practical Laboratory Parasitology.* New York: Medcom Press, 1974.

Markell, E. K., and Voge, M. *Medical Parasitology.* 4th ed. Philadelphia: Saunders, 1974.

Olsen, O. W. *Animal Parasites, Their Life Cycles and Ecology.* 3rd ed. Baltimore: University Park Press, 1974.

U.S. Naval Medical School, National Naval Medical Center. *Medical Protozoology and Helminthology.* Washington, D.C.: U.S. Government Printing Office, 1965.

Unit Two

MICROBIAL METABOLISM AND VARIATION

Chapter 7

Molecules of Microorganisms

After you read this chapter, you should be able to:

1. Compare the major chemical elements of a bacterium and the human body.
2. Describe the structure of a monosaccharide, an amino acid, and a fatty acid.
3. Recognize glycosidic, peptide, and ester linkages.
4. Represent a hexose and a pentose using Haworth formulas.
5. Differentiate between L- and D-forms of monosaccharides and amino acids.
6. Describe configuration and bonding of primary, secondary, and tertiary protein structures.
7. List the major classes of carbohydrates, proteins, and lipids.
8. Differentiate between a saturated and an unsaturated fatty acid.
9. Describe the chemical composition of deoxyribonucleic acid (DNA) and ribonucleic acid (RNA).
10. Describe the role of adenosine triphosphate (ATP) molecules in storing energy.
11. Explain the significance of homology of base pairs in ascertaining evolutionary relationships of microorganisms.

Microorganisms, like other forms of life, consist of a complex mixture of chemical materials contained within a matrix of *protoplasm*. The principal inorganic constituent of protoplasm is water. The major organic compounds are carbohydrates, proteins, lipids, and nucleic acids. The proteins, nucleic acids, and some carbohydrates are classified as *macromolecules* because of their large size. These molecules are made up of only a few kinds of atoms. Six elements, carbon (C), hydrogen (H), oxygen (O), nitrogen (N), phosphorus (P), and sulfur (S), account for most of the mass of both the human body and microorganisms (Table 7-1). The cells also contain some inorganic salts that have various regulatory functions. A continuum of reactions among the molecules of microorganisms permits the primitive cells to generate energy, liberate waste products, carry on photosynthesis, and even cause disease.

Table 7-1 MAJOR ELEMENTS OF A BACTERIUM AND THE HUMAN BODY

ELEMENT	E. COLI	THE HUMAN BODY
Oxygen	65.0%	69.0%
Carbon	18.0	15.0
Hydrogen	10.0	11.0
Nitrogen	3.0	3.0
Phosphorus	1.0	1.2
Sulphur	0.25	0.3

NOTE: Figures represent gross composition of representative cells.

CARBOHYDRATES

Carbohydrates, which are universally distributed among microorganisms, contain carbon (C), hydrogen (H), and oxygen (O). The empirical formula for a carbohydrate is expressed as $(C.H_2O)_n$ in which n is three or greater. Carbohydrates that possess an aldehydic group (HC=O) are called *aldoses*; those that have a keto group (C=O) are called *ketoses*. The simplest aldoses or ketoses are *trioses* in which n is equal to three.

Carbohydrates are commonly classified on the basis of the number of simple carbohydrate units or *monomers* making up the whole molecule. The most abundant monomer in nature is the aldohexose glucose in which n equals six. The monomer is a major energy source for microorganisms and building block of larger carbohydrate molecules. Carbohydrates are characterized by a wide distribution of molecular weights which may vary from 180 to 100,000,000 daltons.

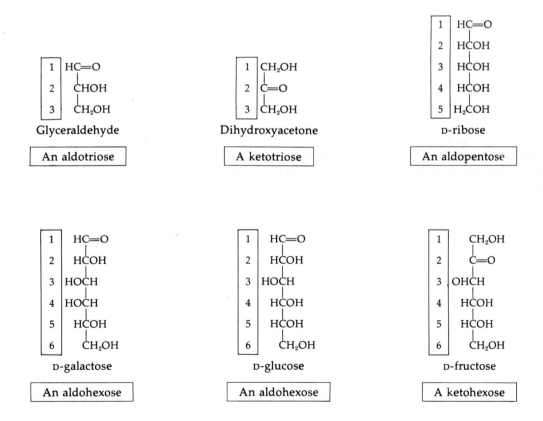

MONOSACCHARIDES

Simple carbohydrates of microorganisms which contain three to seven carbon atoms (C) and either an aldehydic group (HC=O) or a keto group (C=O) are called *monosaccharides*. The aldoses and ketoses shown above are examples of monosaccharides. These products occur as intermediates in the degradation of larger carbohydrate molecules by microorganisms.

One distinguishing property of monosaccharides is that they can exist in either a left-handed (L) or right-handed (D) configuration (Figure 7-1). It can be seen above that monosaccharides have carbon atoms (C) that are bonded to hydrogen atoms (H) or hydroxyl groups (OH). The carbon atoms are numbered from top to bottom. If the carbon atom of position 5 of a hexose or position 4 of a pentose is isolated from the rest of the structure, it can be observed that carbon can be bonded on the left or right with the hydroxyl group. The letter D placed before the name of the monosaccharide indicates that the hydroxyl group is on the right. A mirror image of that portion of a hexose or pentose molecule contains the same atoms with the hydroxyl group on the left; it is designated as the L-form of the monosaccharide.

The D- and L- forms of specific monosaccharides are called *isomers;* they contain exactly the same number and kinds of atoms, but in different spatial arrangements. The D-isomers are the most important in nature and, therefore, are the most significant to microbial life.

In nature the five-carbon monosaccharides (pentoses) and six-carbon monosaccharides (hexoses) occur in ring forms. The closed ring structures occur when bonds are formed between carbonyl (CO) and hydroxyl (OH) groups. In a hexose a bond is formed at carbon number 5; in a pentose at carbon number 4. Formation of the closed ring of aldohexoses or aldopentoses results in a free hydroxyl group at carbon 1, positioned above or below the plane of the ring. Hexoses or pentoses with the hydroxyl group occurring below the plane of the ring are α *isomers;* those with the hydroxyl group occurring above the plane of the ring are β *isomers.* Ketohexoses or ketopentoses form rings with free hydroxyl groups occurring at carbon 2.

The Haworth formulas are most conveniently used to represent cyclic structures of the monosaccharides.

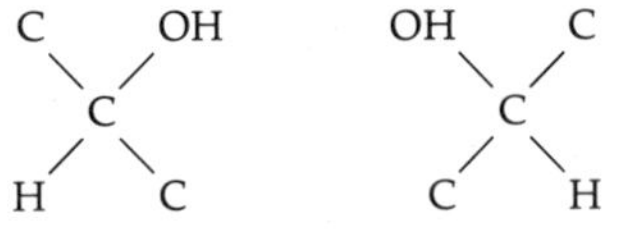

Figure 7-1 An isolated carbon atom of a pentose or hexose showing orientation of carbon-bonding atoms or groups of D- and L-isomers.

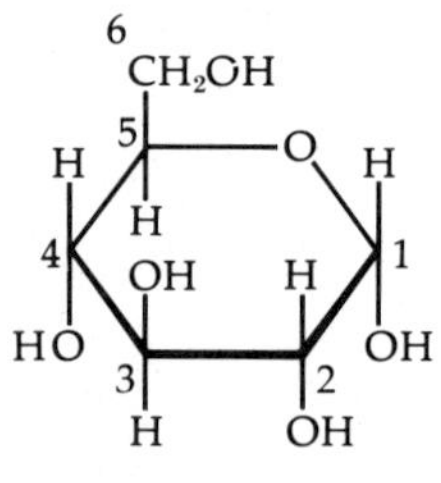

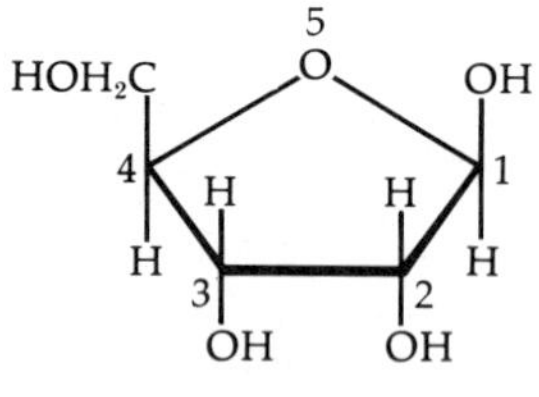

Numbering the carbon atoms of the closed-ring stuctures is helpful in understanding bonding between monomers of carbohydrates. The cyclic structures are sometimes drawn as six- or five-sided structures with only an (O) atom and numbers of the carbon positions identified.

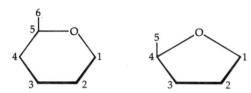

In this chapter simple modified structural formulas are used as much as possible to show positions of bonds or alterations in molecules. The positions of bonds and changes occurring in molecules are important in understanding life-sustaining reactions in microorganisms.

OLIGOSACCHARIDES

A combination of 2 to 10 molecules of monosaccharides with the loss of 1 molecule of water at each bonding site forms an *oligosaccharide*. The monomers of oligosaccharides may be similar or dissimilar. If an oligosaccharide contains two monomers, it is a *disaccharide;* if it contains three monomers, it is a *trisaccharide*. When water is lost as a result of the union of two or three monosaccharides, a *glycosidic linkage* or bond between the monomers is formed at the site of the water loss.

Maltose is a disaccharide which contains two monomers of glucose linked in the one and four positions. The first

molecule of glucose exists in the α form; the second molecule of glucose may have an α or β configuration.

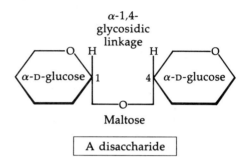

α-1,4-
glycosidic
linkage

Maltose

A disaccharide

Sucrose is a disaccharide which contains a monomer of glucose and a monomer of fructose linked in the α one and the β two positions involving the aldehydic group (HC=O) of glucose and the keto group (C=O) of fructose. In the combined form fructose exists as a five-membered structure or *furanose* ring instead of the usual six-membered or *pyranose* ring.

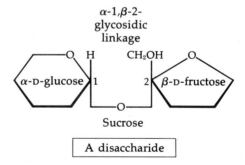

α-1,β-2-
glycosidic
linkage

Sucrose

A disaccharide

Lactose contains a molecule of glucose and a molecule of galactose in a β-1,4-glycosidic linkage. Both monomers exist as pyranose rings.

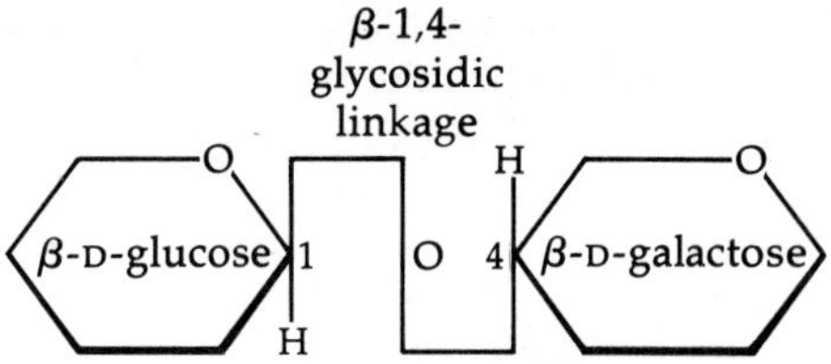

β-1,4-
glycosidic
linkage

Lactose

A disaccharide

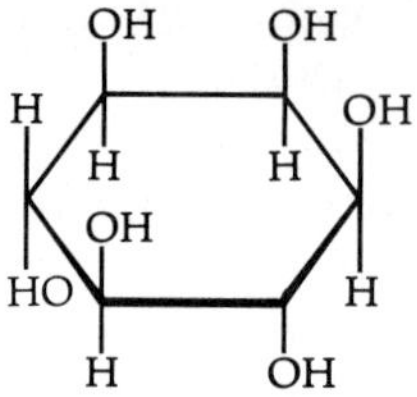

Inositol

A cyclic alcohol sugar

Lactose may be made up of either the L-
or D-forms of glucose and galactose.

DERIVED MONOSACCHARIDES

The aldehydic (HC=O) or keto (C=O)
group of a monosaccharide may be altered by removal or addition of chemical groups. The addition of a molecule
of hydrogen to the aldehydic or keto
groups of trioses, pentoses, or hexoses
produces alcohols. The principal alcohols are glycerol, mannitol, sorbitol,
and ribitol.

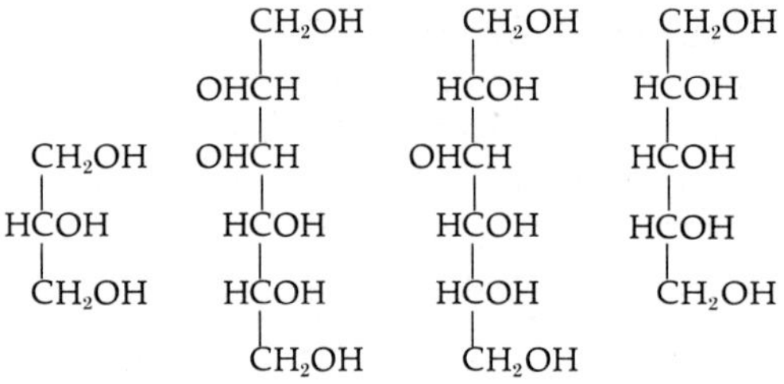

The cell envelopes of all gram-positive bacteria contain *teichoic acids,*
which are polymers of glycerol or ribitol. The ability of some bacteria to use
mannitol, sorbitol, or inositol as a
source of energy provides us with differential characteristics which can be
used to identify particular species.

If monosaccharides are oxidized,
acids such as gluconic or glucuronic
acids are produced. These acids are
commonly found as constituents of
polysaccharides.

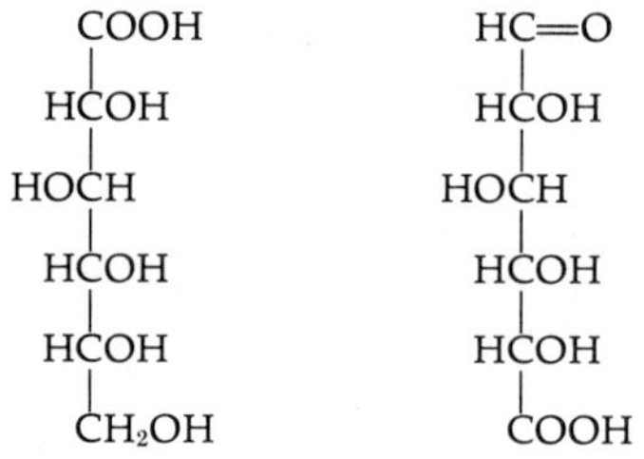

Glycerol   D-mannitol   D-sorbitol   D-ribitol

Alcohol sugars

D-gluconic acid   D-glucuronic acid

Acid sugars

Cyclic formation of an alcohol derivative may form a compound such as
inositol.

The hydroxyl group (OH) of a glucose
or galactose molecule may be replaced
by an amino group (NH$_2$) yielding the

amino acid sugars glucosamine or galactosamine, respectively.

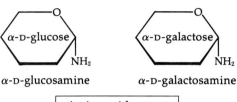

Amino acid sugars

Glucosamine is an important constituent of the lipopolysaccharide component of gram-negative bacteria and the membrane glycoproteins of eucaryotic cells. Glucosamine is also found in the cell walls of some fungi. Galactosamine is found in cartilage, nerve, and spleen tissue.

If an acetylamino group ($NHCOCH_3$) replaces the hydroxyl group (OH) of a glucose molecule, N-acetyl-D-glucosamine (NAG) is formed.

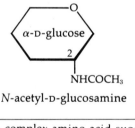

N-acetyl-D-glucosamine

A complex amino acid sugar

A more complex derivative of an amino acid sugar is N-acetylmuramic acid (NAMA) which has a hydroxyl group (OH) connected to a lactic acid molecule.

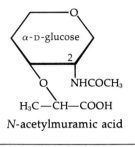

N-acetylmuramic acid

A complex amino acid sugar

The carbohydrate portion of bacterial cell walls is made of N-acetyl-D-glucosamine and N-acetylmuramic acid.

POLYSACCHARIDES

The polysaccharides consist of multiple hexoses or pentoses with numerous glycosidic linkages to form very large molecules. Starch, the form in which carbohydrates are stored in plants, contains an *amylose* and an *amylopectin component*. The amylose unit is composed of α-D-glucose monomers connected linearly by α-1,4-glycosidic linkages; the molecular weight is variable. Amylose constitutes 15 to 25 percent of starch. Amylopectin is a branched molecule containing several thousand α-D-glucose units with α-1,4- and α-1,6-glycosidic linkages; its molecular weight is 500,000 daltons or greater (Figure 7-2).

Cellulose is the most abundant polysaccharide in nature; it is a major constituent of the cell walls of plants. It consists of long chains of glucose units connected by β-1,4-glycosidic linkages. It differs from amylose in that the bonding is arranged differently and the

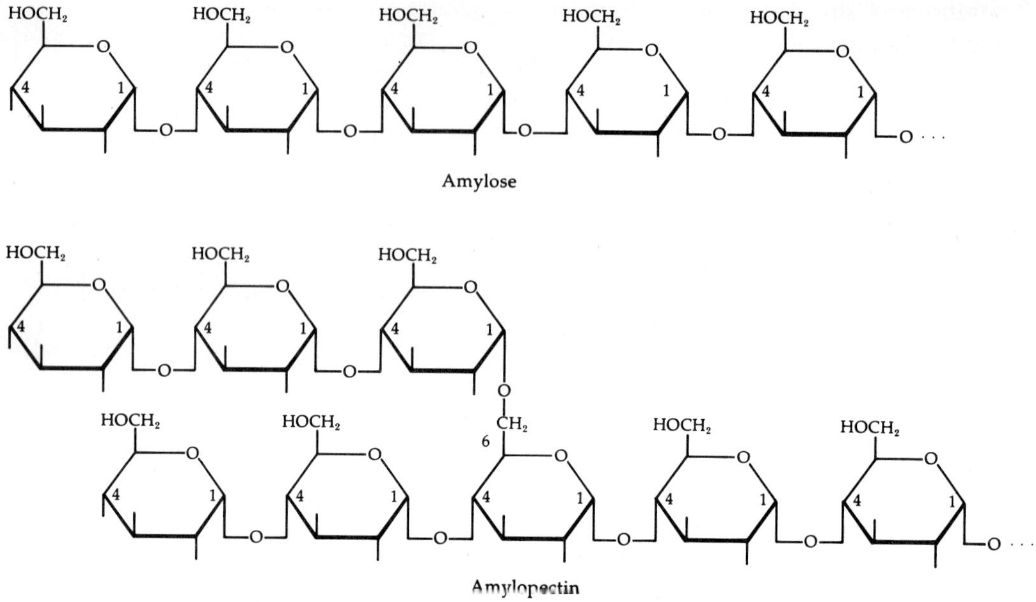

Figure 7-2   The amylose and amylopectin components of a starch molecule showing 1,4- and 1,6-glycosidic linkages.

chains are longer; the molecular weight is approximately 500,000 daltons. The seemingly small difference in bonding makes it impossible for some microorganisms and humans to degrade cellulose as a source of energy. The lack of gastrointestinal enzymes which can act on cellulose allows this polysaccharide to perform the important function of supplying bulk or roughage in the diet. Certain microorganisms, termites, and snails can break cellulose down into glucose monomers which can be easily utilized by many forms of life as a source of energy.

Peptidoglycans are polymers consisting of the amino acid sugars, N-acetyl-D-glucosamine (NAG) and N-acetylmuramic acid (NAMA), joined by α-1,4-glycosidic linkages, and the amino acids L-alanine, D-glutamic acid, D-alanine, and L-lysine or diaminopimelic acid. The molecules of the peptidoglycan polymer are assembled in such a manner as to give extraordinary strength to cell walls of procaryotic cells. The chains of NAG and NAMA are wound around the organism and each turn is reinforced by cross-linkages with chains of amino acids.

Other important polysaccharides include the *mucopolysaccharides* and chitin. One mucopolysaccharide, hyaluronic acid, is a higher molecular weight gelatinous substance containing NAG and glucuronic acid. Hyaluronic acid is the cementing substance between cells of connective tissue. It can be destroyed readily by some microorganisms, a property which permits those organisms to spread rapidly.

Chitin, a polymer of NAG, is both strong and light; it is found in crustaceans, insects, and the walls of some fungi.

PROTEINS

The proteins of microorganisms are macromolecules with molecular weights of 10,000 to 100,000 daltons. They consist of chains of simple monomers called *amino acids.* Amino acids contain carbon (C), hydrogen (H), oxygen (O), nitrogen (N), and sometimes sulfur (S). Different side chains (which are designated R in representations of molecular components) characterize individual amino acids, but all amino acids contain an amino group (NH_2) and a carboxyl group (COOH). Amino acids, like sugars, can be left-handed or right-handed. All naturally occurring amino acids are L-forms with the exception of glycine (Figure 7-3). A few D-amino acids, such as D-glutamic acid and D-alanine, are found in bacterial cell walls. Because of the massive size and complexity of proteins, the configuration of

protein molecules is best understood by consideration of the three sequential arrangements designated as primary, secondary, and tertiary structures occurring in the synthesis of proteins.

PRIMARY STRUCTURE

Amino acids are connected by *peptide linkages* which join a carboxyl group (COOH) of one amino acid with an amino group (NH_2) of another; one molecule of water is lost by a single linkage as in glycosidic bonding.

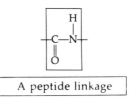

A peptide linkage

Two amino acids joined by a peptide linkage are called *dipeptides;* 3 amino acids bonded similarly are *tripeptides;* a chain of 10 or more amino acids constitutes a *polypeptide.* One molecule each of glycine, alanine, and cysteine make up a tripeptide (Figure 7-4). However, five other possible combinations of the three amino acids could exist. If we use A, B, and C to represent the amino acids, six tripeptides could be formed depending on the orientation of the molecules.

ABC	BCA	CAB
ACB	BAC	CBA

There are 20 commonly occurring amino acids in nature (Table 7-2). It is a curious phenomenon that some di- and tripeptides are better sources of amino acids for some bacteria than are free

Figure 7-3 A representative amino acid showing D- and L-isomers.

D-isomer   L-isomer

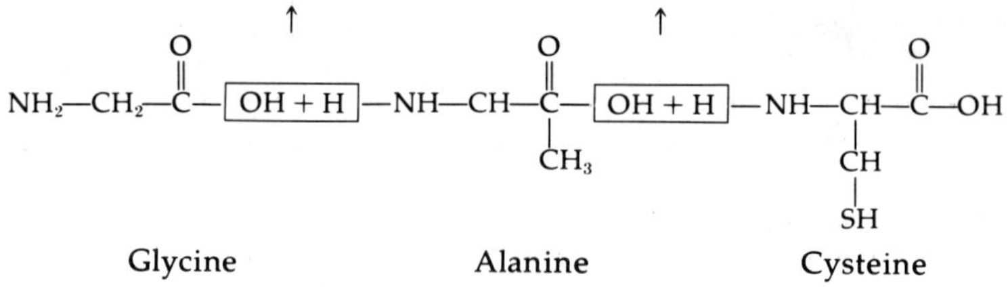

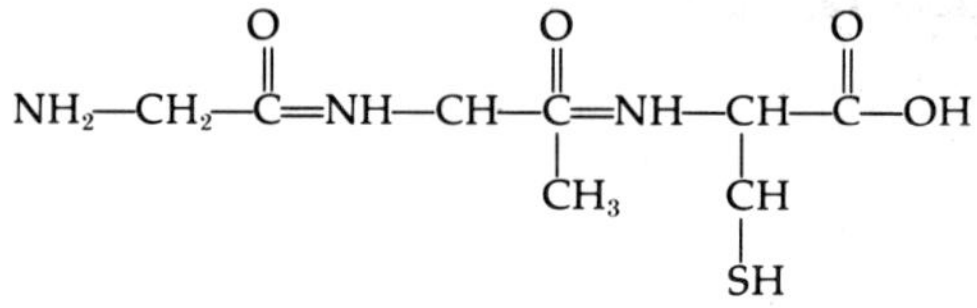

$$NH_2—CH_2—\overset{\overset{\displaystyle O}{\|}}{C}—\boxed{OH + H}—NH—CH—\overset{\overset{\displaystyle O}{\|}}{C}—\boxed{OH + H}—NH—CH—\overset{\overset{\displaystyle O}{\|}}{C}—OH$$

Glycine   Alanine   Cysteine

$$NH_2—CH_2—\overset{\overset{\displaystyle O}{\|}}{C}=NH—CH—\overset{\overset{\displaystyle O}{\|}}{C}=NH—CH—\overset{\overset{\displaystyle O}{\|}}{C}—OH$$

A tripeptide

Figure 7-4   Primary structure of proteins. One molecule each of glycine, alanine, and cysteine forma tripeptide. Carbon and nitrogen atoms are joined by double bonds when water is lost in each peptide linkage.

Table 7-2   TWENTY COMMONLY OCCURRING AMINO ACIDS

AMINO ACID	ABBREVIATION
Alanine	Ala
Arginine	Arg
Asparagine	Asn
Aspartic acid	Asp
Cysteine	Cys
Glutamic acid	Glu
Glutamine	Gln
Glycine	Gly
Histidine	His
Isoleucine	Ile
Leucine	Leu
Lysine	Lys
Methionine	Met
Phenylalanine	Phe
Proline	Pro
Serine	Ser
Threonine	Thr
Tryptophan	Trp
Tyrosine	Tyr
Valine	Val

amino acids. Peptides found in nature include the ubiquitous glutathione (a tripeptide) and vasopressin and oxytocin (octapeptides). If 20 amino acids are used, almost an infinite variety of combinations and chain lengths of amino acids can be envisioned. The variety of polypeptides made possible by combinations of amino acids is responsible for the diversity of both structure and function among living things.

SECONDARY STRUCTURE

If proteins existed merely as long chains of amino acids, clearly the organisms would have to be of extraordinary size to accomodate the molecules. The limitations of a planet like earth to support such life forms are obvious. Instead, long chains of polypeptides tend to

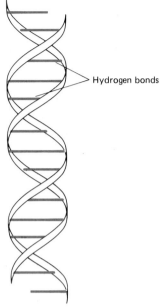

Hydrogen bonds

Helical polypeptide

$$R-\overset{\overset{O}{\|}}{C}-\overset{\overset{H}{|}}{N}-H$$

$$R-\overset{\overset{O}{\|}}{C}-\overset{\overset{H}{|}}{N}-H$$

A hydrogen bond

Figure 7-5 Secondary structure of proteins. Hydrogen bonding between amino acids maintains the formation of a helical protein.

form a helix or to occur in a pleated arrangement. Much of the twisting and pleating is maintained by hydrogen bonds in which the hydrogen (H) of an amino group (NH_2) of one amino acid acts as a bridge to the oxygen (O) of a carboxyl group (COOH) of another amino acid (Figure 7-5). Although a single hydrogen bond is weak, many hundred such bonds collectively provide structural integrity for proteins. Helical proteins include the keratins, myosin, and collagen. Fibroin, a protein found in silk, has a pleated arrangement.

TERTIARY STRUCTURE

The helices or pleats of polypeptides usually undergo additional folding.

During this process hydrophobic or "water-hating" polar side chains are exposed and the hydrophilic or "water-loving" nonpolar side chains are hidden within the molecule. The global structure is stabilized by the formation of additional hydrogen bonds, ionic bonds, or by the oxidation of mercaptan groups (—SH), such as those contained by cysteine, to disulfide bonds (—S—S) (Figure 7-6). The exposed sites determine the properties of particular proteins. Quite clearly, folding does not occur in a random fashion and must be among the most carefully directed processes in nature. All biologically active proteins have global structures. Examples are albumins, globulins, and enzymes. Two globular proteins may join, forming *dimers* which are only

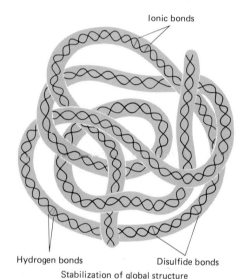

A disulfide bond

An ionic bond

Ionic bonds

Hydrogen bonds   Disulfide bonds

Stabilization of global structure

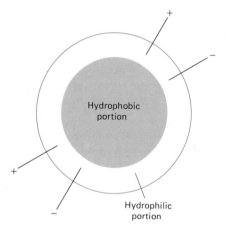

Hydrophobic portion

Hydrophilic portion

Theoretical cross-section of globular protein

active in the dimolecular form (Figure 7-7).

CONJUGATED PROTEINS

A protein combined with a nonprotein, either an inorganic or organic compound, is called a *conjugated protein*. Proteins may be conjugated with carbohydrates (glycoproteins), lipids (lipoproteins), nucleic acids (nucleoproteins), phosphorus (phosphoproteins), or pigments (chromoproteins). Those macromolecules contribute to the integrity of microbial cells and are responsible for specialized transportation functions within cells.

LIPIDS

The lipids of microorganisms consist of a heterogeneous group of compounds containing carbon (C), hydrogen (H), oxygen (O), and sometimes phosphorus (P) and nitrogen (N). All are sparingly soluble in water, but are readily soluble in organic solvents such as ether, acetone, chloroform, benzene, or the alcohols. The molecular weight is usually not more than 1000 daltons. Although some microorganisms can use particular lipids as a source of energy, lipids

Figure 7-6 Tertiary structure of proteins. Global structure results from the folding of a polypeptide helix and is maintained by the formation of hydrogen, ionic, and disulfide bonds. Theoretical cross-section of a protein shows hydrophilic and hydrophobic portions.

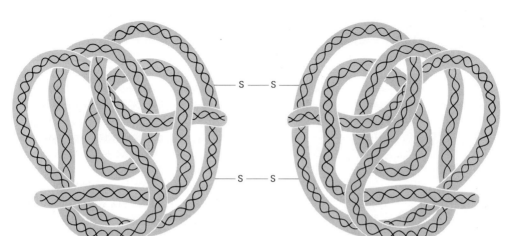

Figure 7-7 A protein dimer containing two similar globular units.

are more important as constituents of cell envelopes of gram-negative bacteria and of some gram-positive bacteria such as *Mycobacterium, Corynebacterium,* and *Actinomycetales.* The lipid composition of many microorganisms merely reflects the lipid content of the culture medium, the age of the organisms, or the temperature of incubation. Because the lipids are such a heterogeneous group and lack distinctive subunits, any classification is somewhat arbitrary.

SIMPLE LIPIDS

Fats, oils, and waxes consist of fatty acids and glycerol or other alcohols. Fatty acids, rarely found free in nature, are straight unbranched hydrocarbon compounds usually containing one carboxyl group (COOH). The most widely distributed fatty acid in nature is oleic acid.

$$CH_3(CH_2)_7CH{=}CH(CH_2)_7COOH$$

Oleic acid

A fatty acid

Fatty acids may possess one to four carbon-to-carbon double bonds (C=C) or only single bonds between carbon atoms. In fatty acids with a single double bond, the double bond usually occurs between carbon atoms 9 and 10. Each carbon atom linked to another carbon atom by a double bond binds one less hydrogen atom than single-bonded carbon atoms. Therefore, fatty acids that contain double bonds are called *unsaturated fatty acids.* Unsaturated fatty acids include oleic, linoleic, linolenic, and arachidonic acids.

Fatty acids having no carbon-to-carbon double bonds possess the maximal number of atoms of hydrogen at carbon-bonding sites and are therefore called *saturated fatty acids.* The most important saturated fatty acids are lauric, myristic, palmitic, and stearic acids. The unsaturated fatty acids are liquid at room temperature. *Saturated fatty acids* with less than 10 carbon atoms are liquids at room temperature; *saturated fatty acids* with chains of more than 12 to 14 carbon atoms are solids.

Instead of learning structural formulas for the fatty acids, it is often convenient and time-saving to use a type of shorthand. The saturated palmitic acid may be written as 16.0, meaning 16 carbon atoms and no double bonds. The polyunsaturated arachidonic acid may be written as 20.4, meaning 20 carbon atoms and 4 double bonds (Table 7-3).

Microorganisms can synthesize monounsaturated fatty acids either aerobically or anaerobically; they do not synthesize polyunsaturated fatty acids. Some mycoplasmas depend entirely on an environmental supply of unsaturated fatty acids.

One group of saturated branched fatty acids, known as mycolic acids, are found in wax of the cell walls of *Mycobacterium*. Waxes are fatty acid esters of long chain alcohols; they have high melting points and are more stable than true fats. The presence of the durable wax contributes to the resistance of those bacteria to staining and heat, and

may partially explain the long time required for their growth. Another high molecular weight component of cell walls of tubercle bacilli, designated as wax D, increases the ability of proteins to stimulate antibody production. Although wax D is not a true wax because it contains carbohydrate and protein moieties, the mycolic acids contribute to its unique properties.

The true fats contain fatty acids and glycerol, a trihydroxyl alcohol derived from a triose. They may alternately be called *glycerides*. The bonding between the hydroxyl group (OH) of glycerol and the carboxyl group (COOH) of a fatty acid is called an ester linkage.

$$O-\overset{\displaystyle \overset{O}{\|}}{C}-C$$

An ester linkage

If a single ester linkage is formed, the compound is a *monoglyceride;* two ester linkages with the same or a different fatty acid form a *diglyceride;* three ester linkages with similar or dissimilar fatty acids form a *triglyceride*. Triglycerides containing mixed fatty acids are more common in nature; they are sometimes called *neutral fats* (Figure 7-8).

Table 7-3 COMMON SATURATED AND UNSATURATED FATTY ACIDS

Saturated Fatty Acids	Abbreviation	Unsaturated Fatty Acids	Abbreviation
Lauric	12.0	Palmitoleic	16.1
Myristic	14.0	Oleic	18.1
Palmitic	16.0	Linoleic	18.2
Stearic	18.0	Linolenic	18.3
Arachidic	20.0	Arachidonic	20.4

$CH_2OCOC_{17}H_{35}$ Stearic acid

$CHOCOC_{17}H_{33}$ Oleic acid

$CH_2OCOC_{15}H_{31}$ Palmitic acid

Figure 7-8 A triglyceride containing dissimilar fatty acids.

COMPOUND LIPIDS

The most important compound lipids of microorganisms are *phospholipids, glycolipids,* and *steroids.* The phospholipids are derivatives of glycerol phosphate. Some contain a nitrogenous base. The nitrogen-containing base may be choline, ethanolamine, or L-serine.

$HO—CH_2—CH_2—N≡(CH_3)_3$ Choline

$HO—CH_2—CH_2—NH_2$ Ethanolamine

$HO—CH_2—CH—NH_2$ L-serine
         |
        COOH

Cytoplasmic membranes of both procaryotic and eucaryotic cells contain phospholipids associated with proteins. Fluidity of membranes is maintained by the presence of phospholipids and unsaturated fatty acids in the inner membranes. The characteristic of fluidity is responsible for physiological properties important in cell growth and integrity. Bacteria appear to have mechanisms to control the synthesis and deposition of selective fatty acids in membranes in response to temperature changes in the environment.

A major component of the outer membranes of gram-negative bacteria is a glycolipid known as *lipopolysaccharide.* Lipopolysaccharides are very large molecules containing sugars, polysaccharides, and a lipid moiety called lipid A. The lipid A fraction of bacteria contains 8 to 10 lipids. The lipopolysaccharides of the gram-negative bacteria are classified as endotoxins.

The glycolipids contain fatty acids and a sugar linked to sphingosine, a nitrogenous base with no glycerol.

$$CH_3(CH_2)_{12}—CH{=}CH—\overset{\displaystyle OH}{\underset{\displaystyle |}{C}}—\overset{\displaystyle NH_2}{\underset{\displaystyle |}{CH}}—CH_2OH$$

Sphingosine

Glycolipids and glycoproteins of cytoplasmic membranes are believed to be responsible for the ability of eucaryotic cells in multicellular organisms to adhere to one another. Alterations in glycoprotein content of host cytoplasmic membranes in cells infected with DNA viruses may affect normal defense mechanisms.

Steroids are a group of structurally complex compounds which have diverse physiological roles in mammalian cells. They have a polycyclic carbon skeleton and contain an alcohol group. Hence, steroids may be called *sterols.* Sterols are not found in the membranes of bacteria, except for some mycoplasmas, but they are universally present in the membranes of eucaryotic cells. The most common sterol is cholesterol.

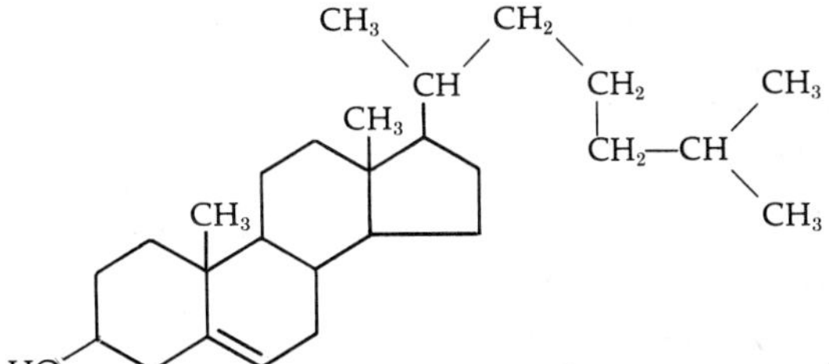

Cholesterol

A steroid alcohol or sterol

The physiological role of cholesterol in eucaryotic and mycoplasma membranes is not well understood, but it may have a role in membrane stability and transport.

NUCLEIC ACIDS

The nucleic acids of microorganisms are deoxyribonucleic acid (DNA) and ribonucleic acid (RNA). They are macromolecules containing carbon (C), hydrogen (H), oxygen (O), nitrogen (N), and phosphorus (P). The names DNA and RNA are derived from the type of sugar contained within the molecules. D-ribose, a pentose, is associated with RNA. The sugar in DNA has one oxygen (O) atom missing in the two position making it 2-deoxy-D-ribose.

D-ribose   2-deoxy-D-ribose

Sugars of nucleic acids

NUCLEOSIDES AND NUCLEOTIDES

The nitrogen-containing portions of nucleic acids are mixtures of basic substances known as *purines* and *pyrimidines*. The major pyrimidines in nucleic acids are *uracil, thymine, cytosine;* they are six-membered ring

structures with minor variations in the numbers of atoms.

Cytosine   Uracil   Thymine
   (C)   (U)   (T)

Nitrogen-containing bases: pyrimidines

The purines are six-membered pyrimidine rings fused to a five-membered imidazole ring. The principal purines in nucleic acids are *adenine* and *guanine*.

Adenine   Guanine
  (A)   (G)

Nitrogen-containing bases: purines

The positions of the carbon atoms (C) in the cyclic structures can be numbered in much the same manner as they are numbered for carbohydrates.

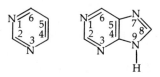

This is often helpful in understanding reactions between the pyrimidine or purine portions of the nucleic acids.

Table 7-4 SUBUNITS OF RNA AND DNA MOLECULES

BASE	NUCLEOSIDES	NUCLEOTIDES
Adenine	adenosine D-adenosine	adenylic acid D-adenylic acid
Guanine	guanosine	guanylic acid D-guanylic acid
Cytosine	cytidine D-cytidine	cytidylic acid D-cytidylic acid
Thymine	D-thymidine	D-thymidylic acid
Uracil	uridine	uridylic acid

The subunits of nucleic acids, formed when a purine or pyrimidine is linked to D-ribose or 2-deoxy-D-ribose, are called *nucleosides* (Table 7-4). In order to differentiate the positions of the carbon (C) atoms of the sugars from those of the nitrogenous bases, a prime (') is used to identify the carbon positions of the sugars. The addition of phosphate (PO_4) to ribose in an ester linkage at position 2', 3', or 5' or to deoxyribose at position 3' or 5' forms a *nucleotide*. Nucleotides are considered the fundamental subunits of nucleic acids.

One of the most important position 5' nucleotides of cells, adenosine triphosphate (ATP), has three phosphate groups (PO_4) at position 5'.

"high energy" bonds

$$Adenine\text{—}ribose\text{—}O\text{—}\underset{\underset{OH}{|}}{\overset{\overset{O}{\|}}{P}}\text{—}O\sim\underset{\underset{OH}{|}}{\overset{\overset{O}{\|}}{P}}\text{—}O\sim\underset{\underset{OH}{|}}{\overset{\overset{O}{\|}}{P}}\text{—}OH$$

Adenosine triphosphate (ATP)

ATP molecules are storage depots for energy in cells. The molecules release energy upon demand yielding a di- or monophosphate molecule which, in turn, can accept energy produced by metabolic activities of cells reforming the triphosphate molecule by combining with one or two inorganic phosphate groups (PO_4).

The nucleic acids consist of very long sequences of nucleotides occurring in double or single strands. DNA exists as a double helical structure in cells, but RNA has multiple forms. In eucaryotic cells approximately 98 percent of the total DNA is bound to proteins called histones; the histone-bound DNA forms the complex chromatin of nuclei. The DNA of mitochondria and chloroplasts occurs as unbound or free DNA in double-stranded form.

DEOXYRIBONUCLEIC ACID

Pyrimidines and purines of double-stranded DNA are joined by hydrogen bonds. Adenine (A) always pairs with thymine (T); guanine (G) always pairs with cytosine (C) (Figure 7-9). This precise pairing of pyrimidines and purines is known as complementarity. DNA has

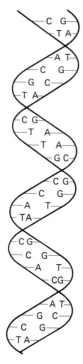

Figure 7-9 A double-stranded DNA molecule showing complementarity. Adenine (A) pairs with thymine (T) and cytosine (C) pairs with guanine (G).

two major functions: to replicate itself and to code for the synthesis of proteins.

The sequence of bases differs somewhat in various species and even in strains of microorganisms. Although molar proportions of guanine to cytosine and adenine to thymine in DNA equal unity, the proportions of G + C residues compared to total base content vary considerably in different organisms. *Escherichia coli* and *Morganella morganii* contain 50 percent G + C; all *Proteus* species contain approximately

37 to 44 percent, and some cells contain as little as 22 percent.

RIBONUCLEIC ACID

Ribonucleic acid (RNA) is distinguished from DNA by the presence of uracil instead of thymine, by the substitution of ribose for deoxyribose, by its location within the cell, and by its specialized functions in the synthesis of proteins. All types of RNA originate from the master blueprint or *template* supplied by DNA. The strands of RNA are complementary to the DNA strands in the same manner that a new strand of DNA is complementary to an unwound strand of DNA except that uracil appears in place of thymine.

The genetic information copied from DNA is contained in three types of RNA. Single strands of RNA having triplet bases or *codons* which are specific for particular amino acids comprise *messenger RNA* (mRNA). Most of the RNA of cells is associated with ribosomes and is called *ribosomal RNA* (rRNA). A third type of low molecular weight RNA, called *transfer RNA* (tRNA), occurs, in part, as a clover leaf conformation with paired bases (Figure 7-10). Triplets of unpaired bases on another part of the molecule are designated as *anticodons*. Anticodons of tRNA are complementary to the triplet bases or codons on the mRNA molecule. Functions for each type of RNA are presented in Chapter 8.

SUMMARY

The major molecules of microorganisms are shared with other forms of life.

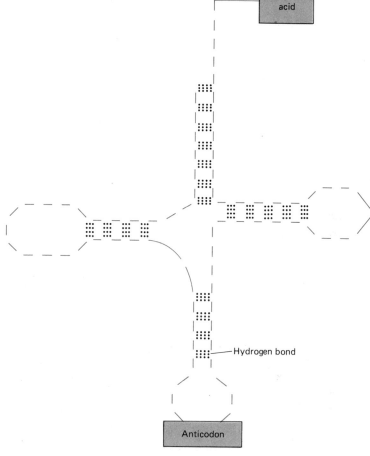

Figure 7-10 A diagrammatic representation of one tRNA. The triplet of bases (anticodon) in the bottom loop is complementary to a triplet of bases (codon) on mRNA.

Atoms of carbon (C), hydrogen (H), oxygen (O), and sometimes nitrogen (N), phosphorus (P), and sulfur (S) are contained both in specific amounts and configurations as the macromolecules of proteins, DNA, RNA, and some polysaccharides, and in the smaller molecular forms of carbohydrates and lipids. Each type of molecule plays a specific role in the structural and functional integrity of the cell. The interactions of microbial molecules are responsible for the properties associated with life.

QUESTIONS FOR STUDY

1. Name the six major elements found in microorganisms.
2. Name the major organic compounds found in all forms of life.
3. Name and describe five carbohydrates or derivatives of carbohydrates which contribute to the structural integrity of microorganisms.
4. Describe the primary, secondary, and tertiary structure of proteins.
5. What is the major function of lipids in microorganisms?
6. Differentiate between nucleosides and nucleotides.
7. Describe the structure of DNA and three types of RNA.

SELECTED REFERENCES

Brenner, D. J.; Farmer, J. J., III; Hickman, F. W.; Asbury, M. A.; and Steigerwalt, A. G. *Taxonomic and Nomenclature Changes in Enterobacteriaceae.* HEW Publication No. (CDC) 78-8356. Atlanta: U.S. Department of Health, Education, and Welfare, 1978.

Conn, E. E., and Stumpf, P. K. *Outlines of Biochemistry.* 3rd ed. New York: Wiley, 1972.

Holum, J. R. *Elements of General and Biological Chemistry.* 4th ed. New York: Wiley, 1975.

Lehninger, A. L. *Biochemistry,* 2d ed. New York: Worth, 1975.

Mahler, H. R., and Cordes, E. H. *Basic Biological Chemistry.* New York: Harper & Row, 1968.

Rose, A. H. *Chemical Microbiology.* 3rd ed. New York: Plenum Press, 1976.

Timberlake, K. *Chemistry.* New York: Harper & Row, 1976.

Toporek, M. *Basic Chemistry of Life.* 2d ed. Englewood Cliffs, N.J.: Prentice-Hall, 1975.

Yudkin, M., and Offord, R. *Comprehensible Biochemistry.* London: Clowes, 1973.

Chapter 8

Microbial Metabolism and Regulation

After you read this chapter, you should be able to:

1. Compare the energy sources of autotrophs and heterotrophs.
2. Recognize the six types of enzyme reactions.
3. Explain the influence of pH, temperature, substrate concentration, and enzyme reactions.
4. Describe two types of enzyme inhibition.
5. Explain the role of coenzymes and cofactors in enzyme reactions.
6. Differentiate between energy-liberating and energy-requiring reactions.
7. Compare the efficiency of aerobic and anaerobic respiration.
8. Differentiate between oxidative and substrate-level phosphorylation.
9. Explain why pyruvic acid is a key intermediate in microbial metabolism.
10. Identify intermediate metabolic products of glycolysis, the citric acid cycle, and the electron transport system.
11. Differentiate between transcription and translation.
12. Describe two major mechanisms which control microbial metabolism.
13. Differentiate between inducible and constitutive enzymes.

Microorganisms exist in animate or inanimate environments as dynamic entities constantly interacting with each other and their environments. The molecules within microorganisms are in a continuous state of flux as energy is released or expended during degradation or synthesis of cellular components (Figure 8-1). The availability of energy is an essential requirement for microbial life. Although structurally diverse, microorganisms share many metabolic pathways and regulatory mechanisms in meeting energy-exchange requirements.

ENERGY RESOURCES

The energy of microorganisms is derived from organic compounds or nonorganic sources. Microorganisms that utilize organic compounds as energy sources are called *heterotrophs*. Nutrients, packaged by nature in the form of carbohydrates, proteins, or lipids, are the major energy-yielding substances for heterotrophs. All pathogens are heterotrophs since they derive energy from their hosts for life-sustaining and disease-producing activities.

Other microorganisms derive energy from absorption of visible light or from inorganic materials such as nitrogen, sulfur, hydrogen, or iron. Algae and a few bacteria employ light energy to reduce atmospheric carbon dioxide to organic compounds in the process of *photosynthesis*. Other bacteria employ energy from inorganic sources, nitrogen, sulfur, hydrogen, and iron, to reduce carbon dioxide to organic compounds in an analogous process known as *chemosynthesis*. Micoorganisms capable of synthesizing their own cellular

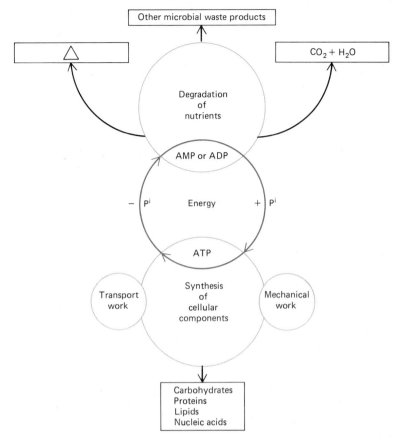

Figure 8-1 Energy flow in microbial metabolism. Energy is released from nutrients and transferred to energy-rich bonds of ATP for use in synthesis of organic compounds. Inorganic phosphate (P^i) is released from ATP to form AMP or ADP and recycled to form ATP as energy is released from nutrients.

requirements from inorganic substances are called *autotrophs*. If light is the source of energy, they are *photoautotrophs;* if inorganic compounds provide the energy, they are *chemoautotrophs.*

ROLE OF ENZYMES

All forms of life contain simple or conjugated proteins known as *enzymes*. Enzymes catalyze chemical reactions by lowering the energy of activation required to start the reaction between two or more chemical components of cells (Figure 8-2). The compounds acted upon by enzymes are called *substrates*. An enzyme reacts with a substrate or a related substrate of similar structure to release energy.

In order to lower the energy of activation, enzymes must associate intimately

167

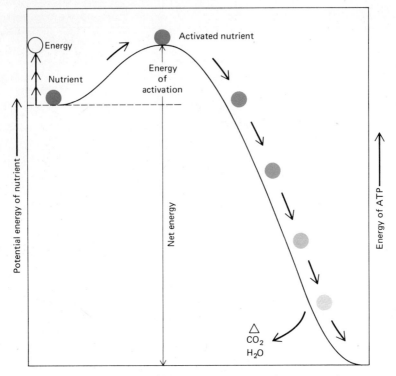

Figure 8-2   The "energy hill." Upon activation of a nutrient by an enzyme, energy is released from the activated nutrient and harnessed by adenosine triphosphate (ATP). Heat (Δ), carbon dioxide (CO_2), and water (H_2O) result from complete degradation of a nutrient.

with substrates. The folding of a protein molecule is hypothesized to provide a particular configuration complementary to the shape of a substrate. The fit between an enzyme and a substrate is analogous to that of a lock and key in which only a key complementary to the lock can open a door. Just as the hand guides a key into position, so attraction of opposite charges on enzyme and substrate promote positioning and binding of substrate at catalytic sites on the enzyme so that subjection to energy forces is maximal. Random energy is converted to coherent energy which polarizes and breaks a susceptible bond during the catalytic cycle. The subsequent change in polarities causes the dissociation of enzyme and product (Figure 8-3). The substrate (S) is bound at three catalytic sites on the enzyme (E) to yield a product (P).

$$ES \rightleftharpoons E + P$$

A second substrate (S_2) can in some cases bind to catalytic sites close to, but

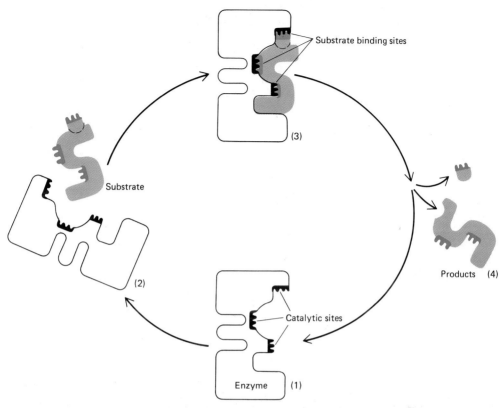

Figure 8-3 The "lock and key" interaction between an enzyme and a substrate. Opposite electrical charges create attraction between enzyme and substrate. Substrate is bound at catalytic sites and a susceptible bond is polarized. The change in polarities causes dissociation of enzyme and product. The enzyme is free to start another catalytic cycle.

separate from, the binding site for an initial substrate (S_1). In that event the reaction yields two products (P_1 and P_2).

$$ES_1S_2 \rightleftharpoons E + P_1 + P_2$$

A conformational change of the enzyme occurs upon binding, during the chemical reaction, and upon separation of enzyme and products.

Some enzymes have nonprotein components, called *prosthetic* groups, which are chemically distinct from the protein portion of the enzyme or *apoenzyme*. A substrate can react, alternately, with a nonprotein moiety of an enzyme.

CLASSIFICATION AND NAMING OF ENZYMES

Enzymes are classified on the basis of the type of reaction catalyzed. All reactions involving degradation or synthesis are catalyzed by one of six types of enzymes. Familiarity with these six types of enzymes and the reactions associated with them is essential for understanding bioenergetics of microbial metabolism. Theoretically, all enzyme reactions are reversible, but, in fact, this is usually not the case.

Oxidoreductases. Oxidation is one of the most available sources of energy for all forms of life. It involves a loss of electrons from highly electronegative atoms and a concomitant gain of electrons by atoms of lesser electronegativity. The loss of electrons is called *oxidation;* the gain of electrons is called *reduction.* The enzymes catalyzing transfers of electrons are *oxidoreductases.* The most active oxidoreductases in microbial systems are *dehydrogenases,* which transport the electrons of hydrogen.

$$AH_2 + B \rightleftharpoons A + BH_2$$

As electrons travel from atoms of greater electronegativity to those of lesser electronegativity, energy is released. The cell traps the energy and stores it immediately in depots of ATP. The loss of electrons and subsequent conserving of energy in phosphate bonds of ATP is a coupled enzyme reaction known as *oxidative phosphorylation.*

Transferases. During degradation and synthesis of compounds in cells, functional groups are frequently transferred from one substrate to another. The groups transferred include amino (NH_2), carboxyl (COOH), methyl (CH_3), glycosyl, and sulfur- or phosphorus-containing groups.

$$AR + B \rightleftharpoons BR + A$$

The enzymes catalyzing transfer of functional groups are *transferases.* The NH_2, COOH, CH_3, glyco-, phospho-, and sulfur transferases are all important in microbial metabolism.

Hydrolases. The degradation of nutrients into soluble substances in the presence of water and enzymes is called *hydrolysis.*

$$AB + H_2O \rightleftharpoons AOH + BH$$

The enzymes catalyzing hydrolytic reactions are called *hydrolases.* They are analogous to the digestive enzymes in animals except in microbial metabolism the hydrolases are secreted into the environment. Nucleases, proteases, lipases, phosphatases, and glycosidases are examples of hydrolases. Although the hydrolase reaction is shown above as reversible, reactions catalyzed by hydrolases are not always reversible.

Lyases. The removal or addition of functional groups from or to a substrate involves the action of *lyases.*

$$AR \rightleftharpoons A + R$$

The primary reaction of photosynthesis, the carboxylation of a pentose, is catalyzed by a lyase. Deamination and decarboxylation are important reactions in the transfer of energy during degradation of nutrients in microbial cells.

Isomerases. The rearrangement of atoms within a molecule causing a change in configuration is called *isomerization*.

$$AB \rightleftharpoons BA$$

The general name of *isomerases* can be applied to enzymes that can promote configurational changes within a molecule. In practice, such conversions may involve intramolecular oxidoreductases, transferases, lyases, racemases, or epimerases. The *racemases* convert L-isomers to D-isomers; *epimerases* alter positions of hydroxyl groups (OH) of sugars. The differences between the monosaccharides relate to the position of the OH groups on the carbon skeletons.

Ligases. The synthesis of microbial polymers involves the action of *ligases* (sometimes still called *synthetases*). Most degradative enzyme reactions are not reversible because the products are not present in sufficient quantities. Microbial syntheses, like those of other biological systems, require energy. Substrates combine with energy-rich ATP in the more complex syntheses yielding ADP and inorganic phosphate (P^i).

$$A + B + ATP \rightarrow AB + ADP + P^i$$

Bacterial growth is the consequence of the synthesis of complex compounds from simple materials.

Naming of Enzymes. Enzymes are named according to the type of reaction catalyzed and the name of the substrate acted upon. A dehydrogenase, for example, is an oxidoreductase which transfers electrons and hydrogen from one substrate to another. The name of the substrate supplying the electrons often precedes the name of the enzyme. For example, a lactic acid dehydrogenase acts upon the substrate, lactic acid, removing electrons and hydrogen. A polymerase is a ligase which catalyzes the combination of monomers into macromolecules. The name DNA polymerase indicates that the molecule synthesized is DNA. When referring to groups of enzymes, the suffix *-ase* is often added to the root of the major class of substrates. Therefore, the enzymes that degrade nutrients may be called *carbohydrases, proteases, lipases,* or *nucleases,* depending on the substrate. In employing group names, the type of reaction or intermediate substrate is not specified.

COENZYMES

Many enzymes require a second molecule to transport functional groups to or from reaction sites. The functional groups or elements transported in this manner are, in essence, passengers on enzyme carrier molecules. The carrier molecules are more frequently called *coenzymes* or coenzyme carriers. Coenzymes are usually relatively small molecules, but their names are often long enough to be so cumbersome that initials are used to designate them (Table 8-1). The structure of many coenzymes includes a vitamin.

Table 8-1   PASSENGER ATOMS OR GROUPS OF COENZYME CARRIERS

CARRIER MOLECULE	PASSENGER ATOMS OR GROUPS						
	ACETYL	AMINO	CARBOXYL	HYDROGEN	FORMYL	METHYL	PHOSPHATE
Adenosine triphosphate (ATP)							x
Biotin			x				
Cobamide						x	
Coenzyme A (Co A)	x						
Flavin adenine dinucleotide (FAD)				x			
Flavin mononucleotide (FMN)				x			
Lipoic acid	x		x	x			
Nicotinamide adenine dinucleotide (NAD)				x			
Nicotinamide adenine dinucleotide phosphate (NADP)				x			
Pyridoxyl phosphate pyridoxamine		x	x				
Tetrahydrofolic acid					x		
Thiamine pyrophosphate (ThPP)			x				

FACTORS INFLUENCING ENZYME REACTIONS

The rate at which enzyme reactions proceed is influenced by a number of environmental factors which include pH, temperature, concentration of the substrate, and concentration of the enzyme. The presence of specific accelerating or inhibiting substances can also affect the rate of enzyme reactions. Individual enzymes, even of a single species of bacteria, respond differently to rate-limiting interference. Therefore, enzymes exhibit not only specificity for substrate binding, but also largely individual responses to environmental factors.

pH

The hydrogen ion concentration, that is, the acidity or alkalinity of the environment, can be a limiting factor in enzyme reactions. The pH of the cellular environment profoundly affects the electrical charges of enzymes and, therefore, the affinities of enzymes for their substrates. Whereas the reactions may proceed over a wide range of pH values, the reaction rate is most rapid at the optimal pH (Figure 8-4). The majority of microbial enzymes are most active at a pH close to 7.0 (neutrality).

TEMPERATURE

The rate of most chemical reactions is increased at higher temperatures. In

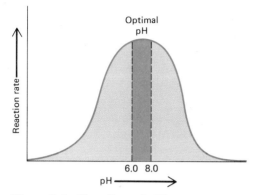

Figure 8-4   The effect of pH on enzyme reactions. The optimal pH for most microbial enzymes is close to 7.0.

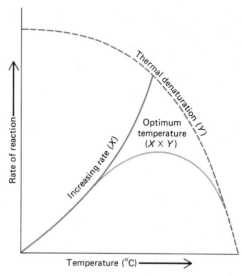

Figure 8-5   Effect of temperature on rate of enzyme reactions. X shows the increasing rate of a reaction as temperature rises. Y shows the decreasing rate of a reaction with thermal denaturation of the enzyme. The optimum temperature ($X \times Y$) depends on the thermal sensitivity of an enzyme. (Adapted from E. C. Conn and P. K. Stumpf, *Outlines of Biochemistry*, 3rd ed., New York, Wiley, 1972.)

microorganisms, as well as in other forms of life, enzymes are inactivated by excessive exposure to heat or cold (Figure 8-5). The mechanisms whereby heat and cold inactivate enzymes are substantially different. Heat renders enzymes inactive by denaturation (the alteration of a substance so that its original properties are changed, diminished, or removed); cold blocks the initiation of protein synthesis and increases the sensitivity of enzyme reactions to end-product control mechanisms. The ability of particular microorganisms to grow within a limited temperature range is a reflection of temperature-dependent enzymes.

SUBSTRATE CONCENTRATION

Increased concentrations of substrate in a substrate-enzyme system with a fixed amount of enzyme increase the velocity or rate of the reaction until active sites on the enzyme are saturated. The

Michaelis-Menton constant expresses the concentration of the substrate which produces one-half of the maximum velocity (Figure 8-6). The lowest concentrations of substrates to yield one-half maximum velocities are the most efficient in energy conservation.

ENZYME CONCENTRATION

Increased concentrations of an enzyme in a substrate-enzyme system with a fixed amount of substrate cause a rapid rise in reaction rate which levels off as all the available substrate is bound to

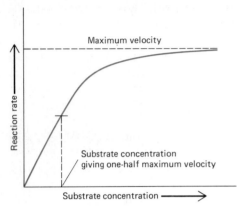

Figure 8-6 The Michaelis-Menten constant. The concentration of substrate that produces one-half of the maximum velocity is a constant for a substrate-enzyme system.

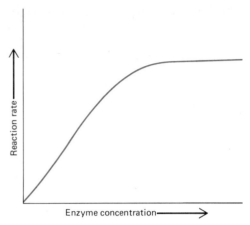

Figure 8-7 Effect of enzyme concentration on enzyme reactions. The rate of the reaction is increased with a fixed amount of substrate until no more substrate is available for binding to reactive sites on enzyme.

active sites on the enzyme (Figure 8-7). The conditions in which enzyme and substrate concentrations are optimal for reaction rate are, quite obviously, of a transient nature in the biochemical continuum of life.

ACCELERATING SUBSTANCES

Some enzyme reactions proceed only in the presence of metals such as iron (Fe), copper (Cu), iodine (I), magnesium (Mg), manganese (Mn), zinc (Zn), molybdenum (Mo), cobalt (Co), or potassium (K). Such metals are often referred to as *cofactors*.

Other enzyme reactions depend on the presence of coenzymes for optimal activity. Two nicotinic acid derivatives, nicotinamide adenine dinucleotide (NAD) and nicotinamide adenine dinucleotide phosphate (NADP), are very important in oxidation-reduction reactions.

INHIBITING SUBSTANCES

A variety of chemical substances can inhibit the rate of enzyme reactions. The effectiveness of the inhibitor depends upon whether it binds in a reversible or irreversible manner with the enzyme. In *competitive inhibition* the inhibiting substance competes with a structurally similar substrate for a position on an active site on the enzyme molecule.

$$E + I \rightleftharpoons EI$$

The rate of the reaction is dependent on the relative concentrations of the substrate and the inhibitor. The inhibition is reversible when the substrate level is increased. One of the most potent of such inhibitors is the organic acid, malonic acid, which competes effectively with another organic acid, succinic acid, for sites on molecules of succinic acid dehydrogenase. When the ratio of malonic acid to substrate is only 1:50, the dehydrogenase enzyme is inhibited by 50 percent.

In *noncompetitive inhibition,* the rate of an enzyme reaction is limited by a chemical combining with the active site or another locus on the enzyme. The inhibition depends only on the concentration of the inhibitor. The inhibition may be reversible or irreversible. If the combining site is other than the active site, it is probable that a conformational change occurs so that the active site no longer is available for reacting with the substrate.

ENERGY-LIBERATING REACTIONS

It is convenient to divide the chemical reactions of microorganisms into energy-liberating reactions (*exergonic*) and energy-requiring reactions (*endergonic*). The sum total of the chemical activities of living things is often called *metabolism.* Energy is liberated by degradation of nutrients into materials which can be employed for synthesis of structural or functional cell components; energy is expended for synthesis.

The term *respiration* is applied to the energy-liberating reactions of cells. The reactions of respiration consist of the transfer of electrons and hydrogen from nutrients by a gradual degradation to a series of compounds with the concom-

itant release of energy. The released energy is stored in high-energy phosphate (PO_4) bonds as ATP is formed from ADP. The nutrients are the *electron donors;* the series of compounds involved in the transfer of electrons and hydrogen are *electron acceptors.* Oxygen is the final electron acceptor in aerobic respiration. Nitrates (NO_3), sulfates (SO_4), or carbon dioxide (CO_2) may act as final electron acceptors in anaerobic respiration.

Some bacteria are *obligate* aerobes or anaerobes, that is, able to live only in atmospheric concentrations of oxygen, in the former case, or only in the complete absence of oxygen, in the latter case. Other bacteria are *facultative* in that they can exist with or without oxygen. Bacteria that grow best under conditions of reduced oxygen tension are described as *microaerophilic* organisms. There are pathogens representative of all groups, although a majority are aerobic and only facultatively anaerobic.

ANAEROBIC PATHWAYS

The initial means whereby energy is released is similar in both aerobic and anaerobic organisms. The first stage of respiration in both aerobic and anaerobic microorganisms involves the release of energy from the hydrolytic products of carbohydrates, proteins, and lipids.

Glycolysis, the step-by-step breakdown of glucose, and concomitant release of energy, is a major metabolic pathway. During glycolysis atoms of hydrogen (H), oxygen (O), and carbon (C) are regrouped to form pyruvic acid.

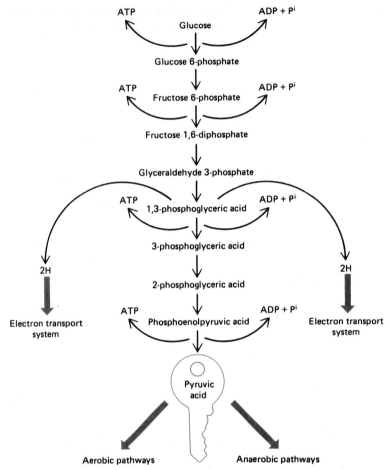

Figure 8-8   Degradation of glucose to the key intermediate pyruvic acid by glycolysis. The two pairs of electrons enter the electron transport system. Pyruvic acid enters aerobic or anaerobic pathways. Enough energy to form two molecules of ATP is released by glycolysis.

$$C_6H_{12}O_6 \longrightarrow 2CH_3COCOOH$$

Glucose   Pyruvic acid

The complete sequence of reactions for the conversion of glucose to pyruvic acid makes up the *Embden-Meyerhof pathway* (Figure 8-8).

Pyruvic acid is an intermediate meta-

bolic product which can be converted into a variety of compounds. In anaerobic respiration of muscle cells the pyruvic acid is reduced to lactic acid.

$$2CH_3COCOOH + 4H \longrightarrow 2CH_3CHOHCOOH$$

Pyruvic acid   Lactic acid

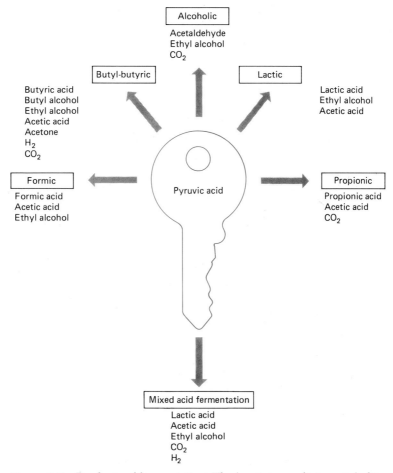

Figure 8-9 Products of fermentation. The key intermediate metabolite pyruvic acid can be converted to a variety of end products.

Fermentation is a sequence of reactions in the metabolism of pyruvic acid in which the final hydrogen acceptor is an organic compound. In microorganisms the pyruvic acid may be converted by fermentation to a variety of acids or alcohols, aldehyde, or acetone (Figure 8-9). Alcoholic, lactic, propionic, formic, and butyl-butyric fermentations produce one primary end product. The microorganisms capable of carrying out such fermentations are *homofermentative*. Fermentation may produce a mixture of end products; microorganisms capable of such reactions are *heterofermentative*. Often molecular H_2 of CO_2 are additional end products of homo- or heterofermentations.

Although fermentation is a highly efficient process for the production of alcohol from grains and grapes, neither glycolysis nor fermentations are efficient energy-yielding processes. The net energy yield in glycolysis is only two molecules of ATP per molecule of glucose.

Obligate anaerobes lack the enzymes necessary to release the total potential energy from glucose and are extremely sensitive to the presence of atmospheric oxygen. Oxygen is so toxic to strict anaerobes that even brief exposure to the atmosphere kills most organisms. Anaerobes must depend, instead, on other electron acceptors.

$$4H_2 + CO_2 \rightarrow CH_4 + 2H_2O$$
$$NaNO_3 + H_2 \rightarrow NaNO_2 + H_2O$$
$$Na_2SO_4 + H_2 \rightarrow Na_2SO_3 + H_2O$$

Nitrites (NO_2) may be further reduced to molecular nitrogen (N_2) or ammonia (NH_3).

The denitrifiers are facultative bacteria found in anaerobic portions of soil. In contrast, the sulfur-reducing bacteria and methane producers are obligate anaerobes widely distributed in polluted waters, swamps, and marshes.

AEROBIC PATHWAYS

The cycle of interdependent reactions that transfers the energy of pyruvic acid to ATP in aerobic organisms is the *citric acid cycle* (Figure 8-10). Pyruvic acid, derived from glycolysis, is oxidized by a dehydrogenase with the aid of coenzyme A (Co A) to form an active acetyl group (CH_3CO). In the reaction one carbon atom of pyruvic acid is converted to CO_2.

$$CH_3COCOOH + Co\ A\text{—}SH \longrightarrow$$

Pyruvic acid   Coenzyme A

$$CH_3CO\text{—}S\text{—}Co\ A + CO_2 + 2H$$

Acetyl Co A

Co A is the carrier molecule transporting the CH_3CO group to the citric acid cycle where it is made available to combine with the four-carbon oxaloacetic acid to form citric acid. The reaction between acetyl Co A, oxaloacetic acid, and H_2O is catalyzed by a synthetase.

$$CH_3CO\text{—}S\text{—}Co\ A + O\text{=}C\text{—}COOH + H_2O \longrightarrow$$
$$\underset{\quad}{\overset{\quad}{H_2C\text{—}COOH}}$$

Acetyl Co A   Oxaloacetic
                            acid

$$H_2C\text{—}COOH$$
$$HOC\text{—}COOH + HS\text{—}Co\ A$$
$$H_2C\text{—}COOH$$

Citric acid   Co A

The series of reactions in the citric acid cycle consist of dehydrogenations and decarboxylations yielding electrons, H^+, and CO_2. The CO_2 can be used by micoorganisms with some chemosynthetic ability to make essential metabolites. Small amounts of CO_2 released during respiration are incorporated into products of synthetic pathways since all microorganisms possess limited chemosynthetic ability. Excess CO_2 is excreted in gaseous form into the environment.

The electrons and hydrogen released during the reactions of the citric acid cycle are transported by a series of compounds making up the *electron transport system* or respiratory chain. In eu-

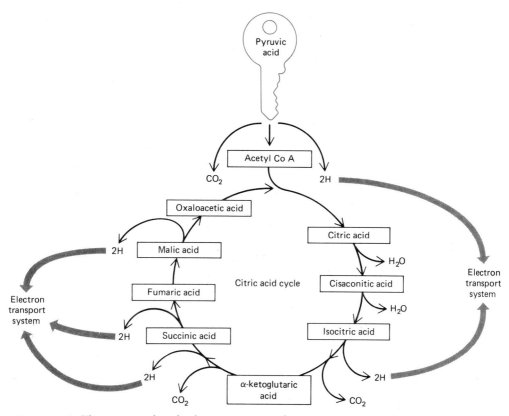

Figure 8-10 The citric acid cycle showing intermediate metabolites yielding carbon dioxide and electrons which enter the electron transport system.

caryotes most of the electron acceptors are contained within the inner membranes of mitochondria, whereas the majority of enzymes of the citric acid cycle are found in the matrix of mitochondria (Figure 8-11). A few carriers are located in the external membranes of mitochondria. In procaryotes enzymes of the citric acid cycle as well as the electron transport system are associated with cell-membrane fragments.

The transport system consists of two coenzymes, NAD (nicotinamide adenine dinucleotide) and FAD (flavin ade-nine dinucleotide), a cyclic compound ubiquinone, sometimes called coenzyme Q, and hemoproteins called *cytochromes*. The electrons proceed in succeeding steps from carriers with low oxidation-reduction potentials to carriers with increasingly higher potentials and, ultimately, reduce oxygen forming H_2O (Figure 8-12). The electron carriers are reduced when electrons are accepted and oxidized when electrons are lost.

The flow of electrons releases energy at three points for converting ADP

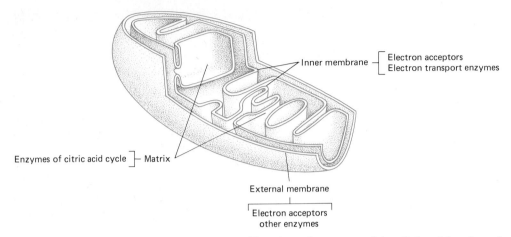

Inner membrane — Electron acceptors
Electron transport enzymes

Enzymes of citric acid cycle — Matrix

External membrane
Electron acceptors
other enzymes

Figure 8-11   Diagrammatic representation of location of enzymes of the citric acid cycle and electron carriers within a mitochondrion. Data is from mammalian mitochondria, since information on microbial mitochondria is meager. (Adapted from A. H. Rose, *Chemical Microbiology*, 3rd ed., New York, Plenum Press, 1976.)

(adenosine diphosphate) and inorganic phosphate (P^i) to ATP (adenosine triphosphate). Phosphorylation occurring in the respiratory chain is *oxidative phosphorylation*, since it is always accompanied by the reduction of molecular oxygen. ATP has a significant role in all cells because it is the compound which links degradative and biosynthetic pathways. ADP serves as an acceptor of phosphate groups (PO_4) and ATP donates PO_4 groups to other acceptor molecules, such as glucose or glycerol, thereby raising their energy content. Uncoupling of oxidative phosphorylation by inhibitors of electron transport limits the formation of ATP and, ultimately, causes a critical energy shortage in cells which often leads to death.

Aerobic respiration is vastly more efficient than anaerobic respiration, yielding 38 molecules of ATP for every molecule of glucose. Most of the energy released during the citric acid cycle is stored in the high-energy bonds of ATP as phosphorylation is coupled with oxidation in the respiratory chain. There are, however, two alternate mechanisms for energy transfer to ATP which do not involve oxidation. In one pathway, energy from molecules containing thioester bonds, that is, bonds between an organic acid group and the S atom of an enzyme complex, is transferred to the bond of a PO_4 recipient other than ATP. There are only two molecules with energy-laden thioester bonds: coenzyme A and lipoic acid. This type of phosphorylation occurs when succinyl Co A phosphorylates guanosine diphosphate (GDP) to form guanosine triphosphate (GTP) in the citric acid cycle.

$$\text{Succinyl Co A} + \text{GDP} + P^i \rightarrow$$

$$\text{Succinic acid} + \text{GTP} + \text{CO A}$$

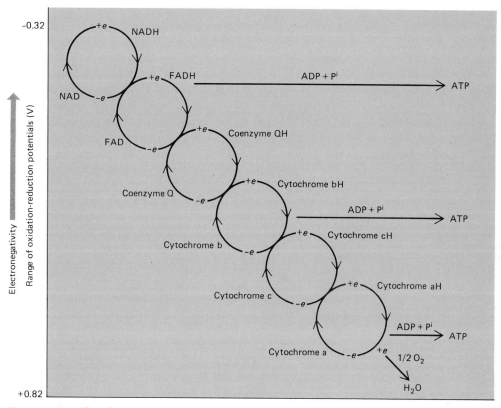

Figure 8-12 The electron transport system. Electrons (*e*) proceed from carriers of low oxidation-reduction potentials to carriers with increasingly higher potentials with oxygen as a final acceptor in aerobic systems. ATP is formed as energy from electrons incorporates inorganic phosphate (P^i) into energy-rich bonds.

The other alternative mechanism is the generation of a high-energy bond by loss of saturation when a molecule of water is removed from a phosphorylated compound. For example, the loss of water from 2-phosphoglyceric acid, in the formation of phosphoenolpyruvic acid during glycolysis, promotes energy storage in a bond adjacent to the double bond. The energy derived from thioester bonds or loss of saturation is ultimately transferred to ATP, but the oxidative process is not involved. Energy generated without concomitant oxidation is called *substrate-level phosphorylation*.

INTERRELATIONSHIPS OF CARBOHYDRATE, PROTEIN, AND LIPID DEGRADATION

The manner in which glucose is broken down to yield energy has been presented, but glucose represents only one

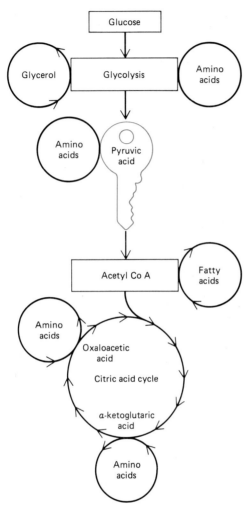

Figure 8-13 Interrelationships in the degradation of carbohydrates, lipids, and proteins.

energy source of microorganisms. The amino acids, derived from hydrolysis, can be deaminated to form pyruvic, oxaloacetic, or α-ketoglutaric acids in reversible reactions. Glycerol can enter the glycolytic pathway after phosphorylation by ATP. Fatty acids are degraded primarily by a process of β-oxidation requiring five enzymes in which each turn of a cycle removes a two-carbon unit. The action of the enzymes requires activation of a fatty acid by ATP to form a fatty acid–Co A complex. The product of β-oxidation is acetyl Co A, which can enter the citric acid cycle after reacting with oxaloacetic acid. Acetyl Co A, derived from carbohydrate or lipid metabolism, is, alternatively, a precursor for many lipids, including fatty acids (Figure 8-13).

The ATP-ADP system is unique in that it is the intermediate link between energy-yielding and energy-requiring reactions. The ATP-ADP energy transport system shuttles PO_4 groups back and forth with incredible speed. The half-life for turnover of the terminal PO_4 groups of ATP is only a few seconds.

ENERGY-REQUIRING REACTIONS

An alternate fate of some of the intermediate products of degradation is in the synthesis of microbial carbohydrates, proteins, lipids, and nucleic acids. It has been estimated that approximately 90 percent of cell energy is expended for synthesis of proteins. The major products of the CO_2-fixing processes of photosynthesis and chemosynthesis are carbohydrates.

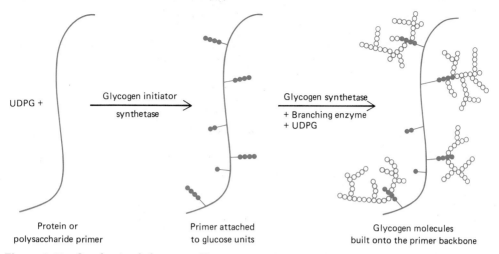

UDPG +

Glycogen initiator
synthetase →

Glycogen synthetase
+ Branching enzyme
+ UDPG →

Protein or
polysaccharide primer

Primer attached
to glucose units

Glycogen molecules
built onto the primer backbone

Figure 8-14 Synthesis of glycogen. Glucose units from uridine diphosphate glucose (UDPG) are added to a polysaccharide or protein primer to form glycogen. (Adapted from W. J. Whelan, *Trends in Biochemical Sciences* 1:13, 1976.)

SYNTHESIS OF CARBOHYDRATES

Glucose derived from nutrition or synthetic processes can enter the Embden-Meyerhof pathway or be packaged in the form of polysaccharides. There are numerous types of sugars in microbial polysaccharides, but the types in a single polysaccharide rarely exceed five. Glucose, galactose, and rhamnose are the most common constituents found in bacterial polysaccharides.

The metabolic pathways for the synthesis of polysaccharides are of particular importance in the production of capsules by some bacteria. Capsular material, containing heteropolysaccharides of glucose, levulose, and galactose, is synthesized at different stages of growth, depending on the organism.

A precursor required for the synthesis of hexoses is uridine diphosphoglucose (UDPG). Other nucleosides participate in the synthesis of other sugars. The energy required for synthesis is obtained from the high-energy phosphate bonds of the nucleosides.

The synthesis of polysaccharides requires, in addition, a primer consisting of a polysaccharide or a protein. In the synthesis of glycogen, glucose units from UDPG are added initially to the primer molecule in the presence of an initiator synthetase. Attachment of additional glucose units to the monomers requires the action of a branching enzyme (Figure 8-14). Thus, the synthetic pathways are not merely the degradative pathways in reverse.

SYNTHESIS OF PROTEINS

The synthesis of proteins is dependent on the transfer of genetic information

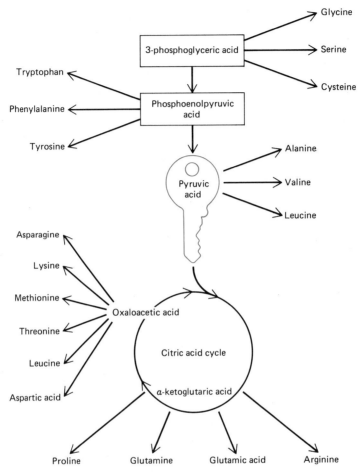

Figure 8-15 Precursors of amino acids. Amino groups are attached to carbon skeletons derived from organic acids.

from DNA to mRNA in a process called *transcription*. The actual specifying of the amino acid content of a protein is done in a process referred to as *translation*.

Microorganisms possess enzymes necessary for synthesis of amino acids not supplied in ample quantities in the environment. The carbon skeletons of most of the amino acids are derived from organic acid intermediates of glycolysis or the citric acid cycle (Figure 8-15).

Amino acids from the cellular pool are activated by ATP and combine with tRNA for transfer to the ribosomes where the synthesis of protein is directed by mRNA. The sequence of

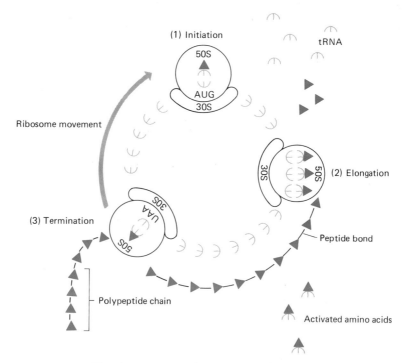

Figure 8-16 The three stages of protein synthesis. (1) Synthesis in procaryotic cells begins with an initiating codon (AUG) which codes for *N*-formylmethionine. (2) Elongation proceeds as activated amino acids are transferred by tRNA to the ribosome and peptide bonds are formed between amino acids. (3) A terminating codon (UAA) provides the signal for release of the polypeptide chain.

amino acids in the polypeptide chains determines the properties of the protein; the amino acid sequence is dependent on the order in which codons appear on the mRNA (Figure 8-16). The bases can exist in 64 different arrangements of triplets providing more than one possible codon for each of the 20 amino acids and some so-called "nonsense" codons which terminate polypeptide chains (Table 8-2). The folding of the polypeptide chains to form globular proteins was discussed in Chapter 8.

SYNTHESIS OF LIPIDS

Microorganisms incorporate fatty acids of the environment into phospholipids of cell membranes. In the absence of fatty acids in the growth medium, fatty acids are synthesized from acetyl Co A by a CO_2-biotin–dependent mechanism (Figure 8-17).

Another major constituent of many bacterial phospholipids is the phosphatide known as ethanolamine. The compound is a derivative of activated gly-

Table 8-2   CODONS FOR THE AMINO ACIDS

	U		C		A		G	
U	UUU	Phe	UCU	Ser	UAU	Tyr	UGU	Cys
	UUC	Phe	UCC	Ser	UAC	Tyr	UGC	Cys
	UUA	Leu	UCA	Ser	UAA	Ochre	UGA	
	UUG	Leu	UCG	Ser	UAG	Amber	UGG	Trp
C	CUU	Leu	CCU	Pro	CAU	His	CGU	Arg
	CUC	Leu	CCC	Pro	CAC	His	CGC	Arg
	CUA	Leu	CCA	Pro	CAA	Gln	CGA	Arg
	CUG	Leu	CCG	Pro	CAG	Gln	CGG	Arg
A	AUU	Ile	ACU	Thr	AAU	Asn	AGU	Ser
	AUC	Ile	ACC	Thr	AAC	Asn	AGC	Ser
	AUA	Ile	ACA	Thr	AAA	Lys	AGA	Arg
	AUG	Met	ACG	Thr	AAG	Lys	AGG	Arg
G	GUU	Val	GCU	Ala	GAU	Asp	GGU	Gly
	GUC	Val	GCC	Ala	GAC	Asp	GGC	Gly
	GUA	Val	GCA	Ala	GAA	Glu	GGA	Gly
	GUG	Val	GCG	Ala	GAG	Glu	GGG	Gly

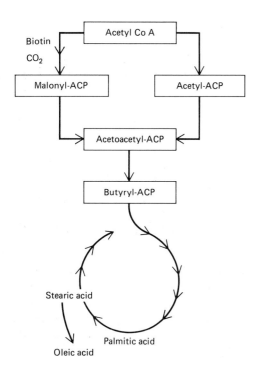

cerol and contains two ester linkages between fatty acids (Figure 8-18). The synthesis of phosphatidyl ethanolamine proceeds in 15 steps; seven high-energy bonds of ATP are required to complete a single molecule of the phospholipid.

Activated glycerol can also combine with fatty acids to form triglycerides, which are important reserve energy sources for fungi (Figure 8-19). Bacteria do not store triglycerides, but instead accumulate poly-β-hydroxybutyric acid (PHB) as a major energy reserve. The storage product can be hydroxylated

Figure 8-17 Synthesis of fatty acids. Formation of malonyl-ACP involves fixation of CO_2 activated by biotin. Fatty acid chains are lengthened as acetyl groups are reduced and added.

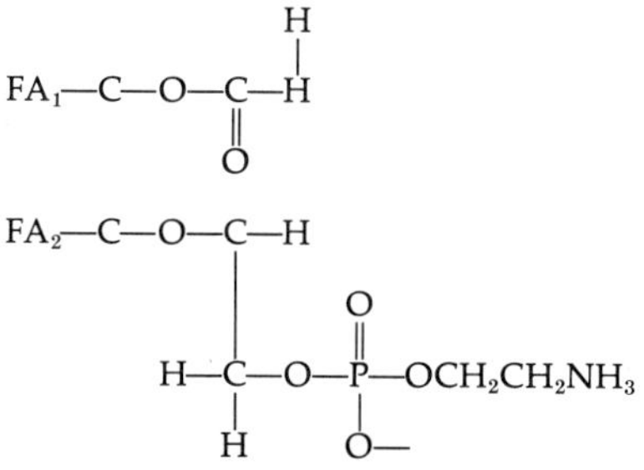

$$FA_1—C—O—C—H$$

$$FA_2—C—O—C—H$$

$$H—C—O—P—OCH_2CH_2NH_3$$

Figure 8-18 General structure of ethanolamine.

from butyryl-ACP of the fatty acid synthetic pathway or originate from a fermentative product of pyruvic acid.

Some microbial lipids are polymers of the five-carbon hydrocarbon isoprene.

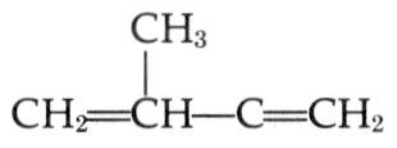

$$CH_2{=}CH—C{=}CH_2$$
$$\text{with } CH_3$$

Isoprene

Chlorophyll, carotenoids, bactoprenols, coenzyme Q, and cholesterol are all derived from isoprene subunits. The

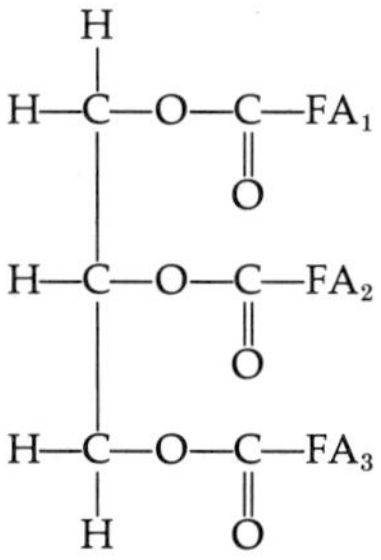

$$H—C—O—C—FA_1$$
$$H—C—O—C—FA_2$$
$$H—C—O—C—FA_3$$

Figure 8-19 General structure of a triglyceride, showing the three fatty acids (FA).

synthetic pathway begins with acetyl Co A and proceeds by way of an important intermediate known as mevalonic acid.

SYNTHESIS OF NUCLEIC ACIDS

The carbon and nitrogen atoms of purines and pyrimidines come from amino acids, formic acid, carbon dioxide, and pentoses (Figure 8-20). Phosphorylation of the pentoses is a prerequisite for the synthesis of both purines

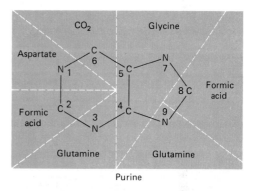

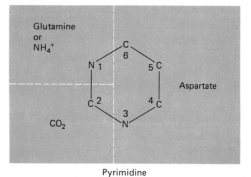

Figure 8-20 Origin of atoms of a purine and a pyrimidine. (Adapted from J. Mandelstam and K. McQuillen, *Biochemistry of Bacterial Growth*, New York, Wiley, 1968.)

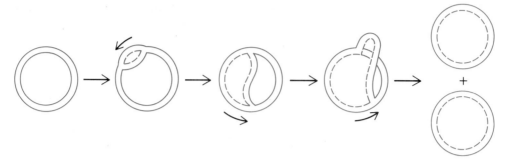

Figure 8-21   Semiconservative replication of DNA. Strand separation and synthesis proceed concurrently. (From M. J. Pelczar and R. D. Reid, *Microbiology,* New York, McGraw-Hill, 1972.)

and pyrimidines. Each nucleotide unit of a nucleic acid consists of a purine or pyrimidine base linked to a phosphorylated pentose. The pentose of DNA is deoxyribose; the sugar of RNA is the five-carbon ribose. A base with a keto group (C=O) always lines up opposite an amino group (NH$_2$) on carbon number 6. The lactic acid bacteria are exceptional in that they lack the ability to synthesize purines or pyrimidines and depend on environmental sources.

The immediate precursors for synthesis of double-stranded DNA are nucleotides activated by three PO$_4$ groups from ATP. Following strand separation, each strand of DNA acts as a template for the replication of a new strand of DNA or RNA using the activated nucleotides (Figure 8-21). Bases line up in positions complementary to the parental DNA strand and are polymerized through the action of DNA or RNA polymerases. The end products consist of one parental strand and one newly synthesized strand—a principle called *semiconservative replication.*

CONTROL MECHANISMS

The many chemical reactions involved in both energy-yielding and energy-requiring processes are subject to both fine and coarse control mechanisms. The number of molecules of a typical *E. coli* cell is a small indication of the amount of "policing" necessary to start or stop the flow of information in maintaining cellular integrity (Table 8-3). Control mechanisms prevent synthesis

Table 8-3   MAJOR MOLECULES OF A CELL OF *ESCHERICHIA COLI*

TYPE OF MOLECULE	NUMBER OF MOLECULES
DNA	1
RNA	15,000
Protein	1,700,000
Lipid	15,000,000
Polysaccharide	39,000

SOURCE: A. L. Lehninger, *Bioenergetics,* 2d ed. (Menlo Park, Calif.: W. A. Benjamin, 1973).

of enzymes by direct action on a metabolic pathway or at the level of transcription.

FEEDBACK INHIBITION

One fine control mechanism, operating at the level of the end product in a series of enzyme reactions, is called *feedback inhibition*. In a simple feedback mechanism the end product inhibits the first enzymatic step in a pathway. Inhibition of syntheses of amino acids provides many examples of simple feedback mechanisms.

$$A \rightarrow B \rightarrow C \rightarrow D \rightarrow E$$

Often however, more than one enzyme is inhibited. Multiple enzyme inhibition takes place in branched pathways. The end products of a branched pathway affect the first enzyme of the common portion of a pathway and enzymes at the branching points.

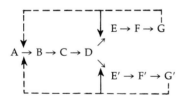

One example of multiple enzyme inhibition takes place in the synthesis of lysine. Lysine interferes with aspartate kinase which converts aspartate to aspartyl-phosphate and a condensing enzyme which converts aspartate semialdehyde to dihydropicolinic acid (Figure 8-22). The regulation of amino acid synthesis is complex because of the multiple connecting pathways. The

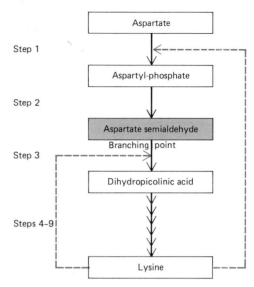

Figure 8-22 Multiple feedback inhibition. Steps 1 and 3 in the synthesis of lysine are inhibited by an accumulation of the end product. Aspartate semialdehyde is the branching point for the synthesis of lysine, isoleucine, and methionine.

mechanisms of feedback inhibition constitute a nitrogen-conserving device for cells.

Enzymes subject to feedback inhibition are called *allosteric* enzymes. An allosteric enzyme has, in addition to an active site, a second or allosteric site to which the end product can bind. Upon binding, the conformation of the enzyme changes so that the active site is no longer available for binding with the substrate (Figure 8-23). Both degradative and synthetic pathways are subject to feedback inhibition. It is, in essence, an energy-conserving mechanism, for the blocking of reactions prevents the expenditure of energy for unneeded materials.

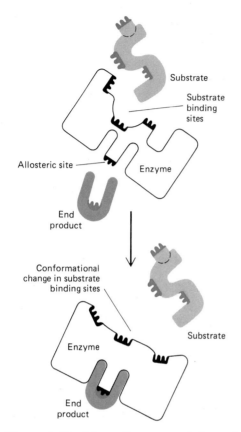

Substrate

Substrate binding sites

Allosteric site

Enzyme

End product

Conformational change in substrate binding sites

Substrate

Enzyme

End product

Figure 8-23 Schematic representation of allostery. When an end product combines with an enzyme, a conformational change makes the active site no longer available for binding with the substrate. (Adapted from J. Mandelstam and K. McQuillen, *Biochemistry of Bacterial Growth*, New York, Wiley, 1968.)

GENETIC REPRESSION AND INDUCTION

Rather than acting directly as an inhibitor, an end product can activate a repressor substance which blocks or activates transcription. The repressor acts on a key gene of a cluster of genes responsible for enzymes of one metabolic pathway. The complete series of genes in the cluster is called an *operon*. The concept of an operon, containing a regulatory gene and structural genes, was first proposed by Jacques Monod and Francois Jacob. They identified a repressor of lactose fermentation in *E. coli* as a protein making up 0.002 to 0.02 percent of cell protein (Figure 8-24). The process of repressor inactivation is more frequently called *induction*. The inducers are substrates and the enzymes produced as a result of protein-repressor inhibition are *inducible* enzymes. Those enzymes, synthesized in the absence of specific substrates, are called *constitutive* enzymes.

CATABOLITE REPRESSION

Another and less specific type of repression occurs when an intermediate of glucose degradation interferes with transcription. It appears that the intermediate metabolite lowers cyclic adenosine monophosphate (AMP) levels in some manner. Cyclic AMP apparently affects a variety of metabolic pathways in bacteria. The glucose effect is correctable by the addition of cyclic AMP to cultures.

SUMMARY

The energy of microorganisms is transferred from nutrients to the intermediate compound ATP by a process of degradation and from energy-rich depots of ATP to structural and functional molecules by synthetic processes.

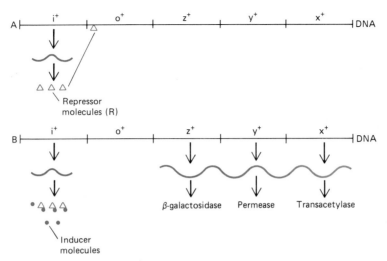

Figure 8-24   Jacob and Monod's operon concept. *A,* Repressor molecules attach to the operator gene and prevent transcription by structural genes z, y, and x which code for enzymes of lactose fermentation. *B,* Inducer molecules inactivate repressor molecules and allow structural genes to function. (Adapted from J. Mandelstam and K. McQuillen, *Biochemistry of Bacterial Growth,* New York, Wiley, 1968.)

The degradation of nutrients and synthesis of polysaccharides, proteins, lipids, and nucleic acids are catalyzed by enzymes. Initial degradative pathways are similar in aerobic and anaerobic microorganisms but the intermediate metabolites and final electron acceptors differ. Aerobic respiration is more efficient than anaerobic respiration, yielding 38 molecules of ATP for every molecule of glucose broken down. The synthetic pathways are not merely reverse degradative pathways, but consist of highly specific reactions requiring energy, precursors, enzymes, coenzymes, and cofactors. Metabolic activities of microorganisms are controlled by a direct action on a metabolic pathway or at the level of transcription.

QUESTIONS FOR STUDY

1. Define autotroph, heterotroph, photosynthesis, and chemosynthesis.
2. Name six factors which influence enzyme reactions.
3. Identify the type of phosphorylation occurring in each of the following energy-generating processes:
   glycolysis
   citric acid cycle
   electron transport system

4. Give three examples which show interrelationships of carbohydrate, protein, and lipid metabolism.

5. List one raw material required for the synthesis of each of the following:

   fatty acids   cholesterol
   glycogen   adenine
   ethanolamine   glucose

6. Of what importance are allosteric enzymes in the control of microbial metabolism?

SELECTED REFERENCES

Brock, T. C. *Biology of Microorganisms.* 2d ed. Englewood Cliffs, N.J.: Prentice-Hall, 1974.

Conn, E. E., and Stumpf, P. K. *Outlines of Biochemistry.* 3rd ed. New York: Wiley, 1972.

Holum, J. R. *Elements of General and Biological Chemistry.* 3rd ed. New York: Wiley, 1972.

Kwapinski, J. B. G.; Bradley, S. G.; Brown, E. R.; Burton, P. R.; Fraenkel-Conrat, H.; Kordova, N.; O'Learcy, W. M.; Reithel, F. J.; Salton, M. R. J.; Storck, R.; and Woodside, E. E. *Molecular Microbiology.* New York: Wiley, 1974.

Lehninger, A. L. *Biochemistry.* 2d ed. New York: Worth, 1975.

Lehninger, A. L. *Bioenergetics,* 2d ed. Menlo Park, Calif.: W. A. Benjamin, 1973.

Levy, J.; Campbell, J. J. R.; and Blackburn, T. H. *Introductory Microbiology.* New York: Wiley, 1973.

Mandelstam, J., and McQuillen, K. *Biochemistry of Bacterial Growth.* New York: Wiley, 1968.

Rose, A. H. *Chemical Microbiology.* 3rd ed. New York: Plenum Press, 1976.

Thimann, K. V. *The Life of Bacteria.* 2d ed. New York: Macmillan, 1963.

Chapter 9

Microbial Growth

After you read this chapter, you should be able to:

1. Differentiate between physical and chemical microbial growth requirements.
2. List seven growth requirements for bacteria.
3. Explain the relationship between cell mass and cell number under conditions of steady-state growth.
4. Differentiate between growth rate and generation time.
5. Identify the phases of growth on a normal growth curve.
6. Describe eight methods for measuring growth of bacteria.
7. Contrast the advantages or disadvantages of direct and indirect estimations of microbial populations.
8. Describe the bases for classifying microbiological culture media.
9. List three methods for isolating bacteria or fungi on solid media.
10. Identify growth patterns of bacteria in broth and on agar slants.
11. Describe the purposes for which continuous and synchronized cultures are used.
12. Compare formation and germination of endospores.

Microbial growth consists of a uniform increase in components of the cell culminating in an orderly process of cell division to produce two daughter cells. Most bacteria divide by binary fission when sufficient amounts of deoxyribonucleic acid (DNA), ribonucleic acid (RNA), protein, and peptidoglycan are available to support metabolic processes of two cells. An organism capable of carrying out metabolic functions, including cell division, is considered to be viable. The time required for growth and division is known as the doubling or *generation time*.

The term growth is most usually applied to populations of microorganisms rather than to individual organisms, in much the same manner as one speaks of the growth in population of a particular geographic area. Bacterial growth can be measured in terms of *cell mass* or *cell number*.

PHYSICAL REQUIREMENTS

The microcosms in nature reveal a great diversity in physical environments. Microbial populations are a reflection of conditions found in the immediate surroundings. An environmental factor required by one microorganism may be detrimental to the growth of another. Some organisms can tolerate extremes of temperature, high osmotic pressure, and a wide range of atmospheric conditions, while others have a very limited range in which they can grow and reproduce. Most microorganisms, however, with the exception of a stage in the life cycle of spore-formers, are dependent on the presence of water in the environment.

Pathogenic bacteria are as a rule much more restricted in survival capacity than saprophytic species. Most disease-producing organisms grow best under conditions optimal for growth of their mammalian hosts.

TEMPERATURE

The temperature requirements for growth are stable characteristics of bacteria and are often important in the isolation and identification of microorganisms grown under laboratory conditions. Almost all bacteria grow over a broad range of temperatures, but optimal growth of an organism is obtained over a relatively narrow range. The lowest temperature supporting growth of an organism is the *minimal growth temperature;* the highest temperature supporting growth is the *maximal growth temperature.*

The *optimal growth temperature* for most bacteria ranges between 20° and 45°C (Figure 9-1). Bacteria whose enzymes react maximally within that temperature range are *mesophiles.* Large numbers of mesophiles, both pathogenic and nonpathogenic, are found in or on warm-blooded animals, including humans. Most vegetative forms of bacterial pathogens cannot withstand extremes of heat or cold.

Bacteria that grow best at temperatures of 45°C or above are called *thermophiles* (heat-loving). In nature thermophiles occur in hot springs, tropical soil, composts, and hay stacks. The spontaneous combustion of stacked hay is caused, in part, by thermophilic action producing temperatures as high as 75°C. Thermophiles can cause food to spoil in heat-processed cans if spores survive heat treatment.

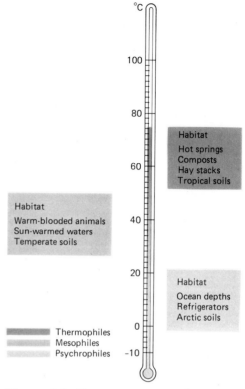

Figure 9-1 Temperature growth ranges and habitats of psychrophiles, mesophiles, and thermophiles.

Bacteria which remain metabolically active at −5° to 20°C are called *psychrophiles* or *cryophiles* (cold-loving). These organisms are found in depths of oceans or in soil of areas having cold climates. The presence of psychrophiles in foods can cause spoilage at refrigerator temperatures.

OSMOTIC PRESSURE

The osmotic pressure of an environment is dependent on the concentration of dissolved salts. A variety of dissolved salts, including sodium chloride (NaCl), is found in most natural environments. Almost all bacteria can withstand concentrations of NaCl of 1 to 2 percent, and some are able to grow in concentrations of 15 to 30 percent. The salt-loving bacteria are called *halophiles*. Marine forms require a salt concentration of approximately 3.5 percent for growth.

The ability to tolerate high NaCl concentrations is the basis of some selective culturing procedures. An interesting relationship exists between temperature and salt requirements in some lactic acid bacteria and halophiles. In general optimal temperatures are higher as NaCl concentrations in the environment are increased.

The mechanism whereby osmotic pressure limits growth of some bacterial species is not well understood. It has been established that osmotic pressure exerts a pronounced effect on phagocytic capability of white blood cells by interfering with respiratory activity.

ATMOSPHERIC CONDITIONS

The gas content of the atmosphere influences the growth of microorganisms. *Obligate aerobes* grow only in the presence of oxygen. *Obligate anaerobes* grow only in the absence of oxygen. The presence of oxygen not only inhibits growth, but is highly toxic to some obligate anaerobes, such as clostridia. The reason for extreme oxygen sensitivity is not well understood, but it may be related to the anaerobes' inability to destroy a free radical form of oxygen,

superoxide. The destruction of superoxide requires the enzyme superoxide dismutase, which is found only in aerotolerant organisms. The extreme sensitivity of strict anaerobes to oxygen must be considered in obtaining, transporting, and culturing clinical specimens suspected of containing anaerobes (Figure 9-2).

A large number of microorganisms grow under aerobic or anaerobic conditions; they are called *facultative anaerobes*. Many yeasts and enteric bacteria can utilize fermentative or oxidative pathways. In nature the facultative anaerobes have great survival capacity, for they can shift "metabolic gears" in response to atmospheric conditions.

Anaerobic conditions may be obtained by using a sealed jar containing a pack that generates hydrogen and carbon dioxide in the presence of a platinum calalyst (Figure 9-3). Atmospheric oxygen is eliminated in the sealed jar when it combines with hydrogen to form water. A reducing agent, such as thioglycollic acid, can also create anaerobiosis when it is added to a liquid medium. If a tube of the broth is boiled to remove oxygen before it is inoculated, anaerobic growth will occur in the bottom of the tube. Facultative organisms will grow throughout the medium, but growth of aerobic organisms will remain limited to the surface.

Bacteria requiring oxygen in quantities less than that found under ordinary atmospheric conditions are called *microaerophilic*. Microaerophiles grow below the surface of broth containing a reducing agent where there is a small

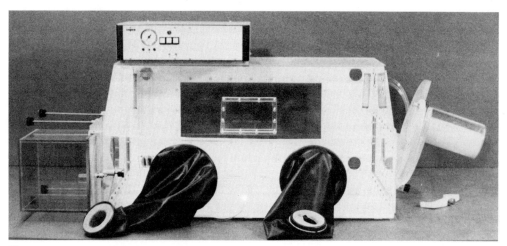

Figure 9-2 An anaerobic chamber which maintains an oxygen-free atmosphere. Hands and arms are placed through glove ports to inoculate media. (Courtesy, Capco, Sunnyvale, California.)

quantity of residual oxygen. Bacteria requiring carbon dioxide in quantities greater than that found under ordinary atmospheric conditions are called *capneic*. Meningococci, gonococci, and mycobacteria are stimulated by increased concentrations of carbon dioxide. Sufficient elevations of carbon dioxide can be obtained using a candle jar or a special incubator. In a candle jar a candle is permitted to burn in a closed container until the flame goes out. In a carbon dioxide incubator the atmospheric concentration is controlled by a gauge connected to a gas tank.

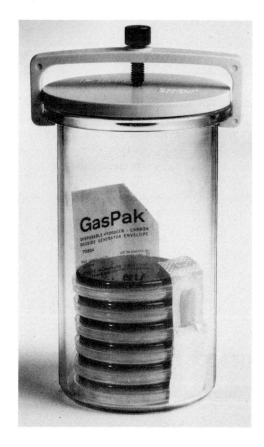

Figure 9-3 Anaerobic culture jar containing a GasPak envelope. (Courtesy, BBL Microbiology Systems, Cockeysville, Md.)

CHEMICAL REQUIREMENTS

The chemical requirements of particular bacteria differ even more substantially than their physical needs. Some bacteria require only inorganic salt solutions to sustain growth since they synthesize their own energy sources; other bacteria require highly complex carbon or nitrogen sources. Large numbers of bacteria will grow in nutrient broth, but some pathogens require enrichment.

pH

Almost all bacteria grow best at a pH approximating neutrality, but tolerate mild acidic or alkaline environments (Figure 9-4). The producers of acetic acid (*Acetobacter*) and sulfuric acid (*Thiobacillus*) are remarkable exceptions, having a capacity to live at a pH of 1.0 or below. Such bacteria have developed adaptive mechanisms for preventing hydrogen (H^+) from entering cells. A few bacteria, most notably the cholera vibrio, grow at a pH of 8.5 or greater. Fungi are acid tolerant and grow best at a pH of 5.0 to 6.0. Differing requirements for pH can be used in selecting for growth of particular microorganisms.

The pH of culture media is controlled by the addition of buffers, substances which resist changes in pH. The buffers stabilize pH by combining either with H^+ ions of strong acids to produce weak acids or with the hydroxyl (OH^-) ions of strong bases to form weak acids and water.

$$H^+ + HPO_4^{2-} \rightarrow H_2PO_4^-$$
$$OH^- + H_2PO_4^- \rightarrow HPO_4^{2-} + HOH$$

Disodium phosphate (Na_2HPO_4) and monosodium phosphate (NaH_2PO_4) are often used in combination to obtain a final pH of 7.0 in culture media. Depletion of buffers allows acid or alkaline metabolites to accumulate and limits growth of bacterial populations.

H$^+$ ion concentration (moles per liter)		pH	
1.0	10^0	0	
0.1	10^{-1}	1	
0.01	10^{-2}	2	
0.001	10^{-3}	3	
0.0001	10^{-4}	4	
0.00001	10^{-5}	5	
0.000001	10^{-6}	6	Neutral
0.0000001	10^{-7}	7	
	10^{-8}	8	
	10^{-9}	9	
	10^{-10}	10	
	10^{-11}	11	
	10^{-12}	12	
	10^{-13}	13	
	10^{-14}	14	

Increasing acidity → Increasing alkalinity

Figure 9-4   Relationship of pH and H$^+$ ion concentration. The number on the pH scale represents the negative logarithm of the H$^+$ ion concentration.

INORGANIC IONS

Bacteria require phosphate (PO_4^{3-}), potassium (K^+), magnesium (Mg^{2+}), ammonium (NH_4^+), and frequently sulfate (SO_4^{2-}) for growth. K^+ and Mg^{2+} are essential for protein systhesis, NH_4^+ serves as a nitrogen source, and PO_4^{3-} and SO_4^{2-} are needed for a variety of metabolic activities. In addition, certain trace elements participate in enzyme reactions. Divalent iron (Fe^{2+}) and trivalent iron (Fe^{3+}) are needed for synthesis of hemoproteins, such as cytochromes and the enzymes catalase and peroxidase. Zinc (Zn^{2+}) and manganese (Mn^{2+}) activate certain hydrolytic enzymes. Calcium (Ca^{2+}) is an important component of bacterial spores. Cobalt (Co^{2+}) and molybdenum (Mo^{2+}) are required for vitamin B_{12} synthesis and nitrogen reduction, respectively.

ENERGY SOURCES

The requirement for energy in microorganisms can be met by an exogenous carbon source in heterotrophs. Using light energy, autotrophs convert atmospheric CO_2 into an endogenous carbon source or use inorganic compounds, such as hydrogen (H_2), hydrogen sulfide (H_2S), nitrite (NO_2), or ammonia (NH_3), as sources of energy. There are relatively few species of bacteria which can degrade complex polysaccharides, but microorganisms possess greater diversification in carbohydrases than do mammals. Many bacteria and fungi can digest starch; some soil bacteria and fungi can break down cellulose; and a few marine microorganisms can use the polysaccharide agar as a source of energy.

Any material that can be broken down by some form of life, usually microorganisms, is called *biodegradable*. Unfortunately, some products developed in the last few decades cannot be degraded by microorganisms. The proliferation of nondegradable products, no matter how convenient to use, interferes with recycling of elements vital to life.

GROWTH FACTORS

Growth factors consist of small organic compounds and include vitamins, amino acids, purines, and pyrimidines. Particular strains of bacteria require specific growth factors. For example, with some species of *Lactobacillus* growth is proportional to the amount of vitamin B_{12} in the medium. The need for specific growth factors is the basis of a technique known as a *microbiological assay* (Figure 9-5). The concentration of a required vitamin or amino acid can be determined from the amount of growth obtained.

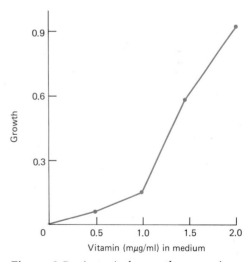

Figure 9-5 A typical growth curve in a microbiological assay. Growth is proportional to the amount of vitamin in the medium.

METHODS OF MEASURING GROWTH

It is often pertinent to ascertain numbers as well as types of bacteria present in milk, water, food, soil, or a clinical specimen, particularly urine. Growth can be measured by determining the numbers of cells in such samples. Measurement of cell mass is more meaningful in studying the biochemistry of cells. Both cell numbers and cell mass are related to the availability of nutrients. The rate of growth in cell number exceeds that of cell mass in young cultures, but both increase until a nutrient is depleted or a toxic metabolite accumulates. Although cell division may be severely limited, and viable cells decreased, cell mass remains constant as long as cells remain intact physically.

The rate of growth under optimal conditions is a function of the generation time, the time required for a cell to grow and divide. The cell number doubles with each generation (Table 9-1). Since we usually transfer at least 10^6 cells with a bacteriological loop, only 20 generations produce $1,048,576^6$ cells! Sometimes it helps to gain perspectives of microbial growth to realize that it takes very large populations of bacteria to produce observable results in laboratory tests.

A logarithmic scale is used to represent growth phases during time intervals (Figure 9-6). There is an identifiable *lag phase* when a culture medium is first inoculated. It takes from one to several hours for cells to increase in number. The lag phase is followed by an *exponential phase* in which growth is proportional to time. During this phase total and viable counts are nearly the same. With time, however, a number of factors limit growth. An essential nutrient may be depleted or products of metabolism, such as acids or alcohols, may be inhibitory. Often, lack of oxygen is the limiting factor. Ultimately, a *stationary phase* is reached in which growth stops rather suddenly and cell size decreases. The stationary phase varies in time with the bacterial species from a few hours to several days, after which the cells begin to die. A fourth phase is sometimes referred to as the *death phase;* it continues until most, if not all, microorganisms are unable to sustain life. In some species a few bacteria demonstrate remarkable resistance

Table 9-1   INCREASE IN CELL COUNT AS A RESULT OF BINARY FISSION

GENERATION NUMBER	CELL COUNT
0	1
1	2
2	4
3	8
4	16
5	32
6	64
7	128
8	256
9	512
10	1024
20	1,048,576

SOURCE: J. R. Sokatch, and J. J. Ferretti, *Basic Bacteriology and Genetics.* (Chicago: Year Book Medical Publishers, 1976).

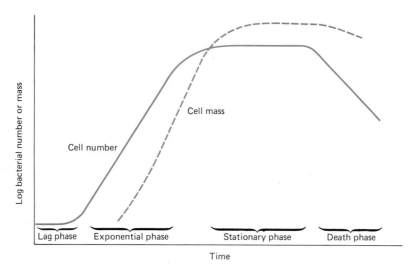

Figure 9-6   A typical bacterial growth curve showing four phases and relationship between cell mass and cell number. (From B. D. Davis et al., *Microbiology*, 2nd ed., New York, Harper & Row, 1973.)

to the accumulative effects of growth and will survive if transferred to a new culture medium.

TURBIDIMETRIC MEASUREMENT

Growth of bacteria in a liquid medium causes visible turbidity which can be measured in a colorimeter or spectrophotometer. The amount of light permitted to pass through the liquid gives a reading of the *optical density* (Figure 9-7). The greater the cell mass, the less light will pass through it and the higher the optical density. The optical density is proportional to cell mass between 0.01 mg and 0.5 mg dry weight. Measurement of very dense

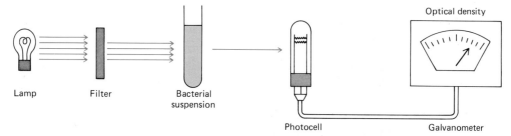

Figure 9-7   Simplified diagram of a spectrophotometer. The amount of light which hits the galvanometer is proportional to the mass of cells in the bacterial suspension.

populations of bacteria requires dilution in order to obtain accurate estimates of cell mass.

GRAVIMETRIC MEASUREMENT

Cell mass can be determined in terms of dry or wet weight, after harvesting cells by centrifugation. Dry weight measurements, while more time consuming, are a more accurate estimation of cell mass since amounts of water in cells may not be directly related to protoplasmic content. Wet weights usually exceed dry weights by 20 or 25 percent.

Dry weights of procaryotic cells average about 10^{-13} gm, while eucaryotic microorganisms weigh approximately 10^{-10} gm. Average weights can be obtained by dividing weight of a population of cells by total number of cells estimated by direct microscopic- or electronic-device counts. Gravimetric techniques are not practical unless one is dealing with massive populations of cells.

DIRECT CELL COUNTS

Total cells can be counted in a specially designed slide known as the *Petroff-Hausser counting chamber* (Figure 9-8). The slide contains a grid of 25 small squares within 1 mm². The space between the cover slip and slide is 1/50 mm. A bacterial suspension is added carefully so that it covers the grid completely, but does not overflow the chamber. Several squares are counted and the average is used to calculate the number of cells per milliliter.

$$N = \text{average cells} \times 25 \times 50 \times 10^3$$

Cells may also be counted by a stained-smear technique. A measured amount of a bacterial suspension is spread over a square centimeter on an ordinary glass slide, dried, stained, and counted. Several randomly selected fields are usually counted. The number of fields in the square centimeter can be ascertained by using a stage micrometer. The number of fields multiplied by the average number of cells per field times 100 equals the number of cells per milliliter of sample. Both the counting-chamber and stained-smear techniques are subject to many technical errors.

Estimation of total cells by an electronic cell counter eliminates some of the human error and gives rapid results. A small volume of a dilute bacterial suspension is allowed to flow past a pair of electrodes. Interruption in the current by the cells is recorded as a pulse on an electronic device. The total cell count may not be the same as a viable cell count.

Direct microscopic and electronic counts have additional limitations.

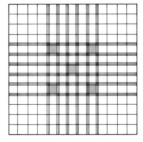

Figure 9-8 The grid of a Petroff-Hausser counting chamber. Several small squares are counted, averaged, and multiplied by a dilution factor to calculate the number of cells in a milliliter of sample.

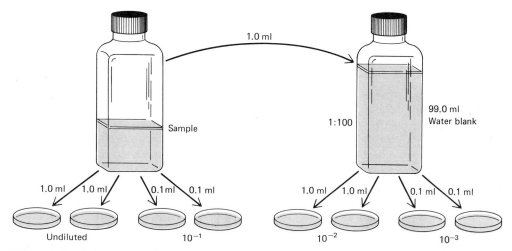

1.0 ml

Sample

1:100

99.0 ml
Water blank

1.0 ml 1.0 ml 0.1 ml 0.1 ml

1.0 ml 1.0 ml 0.1 ml 0.1 ml

Undiluted 10^{-1}

10^{-2} 10^{-3}

Figure 9-9 A diagrammatic representation of the technique employed in the standard plate count to obtain colony-forming units (CFU) per milliliter.

Sometimes two cells adhere to each other and are recorded as a single unit by electronic cell counters. In direct microscopic counts it is often difficult to distinguish bacteria from debris. As a rule, chamber or slide counts are applicable only to populations of cells which exceed 10^6 organisms per milliliter.

STANDARD PLATE COUNT

One of the most practical methods for determining numbers of viable cells employs small volumes of a series of 10-fold (10^{-1}) or 100-fold (10^{-2}) dilutions of bacterial suspensions (Figure 9-9). Measured amounts of each dilution are added to each of two sterile Petri plates. Fifteen to 20 ml of melted and cooled agar medium is added to each plate. The contents of each plate are mixed by gentle swirling. The technique is based on the premise that single organisms

will give rise to colonies during an incubation period of 24 or more hours at 35°C. Duplicate plates of the same dilution of sample having 30 to 300 colonies are selected for counting, for within that range accuracy is the greatest. The number of colonies can be counted on a Quebec colony counter or an electronic device which provides an instant digital readout (Figure 9-10). Petri plates are placed directly on an illumination platform in a Quebec colony counter. An adjustable lens with a magnification of 1.5× permits one to see and count colonies. The electronic colony counter saves time when large numbers of counts are performed.

The average number of colonies on duplicate plates of the same dilution of sample is multiplied by the dilution factor to obtain the number of colony-forming units (CFU) per milliliter. If two plates of a 10^{-2} dilution were found

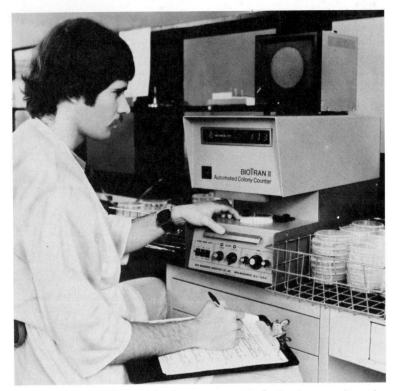

Figure 9-10   An electronic colony counter and viewing monitor. An integrated video camera scans the culture plate and the colony count appears on a digital readout. (Courtesy, New Brunswick Scientific Co., Inc., Edison, New Jersey.)

to have 230 and 220 CFU, respectively, the average is multiplied by 10^2.

$$225 \times 10^2 = 22,500 \text{ CFU/ml}$$

It must be remembered that some bacteria have a tendency to aggregate so that CFU's may not actually represent numbers of cells in the original sample. With mixed populations it is doubtful that all organisms would grow on a single plating medium and at a single temperature of incubation. However, since many mesophiles, including some pathogens, grow on nutrient agar and at 35°C, the technique does detect most bacteria of interest to medical and public health microbiologists. Appropriate use of dilutions makes the standard plate count applicable over a wide range of bacterial populations.

MEMBRANE-FILTER COUNT

A modification of the standard plate count employs a membrane filter. Bacteria are trapped by the filter as samples

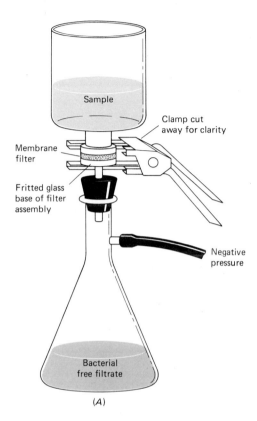

(A)

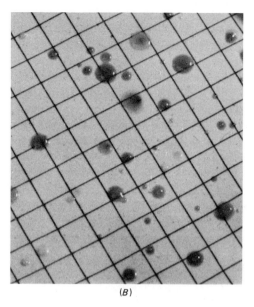

(B)

Figure 9-11 Membrane-filter technique. (A) Bacteria are trapped on membrane filter when negative pressure is applied. (B) Bacteria develop into colonies after saturation in medium and an overnight incubation period. (Reprinted with permission of Millipore Corporation, Bedford, Massachusetts.)

of water or other liquids are passed through it (Figure 9-11). The membrane filter is then placed in a plate containing a pad saturated with a desired medium. The medium diffuses into the membrane filter; trapped bacteria develop into colonies after an overnight incubation period. CFU's per milliliter can be determined by multiplying numbers of colonies detected on a Quebec or electronic colony counter by the amount of the sample subjected to filtration.

The use of a medium conducive to the growth of particular microorga-

nisms can give qualitiative information in addition to the quantitative count. For example, in a water analysis to determine the presence of gram-negative lactose-fermenting bacteria, a selective medium, such as MF-Endo agar, is employed.

MOST PROBABLE NUMBER

Another technique which provides qualitative and quantitative information in water analyses is the most probable number (MPN) technique. More than two organisms of *Escherichia coli* per 100 ml of a water supply is considered evidence of fecal pollution. The *E. coli* may be innocuous, but its presence could mean that pathogenic bacteria, protozoa, or viruses of fecal origin also could be contaminants. In the MPN technique three sets of lactose fermentation tubes are inoculated with water samples. One set of five tubes is inoculated with 0.1 ml amounts of the water sample; the second set receives 1.0 ml amounts of the sample; and the third set receives 10 ml amounts. After a 24- to 48-hour incubation period at 35°C,

Table 9-2   MOST PROBABLE NUMBERS OF COLIFORMS

POSITIVES WITH 10 ML	1 ML	0.1 ML	PROBABLE NO. PER 100 ML	POSITIVES WITH 10 ML	1 ML	0.1 ML	PROBABLE NO. PER 100 ML	POSITIVES WITH 10 ML	1 ML	0.1 ML	PROBABLE NO. PER 100 ML	POSITIVES WITH 10 ML	1 ML	0.1 ML	PROBABLE NO. PER 100 ML
2	0	0	4.5	3	0	0	7.8	4	0	0	13.0	5	0	0	23.0
2	0	1	6.8	3	0	1	11.0	4	0	1	17.0	5	0	1	31.0
2	0	2	9.1	3	0	2	13.0	4	0	2	21.0	5	0	2	43.0
2	0	3	12.0	3	0	3	16.0	4	0	3	25.0	5	0	3	58.0
2	0	4	14.0	3	0	4	20.0	4	0	4	30.0	5	0	4	76.0
2	0	5	16.0	3	0	5	23.0	4	0	5	36.0	5	0	5	95.0
2	1	0	6.8	3	1	0	11.0	4	1	0	17.0	5	1	0	33.0
2	1	1	9.2	3	1	1	14.0	4	1	1	21.0	5	1	1	46.0
2	1	2	12.0	3	1	2	17.0	4	1	2	26.0	5	1	2	64.0
2	1	3	14.0	3	1	3	20.0	4	1	3	31.0	5	1	3	84.0
2	1	4	17.0	3	1	4	23.0	4	1	4	36.0	5	1	4	110.0
2	1	5	19.0	3	1	5	27.0	4	1	5	42.0	5	1	5	130.0
2	2	0	9.3	3	2	0	14.0	4	2	0	22.0	5	2	0	49.0
2	2	1	12.0	3	2	1	17.0	4	2	1	26.0	5	2	1	70.0
2	2	2	14.0	3	2	2	20.0	4	2	2	32.0	5	2	2	95.0
2	2	3	17.0	3	2	3	24.0	4	2	3	38.0	5	2	3	120.0
2	2	4	19.0	3	2	4	27.0	4	2	4	44.0	5	2	4	150.0
2	2	5	22.0	3	2	5	31.0	4	2	5	50.0	5	2	5	180.0
2	3	0	12.0	3	3	0	17.0	4	3	0	27.0	5	3	0	79.0
2	3	1	14.0	3	3	1	21.0	4	3	1	33.0	5	3	1	110.0
2	3	2	17.0	3	3	2	24.0	4	3	2	39.0	5	3	2	140.0
2	3	3	20.0	3	3	3	28.0	4	3	3	45.0	5	3	3	180.0
2	3	4	22.0	3	3	4	31.0	4	3	4	52.0	5	3	4	210.0
2	3	5	25.0	3	3	5	35.0	4	3	5	59.0	5	3	5	250.0
2	4	0	15.0	3	4	0	21.0	4	4	0	34.0	5	4	0	130.0
2	4	1	17.0	3	4	1	24.0	4	4	1	40.0	5	4	1	170.0
2	4	2	20.0	3	4	2	28.0	4	4	2	47.0	5	4	2	220.0
2	4	3	23.0	3	4	3	32.0	4	4	3	54.0	5	4	3	280.0
2	4	4	25.0	3	4	4	36.0	4	4	4	62.0	5	4	4	350.0
2	4	5	28.0	3	4	5	40.0	4	4	5	69.0	5	4	5	430.0
2	5	0	17.0	3	5	0	25.0	4	5	0	41.0	5	5	0	240.0
2	5	1	20.0	3	5	1	29.0	4	5	1	48.0	5	5	1	350.0
2	5	2	23.0	3	5	2	32.0	4	5	2	56.0	5	5	2	540.0
2	5	3	26.0	3	5	3	37.0	4	5	3	64.0	5	5	3	920.0
2	5	4	29.0	3	5	4	41.0	4	5	4	72.0	5	5	4	1600.0
2	5	5	32.0	3	5	5	45.0	4	5	5	81.0	5	5	5	1800.0 +

SOURCE: *Standard Methods for the Examination of Dairy Products,* 13th ed. (New York: American Public Health Associations, 1972).

the number of coliforms per 100 ml of water is determined by observing the number of tubes in each set which show the presence of gas. The numbers are compared with values on a statistical chart (Table 9-2). Determination of MPN's is more time consuming than a membrane-filter count, but the technique is extremely reliable when performed under standardized conditions.

INDIRECT MEASUREMENTS

Less specific methods for estimating numbers in a bacterial population depend on the ability of microorganisms to reduce dyes incorporated into culture media or to produce a measurable end product from particular substrates. In the methylene blue reduction test a change in color of the dye from blue (the oxidized state) to a colorless compound (the reduced state) is the basis for determining relative numbers of bacteria. The test is limited in that reduction of methylene blue by mixed flora may represent varying degrees of metabolic activity, but it is generally considered a reliable, indirect, semiquantitative method for the specific application of grading milk. In dairy bacteriology milk which retains the blue color after an incubation period of six hours at 35°C is considered to be of good quality.

Under carefully controlled conditions, the amount of an end product yielded by a specific metabolic reaction is proportional to the density of a bacterial population. Quantitative determinations of end products, such as ammonia, reducing sugars, or acids, are usu-

ally reserved for studies on pure cultures.

CULTIVATION OF HUMAN PATHOGENS

The successful cultivation of human pathogens depends on the availability of appropriate nutrients and environmental conditions. Nutrients are supplied in the form of mixtures known as culture *media*. Nature provides a number of environments favorable for microbial growth. Rivers, ponds, oceans, lakes, and the snow cover of mountains all contain varying degrees of supportive nutrients. Some soils, marshes, and compost heaps are especially rich in energy sources. Bacteria, themselves, commonly serve as a food supply for protozoa in nature. Fluids, such as blood, cerebrospinal fluid (CSF), urine, and the skin of vertebrate hosts, including humans, make excellent culture media. The life-supporting nutrients of such abiotic or biotic environments constitute *natural* media (Figure 9-12).

The mixtures compounded in the laboratory to meet nutritional needs of microorganisms constitute *artificial* media. All artificial culture media must contain available sources of carbon, nitrogen, water, and inorganic salts. A few fastidious organisms require vitamins or other growth factors. Culture media containing supplemental growth factors are called *enrichment* media (Table 9-3).

Artificial media may consist of ill-

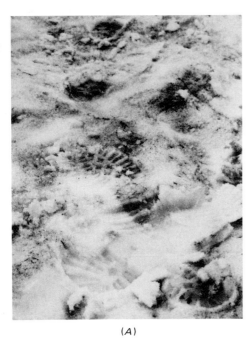
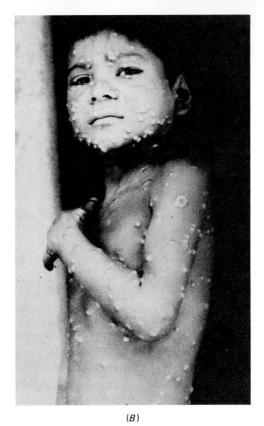

(A)   (B)

Figure 9-12 Abiotic and biotic habitats of microorganisms. (*A*) Red algae growing on the snow cover of a Colorado mountain slope. (Courtesy, R. Bigelow, Van Nuys, California.) (*B*) Smallpox virus lesions on a 7-year-old boy who had one of the last cases of smallpox. (Courtesy, World Health Organization, Geneva.)

Table 9-3 EXAMPLES OF ENRICHMENT MEDIA

MEDIUM	ENRICHMENT	RECOMMENDED USE
Blood agar	sheep blood	good general purpose medium for isolation of human pathogens
Bordet-Gengou agar	potato, glycerol, blood	isolation of *Bordetella pertussis*
Charcoal yeast extract	yeast extract	isolation of *Legionella pneumophila*
Chocolate agar	hemoglobin, yeast extract	isolation of *Neisseria* and *Haemophilus* species
Loeffler's medium	beef serum	isolation of *Corynebacterium diphtheriae*
Nagler agar	egg yolk	isolation of *Clostridia* species
Mueller-Hinton agar	starch	antimicrobial susceptibility tests
Thayer-Martin agar	hemoglobin, isovitalex	isolation of *Neisseria* species

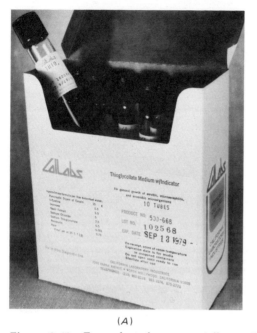
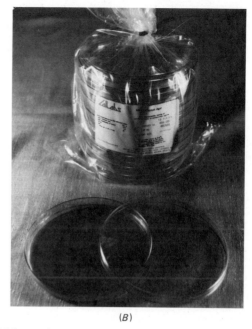

Figure 9-13 Examples of commercially available media. (*A*) Broth medium dispensed in screw capped test tubes. (*B*) Solid medium dispensed in Petri plates. (Courtesy, Cal Labs, Van Nuys, California.)

defined mixtures of ingredients that supply essential nutrients or be made up of only chemicals of known purity in exact quantities. The ingredients of an artificial culture medium and atmospheric conditions can be adjusted to meet growth requirements of particular organisms. Since optimal growth is obtained on culture media with a particular pH, care must be taken to keep the pH relatively constant during growth. This is accomplished by the addition of buffers which have been described earlier in this chapter. At times, depending on the origin of the specimen sent to the laboratory for culturing, it is necessary to supply more than one temperature and both aerobic and anaerobic conditions.

A variety of artificial culture media are available commercially in dehydrated form. Water is added to carefully weighed amounts of the powdered products. Frequently, heat must be applied to solubilize ingredients before dispensing them in suitable tubes, bottles, or Petri plates. Media must be sterile, that is free of microbial contamination, if only organisms from the human host are to be grown. Sterilization is accomplished by autoclaving, by exposure to flowing steam for intermittent periods, or by filtration processes described in Chapter 26.

Many laboratories find it more convenient to purchase sterile media ready for use (Figure 9-13). Commercially prepared media are subjected to rigid quality control procedures to insure reliability and reproducibility of test results. Depending on work loads, it often saves valuable technical time to purchase ready-made products.

LIQUID, SEMISOLID, AND SOLID MEDIA

Components of culture media may be supplied in tubes or bottles as *liquid* media called broth. The consistency of a liquid medium may be modified by the addition of a solidifying agent, such as agar or gelatin, to change it to a *semisolid* or a *solid* medium. Semisolid media are usually dispensed in tubes, but solid media are dispensed in Petri plates or slanted in tubes or bottles to provide maximal surfaces for growing bacteria or fungi. Patterns of growth obtained in broth or on agar slants are useful identification criteria when applied to bacteria (Figure 9-14).

SELECTIVE AND DIFFERENTIAL MEDIA

Dyes, salts, or antimicrobial agents can be added to media to inhibit the growth of particular organisms. Such media are called *selective* media because by inhibiting the growth of some organisms, they allow other organisms to grow.

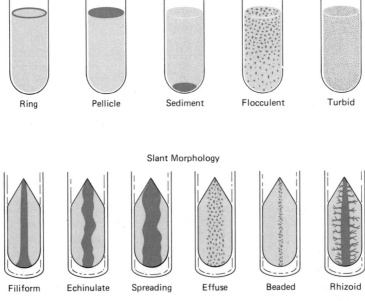

Broth Morphology

Ring   Pellicle   Sediment   Flocculent   Turbid

Slant Morphology

Filiform   Echinulate   Spreading   Effuse   Beaded   Rhizoid

Figure 9-14 Growth patterns of bacteria on two types of media: broth cultures and agar slants.

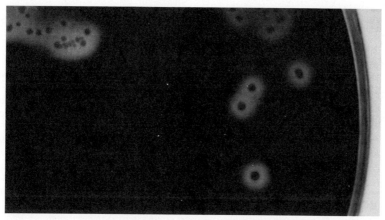

Figure 9-15 Beta hemolysis on a blood agar plate. Clear zones surrounding colonies indicate complete dissolution of red blood cells. (Courtesy, C. Luckenbach, Van Nuys, California.)

Selective media are useful in isolating bacteria or fungi from specimens containing more than one organism, or those contaminated with indigenous microorganisms.

Media designed to separate organisms based on type of growth or end products of metabolic reactions are called *differential* media. Differential media contain particular substrates, dyes, salts, or pH indicators which make it possible to divide organisms into two or more groups. Sometimes it is necessary to add chemical reagents to culture media after an appropriate time of incubation to detect end products of metabolism.

Enrichment and selective media can be classified as differential media as well if they make it possible to differentiate between two or more groups of organisms. For example, blood agar permits the more fastidious organisms to grow, but also differentiates organisms based on the type of hemolysis (dissolution of red blood cells) produced surrounding colonies. A green zone of discoloration around colonies indicates partial dissolution of red blood cells and is called *alpha* hemolysis. A clear zone around colonies indicates complete dissolution of red blood cells and is called *beta* hemolysis (Figure 9-15).

Indicators added to lactose media to inhibit the growth of gram-positive bacteria permit the differentiation of lactose-fermenting organisms from non-lactose-fermenting organisms. Lactose-fermenting bacteria typically produce colored colonies on a medium, such as eosin methylene blue (EMB); non-lactose fermenters form colorless colonies on the same medium. Table 9-4 contains representative examples of selective media which are used in the microbiology laboratory. These media will be referred to later in the text in sections entitled "Laboratory Diagnosis"

Table 9-4   EXAMPLES OF SELECTIVE MEDIA

Medium	Selective Agent	Recommended Use
Eosin methylene blue agar (EMB)	eosin Y, methylene blue	isolation of gram-negative bacilli
Desoxycholate citrate agar	sodium desoxycholate, sodium citrate	isolation of gram-negative bacilli
Hektoen enteric agar (HE)	bile salts	isolation of gram-negative bacilli
MacConkey agar	bile salts, crystal violet	isolation of gram-negative bacilli
Phenylethyl alcohol blood agar	phenylethyl alcohol	isolation of gram-positive aerobic bacilli and cocci, isolation of gram-positive anaerobic cocci and non-spore-forming bacilli
Mannitol-salt agar (MS)	sodium chloride	isolation of *Staphylococcus aureus*
Sabouraud dextrose agar	pH	isolation of fungi
SS agar	bile salts, brilliant green, sodium citrate	isolation of *Salmonella-Shigella* species
Thioglycolate broth	thioglycolic acid, L-cystine, agar	isolation of anaerobes

under infectious diseases of the human presented in Chapters 16 through 24.

The study of metabolic activities of microorganisms requires the subculturing of pure colonies to a variety of substrates. The ability or inability to use certain substrates included in a panel of biochemical tests, or to produce specific end products of degradation, is the basis for species identification. The number of tests required for speciation are often both time consuming and costly.

An alternative to the use of tubed media and reagents is a number of rapid identification systems in which substrates and reagents have been applied to filter-paper strips or in wells of plastic trays (Figure 9-16). A large number of self-contained units are commercially available for the identification of gram-negative bacilli belonging to the family *Enterobacteriaceae*. Some units are designed so that results can be read in as little as four hours of incubation at 35°C. Specific tests required for the identification of particular species of human pathogens are included in sections entitled "Laboratory Diagnosis" in Chapters 16 through 24.

PURE-CULTURE TECHNIQUES

The identification of bacteria depends on isolating pure colonies, that is colonies containing a single species of an organism. Isolation can be accomplished by use of three techniques: a *streak plate*, a *pour plate*, or a *spread plate*.

The streak-plate technique employs an inoculating loop for implanting bac-

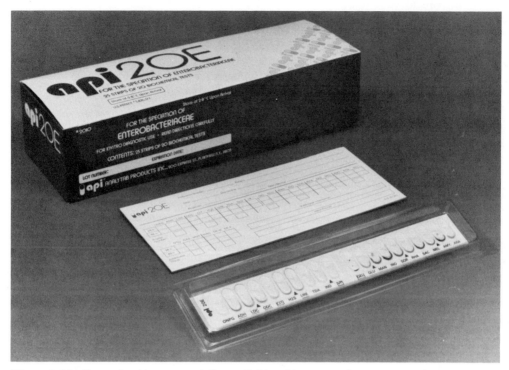

Figure 9-16 Example of a commercially available self-contained unit containing 20 biochemical tests for the identification of the *Enterobacteriaceae*. (Courtesy, Analytab Products, Plainview, New York.)

teria on the surface of agar in a process called *streaking*. Patterns of streaking vary, but the purpose is to disperse the original inoculum so that isolated colonies are obtained after an appropriate period of incubation (Figure 9-17).

In the pour-plate technique, bacteria are inoculated into a tube of melted agar cooled to a temperature of 45° to 47°C, mixed, and poured into a sterile

Bacterial Streak-Plate Technique

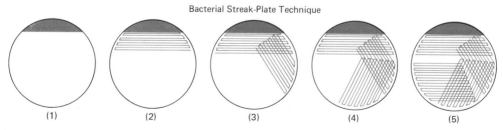

(1) (2) (3) (4) (5)

Figure 9-17 The "clock-plate" method of streaking.

Pour plate

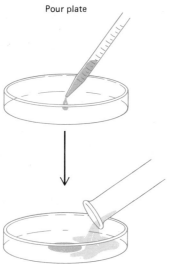

Spread plate

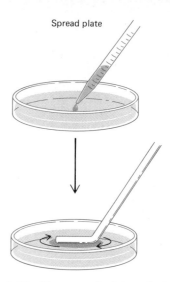

Figure 9-18 The pour-plate technique.

Figure 9-19 The spread-plate technique.

Petri plate (Figure 9-18). An alternate procedure is sometimes used in which dilutions of milk, water, food, or soil samples are placed directly into sterile Petri plates before adding melted and cooled agar.

Preparation of spread plates requires that surfaces of plates be dry before inoculation. Approximately 0.05 ml of a liquid inoculum is placed in the center of the plate and spread over the surface with a sterile bent glass rod in circular

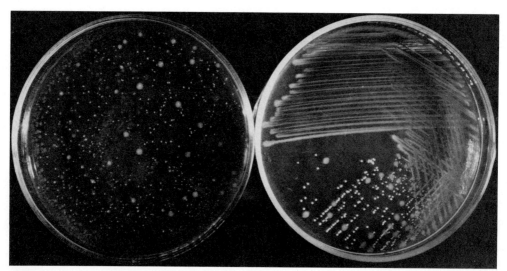

Figure 9-20 Appearance of colonies on a pour plate (left) and on a streak plate (right). (Courtesy, C. Luckenbach, Van Nuys, California.)

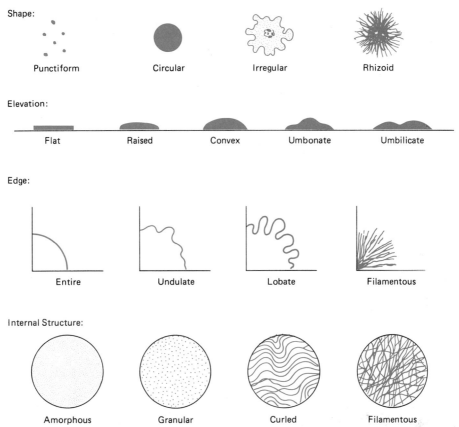

Colonial Morphology

Shape:

Punctiform　　　Circular　　　Irregular　　　Rhizoid

Elevation:

Flat　　　Raised　　　Convex　　　Umbonate　　　Umbilicate

Edge:

Entire　　　Undulate　　　Lobate　　　Filamentous

Internal Structure:

Amorphous　　　Granular　　　Curled　　　Filamentous

Figure 9-21 Morphology of bacterial colonies. Observations of shape and elevation are made with the unaided eye. Observations of edge and internal morphology are made under low power of a bright-field microscope.

movements while rotating the plate (Figure 9-19). Plates must be allowed to dry an hour or two before incubating.

It is important that all inoculated plates be incubated in an inverted position, that is with the bottom agar-containing portion of the Petri plate on top. Positioning of plates in this manner prevents condensed moisture from dripping onto the surface of the plates, and subsequent spreading of growth into confluent patterns which would obliterate isolated colonies. Inverting Petri plates also minimizes the risk of contamination by inadvertent removal of Petri-plate covers when taking plates from the incubator.

Incubated pour plates contain both surface and subsurface colonies; streak plates and spread plates, if inoculated properly, contain only surface colonies (Figure 9-20). Colonies obtained by any of the techniques must be examined for colony morphology (Figure 9-21). Only carefully selected colonies should be subcultured.

SPECIAL CULTURE TECHNIQUES

Sometimes it is necessary to employ special culture techniques in qualitative or quantitative microbiology. Cultivation techniques for viruses were presented in Chapter 5. Rickettsiae, like viruses, may be grown in embryonated eggs or tissue from a variety of animal or human sources. Growth media for tissue cultures consists of balanced salt solutions enriched with sera, amniotic fluids, tissue extracts, or protein hydrolysates.

Cells to be used for culturing viruses or rickettsiae are usually allowed to grow until a single layer of cells known as a *monolayer* is obtained before material suspected of containing the microorganisms is added. Cultures require replacement of media and rinsing at periodic intervals to maintain optimal growth conditions. Specific cytopathic effects (CPE) observable in host cells with a bright-field microscope were discussed in Chapter 5. Tissues infected with rickettsiae can be stained directly using Giemsa's stain and examined with a bright-field microscope, or be allowed to react with tagged antibodies, for examination by fluorescent microscopy.

Cultivation of protozoa and helminths is time consuming and requires both special materials and equipment. It is, therefore, not practical for most laboratories to attempt to grow those parasites. The only culture methods in general use are those used for the isolation of amebas and a few flagellates.

CULTURE OF ANAEROBES

Anaerobes exhibit varying degrees of aerotolerance. Some are destroyed by even brief exposure to oxygen. Anaerobic conditions described earlier in this chapter must, therefore, be supplied to accommodate their growth requirements.

ANIMAL INOCULATION

When microbiology was in its developmental stages, animals were used to confirm the pathogenicity of bacteria isolated from cases of human disease. Guinea pigs continued to be injected routinely in the diagnosis of tuberculosis for many years and are, sometimes, still used for that purpose. Mice are injected intraperitoneally with exudates, fluids, or suspensions of tissue from some patients with suspected viral or fungal infections. Mice or guinea pigs are used to demonstrate the presence of specific toxins, such as those produced by the etiological agents of botulism and diphtheria.

Generally, only large medical centers or public health laboratories have animal quarters for use in diagnostic microbiology. Regulations for care of laboratory animals are rigid. Not only must separate quarters be maintained for animals, but adequate personnel must be available for care and feeding of animals. Most hospital laboratories send cultures of microorganisms requiring animal inoculation to a regional public health or reference laboratory.

CONTINUOUS AND SYNCHRONIZED CULTURES

Overnight cultures are usually employed in most hospital and public health laboratories, but continuous culture techniques are used in industrial and research laboratories to produce large amounts of bacteria or their products. In addition, sometimes it is necessary to synchronize growth in studying details of particular cell cycles so that populations can be studied at the same stages of their life cycles.

CONTINUOUS CULTURE

Provision for continuous culture can be made in a growth chamber known as a chemostat (Figure 9-22). Fresh nutrients are supplied and the effluent is removed at a constant rate. Under carefully controlled conditions cells in the open system remain in the exponential phase of growth. The increase in cell population is described as *steady-state growth*. During steady-state growth cell mass and cell number are proportional.

SYNCHRONIZED CULTURE

Synchronized growth can be obtained by physiological or mechanical selection procedures. Physiological selection is based on control of specific requirements for growth. DNA replication can be inhibited by a reduction in temperature or deprivation of an essential nutrient such as thymine. Growth will

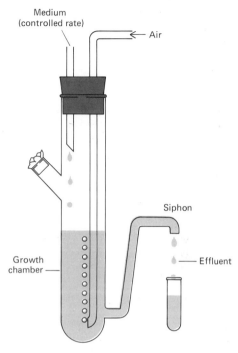

Figure 9-22 A simplified version of a chemostat. Bacteria in the growth chamber remain in the exponential phase of growth.

start again when the temperature returns to 35°C or the missing nutrient is made available. Growth is synchronized by controlled restoration of requirements.

Mechanical selection, either by employing a series of filter papers or by periodic flushing of a membrane filter through which a random culture has been poured, releases cells in the same stage of the cell cycle. Continuous flushing releases progeny of cells trapped by the membrane filter.

Cells become asynchronous after three or four generations, presumably because of individual differences in

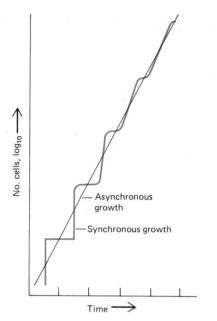

Figure 9-23 Synchronous and asynchronous growth compared. Cells become asynchronous after three or four generations.

partition of cytoplasm during cell division (Figure 9-23).

ENDOSPORES

FORMATION OF ENDOSPORES

Endospore formation appears to be a special type of internal membrane-dependent cell division occurring as a part of the life cycle in certain bacteria. Depletion of an essential nutrient triggers an internal reorganization process leading to formation of an endospore. The internal reorganization of the cell begins with the condensation of nuclear material and the unfolding of the cytoplasmic membrane to form a double-layered structure known as a *forespore* (Figure 9-24). DNA, RNA, and protein synthesis cease at this point and the cell is now "committed" to spore formation. A layer known as the *cortex* subsequently develops between

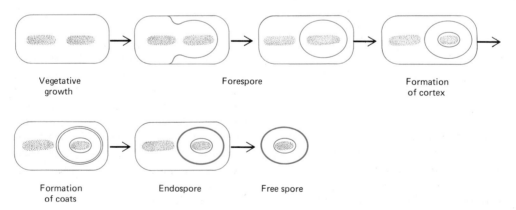

Figure 9-24   Stages of sporulation.

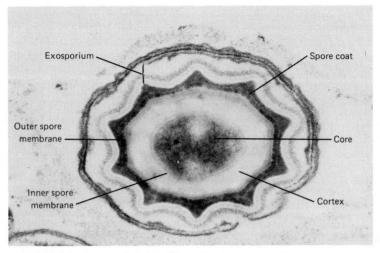

Figure 9-25   A mature spore of *Bacillus macerans* showing integuments and core. (Courtesy, S. Decker, Cincinnati, Ohio.)

the two layers of the forespore. The cortex can be considered a cell wall for it encloses the protoplast of the spore. A layer peripheral to the outer forespore membrane, known as the *spore coat*, surrounds the entire cell. A less dense outermost layer, known as an *exosporium*, completes the extra integuments formed during sporulation. The innermost portion or *core* contains a membrane enclosing the cytoplasmic constituents (Figure 9-25).

During this unusual type of cell division the condensation of protoplasm causes the cell to lose 20 to 30 percent of its water. The dehydrated cell contains large amounts of calcium and dipicolinic acid, an uncommon amino acid found no other place in nature. The spores are grossly deficient in enzymes, containing only minimal amounts of enzymes required for translation, transcription, and respiration.

The resistance of mature spores to heat, cold, and disinfectants is presumably explained by the protection afforded by the structural compactness of the spore coat. Spores of bacilli belonging to the genera *Bacillus* and *Clostridium* can survive in the dormant state for hundreds of years.

GERMINATION OF ENDOSPORES

Germination, that is, the conversion to a vegetative form capable of metabolic activity, occurs when the endospore is placed in an environment conducive to growth. Activation of the endospore precedes actual germination. An activating agent, such as aging, heat, low pH, or a sulfhydryl compound promotes the rupture of the integuments of endospores. Germination requires water and a triggering agent, such as

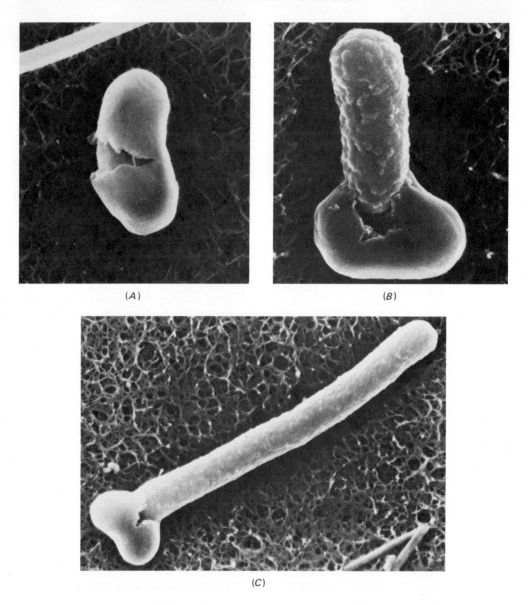

(A)

(B)

(C)

Figure 9-26 Germination of spore of *Bacillus subtilis* after triggering by heat at 60°C and growth at 37°C on thin layer agar. (*A*) Disruption of spore wall and emergence of spore at 60 minutes. (*B*) Initial stage of outgrowth at 120 minutes. (*C*) Terminal stage of outgrowth at 150 minutes. (Courtesy, A. Amako, Fukuoka, Japan. From K. Amako and A. Umeda, *J. Ultrastr. Research* 58:34, 1977.)

alanine or Mn^{2+}, which penetrates the coat damaged by the activating agent. The accompanying changes are rapid. Fragments of peptidoglycan and calcium dipicolinate are released spontaneously; water, K^+, and Mg^{2+} are taken up with the disappearance of the cortex. Refractility and resistance to heat, light, drying, and chemicals are lost.

If the germinated cell is in a suitable nutrient-rich environment, outgrowth occurs (Figure 9-26). Outgrowth is a gradual process requiring several hours for resumption of vegetative cell activities. In the absence of supporting nutrients in the environment, the germinated cell is unable to resume metabolic activity.

SUMMARY

In the study of microorganisms the term growth usually refers to increases in populations of cells. An organism capable of carrying out metabolic functions, including cell division, is considered to be viable. Under optimal growth conditions of temperature, moisture, osmotic pressure, atmospheric gases, pH, and availability of an energy source and nitrogen, bacteria undergo four distinct growth phases: a lag, an exponential, a stationary, and a death phase. Bacterial growth is usually measured as cell mass or cell number. The successful isolation, cultivation, and identification of microorganisms causing disease in the human host require specialized techniques and a variety of substrates available in culture media. Large yields of organisms or their products are obtained by synchronizing growth and using special growth

chambers. Some bacteria possess a unique ability to undergo an alteration in morphological and physiological states to form endospores. Formation of endospores constitutes an interruption in vegetative status which may last hundreds of years.

QUESTIONS FOR STUDY

1. How can the detrimental effect of acidic or basic waste products resulting from microbial growth be controlled in culture media?
2. Explain why facultative anaerobes have a survival advantage over obligate anaerobes.
3. What measurements are necessary to determine growth rate and generation time of a bacterial species?
4. How does the most probable number technique provide both quantitative and qualitative information?
5. Explain how it is possible for a medium to be both selective and differential.
6. Why is it necessary to obtain pure cultures before studying metabolic characteristics of an organism?
7. Describe the environmental circumstances which trigger endospore formation and germination.

SELECTED REFERENCES

Brock, T. D. *Biology of Microorganisms.* 2d ed. Englewood Cliffs, N.J.: Prentice-Hall, 1970.

Davis, B. D.; Dulbecco, R.; Eisen, H. N.; Ginsberg, H. S.; and Wood, W. B., Jr. *Microbiology.* 2d ed. New York: Harper & Row, 1973.

Deibel, R. H. Utilization of arginine as

an energy source for the growth of *Streptococcus faecalis*. *J. Bacteriol.* 87:988, 1964.

Goldman, M.; Deibel, R. H.; and Niven, C. F., Jr. Interrelationship between temperature and sodium chloride on growth of lactic acid bacteria isolated from meat-curing brines. *J. Bacteriol.* 85:1017, 1962.

Sbarra, A. J.; Shirley, W.; and Baum-stark, J. S. Effect of osmolarity on phagocystosis. *J. Bacteriol.* 85:306, 1963.

Sokatch, J. R., and Ferretti, J. J. *Basic Bacteriology and Genetics*. Chicago: Year Book Medical Publishers, 1976.

Wistreich, G. A., and Lechtman, M. D. *Microbiology and Human Disease*. 2d ed. Beverly Hills, Calif.: Glencoe Press, 1976.

Chapter 10

Microbial Genetics

After you read this chapter, you should be able to:

1. Differentiate between the genotype and phenotype of a microorganism.
2. Explain causes of environmentally- and genetically-induced alterations in phenotype.
3. Define mutation rate and mutation frequency.
4. Describe six types of mutations.
5. Differentiate between an auxotroph and a prototroph.
6. Describe three methods for detecting the presence of mutants.
7. Describe the possible effects of point, deletion, or insertion mutations.
8. Contrast the three methods of genetic recombination in procaryotic cells.
9. Explain the significance of generalized, specialized, and abortive transduction.
10. Compare efficiency of chromosomal and fertility factor transfer in crosses between F⁺ and F⁻ and Hfr and F⁻ strains of *Escherichia coli*.
11. Differentiate between plasmids and episomes.
12. Explain the basis of *in vitro* recombination experiments.
13. Contrast the two types of genetic recombination in eucaryotic cells.

Classical genetics, which is concerned with inheritable characteristics of macroorganisms, began in the middle of the nineteenth century when the Austrian monk Gregor Mendel studied characteristics of pea plants. Mendel introduced the concept of structural units called *genes* as the agents responsible for heredity. The contributions of Mendel have been invaluable in the understanding of inheritable variance in multicellular plants and animals. Until 1944 geneticists believed that genes were composed of proteins. In that year the genetic specificity was demonstrated to reside within DNA molecules. In 1953 James Watson and Sir Francis Crick elucidated the structure of DNA and provided a foundation for the development of molecular genetics.

The study of microbial genetics during the past two decades has advanced the understanding of certain universal genetic principles. A gene is now recognized as a unit of structure and function on a segment of DNA. It consists of a particular base sequence and contains approximately 1000 bases (Figure 10-1). The major function of genes is to direct the synthesis of proteins.

More recent efforts to isolate and rejoin segments of DNA *in vitro* have created new types of biologically active recombinant DNA in the form of small units known as *plasmids*. Both the artificially produced plasmids and those which occur naturally are capable of replication independent of their host cells. The potential use of artificially constructed recombinant DNA molecules to alter the course of evolution has stirred one of the greatest biological controversies of the twentieth century.

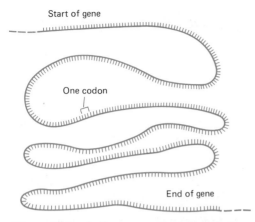

Start of gene

One codon

End of gene

Figure 10-1 A diagrammatic representation of a gene. Each short line stands for one base. No break occurs where one gene begins and another gene ends. (From F. H. C. Crick, *Proc. of Sixth Internal. Cong., Biochemistry Plenary Sessions* 33:109, 1964. Copyright The American Society of Biological Chemists, Inc.)

ALTERATIONS IN CHARACTERISTICS OF ORGANISMS

The sum total of genetic material of an organism is called the *genotype*. Alterations in genotype occur as a result of a sudden, inheritable change in genes known as a *mutation* or by genetic recombination with foreign DNA. Mutations occur spontaneously in nature, but can also be induced in the laboratory by the application of specific chemical or physical *mutagens*.

The genes determine all the observable characteristics of an organism, but not all genes are expressed. The sum total of observable characteristics of an organism is known as the *phenotype*. Since genetic material, if expressed, produces a variation in phenotype, such variation is said to be *genetically induced*.

Variations in phenotype may also be *environmentally induced*. An organism may have a gene for a particular characteristic which is expressed only under certain environmental conditions. Environmental factors, such as temperature, available nutrients, and the physical state of a culture medium, influence the phenotype of some bacteria. For example, pigmentation of *Serratia marcescens* is temperature dependent. Strains of that organism have a gene for pigment production. However, while they exhibit a brick-red pigment at room temperature, they exhibit little or no pigment at 35°C. Production of the enzyme β-galactosidase occurs in some strains of *Escherichia coli* only when lactose is present in the medium. The dimorphic fungi tend to grow as yeasts at 35°C, but as molds at room temperature (Figure 10-2).

Depletion of nitrogen causes *Bacillus* species to sporulate; an excess of calcium inhibits endospore formation. Some bacteria produce capsules only when supplied with a growth factor found in milk. Cultivation on a dehydrated medium may suppress formation of flagella in certain gram-negative bacilli. Most microorganisms grown in broth are discernibly larger than those cultivated on an agar-base medium. In all instances the genetic information is

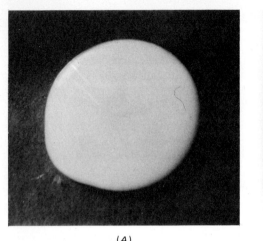
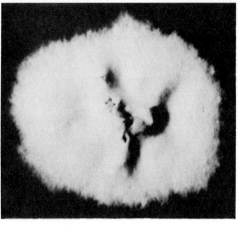

(A)   (B)

Figure 10-2   Dimorphism expressed by a fungus at different temperatures. (A) A typical yeast colony at 37°C. (B) A typical mold colony at room temperature. (From *Clinical Laboratory Mycology*, Part II, Slide Illustrations © copyright by MedCom Inc., New York, 1971.)

present in the microbial cells, but expression of the genes is influenced by the environment.

GENETIC VARIABILITY IN MICROORGANISMS

Unlike environmentally induced alterations, which affect entire populations of microbial cells, a spontaneous mutation is a rare event usually affecting not more than one in 10^6 cells. Some nucleotide pairs are highly mutable, but the reason for such "hot spots" is unclear. Mutations occurring over hundreds of years are responsible in part for the great diversity of microbial forms and metabolism.

MUTATION RATE AND MUTATION FREQUENCY

The *mutation rate* is the probability that a particular mutation will occur, expressed as the average number of mutations per cell per generation. A mutation rate of 10^{-6} would mean that when 10^6 cells divided to form 2×10^6 cells, 1 mutant cell occurred. The probability that two mutations would occur simultaneously in the same cell is equal to the product of the individual probabilities.

Much of our information on mutation rates comes from studying drug-resistant mutants. If the mutation rate for resistance to chloramphenicol is 10^{-8}/cell/generation and the mutation rate for resistance to streptomycin is 10^{-10}/cell/generation, the probability that both mutations will occur in 1 cell simultaneously is 10^{-18}/cell/generation.

The *mutant frequency* is the number of mutants in a particular population. A mutant frequency of 10^{-5} means that there is 1 mutant in a population of 100,000 cells.

TYPES OF MUTATIONS

Any characteristic of an organism can be altered by a spontaneous or induced mutation. Bacterial mutants requiring specific amino acids, vitamins, purines, or pyrimidines for growth are common. Nutritional mutants are called *auxotrophs;* the wild types, from which they are derived, are called *prototrophs.* Fermentative mutants are those which have lost the ability to ferment a particular carbohydrate. Antigenic mutants no longer have the ability to produce specific flagellar, capsular, or somatic antigens. Mutant strains of bacteria and yeast sometimes exhibit rough colonies in direct contrast to the smooth colonies of wild types. Some mutations are conditionally lethal. Temperature-sensitive mutants, for example, will grow at room temperature, but not at higher temperatures.

The most important bacterial mutants in microbial populations of the hospital environment are those which demonstrate increased virulence or resistance to antimicrobial agents. The widespread use of antimicrobial agents is a selective pressure which permits resistant strains to survive. Diseases caused by strains exhibiting multiple drug resistance are particularly difficult to treat.

It is important to be able to identify mutant strains of microorganisms so

names are assigned to them. A streptomycin-resistant mutant is designated as *str⁻ʳ*. A histidine-requiring mutant is designated as *his⁻* because it cannot synthesize histidine. A histidine- and proline-requiring mutant would be designated as *his⁻ pro⁻*. A *lac⁻* strain lacks the ability to ferment lactose.

DETECTION OF MUTANTS

Since mutation rates are so low, it is to be expected that mutants are difficult to detect. Under ordinary cultural techniques mutants may go unnoticed — just one of a crowd in a population of a million or more cells. Therefore, it is necessary to use cultural techniques designed to select for the presence of mutants.

Replica Plating. A technique known as replica plating is uniquely applicable for separating mutants from a mixed population of cells. The selection technique employs a master plate, containing colonies of both prototrophs and auxotrophs, and a minimal agar plate, upon which auxotrophs will not grow. Particular auxotrophs can be selected for by supplementing minimal agar with specific growth factors. The minimal agar plates are inoculated with minute amounts of colonies picked up from the master plate by sterile velveteen, placed over a cylindrical carrier. When the velveteen is pressed against the minimal agar plates colonies of parent cells grow on minimal agar in the exact positions as on the master plate. Colonies of auxotrophs are conspicuously absent on minimal agar

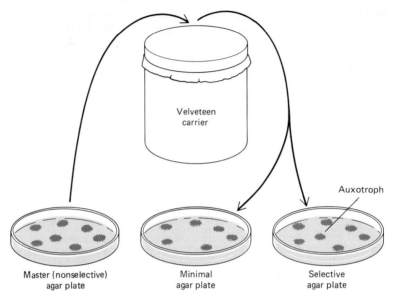

Figure 10-3   Replica-plating technique. Sterile velveteen on a cylindrical support carrier is used to pick up portions of colonies from a master plate containing a nonselective medium. The imprint of colonies is stamped onto the surface of a plate of minimal agar and a plate of selective agar (minimal agar plus the growth factor being selected for). After overnight incubation auxotrophs are absent from minimal agar plate, but appear on the selective medium.

alone, but appear on minimal agar plates supplemented with the particular growth factor affected by the mutation (Figure 10-3).

Penicillin Selection. An alternate method for detecting auxotrophs consists of subjecting a mixed population to the selective action of penicillin (Figure 10-4). Penicillin rapidly kills metabolizing cells of gram-positive and some gram-negative bacteria. If a mixture of wild-type and mutant cells are grown in a minimal broth containing a lethal concentration of penicillin, prototrophs will be destroyed as they begin

to grow. Any auxotrophs will be unable to grow, but will remain viable and can be transferred to specific selective media.

Antibiotic Supplements. Antibiotic-resistant mutants can be detected by plating a mixed population on an agar containing the antibiotic or by use of a disc-susceptibility test in which a small disc containing the antibiotic is placed in the center of a plate to create a zone in which prototrophs cannot grow. Mutants will grow on antibiotic-containing agar or within the zone of inhibition surrounding a disc (Figure 10-5).

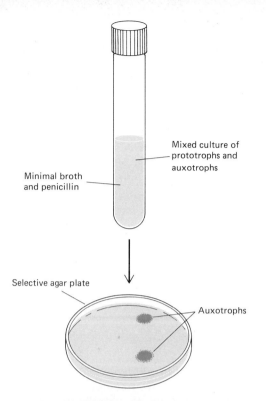

Minimal broth and penicillin

Mixed culture of prototrophs and auxotrophs

Selective agar plate

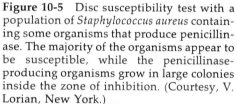

Auxotrophs

Figure 10-4 Penicillin-selection technique. Penicillin kills metabolizing cells in minimal broth. After overnight incubation auxotrophs grow on selective agar.

Figure 10-5 Disc susceptibility test with a population of *Staphylococcus aureus* containing some organisms that produce penicillinase. The majority of the organisms appear to be susceptible, while the penicillinase-producing organisms grow in large colonies inside the zone of inhibition. (Courtesy, V. Lorian, New York.)

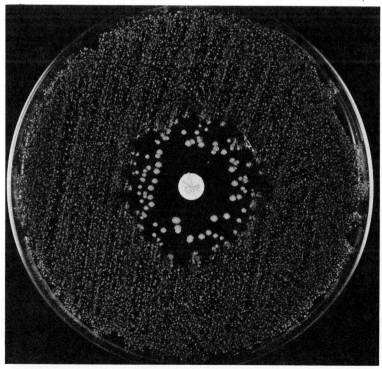

229

THE MOLECULAR BASIS OF MUTATION

In 1953 James Watson and Francis Crick described DNA as a structure of two chains of nucleotides coiled around each other and held together by hydrogen bonds in the now famous helical configuration. However, continuing studies on large numbers of microorganisms, including bacteria and viruses, have revealed that DNA does not have to be double-stranded; the nucleic acids of some viruses are single-stranded. Also, the nucleic acids of several viruses and bacteria have been shown to be circular. The chromosome of a typical bacterium is circular, double-stranded DNA (Figure 10-6). The amount of coil-

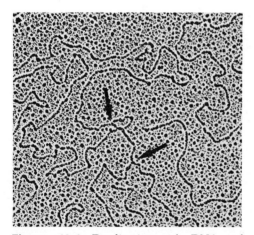

Figure 10-6 Duplication of DNA of *Escherichia coli,* strain K-12. Arrows show loops formed from duplicate strands. (Courtesy, H. Saedler, Freiburg, Germany.)

ing can be appreciated when one considers that the estimated length of DNA in *Escherichia coli* is approximately 1000 times as long as the length of the cell.

The strands of DNA do not fully unwind to begin the copy process. Only a small part of the chromosome appears to be single-stranded at any one time. Autoradiographic pictures of the circular chromosome of DNA suggest that the new strands of a double helix appear in opposite directions after replication—a phenomenon called the *Y mechanism* (Figure 10-7). When two sets of hereditary instructions are completed, the cell divides in such a manner that each set becomes the chromosome of a daughter cell.

The specific sequences of trinucleotides on the gene transfer instructions to mRNA for coding of particular amino acids. Since a gene and its protein are colinear, any alteration in structure of the DNA molecule will be reflected in the same relative position on the protein molecule (Figure 10-8). Mutagens promote an alteration of DNA during replication or have a direct effect on resting DNA.

POINT MUTATIONS

A *point mutation* involves a change in a single base of a nucleotide. One base may be replaced by another base or a base may be deleted when a chemical agent strips the backbone of DNA. When a purine replaces another purine or a pyrimidine replaces another pyrimidine, the substitution is called a *transition*. When a purine is replaced by a pyrimidine or a pyrimidine is replaced

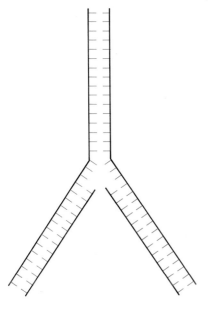

Figure 10-7 A diagrammatic representation of the Y mechanism showing direction of rotation, parent molecule, and two daughter molecules.

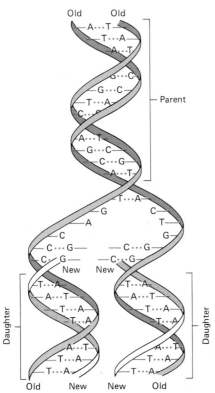

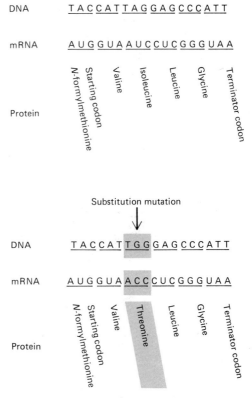

DNA   T A C C A T T A G G A G C C C A T T

mRNA   A U G G U A A U C C U C G G G U A A

Protein   Starting codon / N-formylmethionine   Valine   Isoleucine   Leucine   Glycine   Terminator codon

Substitution mutation ↓

DNA   T A C C A T T G G G A G C C C A T T

mRNA   A U G G U A A C C C U C G G G U A A

Protein   Starting codon / N-formylmethionine   Valine   Threonine   Leucine   Glycine   Terminator codon

Figure 10-8 Colinearity of part of a gene and the amino acids of the protein molecule for which it codes. A substitution of cytosine (C) for uracil (U) causes threonine instead of isoleucine to be specified in the polypeptide chain.

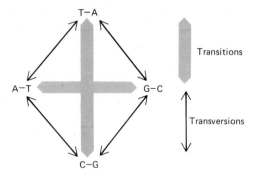

Figure 10-9 Possible alterations in a single nucleotide. Replacement of a purine with a purine or a pyrimidine with a pyrimidine is a transition. Substitution of a purine for a pyrimidine or a pyrimidine for a purine is a transversion.

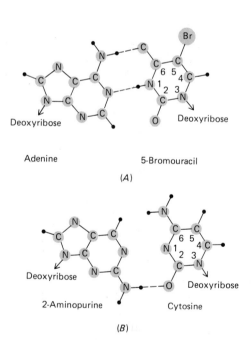

Figure 10-10 Transitions in base analogs. (A) 5-bromouracil replaces thymine. (B) 2-aminopurine replaces guanine.

by a purine, the substitution is called a *transversion* (Figure 10-9).

Transitions may be produced by *base analogs* which are nitrogen-containing compounds resembling the bases of nucleic acids except in the distribution of hydrogen atoms. Potent mutagens among the base analogs include 5-bromouracil (5-BU), which resembles thymine, and 2-aminopurine (2-AP), which is much like adenine (Figure 10-10). Incorporation of base analogs into DNA provides an increased probability for *errors in pairing*. A mistake in pairing can occur during incorporation of the analog into DNA or during subsequent replication of DNA.

Some chemical mutagens, chiefly nitrous acid, promote transitions by acting upon resting DNA. Nitrous acid deaminates adenine, guanine, or cytosine. The deaminated products do not pair with purines or pyrimidines complementary to the original bases. Deamination of adenine produces hypoxanthine which pairs with cytosine instead of thymine, causing an AT⟶GC transition. Hydroxylamine acts in a manner similar to nitrous acid except that its mutagenic action is directed against cytosine only. The effect of deamination is the introduction of a copy error.

The alkylating agents, such as the nitrogen mustards and ethylene oxides, promote transitions or transversions. When guanine is alkylated, it pairs with thymine instead of cytosine.

A single base substitution can cause the formation of a codon specifying for a different amino acid. However, more

Amino acid sequence from N-terminal end

	1	2	3	4	5	6	7	8
Hemoglobin A (normal)	val	his	leu	thr	pro	glu	glu	lys ...
Hemoglobin S	val	his	leu	thr	pro	val	glu	lys ...

Figure 10-11 Amino acid sequences in first part of beta chains of hemoglobin A (normal) and hemoglobin S (sickle cell anemia). (Adapted with permission from J. R. Sokatch and J. J. Ferretti, *Basic Bacteriology and Genetics.* Copyright © 1976 by Year Book Medical Publishers, Inc., Chicago, Illinois.)

than one triplet nucleotide can code for an amino acid (a phenomenon known as *degeneracy*). Therefore, if a codon is changed by the substitution of one base for another, the codon could still contain instructions for the same amino acid. In that event the protein molecule would remain unchanged even though a point mutation had occurred. Such mutations are called *silent mutations*.

The consequence of a point mutation may be negligible or may be so serious as to be harmful, or even lethal, to microorganisms as well as higher forms of life. A single substitution of an amino acid can alter the properties of a protein molecule significantly. For example, the hemoglobin molecules of persons with sickle cell anemia contain valine instead of glutamic acid on two parts of the molecules (Figure 10-11). The change in sequence of the amino acids produces a hemoglobin variant with a lesser affinity for oxygen than normal hemoglobin. The production of a completely functionally inactive protein as a result of a mutation could be lethal to an organism. If a single base substitution

resulted in the formation of the nonsense codons (UAA, UAG, or UGA) which specify for no amino acids on mRNA, protein synthesis would be terminated.

DELETIONS OR INSERTIONS

Distinct chromosomal breaks may cause the *deletion* or *insertion* of one or more nucleotides of a gene. The consequence of the loss or addition of a single base can be appreciated by considering the subsequent alteration in mRNA after transcription (Figure 10-12). The deletion or insertion of a single base causes a *reading frameshift* of nucleotide sequences. Deletion or insertion of three nucleotides, or a multiple of three, does not shift the reading frame, but can result in the synthesis of nonfunctional proteins.

Small deletions occur spontaneously, but loss of extended segments results from exposure to ultraviolet (UV) radiation, X rays, nitrogen mustards, or ethylene oxides. Radiation promotes the formation of a loop which is not copied

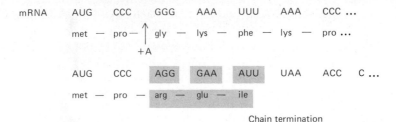

Figure 10-12 Reading frameshift. Insertion of base (+A) shifts the reading frame, producing amino acid substitutes (*arg, glu, ile*) and a nonsense code (UAA) terminating the polypeptide chain. (Adapted with permission from J. R. Sokatch and J. J. Ferretti, *Basic Bacteriology and Genetics.* Copyright © 1976 by Year Book Medical Publishers, Inc., Chicago, Illinois.)

during replication (Figure 10-13). Production of nonsense codons or elimination of termination signals results when an acridine dye, such as proflavin or 5-aminoacridine, binds to DNA between adjacent base pairs.

Substances known to be mutagenic (with less-well-understood action) are hydrogen peroxide, organic peroxides, manganous chloride, and N-methyl-N^1-nitro-nitrosoguanidine (NTG). NTG is an extremely efficient mutagen. In

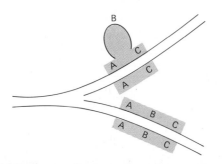

Figure 10-13 Mechanism of deletion for extended segment of DNA. A loop containing marker B is produced and deleted during replication. (Adapted with permission from J. R. Sokatch and J. J. Ferretti, *Basic Bacteriology and Genetics.* Copyright © 1976 by Year Book Medical Publishers, Inc., Chicago, Illinois.)

populations of cells subjected to NTG, mutation yields in excess of 10 percent can be obtained.

REVERSIONS

Some mutants can revert to wild-type phenotypes in a process known as *back mutation* or *reversion*. The restoration in phenotype can occur by a variety of mechanisms. The base sequence can be changed back to the original sequence when chemical mutagens promote transitions in both directions.

Alternately, a mutation at another location on the DNA molecule could function in a manner similar to the original altered gene. When a second mutation inhibits expression of an initial mutation, it is called a *suppressor mutation*. Revertants arising from suppressor mutations grow more slowly than other revertants or wild types.

Some bacteria have special enzymes which restore the integrity of genes altered by exposure to ultraviolet light. These repair mechanisms will be examined in Chapter 26. Back mutations to the normal gene arrangement does not occur if DNA is severely impaired by any mutagens.

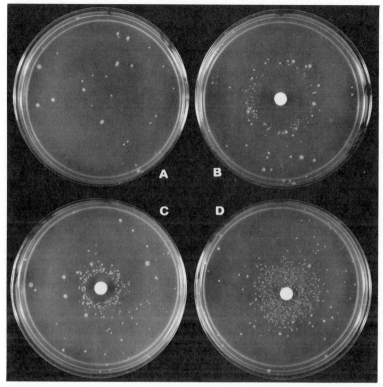

Figure 10-14 The Ames spot test. Each plate contains a tester strain of *Salmonella typhimurium;* plates C and D contain liver homogenate. Spontaneous revertants appear on plate *A.* Revertants surround furylfuranide, AF-2 (1 μg) on plate *B;* aflatoxin, B₁ (1 μg) on plate C; and 2-aminofluorente (10 μg) on plate *D.* (From B. N. Ames, J. McCann, and E. Yamasaki, *Mutation Res.* 31:347, 1975.)

DETECTION OF CHEMICAL MUTAGENS

The Ames spot test is a simple, sensitive method for detecting chemical mutagens causing base-pair substitutions and various kinds of frame-shift mutations. The method employs mutant strains of the gram-negative bacillus *Salmonella typhimurium*, which is deficient in the ability to synthesize histidine, and rat-liver homogenates, which are a source of activating enzymes. DNA of the mutant bacterial strains is repaired in the presence of a chemical mutagen and the rat-liver homogenates. If discs containing the suspected mutagenic agents are placed on the surface of histidine-deficient agar plates seeded with tester strains of *S. typhimurium*, colonies of reverted bacteria grow in the immediate areas surrounding the discs (Figure 10-14). The number of colonies is related to the degree of mutagenicity.

The Ames spot test has been used as

a screening procedure for potential carcinogenic agents. It is believed that most chemicals causing cancer do so by promoting cellular mutations. In most instances agents shown to be mutagenic by the Ames spot test have been demonstrated to cause cancer in laboratory animals. An exception appears to be the dye acridine. The use of bacterial mutants in an *in vitro* test system to detect potential carcinogens is both more economical and more efficient than wide-scale animal studies.

GENETIC RECOMBINATION IN PROCARYOTIC CELLS

Procaryotes acquire new genetic material in nature not only by mutation, but also by genetic recombination, following the transfer of DNA from one bacterium to another. *Transformation* is the transfer of genes from one bacterium to another under some rather specialized conditions. *Transduction* is the transfer of genes by a bacteriophage. *Conjugation* requires cell-to-cell contact to initiate gene transfer.

Recently devised techniques have made it possible to make recombinant DNA particles from eucaryotic cells *in vitro* which can be taken up by procaryotic cells. Regardless of the mechanism of transfer, the recipient bacterium becomes partially diploid until cell division occurs. The *diploid* state is characterized by two chromosomes in bacteria; the *haploid* state is characterized by a single chromosome. A cell is partially diploid when it contains duplication of some genes. The genetic material of the donor bacterium is segregated into a haploid state when it crosses over and recombines with homologous portions of the DNA molecule of the host bacterium (Figure 10-15).

TRANSFORMATION

The process of transformation was first observed by the British bacteriologist Fred Griffith in 1928. It involves the transfer of a small amount of cell-free DNA from one bacterium to another. Griffith inoculated one group of mice with a mutant avirulent, nonencapsulated strain of pneumococcus, now known as *Streptococcus pneumoniae*. He inoculated a second group of mice with a heat-killed virulent, encapsulated strain of the same organism. A third group of mice received a mixture of heat-killed encapsulated and living nonencapsulated pneumococci. Only the mice receiving the mixture of dead encapsulated and living nonencapsulated organisms got fatal pneumonia (Figure 10-16). Virulent, encapsulated pneumococci were isolated from the dead animals. In some manner the avirulent, nonencapsulated bacteria had been "transformed" into disease-producing, encapsulated organisms. Oswald Avery, Colin MacLeod, and Maclyn McCarty did not identify the transforming substance as DNA until 1944. The mice were merely a means of selecting for the new characteristic of virulence and not necessary for transformation to take place. Transformation

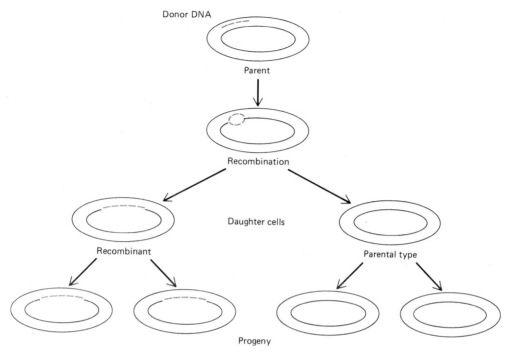

Figure 10-15 Recombination and segregation. Donor DNA crosses over and recombines with homologous portions of host DNA. Recombinant DNA occurs in a single daughter cell and progeny with small pieces of donor DNA.

does occur in nature to some extent, but the process has also been a powerful tool for manipulating the genetic makeup of bacterial cells in the laboratory. A number of factors including physiological state, strandedness, concentration of DNA, and size of DNA molecules influence the uptake of DNA in transformation.

Although double-stranded DNA can be bound to bacterial surfaces, it appears that only a single strand enters the cell. The single strand becomes integrated into the chromosome of the recipient cell. It has been hypothesized

that mesosomes may produce enzymes necessary for breaking down double-stranded DNA and incorporating single strands into the chromosome.

CONJUGATION OR SEXUAL RECOMBINATION

Conjugation involves transfer of genetic material during cell-to-cell contact between mating types of bacteria. The process was first demonstrated by Joshua Lederberg and Edward Tatum in 1946. It was the outcome of the ability to select for the presence of specific mu-

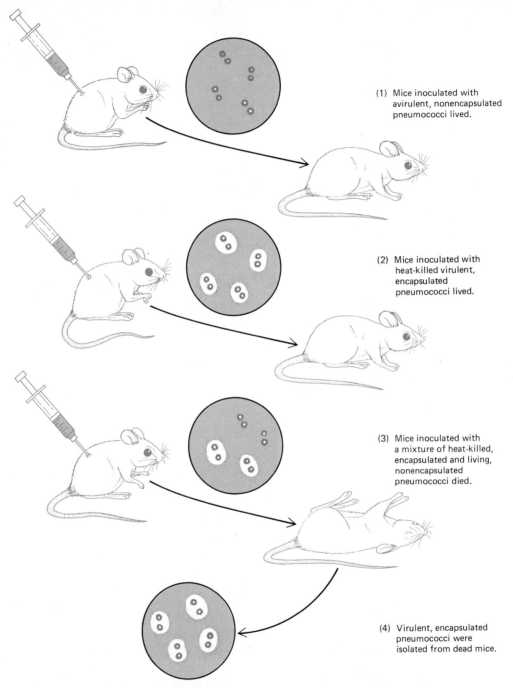

(1) Mice inoculated with avirulent, nonencapsulated pneumococci lived.

(2) Mice inoculated with heat-killed virulent, encapsulated pneumococci lived.

(3) Mice inoculated with a mixture of heat-killed, encapsulated and living, nonencapsulated pneumococci died.

(4) Virulent, encapsulated pneumococci were isolated from dead mice.

Figure 10-16 Griffith's experiment which "transformed" avirulent pneumococci into disease-producing organisms.

tants of *E. coli*, K-12, by replica plating. Donor cells contain a fertility factor (F), which can be transmitted independently or as a part of the transfer of the entire chromosome during cell-to-cell contact (Figure 10-17). Cells lacking the F factor are designated as female or F⁻ cells; cells with the factor are male or F⁺. In nature F⁻ strains are more prevalent than F⁺ strains since the sex factor is quite sensitive to temperatures above 42°C. Transfer of the F factor in crosses between F⁺ and F⁻ strains approaches

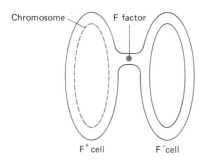

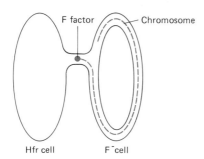

Figure 10-17 Transmission of cytoplasmic and chromosomal fertility factor (F). The F factor is transmitted independently from the F⁺ cell to the F⁻ cell and with the entire chromosome from the Hfr cell to the F⁻ cell.

100 percent, but transfer of segments of chromosome and subsequent recombination occur in only 1 in 10^4 or 10^5 cells.

Certain donor strains, designated as Hfr (high frequency of recombination), transfer chromosomal material with greater efficiency, but rarely transfer the F factor. Recombinants can be demonstrated in approximately 1 in 10^2 cells after a cross between an F⁻ and an Hfr strain. The Hfr cells are derived from F⁺ cells in which the F factor has become integrated into the chromosome.

By periodic interruptions in matings, François Jacob and Elie Wollman demonstrated that Hfr cells transfer genetic material to recipient F⁻ cells in an oriented fashion. The sequence of their entry depends on the order of arrangement on the chromosome. The entire chromosome of *E. coli* enters in 90 minutes, if mating is not interrupted.

Studies on conjugation have been valuable in elucidating the nature of the bacterial chromosome. The circular nature of the bacterial chromosome was first established by conjugation experiments and later confirmed by radioautography. Conjugation has made it possible to map the chromosome of *E. coli* (Figure 10-18). Some limited interspecies transfer between gram-negative bacilli has been demonstrated during conjugation experiments.

TRANSDUCTION

The phenomenon of transduction was discovered by accident in 1951 when Joshua and Esther Lederberg, working

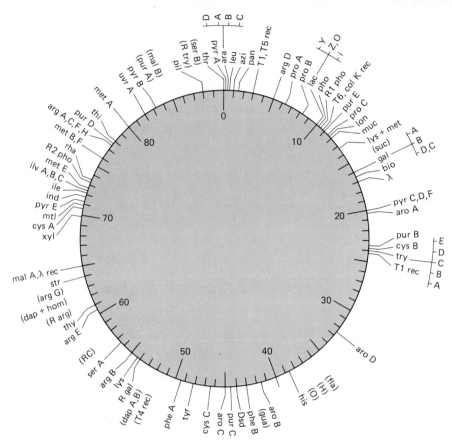

Figure 10-18 Chromosome of *E. coli*, strain K-12, mapped according to time in minutes required for transfer of markets. (From A. L. Taylor and C. D. Trotter, *Bacteriol. Rev.* 36:504, 1972.)

with Norton Zinder, were attempting to demonstrate conjugation in mutant strains of *Salmonella typhimurium*. During the course of their studies recombinants were produced when the culture of one mutant was exposed to a cell-free extract of another mutant. The transducing agent was subsequently found to be a bacteriophage, now commonly called P22.

Susceptible bacteria and a phage-infected culture are necessary to promote transduction. The size of DNA fragments transduced is approximately 1/100 that of the bacterial chromosome. Only about 10^{-5} to 10^{-7} of a phage population carrying donor DNA can successfully transfer the genetic material for a particular marker. Some phages transfer a restricted set of host genes. The transfer of unrestricted DNA is called *generalized transduction*; the transfer of restricted markers is called *specialized transduction*.

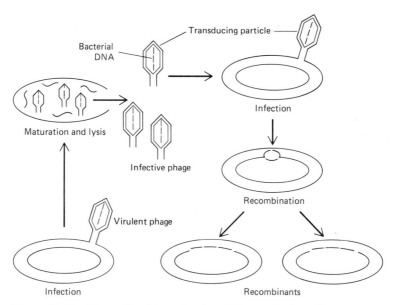

Figure 10-19 Generalized transduction. When a virulent phage enters a bacterium, a lytic infection is established. If a piece of bacterial DNA is accidentally assembled and packaged in the protein coat of a phage, it gives rise to a transducing particle. When the bacterial DNA of a transducing particle enters a bacterium, recombination can occur during cell division if donor and recipient DNA fragments are homologous. The progeny are called recombinants.

In generalized transduction a piece of bacterial DNA accidentally is assembled and packaged as part of the phage DNA during a lytic infection. When the bacterial cell lyses, the *transducing particles* are released along with infective phage (Figure 10-19). Because the transducing particles cannot promote an infection in a new host, they are also called *defective particles*. Only a single defective particle is released for approximately every 10^5 phages. Integration depends on homology between the donor and recipient fragments of DNA and the amount of donor DNA. Actual incorporation into the

chromosome of the recipient occurs during cell division.

Transducing particles may also arise by induction of lysogenic cells (Figure 10-20). Induction takes place when the integrated phage DNA, called *prophage*, is converted to vegetative phage. It can occur spontaneously or be induced by ultraviolet light, alkylating agents, and some carcinogens. The return to the vegetative state is aptly called *zygotic induction*. The prophage is excised from bacterial DNA, multiples, and promotes lysis of the host cell.

Abortive transduction occurs when a fragment of DNA from a transducing

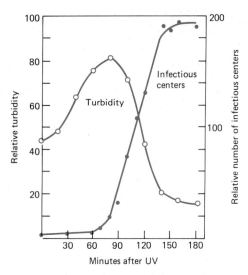

Figure 10-20 Induction of the prophage of lysogenic *E. coli,* strain K12, by ultraviolet light. (From J. Jacob and C. R. Fuerst, *J. Gen. Microbiol.* 18:518, 1958. Cambridge University Press.)

phage fails to multiply, but is transferred in a unilinear fashion (Figure 10-21). During cell division the abortive fragment is transferred to only one daughter cell. Since the fragment is functionally active, its products may be synthesized by several generations of daughter cells.

DNA of viral origin can also be transferred to bacteria. Nontoxigenic strains of *Corynebacterium diphtheriae* can be converted to toxigenic strains and rendered immune to lytic infection by phage derived from a virulent, toxigenic strain. Nontoxigenic strains of *Clostridium tetani* and *Streptococcus pyogenes* can be converted to exotoxin-producing strains. The process is called *phage conversion.* The study of such bacterium-phage interrelationships may one day demonstrate an even larger role of viruses in virulence of bacteria associated with human disease.

Although less genetic material is transferred by both transformation and transduction than by conjugation, both processes have also been valuable in mapping chromosomes. Bacteria containing recombinant DNA, regardless of the mechanism of transfer, often have survival advantages. Newly acquired traits are frequently protective or provide organisms with the capability of using a greater variety of energy sources. Bacteria in which transformation, conjugation, or transduction have been demonstrated are listed in Table 10-1.

Table 10-1   GENERA OF BACTERIA IN WHICH GENETIC TRANSFER BY CONJUGATION, TRANSDUCTION, OR TRANSFORMATION HAS BEEN DEMONSTRATED TO OCCUR

CONJUGATION	TRANSDUCTION	TRANSFORMATION
Escherichia	*Salmonella*	*Neisseria*
Salmonella	*Escherichia*	*Haemophilus*
Pseudomonas	*Pseudomonas*	*Streptococcus*
Vibrio	*Staphylococcus*	*Staphylococcus*
Streptomyces	*Bacillus*	*Bacillus*
	Proteus	*Acinetobacter*

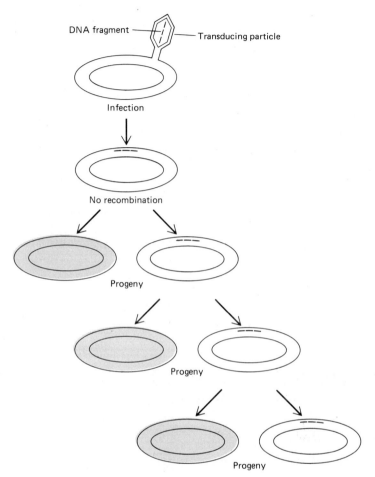

DNA fragment

Transducing particle

Infection

No recombination

Progeny

Progeny

Progeny

Figure 10-21   Unilinear transmission of genetic factor in abortive transduction. The shaded cells are parental types.

EXTRACHROMOSOMAL INHERITANCE

The autonomous nature of the sex factor in F⁺ cells led to the discovery of other DNA self-replicating entities, which exist independently, in the cytoplasm of bacterial cells. If the entity exists only in the cytoplasm, it is called a *plasmid* (Figure 10-22). If the entity can exist as a chromosomal or cytoplasmic factor, like the sex factor, it is referred to as an *episome*. One writer has described plasmids as "genetic loose change."

Plasmids have been studied extensively in gram-negative bacilli, but the entities are found in other organisms as well. Cells can contain as many as 20 to

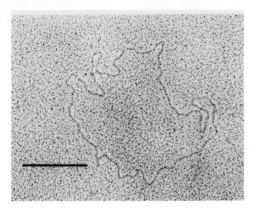

Figure 10-22   An electron microphotograph of the DNA of a circular plasmid of *Bacillus subtilis*. Bar corresponds to a molecular weight of 0.5×10^6. (From T. Tanaka, M. Kuroda, and K. Sakaguchi, *J. Bacteriol.* 129:1487, 1976.)

30 plasmids per cell. Very large plasmids have as many as 250 genes. Plasmids responsible for the synthesis of bactericidal agents known as *colicins* are present in some strains of *Salmonella*, *Shigella*, and *Escherichia*. Colicins adsorb to specific receptors on the surfaces of susceptible cells. Colicin-producing organisms are immune to the action of their own colicins.

IN VITRO RECOMBINATION

The potential for altering the evolutionary process by genetic engineering, using *in vitro* recombinant DNA, has aroused both enthusiasm and apprehension among scientists. François Jacob has suggested that natural selection works like a tinkerer who does not know what he is going to make, but who employs raw materials at his disposal until a workable object is produced. Marks of tinkering exist at every level in the biological world. Tinkering at the molecular level is most apparent. Despite the tinkering, however, elephants, redwoods, bacteria, and even viruses have similar underlying molecular units. Engineering, unlike tinkering, employs particular raw materials and scientifically tested methodology and tools.

The ability to program cells genetically to perform specific tasks is possible with recombinant DNA techniques (Figure 10-23). Plasmids conferring penicillin resistance upon *Staphylococcus aureus* have been transferred to *Escherichia coli*. Genes of the toad *Xenopus laevis* have been transplanted into the cells of *E. coli*. Recombinant plasmids containing DNA complementary to mRNA from rat islets of Langerhans have been constructed. The clones may lead to a better understanding of insulin biosynthesis and expression in mammalian cells. The successful transplantation of an interferon-producing gene into a bacterium was announced in 1980. It is hoped that the discovery may make available sufficient quantities of the antiviral substance to study its use in treatment of leukemia and other types of cancer.

Some skeptics fear that experimentation with *in vitro* recombinant DNA will lead to the creation of genetically altered microorganisms which could destroy mankind. They are asking such questions as "Do we want to assume the responsibility for life on

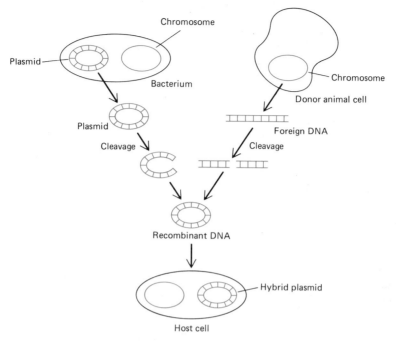

Figure 10-23 Programming of a bacterium with recombinant DNA. Hybrid fragments are assembled *in vitro* and introduced into a host bacterium. (Adapted from G. Wald, *The Sciences* 16:6, 1976.)

this planet?" Supporters of genetic engineering believe that commitment to responsible experimentation may make it possible to replace defective genes with functional genes in mammalian cells or to transfer nitrogen-fixing genes to bacterial cells for mass production of fertilizers. The potential is almost incomprehensible.

SEXUAL RECOMBINATION IN EUCARYOTIC CELLS

Sexual recombination occurring in eucaryotic cells is more complex than in procaryotes because eucaryotes have more than one chromosome contained within a nuclear membrane. Recombinant procaryotic cells remain haploid, but during sexual reproduction in eucaryotes the haploid sex cells fuse to produce the diploid state in the *zygote*.

MEIOTIC RECOMBINATION

During gametogenesis (formation of *gametes* or sex cells) a form of reduction division known as *meiosis* takes place (Figure 10-24). In meiosis homologous chromosomal units pair with each other in a process known as *synapsis*. Each chromosomal unit is composed of the original genetic material and an exact replicate. The subunits, called *chromatids*, are connected at a junction known

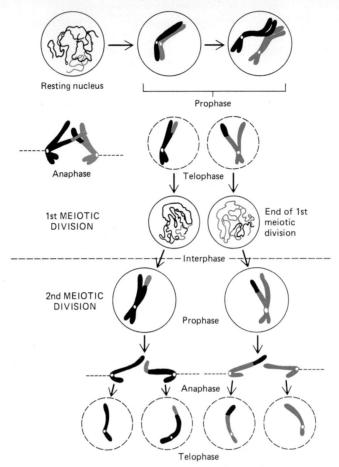

Figure 10-24 Meiosis in sex cells during gametogenesis. Only a single pair of homologous chromosomes is shown within the nucleus. Metaphase has been omitted from the diagram. The daughter cells formed during the 1st meiotic division are diploid, but the daughter cells formed during the 2nd meiotic division are haploid. (Adapted from W. Hayes, *The Genetics of Bacteria and Their Viruses*, 2d ed., New York, Wiley, 1968; Oxford, Blackwell Scientific Publications.)

as a *centromere*. Therefore, when pairing of chromatids occurs, a *tetrad* is formed. The process provides a unique opportunity for crossing-over (interchange of genes) to occur since chromatids of homologous chromosomes become attached to one another at some points. Genes become separated and join others in new linkage associations (Figure 10-25). The greater the distance between genes on a chromosome, the greater is the chance for separation during cross-over. Tetrads line up on a spindle of microtubules and ultimately separate, moving in opposite directions during formation of daughter cells. The newly formed daughter cells undergo subsequent division, maintaining half of the number of chromosomes in the original cell.

MITOTIC RECOMBINATION

Mitosis is a type of asexual nuclear division occurring in eucaryotic cells. The process takes place in gametogenesis following meiosis, but also in other cells during growth processes. Mitosis is accompanied by *cytokinesis*, a simultaneous process of cytoplasmic division. Mitosis and cytokinesis consist of a series of morphological and biochemical events recognizable by distinct changes in the nucleus and cytoplasm. The nuclear and cytoplasmic changes accompanying cell division permit the microscopic identification of four phases of mitosis as *prophase, metaphase, anaphase,* and *telophase* (Figure 10-26). The time required for division varies from several minutes to many months, depending on the type of tissue or species of the biological kingdom.

During prophase chromatin material condenses to form the elongated chromosomal units. The thickened appearance is the result of progressive coiling. No pairing of chromosomes occurs during mitosis. The chromatids are connected at a junction called a *centromere* as in meiosis. The nuclear membrane and nucleolus disappear as a set of spindle fibers develops. In animal cells the fibers originate from cytoplasmic structures known as *centrioles,* which

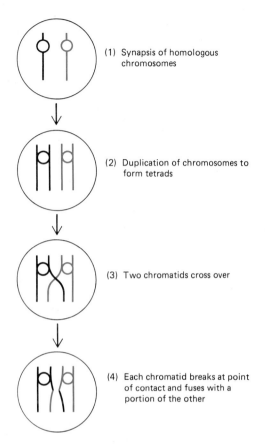

(1) Synapsis of homologous chromosomes

(2) Duplication of chromosomes to form tetrads

(3) Two chromatids cross over

(4) Each chromatid breaks at point of contact and fuses with a portion of the other

Figure 10-25 Separation of genes and formation of new linkages during cross-over. (Adapted from J. D. Watson, *Molecular Biology of the Gene,* 1st edition, Benjamin/Cummings Publishing Company, Menlo Park, Calif., copyright, 1965.)

can be observed in prophase. Centrioles cannot be seen in fungi or typical plant cells.

Metaphase is characterized by an alignment of individual chromosomal units on the spindle at the equator. The chromatids of each chromosomal unit separate and move in opposite directions.

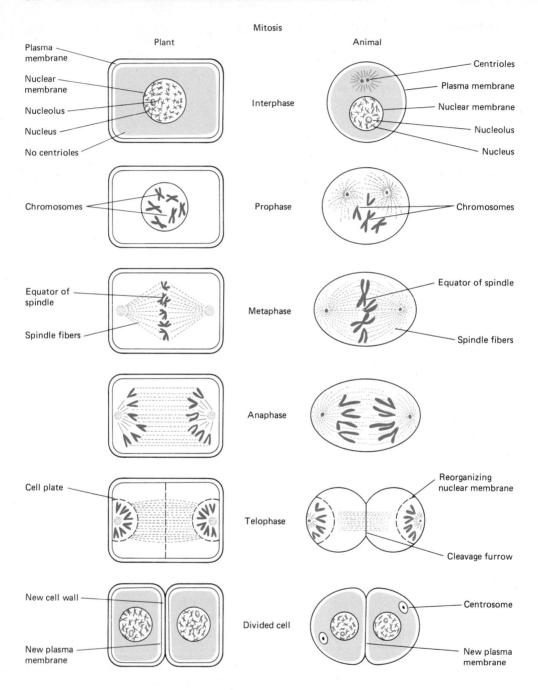

Figure 10-26   Mitosis in plant and animal cells.

During anaphase daughter chromosomes continue to migrate to opposite poles under the influence of the spindle fibers. By late anaphase chromosomes are widely separated. A constriction of cytoplasm occurs at the equator in animal cells; in plant cells formation of a cell plate takes place.

Telophase is characterized by the completed migration of chromosomes to the poles of the cell, a reorganization of the nuclear membrane, uncoiling of chromosomes, disappearance of spindle fibers, and the formation of a new cell boundary. The chromatin material appears in a diffuse state once again at the end of telophase.

Recombination can take place in some fungi during mitosis. The process provides a means for diversity in the fungi which do not reproduce sexually. Some filamentous fungi are multinucleate and nuclei occasionally fuse in a process analogous to formation of a zygote in organisms reproducing sexually. The diploid nuclei can revert to the haploid state. It is during nuclear fusion that crossing-over can occur.

The life cycle of eucaryotic cells can be divided into two periods: the division period described above during which mitosis and cytokinesis occur and the interphase during which the cell grows in size. The interphase period can further be divided into three periods: primary growth stage (G-1); synthesis stage (S), during which DNA replicates; and secondary growth stage (G-2), extending from the end of DNA replication to the actual start of cell division (Figure 10-27).

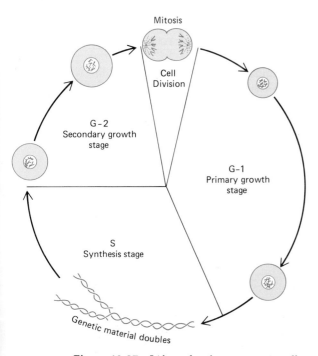

Figure 10-27   Life cycle of a eucaryotic cell.

SUMMARY

Microbial variation may be environmentally induced or arise from alteration of genetic material by mutation or genetic recombination. Mutations are spontaneous, random, and rare events in nature, but can be induced in the laboratory by a variety of physical and chemical agents. Recombination in procaryotes is a consequence of transformation, conjugation, transduction, or uptake of recombinant DNA synthesized *in vitro*. Recombination in eucaryotes is a consequence of crossing-over strands of DNA during meiosis, mitosis, or nuclear fusion. Mutation and recombination are responsible for the immense diversity of genotypic variation in the microbial world.

QUESTIONS FOR STUDY

1. Identify the following character-istics as environmentally or genet-ically induced:
   loss of motility
   inability to grow at body tempera-ture
   resistance to streptomycin
   formation of endospores
   production of rough colonies
2. Name five mutagenic agents.
3. How could one select for the pres-ence of a double auxotroph?
4. Give an example of how phage con-version can affect the ability of a bacterium to cause disease.
5. Name and describe the four phases of mitosis.
6. Name and describe three stages of interphase.
7. Formulate an argument for or against experimentation involving genetic engineering.

SELECTED REFERENCES

Crick, F. H. C. The biochemistry of genetics. *Proc. Sixth Intern. Cong. Bio-chem.* I.U.B. Vol. 33:109, 1964.

Hayes, W. *The Genetics of Bacteria and Their Viruses.* 2d ed. New York: Wiley, 1968.

Herreid, C. F., II. *Biology.* New York: Macmillan, 1977.

Jacob, F. Evolution and tinkering. *Science.* 196:1161, 1977.

Jacob, F. and Wollman, E. L. *Sexuality and the Genetics of Bacteria.* New York: Academic Press, 1961.

Sokatch, J. R., and Ferretti, J. J. *Basic Bacteriology and Genetics.* Chicago: Year Book Medical Publishers, 1976.

Tomasz, A. Cellular factors in genetic transformation. *Sci. Am.* 220:38, 1969.

Ullrich, A.; Shine, J.; Chirgwin, J.; Pic-tet, R.; Tischer, E.; Rutter, W. J.; and Goodman, G. H. Rat insulin genes: construction of plasmids containing the coding sequences. *Science.* 196:1313, 1977.

Watson, J. D. *Molecular Biology of the Gene.* 3rd ed. New York: W. A. Ben-jamin, 1976.

Weinberg, J. H. 'Plasmid' — welcome to the word pool. But what are you? *Sci. News.* 107:404, 1975.

Zinder, N. D. Transduction in bacteria. *Sci. Am.* 105:2, 1958.

Unit Three

HOST-PARASITE RELATIONSHIPS

Chapter 11

Microorganisms Indigenous to the Human Host

After you read this chapter, you should be able to:

1. Describe the factors which favor colonization of microorganisms on the surface of the body.
2. List the genera of the major microorganisms which colonize the skin, mouth, oropharynx, nose, nasopharynx, gastrointestinal tract, and genitourinary tract.
3. List several parts of the body that are free from microbial contamination in health.
4. Trace the postulated pathway of latent herpesviruses and varicella viruses when activated by environmental factors.
5. Explain the environmental circumstances provided by the large intestine which promote colonization by bacteria.
6. List the parts of the male and female genital tracts that constitute reservoirs for microorganisms.
7. Explain how progesterone affects the microbial population of the vagina.
8. Describe the role of lactobacilli in maintaining an acid pH in the vagina.
9. Define the terms pathogen and nonpathogen.

The microorganisms considered indigenous to the human host include even those microorganisms that are able to colonize the human host for only short periods of time. It is increasingly precarious to speak of "normal flora and fauna" when applied to the continuum of changes going on as humans and microorganisms react or as microorganisms react with one another.

The ecological distribution of microorganisms in the human host is related to multiple factors. Alteration in environmental conditions, competition for essential nutrients, and interference in immune responses of a host all play roles in determining the indigenous microbial population at any one time. In general, however, moist areas of the body favor colonization of bacteria, fungi, and some protozoa. The sites where microorganisms abide in the largest numbers include the skin, mucous membranes, oro- and naso-pharynx, lower intestinal tract, and lower genitourinary tract. Generally, no microorganisms are found in the blood, larynx, bronchi, stomach, bladder, ureters, kidneys, prostate gland, or ovaries.

SKIN AND MUCOUS MEMBRANES

The skin and mucous membranes are effective barriers against the penetration of large numbers of microorganisms. As one might expect, however, the skin is exposed to large numbers of organisms, some of which are able to colonize at particular sites. Protected, moist areas, such as the axilla, groin, genitalia, spaces between the toes, and folds under women's breasts, support microbial growth better than do drier areas (Figure 11-1).

Two groups of gram-positive bacteria are the most abundant microorganisms on healthy skin; the aerobic cocci and anaerobic pleomorphic bacilli. By far the most numerous of the gram-positive cocci encountered on the skin are strains of *Staphylococcus epidermidis*. The pathogen *S. aureus* is less frequently recovered from the skin and probably its presence is of a transitory nature.

One representative of fauna which inhabits hair follicles is the mite *Demodex folliculorum* (Figure 11-2). This tiny mite is present on the skin of most adults, but causes no discomfort. The mite is approximately 400 times larger than a bacterium, but is barely visible to the naked eye.

The gram-positive lipophilic anaerobe *Propionibacterium acnes* survives

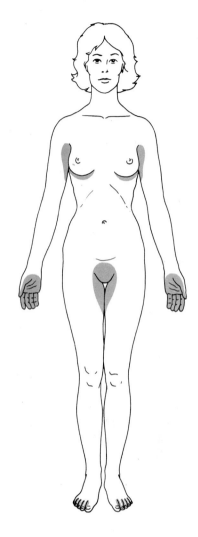

Figure 11-1 Sites of colonization for microorganisms on the skin. The protected, moist areas, such as the axilla, groin, spaces between toes, and folds under breasts, support microbial growth. Hands are highly colonized because of constant environmental exposure.

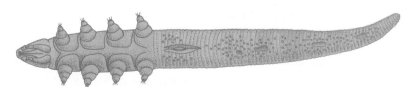

Figure 11-2 Schematic representation of female mite, *Demodex folliculorum*. (Redrawn from H. W. Brown, *Basic Clinical Parasitology*, 4th ed., Englewood Cliffs, N.J., Prentice-Hall, 1975.)

only in subsurface epithelium or sebaceous glands and is for the most part not associated with dermatitis. Streptococcal organisms have been isolated from the skin, but the skin does not represent a major reservoir for pathogenic streptococci. The propensity of the skin to promote colonization of gram-positive bacteria is related to the ability of those organisms to degrade sebaceous gland secretions to unsaturated fatty acids. The odor associated with degradation of sebum results from an accumulation of unsaturated fatty acids in some protected areas.

Most gram-negative bacteria are inhibited by unsaturated fatty acids. One exception to the acids' antimicrobial action appears to be gram-negative bacteria belonging to the genus *Acinetobacter*. Members of that genus can apparently withstand accumulations of the antimetabolites. *Acinetobacter* species are frequently found on the feet of children and adult males. They are usually considered to be opportunists, that is, capable of causing disease only under special circumstances.

Among the transient residents of the skin are several fungi commonly found in soil. In the absence of injury or a suppression of immune mechanisms, most have difficulty in colonizing the skin in any appreciable numbers. Yeasts can frequently be isolated from between the toes and fingers and from dandruff. The most common yeasts isolated from the skin are members of the genus *Candida*. Yeasts typical of the genus *Pityrosporum* more commonly inhabit the scalp.

Certain molds (*Trichophyton mentagrophytes, T. rubrum, Epidermophyton floccosum*) may colonize the skin of the feet in some individuals without detectable evidence of disease. Some believe these agents of "athlete's foot" can remain in a latent state until an environmental circumstance triggers their growth in sufficient numbers to produce an infection.

It is highly probable that viruses reside in cells in the deeper layers of skin with little or no effect on the cells in healthy individuals. Environmental factors appear to trigger viruses to produce skin lesions. Although the herpesvirus that causes fever blisters is not recoverable from asymptomatic individuals, there is strong evidence that the virus remains latent in sensory nerve cells of the trigeminal nerve ganglion between episodes of lesions. Once activated, the virus propagates and spreads by way of cells of sensory nerve sheaths to contiguous epidermal cells where it multiplies and produces blisters (Figure 11-3).

A particularly painful type of facial neuralgia occurs when the herpesvirus proliferates in the sensory fibers of the maxillary or mandibular branches of the trigeminal nerve. For some reason the viruses remain contained within cells of sensory fibers and do not enter surrounding epithelial cells.

The herpesvirus which causes shingles is present only in individuals who have had chickenpox (varicella). The varicella virus remains latent in sensory cells of the dorsal root ganglion. Upon appropriate stimulation the activated virus multiplies and moves along the cells of sensory nerve sheaths.

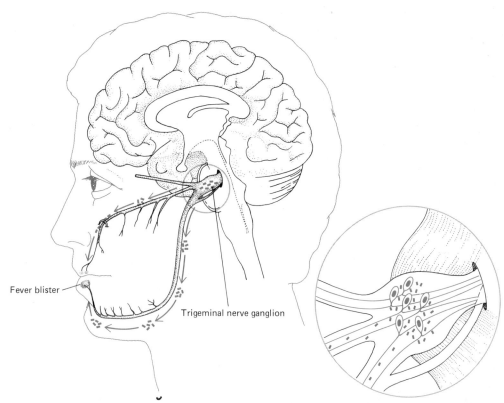

Fever blister

Trigeminal nerve ganglion

Figure 11-3   Postulated reservoir for herpesvirus. The virus remains latent in the sensory nerve cells of the trigeminal nerve ganglion. Upon activation it travels by way of the sensory nerve sheaths to the lip causing typical fever blister.

MOUTH AND OROPHARYNX

Large numbers of microorganisms enter the mouth with food (Table 11-1). Saliva contains solubilized buffers which keep the oral cavity close to neutral despite highly acid or alkaline contents of food. It has been estimated that saliva contains approximately 1 billion bacteria per milliliter. That count does not take into consideration bacteria that attach to epithelial surfaces of the mouth or gingiva or those that prefer the surfaces of the teeth for colonization. Crevices and pits of the teeth provide environments where oxidation-reduction potentials are low enough to support the growth of obligate anaerobes. Both aerobic and anaerobic gram-positive cocci are abundant in the mouth. Gram-negative cocci belonging to the genus *Branhamella* frequently colonize the mucous membranes of the

Table 11-1   SOME MICROORGANISMS OF THE MOUTH AND OROPHARYNX

GRAM-POSITIVE BACTERIA	GRAM-NEGATIVE BACTERIA	MISCELLANEOUS ORGANISMS
Actinomyces israelii	*Bacteroides species*	*Candida albicans*
Alpha streptococci	*Branhamella catarrhalis*	*Endamoeba gingivalis*
Lactobacillus species	*Fusobacterium nucleatum*	Herpesviruses
Nonhemolytic streptococci	*Haemophilus influenzae*	*Treponema species*
Peptostreptococci	*Haemophilus parainfluenzae*	
Proprionibacterium acnes	*Neisseria meningitidis*	
Staphylococcus aureus	*Veillonella alcalescens*	
Staphylococcus epidermidis		
Streptococcus mutans		
Streptococcus pneumoniae		

SOURCE: Adapted from G. P. Youmans, P. Y. Paterson, and H. M. Sommers, *The Biologic and Clinical Basis of Infectious Diseases* (Philadelphia: Saunders, 1975).

oropharynx. Of the anaerobic organisms, species of the genus *Bacteroides* and *Veillonella* are common isolates of oropharyngeal secretions.

Gram-positive bacilli of the genus *Lactobacillus* colonize the oral cavity soon after birth; they may be homofermentative or heterofermentative. The homofermentative strains produce lactic acid, while heterofermentative strains produce alcohol, acetic acid, and carbon dioxide in addition to lactic acid.

Filamentous branched forms of an anaerobe belonging to the genus *Actinomyces* are also common in the oral cavity growing on or near dental plaque. Their numbers are usually few enough to present no difficulty (Figure 11-4).

The oral spirochetes are common inhabitants in adults with normal dentition, but their prevalence increases to nearly 100 percent as gingival recession occurs. A competitive environment keeps the oral spirochetes from attacking mucosa of the oropharynx. Fuso-

bacteria, spirilla, vibrios, and mycoplasmas are common oral residents.

Candida albicans is the most prominent permanent fungal resident of the oral cavity. It occurs in approximately one-half of the general population. It is more common among women than men, but the reason for the preferential predilection is not clear. Colonization of the protozoan *Entamoeba gingivalis* is

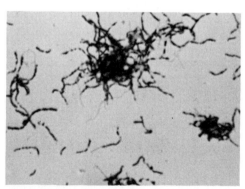

Figure 11-4   Gram stain of an *Actinomyces* species from the oral cavity. Members of the genus are gram-positive, filamentous bacilli. (Courtesy, P. D. Mitchell, Marshfield, Wisconsin.)

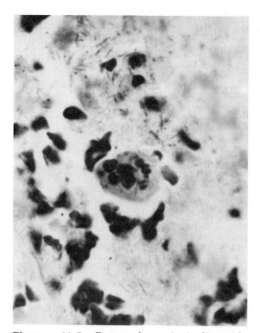

Figure 11-5 *Entamoeba gingivalis.* Although the ameba is found in approximately one-tenth of clean, healthy mouths, the organism can promote periodontal disease. (From D. S. Gottlieb and L. H. Miller, *J. Periodontol.* 42:412, 1971.)

equally prevalent in mouths of men and women; it is found in approximately one-tenth of clean, healthy mouths (Figure 11-5).

Viruses, with the possible exception of the herpesvirus group, are probably transient residents of oropharyngeal cells. During the course of a viral disease and even for considerable periods thereafter, viruses may be shed in oropharyngeal secretions. A cytomegalovirus which causes salivary gland disease probably remains latent in cells of salivary glands with or without clinical manifestation of disease during infancy. Salivary gland involvement by the virus is a frequent consequence of immunosuppressive treatment in adults.

The microorganisms in the mouth contribute to periodontal disease and dental caries. Bacteria accumulate in plaques which adhere to tooth surfaces and nearby epithelial surfaces (Figure 11-6). Products of microbial metabolism

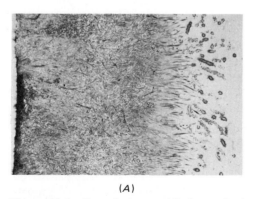

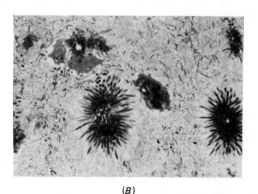

(A)   (B)

Figure 11-6 Dental plaque. (A) Supragingival plaque showing dense, predominantly filamentous bacterial mass in "corncob" formations adherent to the enamel surface. (B) Cross-section through "test-tube" formations of subgingival plaque. The adherent flora is less filamentous than the supragingival plaque. (From M. A. Listgarten, *J. Periodontol,* 47:1, 1976.)

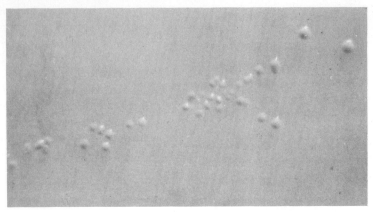

Figure 11-7   Appearance of colonies of *Streptococcus mutans* on a medium selective for salivary streptococci. (Courtesy, H. A. B. Linke, New York.)

can penetrate gingival tissue and cause inflammation. Environmental conditions within plaque vary with growth of bacteria, but cause some predictable shifts in microbial populations. Early plaques contain aerobic organisms, but as negative oxidation-reduction potentials are approached from accumulated glycoproteins, inorganic salts, and bacteria, anaerobic genera persist. Streptococcal species predominate in early plaque; *Actinomyces* species are most abundant in late plaque. Gingivitis is caused by invasion of contiguous epithelial surfaces and concomitant manifestations of cell-mediated immunity directed against plaque organisms.

Dental caries occur when tooth substance of a pit, fissure, or proximal surface is lost. Ingestion of large quantities of sugar-laden foods selects for plaque organisms that form acid capable of increasing the solubility of subsurface layers of enamel. *Streptococcus mutans* is the most common plaque organism im-

plicated in human dental caries, but the numbers and interrelationships of the oral flora make it difficult to eliminate the role of other bacteria (Figure 11-7).

NOSE AND NASOPHARYNX

To some extent the microorganisms of the nose and nasopharynx reflect the microbial population of the skin. The variation in numbers of total flora is probably great in any one individual at different times, but usually nasal washings will yield more than 20,000 organisms per milliliter. Both *S. aureus* and *S. epidermidis* can be recovered with frequency from nasopharyngeal cultures. *S. aureus* is most often a transient resident, although it has been estimated that from 2 to 25 percent of some groups are carriers of the pathogen. Carrier rates for group A streptococci are high among children of school age. Other streptococci and diphtheroids are out-numbered only by staphylococci. *Branhamella* and *Neisseria* species are often abundant in both children and adults; the pathogens *Haemophilus influenzae* and *Streptococcus pneumoniae* frequently inhabit the nasopharynx of adults. Gram-negative bacilli appear irregularly in healthy individuals, but alterations in defense mechanisms can allow the nasopharynx to be permissive for the colonization of a variety of gram-negative species. The causative organisms of the pneumonias caused by gram-negative organisms originate in the nasopharynx.

GASTROINTESTINAL TRACT

Under most circumstances the stomach does not harbor many viable microorganisms. Most bacteria, with the exception of mycobacteria, cannot survive in the acid environment of the stomach. A few organisms can escape the bactericidal action of the gastric juices by being enmeshed in food particles. They may also survive if a reflux of intestinal contents into the stomach because of intestinal obstruction, provides sufficient alkalinity to promote the growth of bacteria of oropharyngeal origin.

Few bacteria colonize the upper part of the intestine, but the numbers increase progressively with distance from the duodenum to the colon. The jejunum may contain streptococci, lactobacilli, and diphtheroids. Small numbers of *Candida* also commonly reside in the small intestine. The yeasts flourish

only when antimicrobials that inhibit the growth of other enteric organisms are given orally. The formation of intestinal pouches, known as *diverticula*, permits proliferation of microorganisms in a protected environment (Figure 11-8). Most individuals with diverticula are asymptomatic. However, diverticulosis can be hazardous should an inflammatory process develop which affects adjacent areas.

The colon constitutes a large fermentation vessel in which numbers of bacteria approximate 100 billion per gram of feces. Anaerobic gram-negative and gram-positive bacteria are the most abundant organisms. *Bacteroides* and *Fusobacterium* species rank high in frequency of gram-negative bacilli found among microorganisms of the gastrointestinal tract (Table 11-2). A gram-positive, anaerobic, spore-forming bacillus, *Clostridium perfringens*, colonizes the large intestine of approximately one-third of healthy individuals with no apparent harm, although this organism commonly causes infection in traumatized tissue. Other *Clostridium* species are easily recoverable from stool specimens and have similar potentials for causing infections.

Both species of *Peptostreptococcus* (anaerobic streptococci) and *Peptococcus* (anaerobic staphylococci) abound in the large intestine. Group D *Streptococcus* (enterococci) are recoverable from stool specimens of all healthy individuals, but *S. aureus* in feces is usually associated with nasopharyngeal carriers. *Candida* species frequently colonize the large intestine. Both *S. aureus* and *Candida* species tend to flourish

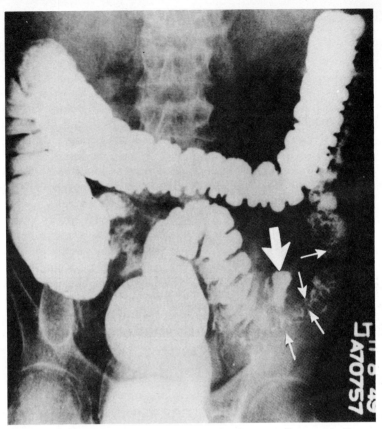

Figure 11-8 Diverticula in the sigmoid colon (small arrows). Extravasation of barium through a perforated diverticulum (large arrow). (From P. D. Hoeprich, *Infectious Diseases*, 2d ed., New York, Harper & Row, 1977.)

Table 11-2 SOME MICROORGANISMS OF THE GASTROINTESTINAL TRACT

GRAM-POSITIVE BACTERIA	GRAM-NEGATIVE BACTERIA	MISCELLANEOUS MICROORGANISMS
Bifidobacterium bifidum	*Bacteroides species*	Bacteriophages
Clostridium species	*Enterobacter species*	*Candida albicans*
Enterococci (group D *Streptococcus*)	*Escherichia coli*	*Chilomastix mesnili*
Eubacterium limosum	*Fusobacterium species*	*Dientamoeba fragilis*
Lactobacillus species	*Klebsiella species*	*Endolimax nana*
Peptococcus species	*Proteus species*	*Entamoeba coli*
Peptostreptococcus species	*Pseudomonas species*	*Enteromonas hominis*
		Giardia lamblia
		Iodamoeba bütschlii
		Retortamonas intestinalis

SOURCE: Adapted from G. P. Youmans, P. Y. Paterson, and H. M. Sommers, *The Biologic and Clinical Basis of Infectious diseases* (Philadelphia: Saunders, 1975) and T. Rosebury, *Microorganisms Indigenous to Man* (New York: McGraw-Hill, 1962).

when antimicrobial therapy destroys competing microorganisms.

Although the ratio of facultative, anaerobic, gram-negative bacilli to obligate anaerobes is 1:300 in the large intestine, attention has been focused on the facultative gram-negative bacilli for many years. *E. coli*, for example, is universally recoverable from stool specimens of healthy individuals. *Klebsiella, Enterobacter, Proteus,* and *Pseudomonas* species, all gram-negative bacilli, also can be found in the intestinal microbiota.

During active enteroviral infections and for varying periods thereafter viruses are shed in feces. In health, however, the enteroviruses are only transient residents as far as is known. Bacteriophages that infect intestinal bacteria can be recovered with regularity from stool specimens.

THE GENITOURINARY TRACT

There are no microorganisms normally residing in the kidneys, ureters, or urinary bladder. In both sexes the numbers of bacteria near the distal end of the urethra are relatively few. The flora are largely a reflection of the organisms of the skin, but often include organisms of intestinal origin as well (Table 11-3). Bacteria inhabiting those anatomic sites in both sexes and the vagina in women constitute the reservoirs for organisms causing urinary tract infection.

The microbial flora of the vagina varies with age and even during the menstrual cycle. Microaerophilic lactobacilli, sometimes called Döderlein's bacilli, colonize the vagina shortly after birth, but disappear as effects of maternal progesterone dissipate. They return to populate the vagina again with the beginning of menses. The vaginal lactobacilli tend to be heterofermentative, but maintain the pH of the vagina below 5.0 (Figure 11-9). Coliforms are inhibited by the acid environment, but more tolerant anaerobic *Bacteroides, Clostridium,* and *Peptostreptococcus* species survive and sometimes flourish. In addition, enterococci, staphylococci, and diphtheroids may be recovered with regularity from vaginal secretions.

Table 11-3 SOME MICROORGANISMS OF THE GENITOURINARY TRACT

GRAM-POSITIVE BACTERIA	GRAM-NEGATIVE BACTERIA	MISCELLANEOUS MICROORGANISMS
Aerobic corynebacteria (diphtheroids)	*Bacteroides species*	*Candida albicans*
Bifidobacterium bifidum	*Enterobacter species*	Herpesviruses
Clostridium species	*Escherichia coli*	*Mycobacterium smegmatis*
Enterococci (group D *Streptococcus*)	*Morganella morganii*	Mycoplasma *hominis*
Lactobacillus species	*Proteus species*	*Trichomonas vaginalis*
Peptostreptococcus	*Pseudomonas species*	*Ureaplasmaurealyticum*
Eubacterium limosum		
Staphylococcus aureus		
Staphylococcus epidermidis		
Streptococcus pyogenes, group B		

SOURCE: Adapted from G. P. Youmans, P. Y. Paterson, and H. M. Sommers, *The Biologic and Clinical Basis of Infectious Diseases* (Philadelphia: Saunders, 1975).

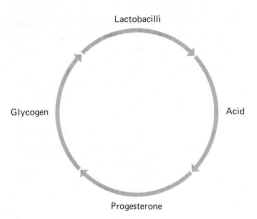

Lactobacilli

Glycogen

Acid

Progesterone

Figure 11-9 Interrelationship of vaginal factors. Progesterone increases the glycogen content of vaginal epithelium. Lactobacilli break down products of glycogen hydrolysis to maintain an acid environment.

The acidity of the vagina is conducive for the growth of *Candida* species. A consequence of the widespread use of birth control pills has been an increase in vaginitis caused by *Candida*. The progesterone-containing pills increase the glycogen content of the vaginal epithelium, supplying a readily fermentable substrate for yeast cells.

Mycoplasmas are ubiquitous inhabitants of male and female genital tracts. Genital mycoplasma colonization increases with the number of sexual partners. *Mycobacterium smegmatis,* an acid-fast bacillus, has been recovered from smegma of the preputial sac or clitoris. The protozoan *Trichomonas vaginalis,* despite its name, may be found in genitourinary tracts of both men and women. Although the organism is most often a resident of the vagina, it is not uncommon to discover it in the bladder, urethra, or vestibular glands.

The cervix may contain a few bacteria, reflecting to a large degree the microbiota of the vagina, but it is often sterile. The vulva contains a mixture of organisms found on the skin and in the vagina.

A herpesvirus, similar to the one which causes fever blisters, has a predilection for the genitalia of both sexes. The virus can cause extensive ulcerative lesions during a primary infection. Its recurrence despite treatment makes it appear possible that it exists in a latent intracellular form, similar to that of the facial herpesvirus.

THE CONCEPT OF PATHOGENICITY

The term *pathogen* is commonly used to refer to a disease-producing organism. It becomes increasingly evident that the ability to produce disease cannot be totally ascribed to an invading organism. The environmental circumstances which permit invasion and proliferation may be of host or microbial origin. The human host presents a continuum of environmental changes, some of which can select for multiplication of one species at the expense of indigenous flora. Characteristics of indigenous microbiota and conditions in particular body parts and surfaces provide quantitative and qualitative stability within healthy individuals. However, alterations in the internal environment can lead to an overgrowth of a particular endogenous organism, which then assumes the posture of a pathogen.

A *nonpathogen* is a microorganism which, under ordinary circumstances, does not produce disease. Since the factors making up the host's defense are in a continuous flux, the ordinary circumstances sometimes elude definition. Therefore, the terms pathogen and nonpathogen are only relative terms and cannot be considered apart from the environment of the host.

SUMMARY

The skin and mucous membranes of the oropharynx, nasopharynx, gastrointestinal tract, and genitourinary tract represent major areas of the body colonized by microorganisms. The indigenous microbiota include a variety of aerobic and anaerobic organisms and often constitute an expression of the immediate environment. The role of indigenous microbiota in health or disease is a function of complex interrelationships between the human host and the microbes and among the indigenous microbiota themselves.

QUESTIONS FOR STUDY

1. Name a microbial habitat on or within the body for each organism.
   Entamoeba gingivalis
   Haemophilus influenzae
   Escherichia coli
   Clostridium perfringens
   Streptococcus mutans
   Actinomyces israelii
   Candida albicans
   Demodex folliculorum

2. What are the most common habitats of viruses on or within the body?
3. How does constipation affect numbers of intestinal bacteria?
4. How does neglect of oral hygiene increase the opportunity for dental disease?
5. Name an effect of each on proliferation and type of microorganisms constituting normal flora.
   moisture generated by exercise
   oral antimicrobial medication
   formation of diverticula
   consumption
      of sugar-laden foods
   use of oral contraceptives

SELECTED REFERENCES

Bockus, H. L. *Gastroenterology.* 3rd ed. Philadelphia: Saunders, 1976.

Burnett, G. W., and Scherp, H. W. *Oral Microbiology and Infectious Disease.* Vol. 3. Baltimore: Williams & Wilkins, 1968.

David, C., and Finland, M. *Obstetric and Perinatal Infections.* Philadelphia: Lea & Febiger, 1973.

Fenner, F.; McAuslan, B. R.; Mims, C. A.; Sambrook, J.; and White, D. O. *The Biology of Animal Viruses.* 2d ed. New York: Academic Press, 1974.

McBride, M. E.; Duncan, W. C.; Bodey, G. P.; and McBride, C. M. Microbial skin flora of selected cancer patients and hospital personnel. *J. Clin. Microbiol.* 3:14, 1976.

Marples, M. J. Life on the human skin. *Sci. Am.* 220:108, 1969.

Pillsburg, D. M., and Rebell, G. The bacterial flora of the skin. *J. Invest. Dermatol.* 18:173, 1952.

Rosebury, T. *Microorganisms Indigenous to Man.* New York: McGraw-Hill, 1962.

Schlessinger, D. *Microbiology—1975.* Washington, D.C.: American Society for Microbiology, 1975.

William, R. E. O. Healthy carriage of *Staphylococcus aureus:* its prevalence and importance. *Bacteriol. Rev.* 27:56, 1963.

Wistreich, G. A., and Lechtman, M. D. *Microbiology and Human Disease.* 2d ed. Beverly Hills, Calif: Glencoe Press, 1976.

Youmans, G. P.; Paterson, P. Y.; and Sommers, H. M. *The Biologic and Clinical Basis of Infectious Diseases.* Philadelphia: Saunders, 1975.

Chapter 12

The Nature of Immunity

After you read this chapter, you should be able to:

1. Differentiate between natural and acquired immunity.
2. Describe the factors which influence natural immunity.
3. Contrast the roles of polymorphonuclear and mononuclear phagocytes in resistance.
4. Explain the basis of species, racial, and individual natural immunity.
5. Differentiate between active and passive immunity.
6. Define antigen, antibody, hapten, adjuvant, anamnestic response, and immunoglobulin.
7. Describe five classes of immunoglobulins.
8. Discuss two types of antigen-antibody binding.
9. Explain the role of T-cell and B-cell lymphocytes in cellular and humoral immunity.
10. Explain why tumor-associated antigens can be expected to initiate an immune response.

Vertebrates have been exposed to infectious agents throughout their existence on earth. Defense mechanisms of vertebrate hosts have evolved which herald the presence of invading microorganisms and attempt to destroy them. Microorganisms, however, have developed their own defense mechanisms to ward off the responses of their hosts. The persistence of infectious agents as causes of disease is evidence that microorganisms have been successful in overcoming defense mechanisms of their hosts.

NATURAL IMMUNITY

The ability of a vertebrate host to resist infectious disease without previous contact with the causative agent is called innate or *natural immunity*. It de-

pends on nutritional status, age, stress factors, environmental factors, phagocytic activity, and certain nonspecific resistance factors present in cells or fluids of the host.

NUTRITIONAL STATUS

It is not always possible to separate effects of malnutrition from socioeconomic factors. The undernourished are often the products of an environment where crowding, inadequate housing, and poor hygiene also prevail. The incidence of communicable disease is high in developing countries where a severe form of protein deficiency, known as kwashiorkor, is common (Figure 12-1). Deficiencies of vitamins A, B, and C affect the integrity of mucosal surfaces and increase susceptibility to infections. Protein deficiency interferes with production of both specific and nonspecific resistance factors.

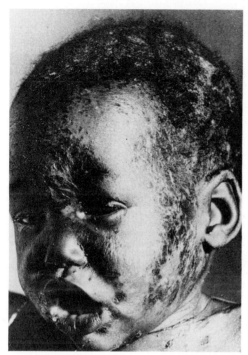

Figure 12-1 A victim of severe kwashiorkor. Classical symptoms include blotchy, discolored, or scaly skin. (Courtesy, World Health Organization, Geneva.)

AGE

Susceptibility to infectious agents is greater in the very young and the very old. In infants the ability to combat the effects of infectious agents has not been fully developed. Moreover, the bronchial airways of infants are narrow and easily blocked. In addition, vomiting or diarrhea can be very serious in infants as it often leads to acid-base imbalances. The buffering capacity of the blood is exhausted by any prolonged loss of fluids.

In persons of advanced age the efficiency of immune responses often suffers a decline. It is sometimes difficult to separate age and nutritional factors as contributory factors in infections in the elderly because anorexia (loss of appetite) and malabsorption syndromes are common.

STRESS FACTORS

Infection in itself constitutes stress for the vertebrate host. Stress of any nature is known to stimulate the release of hormones known as corticosteroids from the adrenal glands. Any persistent increases in circulating levels of corticosteroids, mediated by stress, can probably trigger opportunistic microorganisms to promote infections. For example, the bacillus of tuberculosis proliferates rapidly if corticosteroids are administered.

ENVIRONMENTAL FACTORS

The environment of any vertebrate host is complex and it is difficult, if not impossible, to incriminate one particular factor as predisposing to infectious disease. An exception is, however, the association of silica particles with respiratory disease. Silica particles occur in sandstone, granite, shale, and other irritants sometimes encountered by miners. Alveolar macrophages become destroyed or damaged following phagocytosis of silica particles. Nodules of debris accumulate and often interfere with oxygenation in the lung and drainage of lymph by blocking capillaries and lymphatic vessels. The lack of functioning macrophages, hypoxia, and inadequate drainage of lymph causes increased susceptibility to both pneumonia and tuberculosis.

PHAGOCYTIC ACTIVITY

Phagocytes are quick to respond once microorganisms invade tissue. There are two types of phagocytes: polymorphonuclear white blood cells and mononuclear macrophages. The polymorphonuclear and mononuclear phagocytes, despite their diversity of location, comprise the reticuloendothelial system (RES).

Among the most active polymorphonuclear white blood cells (PMN's) are the *neutrophils* which make up 50 to 70 percent of the total circulating leukocytes. The cytoplasm of neutrophils has large numbers of *lysosomes*, which contain many types of hydrolytic enzymes. The neutrophils are often the first cells to appear in areas of the body invaded by microorganisms (Figure 12-2). *Eosinophils*, another type of leukocyte, are not as effective as neutrophils in destroying microorganisms, but are able to phagocytize antigen-antibody complexes. The role of *basophils* in infections is less well understood. The ingestion of particles is facilitated by *opsonin*, a serum component which promotes adherence of invaders to the surface of the phagocytes.

The macrophages include the monocytes, their precursor cells in bone marrow, and cells found in certain tissues of the body. Macrophages are divided into two groups: wandering and fixed (sessile) cells. The wandering cells circulate in peripheral blood and accumulate in large numbers in infected tissues in later stages of inflammation. The fixed cells reside permanently in various tissues. Macrophages of connective tissue are more specifically designated as *histiocytes*. Macrophages of the liver, bone, and nerve tissue are known as *Kupffer cells, osteoclasts,* and *microglial cells,* respectively.

Phagocytosis is not specifically directed against microorganisms since worn-out cells are also ingested by macrophages. Particles ingested by phagocytes are broken down by enzymes or processed in such a manner that they stimulate other white blood cells, the *lymphocytes,* to produce substances which further enhance the action of macrophages. The physiologically active substances made by lymphocytes

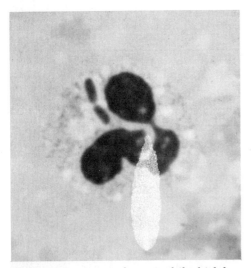

Figure 12-2 A typical neutrophil which has engulfed two cells of *Clostridium perfringens.* (Courtesy, M. R. Talluto, Rochester, New York.)

in response to processed particles are called *lymphokines*.

NONSPECIFIC RESISTANCE FACTORS

A variety of nonspecific factors associated with cells or fluid of vertebrate hosts contributes to resistance. The mechanism of action for some nonspecific resistance factors is well known; the exact protective role of other factors is less clear.

Lysozyme. The enzyme lysozyme is abundant in biological fluids, such as tears, mucus, saliva, and in granules of phagocytes. The antimicrobial action of lysozyme is related to the ability of the enzyme to destroy cell walls of susceptible gram-positive bacteria. The enzyme splits the linkages between amino acids and *N*-acetylmuramic or *N*-acetylglucosamine components of the walls. The lipopolysaccharide component of gram-negative bacteria enables those organisms to resist the action of lysozyme.

Complement. Complement consists of at least 11 proteins present in normal serum. Complement is bactericidal for gram-negative bacteria. The major function of complement is to activate successive proteins in a cascade of enzyme reactions (Figure 12-3). Component C1 is activated when it combines with antigen-antibody complexes. The newly formed alliance causes C3 to attract polymorphonuclear leukocytes and promotes the release of histamine. The binding of the C3 component to the white blood cells enhances phagocytic activity. Phospholipase, an enzyme activated later in the chain of complement events, damages membranes of microorganisms causing them to lyse.

Properdin. Properdin consists of at least four proteins, distinct from the complement system, which also serve to enhance inflammatory and phagocytic responses. Properdin is active against some viruses and gram-negative bacteria. Properdin activates C3 by an alternate pathway when it reacts with the surfaces of microorganisms.

Interferons. Interferons are small molecular weight proteins produced by virus-infected cells. An interferon acts on surrounding cells protecting them from subsequent viral infection by inducing the synthesis of an antiviral protein (Figure 12-4). Interferons are species specific, that is, act only upon cells of the same species, but are not virus specific. The rapidity with which interferons are produced in virus-infected cells limits the spread of viruses while more specific defense factors are being readied for battle.

Indigenous Flora. The indigenous microbiota of many parts of the body inhibit colonization of pathogens by competing for food, altering physical factors in the immediate environment, or producing antimicrobial substances. Moreover, the presence of indigenous flora appears to keep vertebrate hosts primed to produce antibodies swiftly when they are invaded by foreign microorganisms.

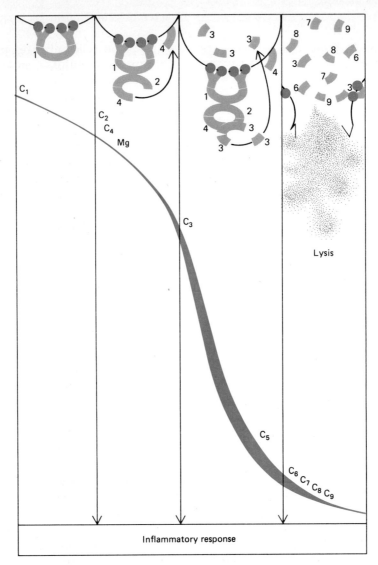

Figure 12-3 Sequential activation of complement components in production of the inflammatory response.

TYPES OF NATURAL IMMUNITY

If nonspecific factors were not so successful in providing resistance to infectious agents, the human host would succumb to their devastating influences before antibodies, with their greater specificity, could be synthesized. Despite exposure to potential pathogens, some persons do not become ill. There are many examples in which the natural

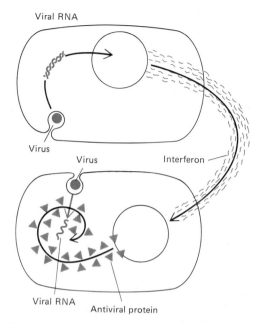

Viral RNA

Virus

Virus   Interferon

Viral RNA

Antiviral protein

Figure 12-4 Mechanism of interferon induction and action. Double-stranded viral RNA initiates production of interferon which is released by the cell. Interferon initiates production of antiviral protein which blocks replication of unrelated viral RNA.

immune mechanisms provide resistance, but they can usually be classified as types of *species, racial,* or *individual* immunity.

Species Immunity. Microorganisms demonstrate varying degrees of host specificity. Some bacteria, like the anthrax bacillus, affect most herbivorous animals and humans; other bacteria, such as the causative agents of gonorrhea, syphilis, and measles, cause disease only in the human host. One of the characteristics of most viruses is host specificity. The specificity is so advanced in bacteria-phage systems that a single species of a bacterium can be divided into multiple phage types.

Racial Immunity. It is difficult, if not impossible, to substantiate examples of immunity on a purely genetic basis. Socioeconomic factors contribute immeasurably to the incidence of infectious disease among the races. For example, the incidence of tuberculosis is higher in blacks and American Indians than in whites. Dark-skinned individuals are more susceptible to the disseminated form of coccidioidomycosis than light-skinned individuals. However, the reasons for these differences may be environmental rather than genetic in origin.

A clear example of genetically related immunity is the resistance of blacks with sickle cell anemia to the protozoan causing malaria. Red blood cells containing sickle cell hemoglobin instead of normal hemoglobin cannot adequately support the oxygen requirements of malarial organisms.

Individual Immunity. Individual resistance can probably be explained by both nonspecific and specific factors. Some persons, for example, appear particularly prone to respiratory infections, while others rarely even have a cold. Resistance to specific infectious agents also occurs in individuals. It is believed by most that such persons may have had an unrecognized form of a particular infectious disease to which they appear immune. Even in the absence of symptoms, sufficient stimulation of antibody-producing cells could supply subsequent protection. It has been established that immune responses are genetically determined, but mechanisms governing responsiveness are complex and not well understood.

ACQUIRED IMMUNITY

The ability of a vertebrate host to resist infectious disease as a result of previous contact with the causative organism is called *acquired immunity*. Such immunity may be acquired *naturally* through placental transmission or by having the disease. It may be acquired *artificially* by vaccination. Naturally or artificially acquired immunity may be *active*, that is, derived from the host's

responses to the infectious agent, or *passive*, that is, received by the host in the form of ready-made substances (Table 12-1).

If a susceptible individual is exposed to most bacteria or certain products of bacterial metabolism, the body's response is the production of antibodies which will afford protection against subsequent exposures. Such immunity is naturally acquired and is active because of the participation by the host. The antibodies are the basis of *humoral immunity*.

If a susceptible individual is exposed to fungi or some viruses, one type of lymphocyte is sensitized and produces lymphokines. The resulting immunity is also naturally acquired and active. The sensitized lymphocytes and their

Table 12-1 EXAMPLES OF ARTIFICIAL ACTIVE AND PASSIVE IMMUNIZATION

DISEASE	FORM OF IMMUNIZATION	TYPE OF PREPARATION
Diphtheria Pertussis Tetanus	active	DPT*
Measles Mumps Rubella	active	combined vaccine
Polio	active	TOPV†
Typhoid	active	vaccine
Cholera	active	vaccine
Smallpox	active	vaccine
Infectious hepatitis	passive	hyperimmune globulin
Rh hemolytic disease	passive	anti-Rho globulin
Tetanus	passive	TAT‡

* DPT—diphtheria and tetanus toxoid with pertussis vaccine.
† TOPV—trivalent oral polio virus vaccine.
‡ TAT—tetanus antitoxin.
NOTE: See Appendix C for recommended immunization schedules for children and adults in the United States.
SOURCE: Adapted from B. H. Park and R. A. Good, *Principles of Modern Immunology: Basic and Clinical* (Philadelphia: Lea & Febiger, 1974).

products, the lymphokines, are the basis of *cellular immunity*.

If, instead, an individual is vaccinated with killed or attenuated bacteria or their products, antibodies are produced, but without the trauma and risk of having an infection. The resulting immunity is also active, but is artificially acquired. The host participates in producing antibodies, but in response to an artificial situation made possible by forced contact with the organisms or their products. The antibodies formed afford protection in the event of subsequent exposure to the organisms in a manner not unlike those antibodies produced as a result of actually having the disease. Similarly, a vaccine of killed or attenuated viruses sensitizes lymphocytes and stimulates production of lymphokines. The resulting active cellular immunity is artificially acquired, rather than naturally acquired through infection by the viruses.

The acquisition of ready-made antibodies is passive immunity. Placental transmission of maternal antibodies is an example of naturally acquired passive immunity; the infant does not contribute to the antibody-making process. Ready-made antibodies may also be administered artificially to protect individuals from particular diseases. Inoculation with an immune globulin after possible contact with the viruses of hepatitis is an example of artificially acquired passive immunity. Antibodies acquired passively are immediately available for use in the host's defense against an invading organism, but do not provide protection which lasts as

long as that afforded by contact with the actual microorganisms or their products.

The administration of an extract of human blood lymphocytes, known as *transfer factor*, in cell-mediated deficiency states also constitutes a means of supplying ready-made products important in cellular immune mechanisms and is, therefore, also a form of artificially acquired passive immunity.

IMMUNE RESPONSES

The study of immune responses in microbiology is concerned with natural biologic substances of microbial origin and products of the host developed in response to microbial invasion. Contact with certain pathogens causes little or no immunologic response. The immunity promoted by exposure to other pathogens endures for a lifetime. Differences in immune responses by humans can be explained by both the nature of the contributions made by microorganisms and those made by the host.

THE NATURE OF ANTIGENS

Materials foreign to a host, including microorganisms, that can initiate production of antibodies are called *antigens*. Antigens are substances with molecular weights of 10,000 daltons or higher. Proteins are the most effective antigens, but polysaccharides and lipoproteins can also initiate antibody response. Many components or products of microorganisms are antigenic. Antigens may be associated with components of cell walls, cell membranes, capsules, chromosomes, pili, or flagella. In addition, certain products of microbial metabolism are capable of stimulating antibody production. Some substances of low molecular weight are capable of invoking antibody response only if they are bound to a carrier protein. Such substances are called incomplete antigens or *haptens*. Antigens may be *particulate*, that is, contained on a particle, such as a bacterium or virus, or *soluble*, that is, exist in a dissolved state in body fluid. All naturally occurring antigens are *multivalent*, meaning that they contain multiple sites for antibody binding.

Antibody production may be enhanced by the simultaneous injection of substances known as *adjuvants*. The materials act in some manner to decrease the solubility of the antigen, enhance immunogenicity (capacity to stimulate an immune response) of the antigen, or promote action of macrophages. Alum, which consists of potassium aluminum sulfate, is an example of an adjuvant used in diphtheria or tetanus toxoids for human immunizations.

Vaccination introduces antigens into the host's body in the form of killed or attenuated microorganisms or their products. Antibodies that act specifically against the antigens used not only are produced in large numbers upon vaccination, but also provide the host with *memory*, so that the ability to make the antibodies is recalled when the host

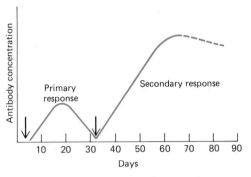

Figure 12-5 Primary and secondary antibody response to injections of antigen.

comes in contact with the antigens again. A subsequent response, known as a secondary or *anamnestic* antibody response, is not only more rapid and greater in magnitude, but the antibodies are longer lasting than those elicited by the primary stimulus (Figure 12-5). The secondary response is the basis of so-called booster shots in immunization programs.

THE NATURE OF ANTIBODIES

Antibodies are high molecular weight plasma proteins, known as *immunoglobulins*, produced in response to the introduction of antigens in an immunologically competent host. The ability to synthesize antibodies in response to antigenic stimulation is unique to vertebrates. Five classes of immunoglobulins, differing in molecular weights, sedimentation constants, and mobility properties in an electric field, have been described (Table 12-2).

The most abundant immunoglobulin is IgG. It is the antibody fraction which

Table 12-2 SOME PROPERTIES OF HUMAN IMMUNOGLOBULINS

	IgG	IgM	IgA	IgD	IgE
Molecular weight	150,000	900,000	170,000	150,000	200,000
Sedimentation constant	7S	19S	7, 9, 11, and 13S	7S	8S
Electrophoretic mobility	γ	slow β	between γ and β	between γ and β	slow β
Serum concentration (gm/100 ml)	1.2	0.4	0.12	0.003	0.0005
Placental transfer	+	−	−	−	−
Carbohydrate content	2.5%	5–10%	5–10%	−	13%
Distribution	blood, body fluids	blood	blood, body fluids, secretions	blood	skin, respiratory and GI tracts, blood

crosses the placenta providing immunity to the newborn. IgM is the largest immunoglobulin molecule. It is usually produced during the primary antibody response. IgG and IgM antibodies are responsible for 85 to 90 percent of the total antibody activity against disease-producing microorganisms or their products. IgA is the predominant immunoglobulin in body secretions, such as tears, saliva, and mucus. IgA appears to be a significant defense mechanism against infections of the respiratory tract. IgD is present in only very small amounts in human plasma. No specific biological role has yet been established for antibodies of this class. IgE also occurs in minute amounts in normal human plasma, but it increases in particular allergies and parasitic diseases of man.

All immunoglobulins have two types of amino acid chains: heavy chains with molecular weights of 55,000 to 75,000 daltons and light chains with molecular weights of approximately 23,000 daltons. Each of the five classes of immunoglobulins has a different heavy chain; a single light chain is common to

all immunoglobulins. Both light and heavy chains have areas of constant and variable amino acid sequences. Constant amino acid sequences are found in carboxyl (COOH) regions of chains; variable sequences are found in the amino (NH_2) regions of chains.

The binding sites of immunoglobulins are located near the end of the four variable chains having terminal NH_2 groups (Figure 12-6). All except IgM contain two binding sites. An IgM molecule is shaped like a star with five identical rays each of which contains

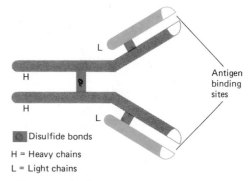

Disulfide bonds
H = Heavy chains
L = Light chains

Figure 12-6 Diagram of light and heavy chains of an IgG molecule connected by disulfide bonds.

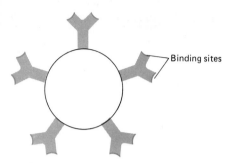

Figure 12-7   Diagram of an IgM molecule. Each ray has two binding sites and resembles the shape of an IgG antibody molecule.

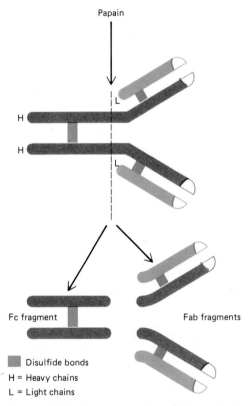

Figure 12-8   Diagram of fragments of IgG molecule produced by treatment with papain. Two Fab fragments with antibody activity and one Fc fragment with no antibody activity are formed.

two binding sites (Figure 12-7). Combining sites of IgG molecules are located on portions known as Fab fragments (Figure 12-8). If IgG is treated with the enzyme papain, it splits the molecule above a connecting point supplied by a disulfide bond that holds the heavy chains together, and three fragments are formed. One piece, the *Fc fragment*, consists of two constant regions of the heavy chain still joined. The other two pieces, the *Fab fragments*, contain all the variable regions of the heavy and light chains. Only the Fab fragments have antibody activity. The enzyme pepsin splits IgG below the same disulfide bond and produces the *F (ab')$_2$ fragment*, that contains two combining sites (Figure 12-9). The Fc fragment is partially digested by pepsin.

Source of Antibodies.   The immunoglobulins are synthesized by B-cell lymphocytes and their progeny, the plasma cells. The name *B-cells* is derived from the term bursa of Fabricius, the lymphoid organ in chickens that is necessary for the development and maturation of the lymphocytes that synthesize antibodies. Although the exact anatomical site responsible for this function in humans has not been determined, it is believed that the bursa equivalent may be lymphoid tissue found in Peyer's patches, tonsils, and the appendix. It is known that B-cells originate from the same stem cell in the bone marrow as thymus-dependent lymphocytes or *T-cells*, which synthesize lymphokines (Figure 12-10).

Biologic Role of Antibodies.   Not all classes of immunoglobulins produced

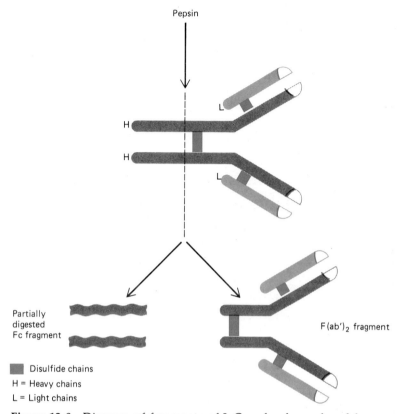

Figure 12-9 Diagram of fragments of IgG molecule produced by treatment with pepsin. One F(ab')$_2$ fragment with antibody activity and a partially digested Fc fragment are formed.

upon antigenic stimulation are protective. Some antibodies, such as antitoxins for diphtheria, tetanus, or botulism, do provide significant protection against diseases, but others are inactive and do not appreciably alter either susceptibility to disease or the course of disease. Still others may be harmful to the host; for example, the antibodies initiated by a streptococcal antigen cross-react with cardiac muscle tissue and cause rheumatic fever. The protective antibodies may be used success-

fully in a number of immunization procedures to guard against infectious diseases.

Antigen-Antibody Binding. The bonds formed between antigens and their antibodies are highly specific, but relatively weak. The "lock and key" model proposed by Ehrlich is useful in describing the specificity of these reactions in general terms, but the molecular forces contributing to the phenomenon are more complex. The two

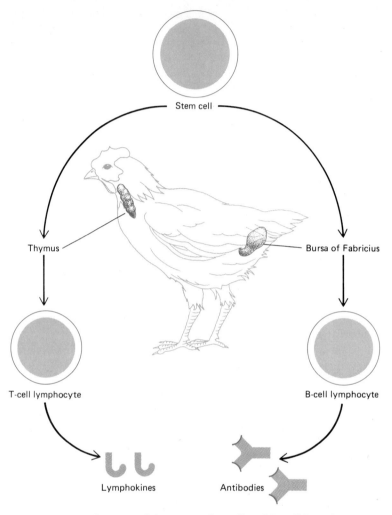

Figure 12-10   Origin and function of T-cell and B-cell lymphocytes in the chicken.

principal weak bonds between antigens and antibodies are formed by electrostatic or van der Waals forces (Figure 12-11). *Electrostatic bonds* occur between oppositely charged particles on the antigen and antibody molecules. The *van der Waals interactions* are caused by attraction between molecules in motion. Large concentrations of molecules reduce the distance between molecules and increase the opportunity for interaction.

Electrostatic and van der Waals forces position molecules in a manner which

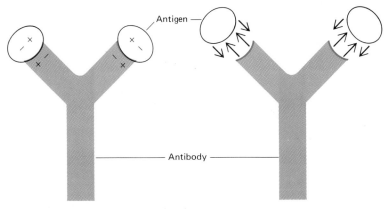

Figure 12-11 Mechanisms of antigen-antibody binding. The electrostatic force is the attraction between oppositely charged particles on the antigen and antibody molecules. The van der Waals force is the attraction between antigen and antibody molecules in motion.

favors hydrogen bonding between *hydrophilic* (hydrogen-loving) groups, such as OH or NH_2 groups, and the hydrogen of a COOH group (Figure 12-12). *Hydrophobic* (hydrogen-hating) groups of antigens and antibodies do not bind with hydrogen in the environment. Since a large amount of hydrogen is associated with water molecules, the greater the number of hydrophobic groups on antigens and antibodies, the

lesser will be the net surface in contact with water. The effect is a close contact or bonding between antigens and antibodies. Antigen-antibody complexes formed in this manner are more susceptible to the action of phagocytes than antigenic material alone. The term *avidity* is used to describe the strength of binding between antigens and antibodies; it is related to the valency of the reactants.

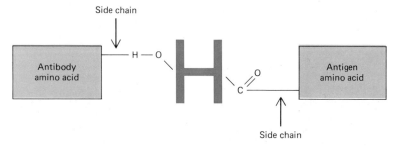

Figure 12-12 Hydrogen bonding between side chains of amino acids of an antigen and an antibody.

Table 12-3 MEDIATORS OF CELLULAR IMMUNITY

LYMPHOKINE	FUNCTION
Migration-inhibitory factor (MIF)	suppresses *in vitro* migration of macrophages
Skin-reactive factor (SRF)	produces an inflammatory reaction in experimental animals
Cytotoxic factor (CF)	destroys target cells *in vitro*
Lymphocyte transforming factor (LTF)	induces nonsensitized lymphocytes to undergo blast-cell transformation
Chemotaxin	attracts macrophages *in vitro*
Macrophage activation factor (MAF)	stimulates macrophage activity *in vitro*

THE NATURE OF LYMPHOKINES

A large number of lymphokines released by or extracted from sensitized lymphocytes have biological activities believed to contribute to cellular immunity (Table 12-3). The activities of lymphokines have been demonstrated largely by employing *in vitro* systems. An exception is the inflammatory skin reaction in guinea pigs, when they are injected with skin-reactive factor (SRF). The role of the lymphokines in cellular immunity *in vivo* is not clear, but individuals with impaired cellular responses are susceptible to chronic infections. The various lymphokines may act synergistically to mobilize phagocytes and lymphocytes at the site of antigen deposition.

The Source of Lymphokines. The lymphokines are synthesized by T-cell or thymus-dependent lymphocytes. The thymus is a small organ found in the young of most vertebrates at the base of the neck or in the upper chest. In humans it is found in the chest cavity of children; it shrinks by the time of puberty and ultimately disappears (Figure 12-13). The thymus is necessary for the development and maturation of approximately 70 to 80 percent of the lymphocyte population. The T-lymphocyte

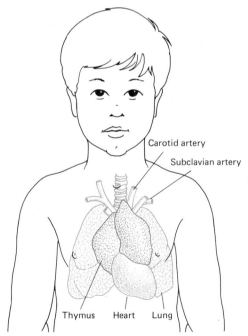

Figure 12-13 Thymus organ in chest cavity of a child. The thymus is located partly behind the lungs, behind the sternum, and in front of the aorta.

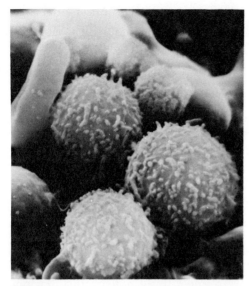

Figure 12-14 A scanning electron micrograph of peripheral blood lymphocytes showing B-cells with large numbers of microvilli and smoother-appearing T-cells with fewer numbers of microvilli. (Courtesy, A. Polliack, Jerusalem, Israel.)

foreign to the host and should induce an immune response. The search for cancer-associated antigens has revealed that cell-surface antigens differing from host antigens are present in Burkitt's lymphoma, malignant melanoma, neuroblastoma, and osteosarcoma. In addition, two antigens have been discovered in tumors of the gastrointestinal tract and the liver. Both these antigens are identical to substances present in fetal life which fall to undetectable levels upon birth. Carcinoembryonic antigen (CEA) is found in neoplasms of the gastrointestinal tract; alpha-fetoprotein is present in the serum of individuals with primary liver cancer. The mechanism which permits synthesis of fetal antigens is not understood.

It has been proposed that escape mechanisms exist which account for the

system monitors the recognition of self from nonself on living cells and also aids B-cells, in some manner, to produce antibodies. In electron microscope studies an abundance of microvilli on the surface of B-cells sometimes gives them a rougher appearance than T-cells (Figure 12-14).

IMMUNOLOGY OF CANCER

Tumor-associated antigens appear on the surface of cancer cells as a result of malignant transformation (Figure 12-15). Tumor antigens are, in a sense,

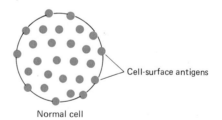
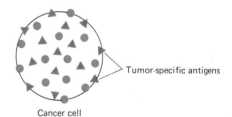

Figure 12-15 Cell-surface antigens. Both normal cell-surface antigens and tumor-associated antigens appear on the cancer cell.

growth of tumor cells. Cancer cells may not be recognized by T-cell lymphocytes during early stages of growth or, in some manner, may resist attacks by the immune system. Alternately, a flood of tumor antigens might tie up available cytotoxic antibodies or receptors on lymphocytes.

There is some evidence that cellular and humoral immunity may sometimes act in an antagonistic manner. For example, some types of tumor growth are enhanced by the presence of blocking antibodies produced in response to tumor-associated antigens. Cellular immune mechanisms may not be able to eliminate a tumor by rejection because of interference by the antibodies. A better understanding of immune responses, including those related to tumors, may lead one day to immunotherapy or immunoprophylaxis for cancer in a manner similar to that which now prevents many devastating infectious diseases.

SUMMARY

Both specific and nonspecific factors provide vertebrates with resistance to invading microorganisms. Immunity may be natural, that is, present without previous contact with the organism, or acquired by contact with an infectious agent or its products or by administration of immune globulins or lymphocyte extracts. Five classes of immunoglobulins, produced by B-cell lymphocytes, are now recognized as the specific factors of humoral immunity. The lymphokines, derived from T-cell lymphocytes, constitute the mediators of cellular immunity. Tumor-associated antigens, occurring on the surface of transformed cells in some types of cancer, stimulate cellular and humoral immune responses. The number of deaths caused by infectious agents has been dramatically reduced by artificial active and passive immunizations. To date, immunotherapeutic agents that can selectively regulate immune responses in cancer are not available.

QUESTIONS FOR STUDY

1. Differentiate between natural and acquired immunity.
2. Name five nonspecific factors which contribute to natural immunity.
3. Name the major phagocytes of the human host.
4. Give an example of each type of immunity.
   naturally acquired
      passive immunity
   artificially acquired
      active immunity
   naturally acquired
      active immunity
   artificially acquired
      passive immunity
5. Differentiate between B-cell and T-cell lymphocytes and explain their role in immunity.
6. Name five classes of immunoglobulins and describe where each is found on the human host.
7. List five *in vitro* reactions of lymphokines.
8. What is the significance of tumor-associated antigens?

SELECTED REFERENCES

Bach, F. H., and Good, R. A. *Clinical Immunobiology*. Vol. 1. New York: Academic Press, 1972.

Good, R. A., and Fisher, D. W. *Immunobiology*. Stamford, Conn.: Sinauer, 1973.

Gordon, B. L., and Ford, D. K. *Essentials of Immunology*. Philadelphia: Davis, 1971.

Humphrey, J. H., and White, R. G. *Immunology for Students of Medicine*. 3rd ed. Philadelphia: Davis, 1970.

Mims, C. A. *The Pathogenesis of Infectious Disease*. New York: Grune & Stratton, 1976.

Park, B. H., and Good, R. A. *Principles of Modern Immunobiology: Basic and Clinical*. Philadelphia: Lea & Febiger, 1974.

Roitt, I. M. *Essential Immunology*. 2d ed. Oxford: Blackwell Scientific Publications, 1974.

Rose, N. R.; Milgrom, F.; and Van Oss, C. J. *Principles of Immunology*. New York: Macmillan, 1973.

Schwartz, R. S. *Progress in Clinical Immunology*. Vol. 2. New York: Grune & Stratton, 1974.

Sell, S. *Immunology, Immunopathology, and Immunity*. New York: Harper & Row, 1972.

van Furth, R. *Mononuclear Phagocytes*. Oxford: Blackwell Scientific Publications, 1970.

Chapter 13

Types of Hypersensitivity Reactions

After you read this chapter, you should be able to:

1. List four basic types of immediate hypersensitivity.
2. Explain the role of histamine and slow-reacting substance of anaphylaxis (SRS-A) in systemic anaphylaxis.
3. Provide names and descriptions of three common types of localized anaphylaxis.
4. Compare the target cells of anaphylactic and cytotoxic hypersensitivity.
5. Define isoagglutinogens, isoagglutinins, and immune isoagglutinins.
6. Identify the isoagglutinogens and isoagglutinins of the major blood groups.
7. Contrast the cause of ABO incompatibility with the cause of Rh incompatibility.
8. Describe the basis for classifying hemolytic anemia, lupus erythematosis, rheumatoid arthritis, rheumatic fever, and acute glomerulonephritis as autoimmune reactions.
9. Give three examples of hypersensitivity mediated by immune complexes.
10. Explain what determines the location of antigen-antibody deposits in immune complex-mediated hypersensitivity.
11. Explain the basis for categorizing one type of hyperthyroidism as a hypersensitivity.
12. Define autograft, syngraft, allograft, and xenograft.
13. Explain the cell-mediated responses involved in the Mantoux skin test, contact dermatitis, graft rejection, and graft-versus-host reactions.
14. Describe four therapeutic approaches to hypersensitivity.

If an individual with humoral antibodies or sensitized lymphocytes produces tissue-damaging reactions upon subsequent exposure to the antigen, the term *hypersensitivity* is applied to the altered response. Some persons are disposed genetically to react in an abnormal way to environmental agents; other individuals acquire an altered state of responsiveness to particular antigens. The antigens are frequently called *allergens* and the state of hypersensitivity may be called an *allergy*. An allergy that appears to have a hereditary basis is called an *atopy*.

Although states of hypersensitivity have classically been categorized as *immediate* or *delayed,* depending upon the time required after exposure to an allergen for symptoms to occur, other differences may be more important. Five types of tissue-damaging reactions have been described. The immediate hypersensitivities (types I, II, III, and V) depend on the interaction of allergens with humoral antibodies. The reactions tend to occur relatively soon after contact with the allergen. A single classification (type IV) is used to categorize delayed hypersensitivities. Type IV reactions involve antibodies on T-cell lymphocytes. Reactions are usually evident several hours to several days after exposure to allergens (Table 13-1).

TYPE I
ANAPHYLACTIC
HYPERSENSITIVITY

Anaphylactic-type reactions involve the release of tissue-damaging agents by mast cells or circulating basophils when allergens combine with membrane-associated antibodies. The mast cells and

Table 13-1   MAJOR CHARACTERISTICS OF FIVE TYPES OF HYPERSENSITIVITY

	I	II	III	IV	V
Antibody	humoral; homocytotropic	humoral; cytotoxic	humoral; soluble	T-cell bound	humoral; tissue-specific
Antigen	exogenous	endogenous	exogenous	exogenous or endogenous	endogenous
Response to intradermal antigen	1/2 hr	none	3–8 hr	24–48 hr	none
Activation of complement	−	+	+	−	−
Release of vasoactive agents	+	−	−	−	−
Transferability	serum	serum	serum	transfer factor	serum
Example	asthma	erythroblastosis fetalis	serum sickness	allograft rejection	thyrotoxicosis

SOURCE: Adapted from I. Roitt, *Essential Immunology*, 2d ed. (Oxford: Blackwell Scientific Publications, 1974).

basophils are called *target cells;* the specific antibodies are called *homocytotrophic* because of their affinity for target-cell surfaces of the species in which they are produced. The antibodies belong to the IgE class of immunoglobulins. They are also sometimes called *reagins*, a name originally given to them because sensitivity can be transferred from the allergic patient to a normal individual by intracutaneous injection of serum. The reactions of allergens and homocytotrophic antibodies on the surface of mast cells and basophils cause an explosive degranulation and secretion of biologically active agents, including vasoactive amines which affect blood vessels (Figure 13-1).

SYSTEMIC ANAPHYLAXIS

A sudden, sometimes fatal, vasomotor collapse occurring upon exposure to an allergen is called *systemic anaphylaxis.* The most important substance released from mast cells and basophils into surrounding tissue is *histamine.* Histamine causes contraction of smooth muscle, principally in the lungs, dilation of capillaries, increased vascular permeability, and, ultimately, collapse due to shock.

Histamine is rapidly degraded after release, but other chemical agents serve to sustain the muscle contraction and capillary dilatation. *Slow-reacting substance of anaphylaxis* (SRS-A) is released from the lungs in IgE-mediated reactions. It is generated only in response to the allergen-antibody reaction on the membrane of mast cells and is not contained in storage depots, like histamine. A number of other biologically active agents such as bradykinin, acetylcholine, and serotonin may have lesser roles in anaphylaxis in some species. Systemic anaphylaxis in humans is

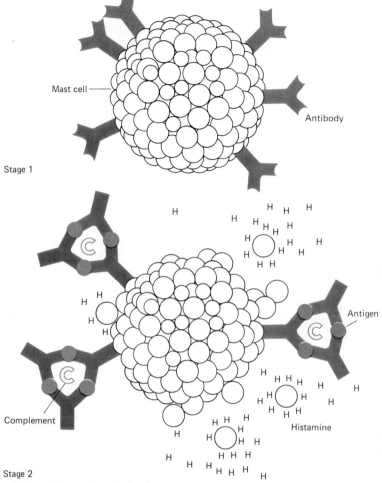

Mast cell

Antibody

Stage 1

Antigen

Complement

Histamine

Stage 2

Figure 13-1 Anaphylactic hypersensitivity (type I). In stage 1 antibodies attach to the surface of a mast cell. In stage 2 histamine is secreted during degranulation of the mast cell in the presence of complement.

quite rare. The ensuing circulatory collapse can be reversed by prompt treatment with epinephrine and antihistamines.

LOCALIZED ANAPHYLAXIS

Asthma, hay fever, and urticaria are examples of IgE-mediated reactions with exogenous allergens. The symptoms are the result of the release of biologically active agents, such as histamine and SRS-A, from mast cells of the involved tissues. The reactions occur in the respiratory, conjunctival, or intestinal mucosa. Asthma and hay fever, particularly, appear to run in families and may be atopic. The homocytotrophic antibodies are reaginic. Common allergens are pollen, animal danders, and ordinary house dust.

Intrinsic asthma, in which no exogenous allergen can be identified, appears to be more complex.

TYPE II
CYTOTOXIC HYPERSENSITIVITY

Cytotoxic-type reactions occur when cell-membrane associated antigens react with humoral antibodies causing cell destruction. The antigens are frequently bound to red blood cells, but may be present on the surface of other somatic cells. The cells containing the surface antigens are also called *target cells,* but should not be confused with the target cells of anaphylactic-type hypersensitivity which have membrane-bound antibodies.

The antibodies are called *cytotoxic* because of their ability to attack cells. The effect of cytotoxic antibodies on target cells is dependent on the ability of the antibodies to promote contact with phagocytes and activate comple-

ment. The complexing of antigen and antibody with complement at a single site causes lysis of a red blood cell, a process designated as *hemolysis* (Figure 13-2). Other somatic cells are more resistant to destruction in this manner and may require activation of complement at several sites on cell membranes for cytolysis to occur.

ISOIMMUNE REACTIONS

The antigens present on red cell membranes permit blood to be classified into four major groups: A, B, AB, and O. The antigens are called *isoagglutinogens* because the reactions with antibodies specific for the blood groups cause *agglutination* or clumping of red blood cells; the antibodies taking part in such a reaction are called *isoagglutinins.* All individuals normally have isoagglutinins to antigens of the ABO system, which are not associated with their own red blood cells (Table 13-2). The isoagglutinins generally belong to immunoglobulin class IgM.

Blood grouping is based on the isoagglutinogen present on red cell membranes. Individuals with A agglutinogens on the surface of red blood cells belong to group A; persons with B

Table 13-2   ISOAGGLUTINOGENS AND ISOAGGLUTININS OF THE MAJOR BLOOD GROUPS

Blood Group	Isoagglutinogen	Isoagglutinin	Percent Frequency in U.S. Caucasians
A	A	anti-B	41
B	B	anti-A	10
AB	A, B	—	4
O	—	anti-A, anti-B	45

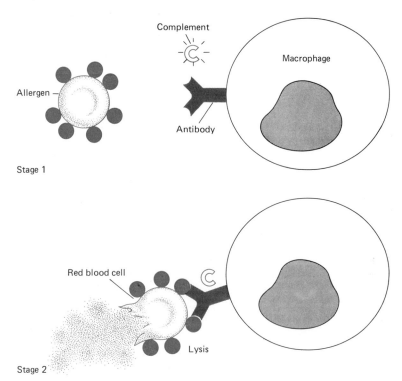

Figure 13-2 Cytotoxic hypersensitivity (type II). In stage 1 antibodies contact macrophages and activate complement. In stage 2 complexing of allergen and antibody with complement causes lysis of target cell.

agglutinogens belong to group B; individuals with both A and B red-cell antigens belong to group AB. If red blood cells have neither A nor B agglutinogens associated with membranes, blood is designated as group O. Group O blood is the most common blood type among Caucasians in the United States.

Isoagglutinins are formed early in life against intestinal flora which have antigenic determinants similar to blood group isoagglutinogens. The *natural* isoagglutinins are designated anti-A and anti-B. An individual will demonstrate tolerance for antigens identical to or very similar to antigens on his own red blood cells. *Immune* isoagglutinins may be produced in response to accidental transfusion with the wrong type of blood or from transfer of fetal antigens across the placenta. In either case severe reactions can occur.

Incompatibilities of Pregnancy. An ABO incompatibility of maternal and fetal red cell isoagglutinogens can promote formation of immune isoagglutinins in the mother. Fetal red blood

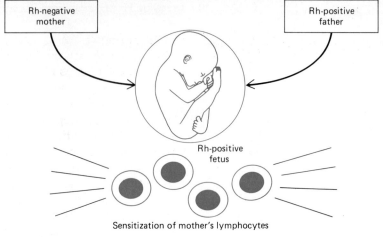

Rh-negative mother

Rh-positive father

Rh-positive fetus

Sensitization of mother's lymphocytes

First pregnancy

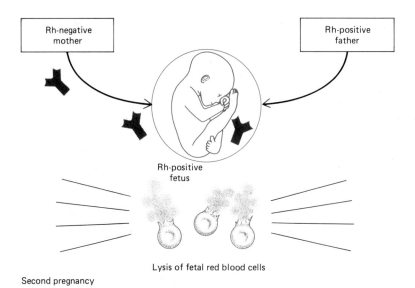

Rh-negative mother

Rh-positive father

Rh-positive fetus

Lysis of fetal red blood cells

Second pregnancy

Figure 13-3 Effect of Rh incompatibility in first and second pregnancies involving an Rh-positive fetus and an Rh-negative mother.

cells enter maternal circulation in greater numbers just before and after delivery. The antibodies produced are primarily of the IgG class and so can readily cross the placenta and promote severe reactions in the fetus or newborn.

ABO incompatibilities that stimulate antibody synthesis sufficiently to cause damage are not as common as Rh antigen incompatibilities. Rh antigens are also associated with red cell membranes. They were first discovered in Rhesus monkeys. There are five major

292

Table 13-3 NOMENCLATURE OF THE FIVE MAJOR RH FACTORS ACCORDING TO THE FISHER-RACE AND WIENER SYSTEMS

FISHER-RACE	WIENER	FREQUENCY IN RH-POSITIVE BLOOD
D	Rh_0	always
C	rh'	often
E	rh"	often
c	hr'	often
e	hr"	often

Rh antigens, but the most important Rh factor involved in isoimmunization by placental transfer is the antigen designated as D (Table 13-3). A person having the D-type Rh antigen is *Rh positive;* the absence of D-type Rh antigen makes one *Rh negative.* Approximately 85 percent of Caucasians in the United States are Rh positive.

Rh incompatibilities occur most frequently when the mother is Rh negative and the fetus is Rh positive (Figure 13-3). Antibodies, sufficient in quantity to produce hemolysis, may be produced in subsequent pregnancies in the absence of intervention by the administration of specific immune serum. The administration of immune serum specific for the Rh factor within 72 hours after delivery prevents mobilization of maternal defense responses by allowing the antigen to complex with specific antibody and be destroyed by proteolytic enzymes (Figure 13-4). Subsequent pregnancies with maternal-fetal Rh incompatibilities are not complicated by the presence of antibodies.

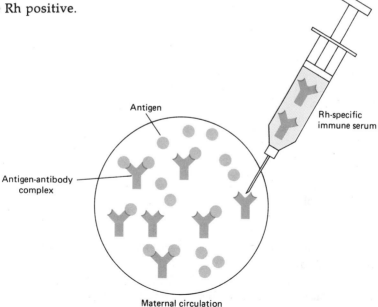

Figure 13-4 Complexing of Rh antigen and antibody following administration of immune serum specific for the Rh factor.

AUTOIMMUNE REACTIONS OF ENDOGENOUS ORIGIN

If antibodies are produced to components of one's own tissues or cells, the cytotoxic consequences are called *autoimmune reactions*. The antibodies are designated as *autoantibodies,* and the lymphocytes that synthesize such antibodies may be called *autoreactive lymphocytes*. Autoantibodies may be produced against antigens of blood, thyroid, kidney, seminiferous tubules, brain, the nuclei of some cells, and even gamma globulin. Autoantibodies are predominantly of the IgG class of immunoglobulins.

Autoimmune Hemolytic Anemia. In autoimmune hemolytic anemia, an individual develops antibodies to his own red blood cell membranes. The disease may be acquired as a consequence of other diseases of the reticuloendothelial system (the system of cells which includes the phagocytic cells of the body) or by exposure to particular viruses, mycoplasmas, or protozoa. The inability of bone marrow to replenish the red cell population destroyed by the autoimmune response makes it necessary to give multiple blood transfusions. Red blood cells from patients with autoimmune hemolytic anemia will survive when transfused into a normal individual, but are destroyed intravascularly in patients with autoantibodies.

Disseminated Lupus Erythematosus. Antinuclear antibodies are produced in a disease known as disseminated lupus erythematosus. The antibodies do not react with intact nuclei of cells, but may complex with antigenic components of damaged cells in the presence of complement. The complexes may be deposited in small blood vessels of the heart, kidneys, lymph nodes, and synovial membranes (membranes of joint, bursa, or tendon sheath which secrete lubricating fluid). The disease occurs mainly in women of child-bearing age and may have, as a concomitant feature, skin lesions consisting of reddish-brown circumscribed soft patches.

Rheumatoid Arthritis. The blood of approximately 90 percent of patients with rheumatoid arthritis contains rheumatoid factor, an autoantibody that reacts with components of IgG molecules. The initial inflammatory process in rheumatoid arthritis occurs in the synovial membrane of joints. Painful joints, limitation of movement, and atrophy of muscles are almost inevitable complications. The cause of rheumatoid arthritis remains an enigma, but it is almost certain that antigen and antibody complex with complement in the joints.

AUTOIMMUNE REACTIONS OF EXOGENOUS ORIGIN

Antibody-induced injury may represent an antibody response to an exogenous agent that persists in a host during or following an infection. The stimulating agents are not natural components of the host, but the reaction is still autoimmune in that the individual is made ill by his own immunologic responses. The injury arises when the exogenous agent accumulates at a particular site. The site depends on predilection of invading microorganisms for particular organs, tissues, or cells.

Rheumatic Fever. Rheumatic fever is an active inflammatory process occurring as a sequela to certain group A streptococcal infections. Antibodies to the streptococcus organism react with cardiac muscle, and damage to the muscle may lead to dysfunction of heart valves and chronic heart failure. Inflammatory responses of the joints may also be involved. Both immunoglobulin and complement have been observed bound to cardiac muscle fibers and smooth muscle of coronary blood vessels. Prompt diagnosis and treatment of group A streptococcal infections are important deterrents to the development of rheumatic fever.

Acute Glomerulonephritis. Acute glomerulonephritis also occurs as a sequela of certain group A streptococcal infections. It is believed that antigen-antibody complexes deposited in the glomerular basement membrane (GBM) or glomeruli cause the severe inflammatory response. At either site immunologic injury affects glomerular permeability and promotes degenerative changes in glomeruli. An increase in glomerular permeability permits protein and sometimes whole red blood cells to escape into the urine. Edema, hypertension, and renal failure may be complications. Only prompt diagnosis and treatment of pharyngitis caused by

group A streptococci can reduce the incidence of the immunological assault.

TYPE III
IMMUNE COMPLEX-MEDIATED HYPERSENSITIVITY

Injurious immune complexes composed of antigen-antibody-complement can form in the presence of excess soluble antigen or antibody. Although differences between some types of cytotoxic antibody reactions, and those occurring in immune complex-mediated hypersensitivity, may be subtle and, indeed, overlap to a degree, reactions of Type III are associated with degranulation of polymorphonuclear leukocytes with release of vasoactive amines (Figure 13-5). In addition platelets may aggregate at the site of immunologic injury. The platelets supply additional vasoactive amines and may occlude blood vessels. Complement may or may not be fixed.

The ratio of antigen to antibody determines the location of antigen-antibody deposits. If antigen is in excess, soluble complexes may be widely deposited; if antibody is in excess, the accumulation occurs at the site of antigen introduction.

ARTHUS REACTION (*ANTIBODY EXCESS*)

A localized response to repeated injections of a soluble antigen caused by a

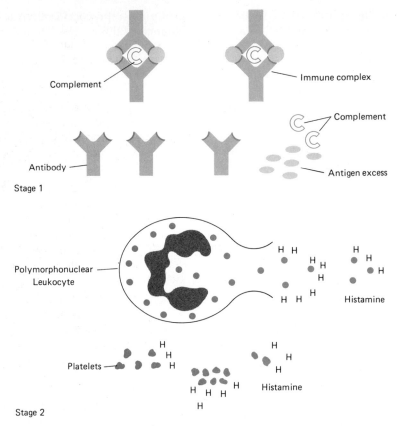

Figure 13-5   Immune complex-mediated hypersensitivity (type III). In stage 1 immune complexes are formed. In stage 2 degranulation of polymorphonuclear leukocytes and aggregations of platelets promote the release of histamine.

precipitating antibody is called an Arthus reaction. It is characterized by hemorrhage and necrosis of the skin at the site of the injections and is believed to be caused by an accumulation of immune complexes followed by invasion of phagocytes. The damage to tissue is probably initiated by neutrophils when enzymes of lysosomes are released.

SERUM SICKNESS (*ANTIGEN EXCESS*)

A more common manifestation of injury caused by circulating immune complexes is seen in serum sickness. When some individuals receive foreign serum containing protective antibodies in a passive immunization procedure, a classical syndrome follows in a week or two. Patients often develop a rash, fever, enlargement of lymph nodes, and edema. A transient proteinuria or hematuria sometimes occurs, but symptoms usually disappear within five days. The immunologic injury is caused by antigen-antibody complexes that circulate, lodge in particular tissues, and set up an inflammatory reaction similar to that seen in a typical Arthus reaction.

SHWARTZMAN REACTION

A localized hemorrhagic necrosis of the skin caused by inflammation and intravascular coagulation associated with injection of endotoxin is called a Shwartzman reaction. It is related to the ability of the lipopolysaccharide molecules of endotoxin to activate complement; activated complement can injure platelets and, thereby, promote intravascular coagulation. The Shwartzman reaction has been studied extensively in experimental animals and may closely approximate the more generalized reactions occurring in bacteremias caused by some gram-negative bacteria in humans.

TYPE IV
CELL-MEDIATED HYPERSENSITIVITY; DELAYED HYPERSENSITIVITY

It is probable that Jenner observed the first delayed hypersensitivity reaction in 1798 when he noted a local inflammatory response to vaccinia virus in an individual who had been previously vaccinated. The inflammatory response was greatest 24 to 72 hours after inoculation and constituted a curious phenomenon, for the expected consequence was a decrease in inflammation in a previously immunized person. Since that first observation of delayed hypersensitivity, many infections caused by viruses as well as bacteria, fungi, and protozoa have been shown to elicit the same phenomenon. The reactions are now known to be cell mediated and to occur in the absence of humoral antibodies. The hypersensitivity response follows stimulation of memory cells by processed antigen. Released lymphokines promote a local inflammation (Figure 13-6). Like other types of hypersensitivity, cell-mediated hypersensitivity represents an altered response, that is, one in which immunity does not follow exposure to antigen.

The classification of some responses to antigenic stimulation is difficult, because an antigen may stimulate only humoral or cellular mechanisms or both. Dermal inoculation of antigen tends to favor T-cell activity. The ability of specific microorganisms to produce erythema (redness) and induration (hardening of tissue) in a previously sensitized individual is the basis of a number of skin tests used for diagnostic purposes (Table 13-4).

THE MANTOUX TEST

One of the most widely used skin tests based on cell-mediated hypersensi-

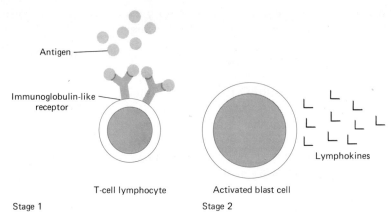

Figure 13-6 Cell-mediated or delayed hypersensitivity (type IV). In stage 1 antigen stimulates T-cell lymphocytes. In stage 2 activated blast cells, transformed from T-cells following the events in stage 1, secrete lymphokines.

Table 13-4 DELAYED HYPERSENSITIVITY DIAGNOSTIC SKIN TESTS

DISEASE	TEST MATERIAL
Brucellosis	filtrate of *Brucella melitensis* or *Brucella abortus*
Candidiasis	*Candida albicans*
Coccidioidomycosis	coccidioidin
Histoplasmosis	histoplasmin
Leprosy	lepromin
Mumps	killed virus
Tuberculosis	tuberculin
Tularemia	protein extract of *Franciscella tularensis*

SOURCE: Adapted from B. H. Park and R. A. Good, *Principles of Modern Immunobiology: Basic and Clinical* (Philadelphia: Lea & Febiger, 1974).

Table 13-5 DOSAGES OF PURIFIED PROTEIN DERIVATIVE (PPD) USED IN TUBERCULIN SKIN TESTING

PPD INJECTED (MG OF PROTEIN)	TUBERCULIN UNITS (TU)	STRENGTH
.00002	1.0	first
.0001	5.0	intermediate
.005	250.0	second

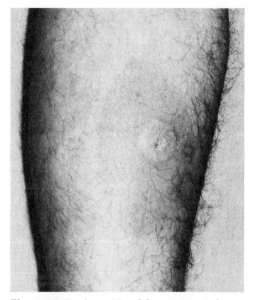

Figure 13-7 A positive Mantoux test showing erythema and induration 48 hours after intradermal inoculation of tuberculin. (Courtesy, Dr. L. Kahana and A/V Services, McMaster University, Hamilton, Ontario.)

tivity is the Mantoux test for tuberculosis. The tissues of an individual who has been exposed to mycobacteria are sensitized to tuberculin, a product of the infectious agent. The standard test dose, designated as *intermediate strength,* is 5 tuberculin units (TU) of a purified protein derivative (PPD) of tuberculin or a dilution of 1:200 of old tuberculin (OT), a product originally introduced by Robert Koch (Table 13-5). For persons suspected of having tuberculosis, a five-fold dilution of the standard test dose or *first strength* is used. A *second strength,* consisting of 250 TU of PPD or a 1:100 dilution of OT, can be used if the standard Mantoux reaction is negative.

Erythema and induration after intradermal inoculation of PPD or OT does not necessarily indicate active tuberculosis, but merely that at one time the individual had been exposed to mycobacteria (Figure 13-7). The reactions are read at 24 and 48 hours. Positive reactions are recorded as follows.

Doubtful (+/−)	Slight erythema and a trace of induration measuring 5 mm or less in diameter.
One plus (+)	Erythema and induration measuring 5 to 10 mm in diameter.
Two plus (++)	Erythema and induration measuring 10 to 20 mm in diameter.
Three plus (+++)	Marked erythema and induration exceeding 20 mm in diameter.
Four plus (++++)	Marked erythema and induration with central necrosis.

A technique known as the *Tine test* employs a disposable steel disc with four needle points containing 5 TU of PPD. In the inoculation procedure the disc is pressed to the skin. The test is read after 48 to 72 hours. The degree of induration is measured. Erythema is ignored. The test is positive if induration measures 10 mm or more.

Tuberculin tests are quite valuable in unvaccinated children, but can be unreliable in adults since cross-reactions in atypical mycobacterial infections do occur. For maximum protection, all individuals with positive Mantoux skin tests should be evaluated carefully by follow-up radiological and cultural studies.

CONTACT DERMATITIS

Some chemical substances may act as allergens or haptens and evoke cell-mediated hypersensitivity reactions. The response to such materials, after initial sensitization, may vary from a mild burning of the skin to distinct skin lesions with or without exudation. One of the most common contact allergens is associated with poison ivy and poison oak. The active agent, urushiol, is absorbed through the skin. Other allergens that can provoke dermatitis are metals, lotions, hair dyes, soaps, perfumes, and lacquers. Widespread contact dermatitis of the elbows and buttocks is reported to have occurred among American soldiers in Japan during World War II. The localization of the rash was curious. It was discovered to be caused by a lacquer applied to bars and toilet seats. The lacquer contained an allergen closely related to urushiol and produced the dermatitis in individuals who had been previously sensitized to poison ivy.

GRAFT REJECTION

Each individual is characterized not only by the antigens of the ABO and Rh systems, but also by histocompatibility (H) antigens found on the surface of cells. The H antigens are glycoproteins and consist of two components. The larger portion has a molecular weight of approximately 45,000 daltons; it is antigenically specific. The smaller portion has a molecular weight close to 11,000 daltons; it is common to all H antigens and is called *B2-microglobulin*. Although immunologic responses to H antigens may involve humoral or cellular mechanisms or both, the rejection of organ or tissue transplants is mainly cell mediated. A skin graft from one site to another site of the same individual is an *autograft*. A transplant from a genetically identical individual, that is, an identical twin, is called an *syngraft*. A transplant from a genetically dissimilar individual of the same species as the recipient is known as an *allograft*.

A tissue graft between different species is designated as a *xenograft*. Most individuals requiring transplants do not have an identical twin, so organ or tissue grafts are almost always followed by rejection phenomena. Fortunately, the most drastic immunological responses to transplants can be avoided by matching antigens of potential donors and recipients and by the judicious administration of immunosuppressive agents. The major H antigens are present on the surface of human white blood cells and are called, therefore, *human leukocyte antigens* or HLA (Table 13-6). Prospective donors and recipients are typed for antigens of the ABO, Rh, and HLA systems. A quantitative estimation of total antigenic disparity may be demonstrated by the

Table 13-6 TWO SERIES OF HUMAN LEUKOCYTE ANTIGENS (HLA)

FIRST SERIES	SECOND SERIES
HLA 1	HLA 5
HLA 2	HLA 7
HLA 3	HLA 8
HLA 9	HLA 12
W 23	HLA 13
W 24	HLA 14
HLA 10	HLA 17
W 25	HLA 27
W 26	W 16
HLA 11	W 20
W 19	W 21
W 29	
W 30	
W 31	
W 32	
HLA 28	

SOURCE: Adapted from B. H. Park and R. A. Good, *Principles of Modern Immunobiology: Basic and Clinical* (Philadelphia: Lea & Febiger, 1974).

mixed leukocyte culture (MLC) test. If lymphocytes of a potential donor and recipient are mixed, the amount of blast cell transformation is proportional to antigenic differences between membrane-bound antigens of the two lymphocyte populations.

GRAFT-VERSUS-HOST REACTIONS

If immunocompetent cells of a graft react against the host in a type of reverse assault, it is called a graft-versus-host (GVH) reaction. A classical syndrome, occurring under experimental conditions when allogenic spleen cells are injected into neonatal laboratory animals, is called *runt disease*. Adult animals develop GVH disease when injected with large doses of allogenic lymphoid cells. Systemic GVH reactions have also been observed in humans. A serious consequence appears to be infections caused by opportunistic pathogens.

Quite clearly, the transplantation of tissues or organs, however desirable to prolong life, is not without some hazard to the recipient. The interest in organ transplants in recent years has stimulated immunological research. The findings may have significance in promoting the understanding of the immunobiology of a number of disease states in which enhancement or suppression of immune responses might be beneficial.

TYPE V STIMULATORY HYPERSENSITIVITY

A category separate from the more common cytotoxic antibodies of autoimmunity appears justified for hypersensitivity caused by an autoantibody that stimulates target cells to secrete large amounts of a normal product.

The immunologic basis of hyperthyroidism known as Graves' disease has only recently been established. It had been known that a long-acting thyroid stimulator (LATS) appears in the serum of some patients with this type of thyrotoxicosis. The immunologic basis was established when LATS was determined to be an IgG immunoglobulin

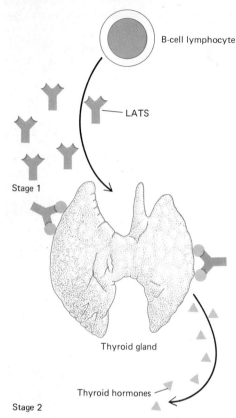

B-cell lymphocyte

LATS

Stage 1

Thyroid gland

Thyroid hormones

Stage 2

Figure 13-8 Stimulatory hypersensitivity (type V). In stage 1 B-cell lymphocytes produce an antibody (LATS). In stage 2 the antibody reacts with antigen on the surface of thyroid cells. The interaction of antigen and antibody stimulates the production of thyroid hormones.

which is thyroid specific. Antigen-antibody reactions on the surface of thyroid cells stimulate thyroid activity in much the same manner as does thyroid stimulating hormone (TSH) from the pituitary (Figure 13-8).

The sera of only approximately 45 percent of patients with Graves' disease demonstrate autoantibodies, so other stimulatory mechanisms must exist.

Whether autoantibodies of a stimulatory nature occur in other hyperactive disease states is not known.

THERAPEUTIC APPROACHES TO HYPERSENSITIVITY

The manifestations of some types of hypersensitivity require relief from symptoms, even if the causative allergen cannot be identified. Quick action on the part of a physician may be necessary, as in systemic anaphylaxis, to save a patient's life. In other instances allergic symptoms are more annoying than debilitating. Increasing numbers of individuals, however, are seeking some form of palliative treatment during severe episodes of wheezing, sneezing, or itching arising from allergic states.

DESENSITIZATION

The subcutaneous administration of repeated injections of allergens to deplete reaginic antibodies or mediators of anaphylaxis is referred to as *desensitization*. Initial doses of a specific allergen are small, but are increased gradually over a period of months or years. It is believed that exposure to the allergen stimulates the synthesis of antibodies of the IgG or IgA classes of immunoglobulins instead of antibodies of the IgE variety. The greater number and avidity of IgG and IgA antibodies allows complexing of the allergens and subsequent destruction. The relief afforded by a desensitizing regimen is sometimes expensive and, unfortunately, temporary.

ANTIHISTAMINES

The effect of vasoactive amines released by mast cells may be modified by treatment with antihistamines. A variety of drugs with antihistaminic activity are used to relieve symptoms of asthma, hay fever, serum sickness, anaphylaxis, and contact dermatitis. The antihistamines are in no way curative, but can be life-saving when manifestations of allergic reactions interfere with physiological functions.

CORTICOSTEROIDS

The ability of corticosteroids to reduce inflammation and act as immuno-suppressive agents makes these drugs of value in many hypersensitive states. The employment of the corticosteroids in organ-transplant recipients has greatly reduced the risks of rejection. However, prolonged use of the drugs is not recommended because the immunosuppression is nonspecific. The immunosuppressive effects must be carefully monitored in individuals receiving allografts because marked depression of humoral and cellular immune mechanisms may predispose persons to infections.

CATECHOLAMINES

Isoproterenol, epinephrine, and norepinephrine are therapeutically useful agents in anaphylaxis or the broncho-spasm and mucosal congestion of asthma. The drugs stimulate the synthesis of cyclic AMP from ATP; the increases in cyclic AMP concentrations inhibit the release of histamine and thereby inhibit the allergic response.

SUMMARY

An altered state of responsiveness to antigenic stimulation known as hypersensitivity may be genetically determined or acquired as a result of some assault on the immunological defense mechanisms. Hypersensitivity states may be divided into five different groups on the basis of reactions caused by complexing of antigen and antibody: anaphylactic, cytotoxic, immune complex-mediated, cell-mediated, and stimulatory. Cell-mediated hypersensitivity is a delayed reaction; the other four are classified as immediate reactions. Immediate hypersensitivity reactions are mediated by antibodies which complex with allergens causing the destruction of tissue or release of vasoactive or other biologically active agents. Delayed hypersensitivity reactions are mediated by lymphokines released by a previously sensitized lymphocyte population. Under certain circumstances hypersensitive states may be both desirable and advantageous to the host. In other instances, the manifestations of hypersensitivity may be harmful and even fatal to the host.

QUESTIONS FOR STUDY

1. Name four types of antibody-mediated hypersensitivity and give an example of each.

2. Give four examples of cell-mediated hypersensitivity.
3. Describe three diseases caused by autoimmune reactions.
4. What are the roles of B- and T-cells in hypersensitivity states?
5. Of what significance are human leukocyte antigens (HLA's) in organ transplants?

SELECTED REFERENCES

Bach, F. H., and Good, R. A. *Clinical Immunobiology*. Vol. 1. New York: Academic Press, 1972.

Golub, E. S. *The Cellular Basis of the Immune Response*. Stamford, Conn.: Sinauer, 1977.

Good, R. A., and Fisher, D. W. *Immunobiology*. Stamford, Conn.: Sinauer, 1971.

Gordon, B. L., and Ford, D. K. *Essentials of Immunology*. Philadelphia: Davis, 1971.

Park, B. H., and Good, R. A. *Principles of Modern Immunobiology: Basic and Clinical*. Philadelphia: Lea & Febiger, 1974.

Roitt, I. *Essential Immunology*. 2d ed. Oxford: Blackwell Scientific Publications, 1974.

Sell, S. *Immunology, Immunopathology and Immunity*. New York: Harper & Row, 1972.

U.S. Department of Health, Education, and Welfare, National Institutes of Health and National Institute of Child Health and Human Development. The biological role of the immunoglobulin E system. *Proc. of a Conference on the Biological Role of the Immunoglobulin E System*. Vero Beach, 1972.

Chapter 14

In Vitro Antigen-Antibody Reactions

After you read this chapter, you should be able to:

1. Define titer, antigenicity, and immunogen.
2. Describe five major antigen-antibody reactions which can be employed *in vitro* for the diagnosis of infectious disease.
3. List five types of agglutination reactions and one test based on each type.
4. Explain the basis of a prozone phenomenon.
5. Contrast single and double diffusion methods of demonstrating precipitation.
6. Identify patterns on Ouchterlony plates as identity, partial, or nonidentity.
7. Explain the principles of immunoelectrophoresis and radioimmunoassay techniques.
8. Compare the direct and indirect methods of immunofluorescence.
9. Explain the basis of complement-fixation tests.
10. Indicate the purpose for which neutralization tests are used.
11. Describe *in vivo* and *in vitro* methods of testing for the presence of neutralizing antibodies.
12. Explain the principles of two enzyme-linked immunosorbent assay methods.

Diseases caused by infectious agents are accompanied by the *in vivo* production of antibodies to a number of antigens associated with microorganisms. The presence of specific antibodies in serum can be detected by permitting them to react with microbial antigens *in vitro*. The initial reaction between antigen and antibody is the formation of an antigen-antibody complex. The formation of large numbers of antigen-antibody complexes is often indicated by specific types of physical evidence. The type of physical evidence is determined by the nature of the antigen and environmental conditions. Reactions between antibodies and insoluble particulate antigens result in agglutination or lysis. Precipitation and complement-fixation are the result of reactions of antibodies with soluble antigens. Some antigen-antibody reactions occur only in the presence of *electrolytes*, that is, substances, such as sodium chloride, which are capable of conducting an electric current in solution.

Not only can the presence of specific antibodies be detected *in vitro*, but a quantitative expression of antibodies known as a *titer* can be obtained by using appropriate dilution techniques. A titer is defined as the reciprocal of the highest dilution of serum producing a visible antigen-antibody reaction. A titer is expressed in antibody units per volume of the original amount of serum used in a test. For example, if 1 ml of serum is used and the highest dilution of that serum promoting a reaction is 1 in 80, the titer would be 80 units per milliliter of serum. Titers have no comparative value between disease states since microbial components differ in *immunogenicity,* that is, the ability to promote antibody production in a host. Differences in titer reflect responses to both numbers and types of antigens associated with infectious agents.

The study of *in vitro* antigen-antibody interactions is called *serology*. Performance of laboratory tests for detection and quantitation of specific antibodies requires patients' sera and purified microbial antigens. A high titer of antibodies to a particular microorganism indicates only that a past infection or vaccination has taken place. It is necessary to show a rise in titer to establish that an infectious disease is being caused by a specific etiologic agent. Titers can sometimes be used to monitor the effectiveness of treatment. A decline in titer usually means that the acute phase of an illness is subsiding.

Another use of serological procedures is for confirming the identification of microorganisms isolated from cases of infectious disease. In such tests serum from inoculated animals is employed as a source of specific antibody. Rabbits, horses, sheep, chickens, and sometimes humans may be inoculated with particular disease agents to produce high titers of antibodies required for the *in vitro* tests. When an antigen is used under controlled conditions to elicit antibody response for the production of high-titer antiserum or specific protective vaccines, the antigen is more appropriately called an *immunogen*.

AGGLUTINATION

Insoluble particulate antigens, such as bacteria, fungi, and red blood cells, combine with homologous antibodies, that is, those having specificity for particular antigenic components. A reaction known as *agglutination* is produced when specific antiserum is added to particulate antigens. Substances which produce agglutination are called *agglutinins*. The reaction is believed to take place in two stages. Antigen and antibody first combine to form a complex. The antibody-coated particles then undergo an alteration in surface charge and are attracted to one another in the presence of an environmental electrolyte, usually sodium chloride. The resultant clumps of particles produce visible agglutination as the clumps settle out of the suspension. The reaction can often be observed macroscopically, depending on particle size and amount of agglutination.

BACTERIAL AGGLUTINATION

Bacterial agglutination tests are of value in a number of febrile diseases (diseases characterized by high fever) including typhoid, paratyphoid, undulant fever, tularemia, and a number of rickettsial diseases. Motile bacteria contain flagellar (H) antigens and somatic (O) antigens which can be distinguished by the type of agglutination produced. Flagellar antigen-antibody complexes are flocculent, that is, loosely aggregated, whereas somatic antigen-antibody complexes are compact and granular (Figure 14-1).

Antimicrobial therapy interferes with reactions of agglutinins, so the test results must be interpreted with some caution if therapy has been started before serum sampling.

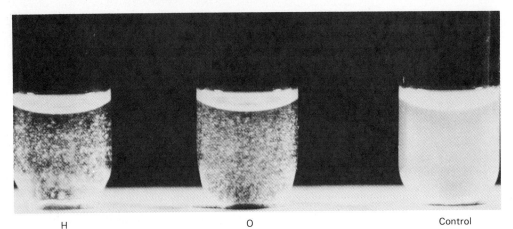

H   O   Control

Figure 14-1   Agglutination of flagellar (H) antigens and somatic (O) antigens of bacteria compared to a nonagglutinated control on the right. (From J. T. Barrett, *Textbook of Immunology*, 2d ed., St. Louis, Mosby, 1974; photo by William Krass.)

NONSPECIFIC HEMAGGLUTINATION

Antibodies known as *cold agglutinins* are often present in the sera of individuals with primary atypical pneumonia and some patients with hemolytic anemia. The antibodies may also be found in the sera of some healthy individuals. They agglutinate group O human red blood cells at temperatures of 0° to 5°C. The reaction is reversible at 37°C.

Another example of hemagglutination is the reaction of heterophil antibodies which increase in sera of patients with infectious mononucleosis. A heterophil antibody is a nonspecific agglutinin in that it reacts with antigens other than the one initiating its production. The heterophil antibodies of infectious mononucleosis agglutinate sheep red blood cells.

PASSIVE AGGLUTINATION

Agglutination reactions may also be used to detect antibodies to soluble antigens even though agglutination does not occur naturally with soluble nonparticulate antigens. Red blood cells, polystyrene latex, or bentonite particles will adsorb nonparticulate antigens to their surfaces upon short-term incubation. Polysaccharides, like those of *Salmonella* O antigens, are easily adsorbed by red blood cells; adsorption of protein antigens requires pretreatment of red blood cells with tannic acid. Antibodies can then react with antigen-coated cells or particles and, in the presence of sodium chloride, produce an observable agglutination (Figure 14-2).

Passive hemagglutination tests have the capacity for yielding positive results with as little as 0.003 μg of antibody ni-

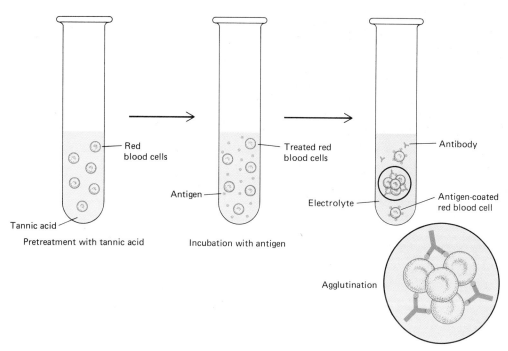

Red blood cells

Treated red blood cells

Antibody

Antigen

Electrolyte

Antigen-coated red blood cell

Tannic acid

Pretreatment with tannic acid

Incubation with antigen

Agglutination

Figure 14-2 Passive agglutination. Red blood cells are treated with tannic acid and then incubated in the presence of antigen. Antibodies react with antigen-coated red blood cells in the presence of an electrolyte producing observable agglutination.

trogen. Three commonly performed passive agglutination techniques are the serologic tests for rheumatoid arthritis, C-reactive protein, and syphilis.

HEMAGGLUTINATION INHIBITION

The role of components of hemagglutination is reversed in certain viral infections so that hemagglutination is actually inhibited in the presence of specific antibody. Some viruses possess reactive sites which combine with receptors on the surface of red blood cells to cause clumping. The addition of specific antibody prevents the attachment of viruses to red cells and thereby prevents agglutination.

Agglutination of human and chicken red blood cells by influenza A and B viruses is suppressed by the presence of influenza antibodies (Figure 14-3). Antibodies to mumps, vaccinia, smallpox, and some viruses that cause encephalitis also inhibit hemagglutination.

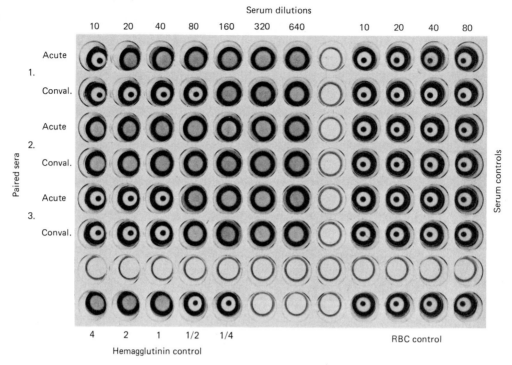

Figure 14-3 Hemagglutination inhibition test of sera of three patients, in acute and convalescent stages. The tests show inhibiting antibody activity on successive two-fold dilutions of sera. A dark center indicates inhibition, whereas uniform distribution of red blood cells indicates hemagglutination. (Courtesy, E. H. Lennette and the Viral and Rickettsial Disease Laboratory, California Department of Health, Berkeley, California.)

PRECIPITATION

Soluble antigens combine with homologous antibodies producing insoluble antigen-antibody complexes in a reaction known as precipitation. It has been postulated that a "lattice" is formed when antigens are linked to antibodies (Figure 14-4). When the antigen-antibody complexes formed exceed a certain level, aggregates precipitate out of solution. The presence of as little as 3 to 15 μg of antibody nitrogen from IgG, IgM, or IgA can be demonstrated. Although less sensitive than most agglutinating antibody reactions, precipitation reactions are particularly valuable in the detection of blood and other body secretions in forensic medicine.

PRECIPITIN RING TEST

If serum containing homologous antibody is layered with soluble antigen in tubes of small diameter, a visible

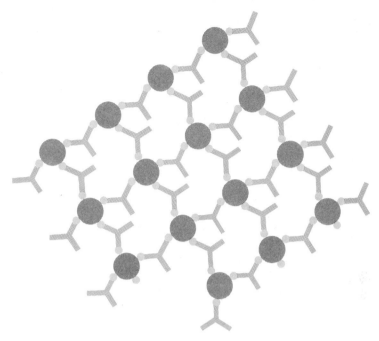

Figure 14-4 Lattice formation. An insoluble framework is formed by antigen-antibody complexes in the presence of an electrolyte.

precipitate forms at the interface in the presence of antibody excess and in the zone of equivalence (Figure 14-5). In the zone of equivalence concentrations of antigens and antibody are such that virtually all of the molecules participate in the reaction. A positive ring can be obtained within 20 minutes at room temperature with a 1:20,000 dilution of human blood and its homologous antiserum. Since blood need not be fresh, dried blood on murder weapons, carpets, or clothing can be identified.

CAPSULAR PRECIPITIN REACTIONS

A variation of the precipitation reaction occurs with encapsulated bacteria and antibodies specific for capsular polysaccharides. When antibody against a specific capsular type is applied to a suspension of organisms, the capsules swell. The reaction is called a *quellung reaction* (from the German *Quellung*, "swelling").

Before the era of antibiotics the quellung reaction was widely employed for typing pneumococci. The only method of treatment was administration of type-specific immune serum. Typing of pneumococci has become less important with the availability of chemotherapy.

The quellung reaction is occasionally helpful in differentiating types of *Haemophilus influenzae*. An advantage of the procedure is that it can be used for direct typing of organisms contained in cerebrospinal fluid.

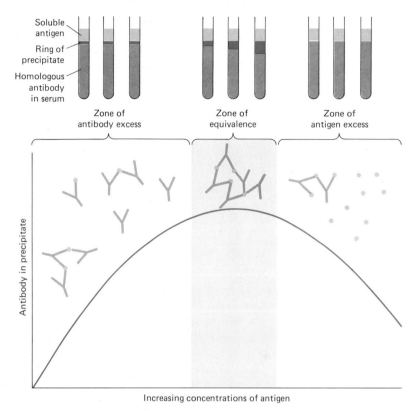

Figure 14-5 Precipitin curve illustrating the effect of increasing antigen concentrations on the amount of antibody precipitated. Only a small amount of precipitate forms in tubes containing homologous antibody in serum layered with soluble antigen in the zone of antibody excess. The amount of antibody precipitated can vary only somewhat in the zone of equivalence, but antigen-antibody complexes are insoluble in the zone of antigen excess.

FLOCCULATION TESTS

Some precipitating antibodies differ from typical precipitins in that insoluble complexes are formed only in the presence of relatively large amounts of antigen over a narrow range of antigen-antibody ratios. The reaction is called *flocculation* to differentiate it from the typical precipitation reaction.

In horses diphtheria and streptococcal toxins stimulate production of antibodies which participate in some *in vitro* flocculation tests. Several popular techniques used in the diagnosis of syphilis are based on flocculation occurring as a result of complexing of the syphilitic antibody, sometimes called reagin, with particles of lipid extracts of beef heart as the antigen. Despite the similarity in name, the syphilitic antibody should not be confused with immunoglobulins of the class IgE.

GEL DIFFUSION

When specific antigen and antibody are solubilized in a semisolid medium, they diffuse toward one another and form a visible band of precipitation at the point of equivalence. The minimal number of antigen-antibody systems is represented by the number of precipitin bands.

A procedure which permits the diffusion of a single component is called *single diffusion in one dimension*. It is known as the *Oudin technique* after its discoverer. An antibody-containing gel is overlayed with a solution of antigen. Antigen diffuses into the agar during refrigeration and a precipitin band forms at the point of equivalence (Figure 14-6).

If antigen and antibody are separated by a layer of clear agar, both antigen and antibody diffuse and form a precipitate in the clear zone (Figure 14-7). The technique is called *double diffusion in one dimension*. A well-defined precipitin band is formed if antigen and antibody are present in equivalent amounts. In the event of an excess of either component, the band migrates slowly away from the excess. The procedure is of particular value for demonstrating the presence of more than one antigen-antibody system.

A somewhat more sophisticated method, known as the *Ouchterlony technique*, gives more quantitative information. The technique provides for *double diffusion in two dimensions*. Solutions of antigen and antibody are placed in separate wells of an agar plate. Lines of precipitin occur where optimal amounts of antigen and antibody meet (Figure 14-8). If excess antigen is

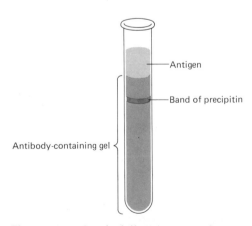

Figure 14-6 Single diffusion in one dimension (Oudin technique). A precipitin band forms at the point of equivalence.

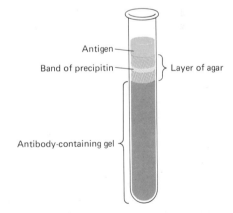

Figure 14-7 Double diffusion in one dimension. A precipitin band forms in the layer of agar as antigen and antibody diffuse.

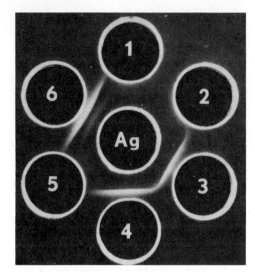

Figure 14-8 Double diffusion in two dimensions by the Ouchterlony technique. Sera placed in wells 2, 3, 4, and 6 gave distinct lines of precipitin when allowed to react with antigen in the center well. No evidence for the presence of specific antibody is observable from wells 1 and 5. (Courtesy, P. C. Smith, Knoxville, Tennessee.)

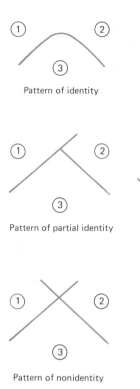

Figure 14-9   Use of Ouchterlony plates in establishing identity. Antigens were placed in wells 1 and 2; antiserum was placed in well 3. The pattern of identity indicates antigens are the same. The pattern of partial identity indicates the presence of common determinants on antigens. The pattern of nonidentity indicates no relationship between antigens.

present, bands of precipitin form near the well containing antiserum; if antibody is in excess, bands form closer to the well containing antigen. The curvature of the precipitin line is a rough indication of molecular weights of the reactants. A straight line indicates that the weights of the reactants are approximately equivalent. If the weights of the reactants differ, the precipitin band curves in the direction of the higher molecular weight.

Ouchterlony plates may be used to establish identity, partial identity, or nonidentity of an antigen in an antigen-antibody system (Figure 14-9). Formation of independent bands of precipitin that cross one another indicates nonidentity or no relationship between antigens. A partial fusion of bands, creating a pattern with a "spur" means the antigens have some common determinants. Fusion of bands with no crossover of lines represents identity or identical antigens.

A modification of the Ouchterlony

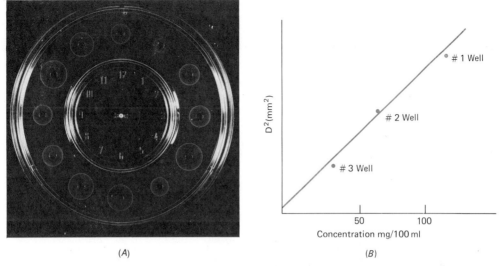

(A)   (B)

Figure 14-10 Estimation of the C3 component of serum complement by radial immunodiffusion. (A) Three different concentrations of a serum protein standard are placed in wells 1, 2, and 3 and aliquots of human sera are placed in wells 5–12. The diameters of the precipitates formed from human sera are measured and squared. (B) Levels of C3 are read from the standard curve prepared by measuring and squaring diameters of precipitates from the protein standards. (From N. J. Bigley, *Immunologic Fundamentals*. Copyright © 1975 by Year Book Medical Publishers, Inc., Chicago. Used by permission.)

method, known as *radial immunodiffusion*, permits quantitation of antigen by incorporating antibody into the diffusing medium. Samples of soluble antigen are placed in wells and examined after a period of incubation for precipitin bands. The concentration of antigen is proportional to the distance of precipitin bands from the wells (Figure 14-

10). Radial immunodiffusion is used to measure complement and immunoglobulin levels.

In *immunoelectrophoresis*, a technique introduced by P. Grabar and F. G. Williams in 1953, antigens mounted in wells cut into agar on a glass slide are allowed to migrate in an electric field according to charge (Figure 14-11). Immunological

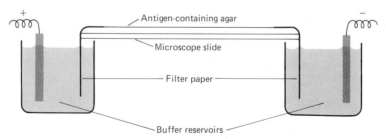

Figure 14-11 Simplified representation of an apparatus used for immunoelectrophoresis.

315

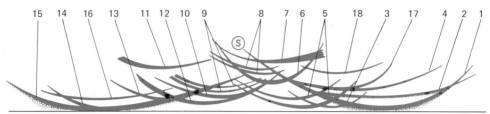

1. Albumin	7. Beta-lipoprotein
2. Orosomucoid	8. Alpha-2 macroglobulin
3. Alpha-1 glycoprotein	9. Heat labile beta-proteins
4. Alpha-1 lipoprotein	10. Unidentified
5. Haptoglobin	11. Beta-2 macroglobulin
6. Ceruloplasmin	12. Siderophilin
13. Gamma-1 globulin
14. Gamma-X globulin
15. Gamma globulin
16. Beta-2-A globulin
17. Heat labile alpha-1 protein
18. Alpha-1 macroglobulin

Figure 14-12 Diagrammatic representation of multiple precipitin bands obtained by immunoelectrophoresis when human serum is allowed to react with rabbit antihuman serum.

identification of antigens is performed in the same gel. For this purpose, a trough is made in the gel parallel to the direction of electrophoretic separation. A solution of antibodies is placed in the trough. Upon subsequent incubation in a cold moist atmosphere, antibodies and antigens diffuse toward each other. Precipitin bands occur at optimal concentrations. If human serum is reacted with rabbit antihuman serum, multiple bands are obtained (Figure 14-12). The technique is important for the detection of atypical types or amounts of serum proteins.

RADIOIMMUNOASSAY

The most sensitive of the assays based on precipitation is the *radioimmunoassay* (RIA), first developed by Solomon Berson and Rosalyn Yalow for measurement of serum insulin. Trace amounts of any antigen or hapten can be detected by the method. The procedure is based on competition for antibodies between radioactively labeled antigen and unlabeled antigen. During incubation of the mixtures at 4°C the unlabeled antigen competes against labeled antigen for binding sites on antibodies. Free antigen is separated from bound antigen by the addition of an adsorbent under carefully controlled conditions. Following a washing procedure, radioactivity of the adsorbent is determined on a gamma counter. The amount of antigen present in a sample is determined by comparing the bound radioactivity with the radioactivity bound in solutions containing known amounts of antigen. The ratio of bound to free antigen is diminished as the concentrations of unlabeled antigen are increased.

RIA techniques are available for assays of viruses, hepatitis B antigen, staphylococcal enterotoxins, type A toxins of *Clostridium botulinum,* and lipopolysaccharides of *Escherichia coli.* The development of RIA methodology has permitted detection of antigens at the millimicrogram (mμg) level. The potential of RIA for diagnostic procedures in microbiology is yet to be realized.

IMMUNOFLUORESCENCE

Immunofluorescence is another technique by which antigens or antibodies can be detected and measured. In the technique antibodies labeled by conjugation with fluorescent dyes such as fluorescein isothiocyanate or tetramethyl rhodamine are allowed to react with antigen. Under ultraviolet radiation both dyes appear fluorescent. Many microscopes can be adapted for fluorescence microscopy by substituting a mercury lamp for the ordinary light illuminator and using appropriate filter systems.

In the *direct method* fluorescent-labeled antibody is allowed to react directly with antigen on a smear prepared from a clinical specimen or imprint of tissue (Figure 14-13). The limited availability of appropriately labeled sera has confined the use of the direct method largely to research or public health laboratories in the United States. Sera is, however, available for separation of B-lymphocytes from T-lymphocytes,

grouping of streptococcal organisms, demonstration of causative organisms of pertussis (whooping cough), and detection of rabies virus in brain tissue imprints from rabid animals.

In the *indirect method* labeled rabbit antiglobulin is allowed to react with antigen-rabbit antibody complexes (Figure 14-14). The method obviates the need for making specific conjugates for large numbers of antigens. The indirect immunofluorescent tests for detection of antibodies in syphilis and lupus erythematosis are the only indirect tests based on immunofluorescence that are routinely used in clinical or public health laboratories. The test for syphilis is not designed as a screening procedure, but rather as a confirmatory test for possible false positives obtained with flocculation tests or as a means of diagnosing late syphilis. Assays for antinuclear antibodies are used to detect active systemic lupus erythematosis. As the quality of fluorescent-labeled antibodies and experience of laboratorians increases, immunofluorescent techniques may have an expanding role in microbiology.

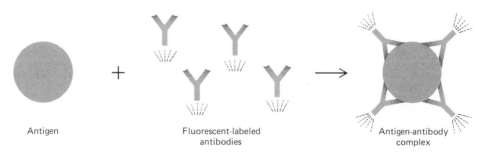

Antigen   Fluorescent-labeled   Antigen-antibody
                              antibodies   complex

Figure 14-13 Schematic representation of direct immunofluorescent method. Antigen unites with antibodies conjugated with a dye which fluoresces under ultraviolet light (radiating lines stand for fluorescence).

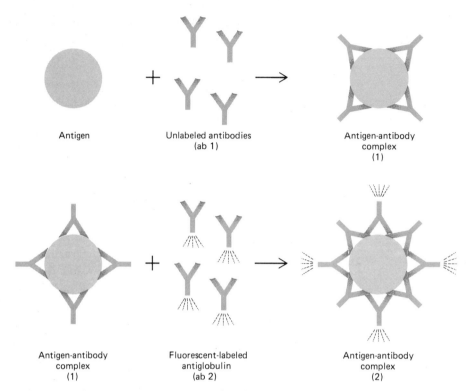

Figure 14-14 Schematic representation of indirect immunofluorescent method. Specific unlabeled antibodies (ab 1) are bound to antigen to form antigen-antibody complex (1). Fluorescent antiglobulins (ab 2) are bound to complex (1) to form antigen-antibody complex (2).

COMPLEMENT FIXATION

Complement participates in the inflammatory response *in vivo* and also takes part in many *in vitro* antigen-antibody reactions. Complement is said to be *fixed* when it combines with specific antibody. Whole bacterial cells, in the presence of complement and homologous antibody, are lysed in a process

appropriately called *bacteriolysis*. If antigens are noncellular, absence of free complement can be detected only by the addition of another complement-fixing antibody and specific antigen as an indicator system. The indicator system commonly employed consists of sheep red blood cells and antibodies to sheep red blood cells (hemolysin), made in rabbits. Hemolysis (the lysis of red blood cells) occurs in the presence of hemolysin and complement when red cell membranes are punctured. The

Step 1: Test system

Step 2: Indicator system

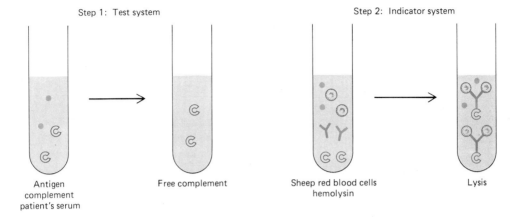

Antigen	Free complement	Sheep red blood cells	Lysis
complement		hemolysin	
patient's serum			

Negative test for complement-fixing antibodies

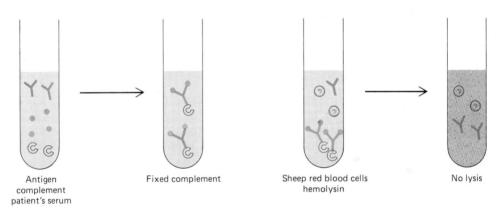

Antigen	Fixed complement	Sheep red blood cells	No lysis
complement		hemolysin	
patient's serum			

Positive test for complement-fixing antibodies

Figure 14-15 Complement-fixation tests. In the absence of specific antibody, complement reacts with the indicator system to produce lysis of red blood cells. In the presence of specific antibody, complement is fixed by the test system and no lysis occurs in the indicator system.

reaction is readily detected, for if lysis occurs, suspensions of red blood cells become clear pink- or red-tinged solutions as cells rupture and release hemoglobin. If complement has been fixed by participation in another antigen-antibody reaction, no hemolysis occurs (Figure 14-15). Complement-fixation tests can be applied to a variety of antigen-antibody systems, but are especially useful for the diagnosis of syphilis, histoplasmosis, coccidioidomycosis, primary atypical pneumonia, and a variety of viral infections.

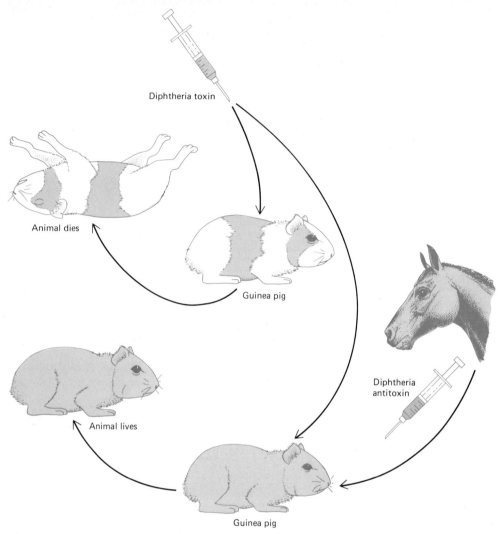

Figure 14-16 Neutralization. Injection of toxin alone causes death of a guinea pig. Injection of antitoxin and toxin neutralizes the toxin and the guinea pig lives.

NEUTRALIZATION

The toxins of some microorganisms, such as strains of diphtheria, botulism, and tetanus organisms, are potent im-

munogens when inoculated into experimental animals. These virulent strains can be identified by demonstration of toxin formation and its neutralization by specific antibody. Injections of cell-free filtrates of toxin-containing broth cause death in laboratory animals. If the toxin is combined with homologous antitoxin effect of the toxin is neutralized, so that inoculated animals are unaffected (Figure 14-16). Neutralization tests can give quantitative information by using several animals and increasing dilutions of specific antitoxin. Most hospital laboratories no longer have animal quarters so that *in vivo* neutralization tests, if necessary, are performed by regional public health or reference laboratories.

An *in vitro* test for toxin-producing strains of diphtheria organisms was introduced by S. D. Elek in 1948. A filter paper strip saturated with diphtheria antitoxin is placed in unhardened agar in a Petri plate. The surface is inoculated with test organisms at right angles to the filter paper strip. Upon overnight incubation at 35°C toxin and antitoxin will form a thin line of precipitate (Figure 14-17). The Elek procedure is less

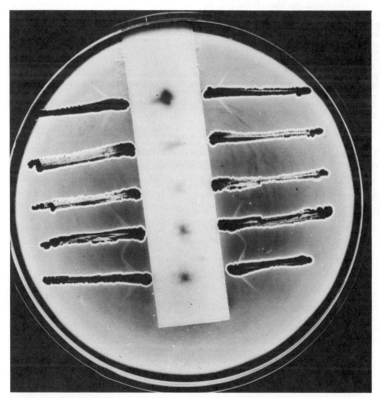

Figure 14-17 *In vitro* test for virulence of causative organism of diphtheria. Antitoxin on filter paper strips reacts with toxin of virulent strains of *Corynebacterium diphtheriae* to produce thin lines of precipitate. (Courtesy, Center for Disease Control, Atlanta, Georgia.)

expensive than *in vivo* tests for virulence and can be adapted to yield quantitative results.

Neutralizing antibodies are produced as a consequence of infections by a variety of viruses, including those of polio, vaccinia, mumps, St. Louis encephalitis, and lymphocytic choriomeningitis. Neutralization of viruses can be tested in chick embryos or tissue culture monolayers, since neutralized viruses do not attach to cells.

ENZYME-LINKED IMMUNOSORBENT ASSAY (ELISA)

The use of ELISA techniques is based on the ability of antigens or antibodies to be linked to an enzyme without altering immunologic or enzymatic activity. Antigens or antibodies have been linked to enzymes such as peroxidase, glucoseoxidase, β-galactosidase, and alkaline phosphatase.

A double antibody sandwich method is used for detection and measurement of antigen. Enzyme-labeled specific antibody is allowed to react with antigen previously reacted with antibody adsorbed on the surface of wells in polystyrene plates. Addition of enzyme substrate, after removal of unreacted material, permits degradation of an amount of substrate proportional to the amount of specific antigen present. In the presence of specific antigen a color change can be observed in wells. The intensity of color can be measured by spectrophotometry. The double antibody sandwich method is used for detection of hepatitis B antigens.

An indirect method in which antigen, instead of antibody, is adsorbed on to a solid surface and allowed to react with serum can be used for detection of antibody. If specific antibody is present, it complexes with antigen. After removal of unreacted material, enzyme-labeled antiglobulin, which attaches to specific antibody, is added to the antigen-antibody complexes. Hydrolysis occurs when enzyme substrate is added to the mixtures. The amount of substrate hydrolyzed is proportional to the amount of antibody present. As in the direct method, the color change which occurs in this case in the presence of specific antibody, is assessed by spectrophotometry. Indirect ELISA methods are applicable for detection of antibodies to a variety of viruses, parasites, and fungi.

SUMMARY

A wide variety of serological tests based on *in vitro* antigen-antibody reactions are available as diagnostic aids for infectious diseases. Particulate antigen reacts with homologous antibody causing agglutination or lysis. Soluble antigen reacts with homologous antibody to form insoluble complexes in a reaction known as precipitation. In addition to lysis and several types of agglutination and precipitation reactions, antigen-antibody reactions involving complement fixation and neutralization of specific antitoxin are used to detect and assay responses of a host to the presence of microbial antigens. Different types of antibodies are formed during the course of an infectious disease so it may be necessary to use more than one serologic method to detect the etiologic agent. Assays of antibodies are expressed in terms of titer. Changes in titer are significant in the diagnosis of an infection and in monitoring the course of a disease.

QUESTIONS FOR STUDY

1. Identify one purpose for which each type of antigen-antibody reaction can be used.
   agglutination
   precipitation
   quellung reaction
   hemagglutination
   hemagglutination inhibition
   passive agglutination
   neutralization
   complement fixation
2. Name two antigen-antibody reactions requiring particulate antigens.
3. What is the role of electrolytes in serological tests?
4. What is the principle upon which radioimmunoassays are based?
5. For what purposes are direct and indirect fluorescent tests used?
6. How has enzyme-linkage been applied to serological test procedures?

SELECTED REFERENCES

Barrett, J. T. Textbook of Immunology. St. Louis: Mosby, 1970.

Bauer, H. Diagnostic applications of the fluorescent antibody method. Amer. Fam. Phys. 13:74, 1976.

Bigley, N. J. Immunologic Fundamentals. Chicago: Year Book Medical Publishers, 1975.

Carpenter, P. L. Immunology and Serology. 2d ed. Philadelphia: Saunders, 1965.

Davidsohn, I., and Henry, J. B. Todd-Sanford Clinical Diagnosis by Laboratory Methods. 14th ed. Philadelphia: Saunders, 1969.

Davis, B. D.; Dulbecco, R.; Eisen, H. N.; Ginsberg, H. S.; and Wood, W. B., Jr. Microbiology. 2d ed. New York: Harper & Row, 1973.

Garvey, J. S.; Cremer, N. E.; and Sussdorf, D. H. Methods in Immunology. Menlo Park, Calif.: W. A. Benjamin, 1977.

Goldman, M. Fluorescent Antibody Methods. New York: Academic Press, 1968.

Good, R. A., and Fisher, D. Immunobiology. Stamford, Conn.: Sinauer, 1971.

Kabat, E. A. Structural Concepts in Immunology and Immunochemistry. New York: Holt, Rinehart and Winston, 1968.

Krueger, R. G.; Gillham, N. W.; and Coggin, J. H., Jr. Introduction to Microbiology. New York: Macmillan, 1973.

Prier, J. E.; Bartola, J.; and Friedman, H. Modern Methods in Medical Microbiology. Baltimore: University Park Press, 1974.

Chapter 15

The Nature of Pathogenicity

After you read this chapter, you should be able to:

1. Describe seven possible responses of the human host to infection.
2. List the four cardinal signs of inflammation.
3. Define purulent exudate, serous exudate, and transudate.
4. Differentiate between a communicable and an infectious disease.
5. Define epidemic, pandemic, and endemic.
6. Describe nine ways in which infections can be classified.
7. Explain the difference between transient and chronic carriers.
8. Differentiate between virulence and pathogenicity.
9. List the microbial factors which contribute to pathogenicity.
10. Explain how enzymes contribute to the ability of microorganisms to invade tissue.
11. Contrast the properties of exotoxins and endotoxins.
12. List five types of exotoxins and their target tissues.
13. List the host factors which provide for colonization or spread of microorganisms within the human host.
14. Differentiate between direct and indirect methods of disease transmission.
15. List the major portals of entry and exit for microorganisms.

The ability of a microorganism to cause disease is called *pathogenicity*. The two characteristics of microorganisms which promote injury to a host are *invasiveness* and *toxigenicity*. When bacteria, protozoa, fungi, viruses, or helminths invade tissue, some damage to the host occurs. The severity of response to the presence of a parasite is dependent on the degree of *virulence* of the parasite and the *degree of resistance* of the host.

RESPONSE OF HOST TO INJURIOUS AGENTS

Some infectious agents promote lymph node swelling. Lymph nodes are located along the course of the larger lymphatic vessels (Figure 15-1). Blind-ended lymphatic capillaries drain all body tissue except that of the central nervous system (CNS), cornea of the eye, striated muscle, bone marrow, cartilage, nails, and hair.

Perhaps the most frequent and familiar response to microbial invasion is fever. It is not always clear if fever is beneficial or harmful to an infected host. Some bacteria actually proliferate more rapidly at temperatures reached in fever.

Infectious agents may also produce enlargement of the liver and spleen. The presence of others may induce hemorrhage or intravascular coagulation.

A local reaction caused by the presence of an irritant of microbial or non-microbial origin is known as *inflammation*. An inflammatory response can occur in any part of the body where an irritant is lodged. To identify a local

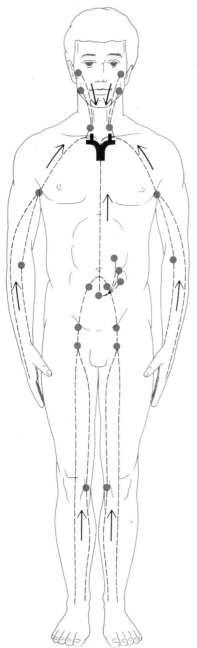

Figure 15-1 Sites of the major lymph nodes and pathways of lymphatic drainage.

inflammation the suffix *itis* ("inflammation of") is added to the name of the organ or body part; thus, the word *dermatitis* is a nonspecific term for an inflammatory response of the skin. The response is a continuum of processes which begins with injury and terminates with healing, if the invading particles do not overwhelm the defense mechanisms of the host. Its gross features or "cardinal" signs are calor (heat), rubor (redness), tumor (swelling), and dolor (pain).

The polymorphonuclear white blood cells (PMN's) respond to the presence of injurious agents by mobilizing at the scene of insult in large numbers. Plasma and PMN's which accumulate constitute fluid known as *exudate,* more commonly called pus. A *purulent exudate* always contains larger numbers of PMN's and bacteria; it has both a high protein content and a high specific gravity. Purulent exudates are usually associated with serious infections. In milder infections a watery fluid, known as a *serous exudate,* containing fewer PMN's and less protein and having a lower specific gravity is produced. Exudates must be distinguished from *transudates,* which are noncellular fluids formed passively by leakage of blood or lymph vessels.

COMMUNICABLE DISEASES

All communicable diseases are infectious, that is, caused by a microbial agent, but all infectious diseases are not communicable. An infection of the gall bladder, for example, is not communicable, whereas the viruses causing upper respiratory infection (URI) are readily passed from one individual to another.

An unusually large number of cases of a particular infection occurring in a community within a short time constitutes an *epidemic*. Childhood diseases, such as poliomyelitis, measles, and mumps, used to occur in epidemic proportions before vaccination programs were instituted. Syphilis and gonorrhea still occur in epidemic proportions in major cities of the United States.

When an epidemic spreads throughout many parts of the world, it is called a *pandemic*. Pandemics of plague are believed to have affected the course of history. During the fourteenth century almost one-third of the world's population died of the disease then known as Black Death.

If a limited number of cases of an infectious disease is present at all times within a geographic area, the disease is said to be *endemic*. A fungal disease, known as coccidioidomycosis, is endemic in the southwestern part of the United States. If a particular disease occurs without regularity in a community, it is described as *sporadic*.

An individual who bears communicable infectious agents but shows no apparent signs of infection is a *carrier*. Some persons are resistant to the organisms themselves, but transmit the infectious agents to susceptible individuals as they move about. In others an infection may be present, but asymptomatic. Unrecognized infections may

be responsible for many cases of individual immunity. Other individuals are reservoirs for infectious agents before symptoms of illness appear and long after symptoms of disease disappear. The microorganisms are shed in body secretions or excreta for varying periods of time. *Transient carriers* shed pathogens for several days or months; *chronic carriers* may transmit infectious agents to susceptible individuals for months or even years.

TYPES OF INFECTIONS

Infections can be classified according to etiologic agent once a definitive diagnosis has been made. Other classifications of infections provide less specific, but important, information which reflects the immune status of the host, virulence of a microorganism, or time sequence in multiple infective states. Unfortunately, in some instances, it is impossible to implicate a particular etiologic agent despite the presence of symptoms of an infection.

PRIMARY AND SECONDARY INFECTIONS

A *primary infection* is the initial disease caused by a microorganism. It can occur on or within any part of the body. If, as a consequence of weakened host defenses or antimicrobial therapy, another infection occurs, it is called a *secondary infection*. Bacteria sometimes follow viruses as secondary invaders.

The bacteria of secondary infections can be of endogenous or exogenous origin.

OPPORTUNISTIC INFECTION

An infection caused by a commensal microorganism, that is, one that usually lives in harmony with its host or that is normally a nonpathogenic organism of the environment, is called an *opportunistic* infection. Opportunistic pathogens can cause primary or secondary infections. Infections caused by normally harmless endogenous or environmental microorganisms are increasing as the classical pathogens are being controlled. Opportunities for infections with commensals are afforded by trauma, manipulative procedures, surgery, chemotherapy, or other interference in homeostasis (the ability of an individual to maintain a consistent internal environment). Opportunistic organisms are often called *superimposed infections* since they are frequently superimposed on underlying diseases.

LATENT INFECTION

If the host's defense mechanisms fail to eliminate a microbial invader completely, the disease may persist as a *latent infection*. Malaria, Brill's disease, and herpes simplex and varicella-zoster infections are examples of latency. Malarial parasites often persist in the liver for many years and cause subsequent attacks of malaria when an individual is subjected to physiological stress. Brill's disease is a mild disease occurring sometime after what appears to be a complete recovery from typhus fever.

The rickettsial organisms can become lodged in lymph nodes or the reticuloendothelial system (RES) following a primary infection of typhus fever. The intracellular parasites are activated by unknown forces. Most individuals harbor herpes simplex and varicella-zoster viruses. It is only when homeostatic mechanisms are compromised, however, that the lesions break out.

Tuberculosis can be a latent infection if viable tubercle bacilli remain within fibrous walls erected by body defense mechanisms to contain them. When the resistance of the host is compromised by malnutrition, irradiation injury, or overlying disease, the organisms may reinfect from within. It is unlikely that many adult infections arise endogenously, but the potential for reactivation of a former tuberculous state does exist.

ACUTE AND CHRONIC INFECTIONS

An *acute* infection is serious, but of relatively short or limited duration. Acute infections are often life-threatening if appropriate treatment is not instituted promptly. Diphtheria is an example of an acute infection causing severe symptoms of pharyngitis and systemic intoxication. It can last as long as six to ten weeks or cause an individual to succumb due to blockage of air passages or effects of toxemia (toxin in blood).

A *chronic* infection is often milder in nature and of less immediate threat, but persists for months or even years. Kuru, a slow virus infection, and athlete's foot, a persistent fungus infection, are examples of chronic infections. Kuru is characterized by progressive brain degeneration and culminates inevitably in death, usually within a year. Sometimes the fungi of athlete's foot are so tenacious as to defy elimination.

Some acute infections turn into chronic infections if a host's defenses cannot be rallied, or if antimicrobial therapy is inadequate to destroy invading microorganisms. Likewise, some chronic infections exhibit acute episodes of disease, so lines of demarcation between the two types of infections are not always absolute.

LOCAL AND DISSEMINATED INFECTIONS

A *local infection* remains contained at a specific site. The nature of the invading agent, the site of the infection, and the immune status of the host contribute to the inability of a microorganism to spread. Most boils are examples of localized infections. If, for any reason, infectious agents are able to spread to other parts of the body, the disease can be described as a *disseminated* infection. Entrance of microorganisms into blood or lymphatic vessels permits widespread dissemination. Coccidioidomycosis exists as a local infection if lesions are confined to the lung. If dissemination occurs, bone, blood, and other organs may be affected.

SPECIFIC AND NONSPECIFIC INFECTIONS

An infection that can be attributed to a particular microorganism or one of its products is called a *specific infection*. For example, tetanus is a specific infection caused by a slender anaerobic bacillus belonging to the genus *Clostridium*. No other bacterium causes such dramatic intoxication of peripheral nerves or the medulla oblongata as the tetanus bacillus.

A *nonspecific infection* is one in which it is not possible to identify a particular microorganism as the causative agent. A nonspecific urethritis sometimes occurs despite the absence of microorganisms other than those comprising the normal flora of the urethra.

INVASIVENESS AND TOXIGENICITY

Microorganisms having invasive or toxigenic properties or both possess a high degree of pathogenicity, a property often called *virulence*. Microorganisms incapable of causing infectious disease, except under unusual circumstances, are described as *avirulent* (without significant pathogenicity). The ability of microorganisms to invade and damage tissues of the human host is associated with both microbial and host factors.

MICROBIAL FACTORS

Microorganisms have both morphological and metabolic characteristics which promote virulence. Many of the metabolic products are enzymes, with the ability to degrade specific substrates of host tissue, but their exact role in causing disease is difficult to assess.

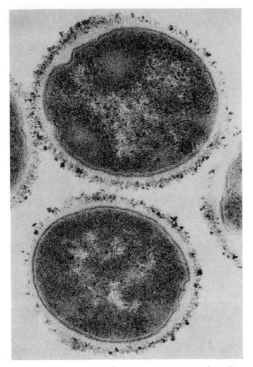

Figure 15-2 An electron micrograph of a section through a streptococcal wall showing location of the M protein on the outer edge. (Courtesy, P. P. Cleary; from W. A. Volk, *Essentials of Medical Microbiology*, Philadelphia, Lippincott, 1978.)

Other products of microbial metabolism are toxins which affect a host in both specific and nonspecific ways.

Morphological Characteristics. Morphological characteristics may promote virulence of microorganisms by providing resistance to phagocytes, motility, or adherence. For example, some bacteria and yeast synthesize capsules made predominantly of polysaccharides. Capsule-forming microorganisms resist the activity of polymorphonuclear and mononuclear phagocytes. Cell envelopes of group A streptococci contain M, T, and R proteins. The M protein, located in a layer of fuzz on the surface of the cocci, has antiphagocytic activity (Figure 15-2).

Other bacteria and some protozoa possess *flagella* which provide them with an advantage in aqueous environments. The success of some motile bacteria in establishing infection is reflected in the ability of flagellated organisms to reach the kidney and cause a number of diseases despite the peristaltic movement of the ureters.

Some gram-negative bacilli attach to epithelial surfaces of the urinary tract by means of flagella or pili (fimbriae), but little is known about the circumstances under which attachment or adherence occurs. The pili of *Streptococcus pyogenes* and *Neisseria gonorrhoeae* similarly aid in promoting adherence to pharyngeal and urethral epithelial cells, respectively.

In natural environments, populated by several kinds of organisms, bacteria produce tangled fibers of polysaccharides which form a *glycocalyx* around individual cells or colonies of cells (Figure 15-3). The glycocalyx is apparent only in a competitive environment, not under the artificial conditions of growth in the laboratory. Thus, bacteria are able to adhere with tenacity to a tooth, the lung, mucous membranes of the urethra, or "brush border" of the intestinal mucosa. The glycocalyx may offer a selective advantage to bacteria trapped in the mesh of fibers by affording the invading organisms protection from both host antibodies and antimicrobial agents.

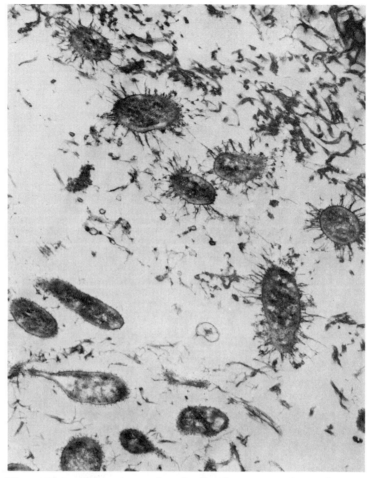

Figure 15-3 Glycocalyx-enclosed cells of gram-negative pathogens from two microcolonies of a floccular mass in urine. (Courtesy, J. W. Costerton, Calgary, Alberta.)

Enzymes. A number of enzymes liberated by bacteria contribute significantly to their virulence. Many gram-positive bacteria secrete *hyaluronidase,* an enzyme which acts on the hyaluronic acid of the connective tissue matrix (Figure 15-4). The enzyme is inducible, that is, produced only in the presence of its substrate, in this case hyaluronic acid. Members of the genus *Clostridium* secrete copious amounts of *collagenase,* an enzyme which acts on a protein of skin, bone, and cartilage known as collagen. The destruction of hyaluronic acid and collagen are not necessary for invasion, but greatly facilitate the spread of organisms in the host.

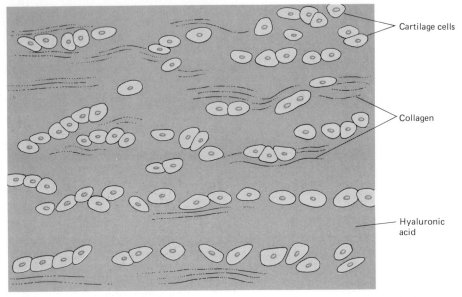

Figure 15-4   Cells of cartilage distributed throughout a matrix containing hyaluronic acid and collagen.

The enzyme *lecithinase,* also known as *alpha toxin,* is associated with virulence of *Clostridium perfringens,* the causative agent of gas gangrene. It can destroy various types of tissue, but seems to have a predilection for red blood cells.

Other enzymes affect blood clotting in the host. *Kinases* dissolve human fibrin by catalyzing the conversion of plasminogen to plasmin. They are called streptokinase or staphylokinase, depending on the source. Virulent staphylococci produce a *coagulase* which promotes, rather than interferes with clotting of plasma, in the presence of a plasma coagulase-reacting factor (CRF). The virulence of staphylococci, however, cannot be explained by coagulase production.

Some enzymes of bacterial origin seem to promote healing or interfere specifically with virulence. The *deoxyribonucleases* of streptococci and staphylococci appear to have a role in liquifying purulent exudates. If some strains of group A streptococci are grown at 37°C, they produce a streptococcal proteinase which specifically attacks the M protein in the outer envelope of the organisms. If strains of the same streptococci are grown at room temperature, the cells contain the M substance. The lack of M-destroying enzyme activity at room temperature serves to point out the temperature dependency of some enzymes.

Exotoxins. A number of exotoxins are secreted into the environment by pathogens. Most exotoxins are general in their lethal effects, but a few have specific destructive effects on particular tissues. *Hemolysins* lyse red blood cells; *leukocidins* degranulate phagocytes; *enterotoxins* act upon a vomiting center in the brain; *exfoliatins* promote generalized exfoliation of epidermal cells. The toxins of both the botulinum and tetanus organisms are selective for nerve cells. The toxin of the diphtheria organism affects both cardiac and nerve tissue.

Ingestion of preformed enterotoxins can cause disease without establishment of an infection. The exotoxins formed in the intestine by strains of *S. aureus* and many gram-negative bacilli are typical enterotoxins.

Endotoxins. Endotoxins are normal components of cell walls of some gram-negative bacteria. Although a few endotoxins are composed solely of protein, most are made up of both proteins and lipopolysaccharides (LPS). The LPS of the gram-negative bacilli, such as *Escherichia*, *Salmonella*, and *Shigella*, consist of a core polysaccharide (common antigen), a specific polysaccharide (O antigen), and a lipid A component.

The lipid A component is a potent endotoxin which causes fever, immunosuppression, and sometimes shock. Very small amounts of endotoxin are detectable in peripheral blood by the Limulus test, a test based on the ability of the endotoxin to cause gelation of a substance obtained from red blood cells of the horseshoe crab, *Limulus polyphemus*.

Differences between exotoxins and endotoxins are summarized in Table 15-1.

HOST FACTORS

The anatomy and physiology of the human host provide means of transportation and advantageous sites for adherence of microorganisms.

Skin and Mucous Secretions. The spread of microbial invaders in the epithelial cells of the epidermis and dermis is relatively slow normally. However, if the skin is moist, infection can spread to parts quite distant from the original site of invasion. Sometimes scratching provides the means for the hands to act as transport vehicles for the dissemination of surface organisms.

Table 15-1 COMPARATIVE CHARACTERISTICS OF EXOTOXINS AND ENDOTOXINS

CHARACTERISTIC	EXOTOXIN	ENDOTOXIN
Major chemical component	protein	lipopolysaccharide
Source	gram-positive and gram-negative organisms	primarily gram-negative organisms
Antigenicity	high	low
Means of release	secretion	lysis of cells
Degree of specificity	high	low

Secretions help to disseminate microorganisms on the mucous membranes of the respiratory and genitourinary tracts. Too much moisture interferes with ciliary action of respiratory epithelium causing microorganisms to escape into lower parts of the respiratory tract. The very acts of coughing and sneezing help to redistribute organisms on mucous membranes.

Adherence Factors. The attachment and adherence of bacteria to mucosal surfaces may be significant factors in pathogenesis. In nature attachment of organisms to a surface results in a higher rate of multiplication than when organisms are free-floating in water. Attachment to epithelial cells of an animal host may provide a selective advantage for microorganisms.

It is difficult to distinguish between contributions of host and microbial factors in the phenomenon of adherence. However, *in vitro* assays have been developed for studying adherence. Using such techniques, it appears that host factors may be responsible for adherence of certain gram-positive bacteria to human epithelial cells. For example, cells of *S. aureus* adhere to nasal mucosal cells with greater tenacity in individuals identified as carriers than in noncarriers (Figure 15-5). Furthermore, studies indicate that individuals who develop rheumatic fever after streptococcal pharyngitis have pharyngeal cells with a particular avidity for adherence to a rheumatic fever-associated strain of streptococci (Figure 15-6). It has been postulated that specific receptor sites may be responsible for the at-

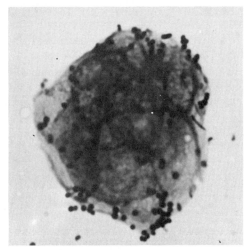

Figure 15-5   Cells of *Staphylococcus aureus* adhering to a nasal mucosal cell in a carrier. (From R. Aly, *Infect. Immun.* 17:547, 1977.)

traction and adherence of gram-positive cocci to selective anatomical sites.

Lymph Vessels and Nodes. Microorganisms or their products enter capillaries of the lymphatic system and reach lymph nodes within minutes. The mouth, lung, and nasopharynx are supplied by a particularly large number of lymph vessels. Phagocytes located in the lymph nodes wage their attack on incoming microorganisms (Figure 15-7). Most microorganisms are trapped and destroyed by phagocytes in the lymph nodes, but some viruses and rickettsiae multiply in the lymph nodes and disseminate freely. Swollen and tender lymph nodes are often the result of host-parasite interactions.

Blood. Blood provides the most efficient transportation system for micro-

Figure 15-6 An electron micrograph of a cell of *Streptococcus pneumoniae*, type 4, adhering to a human epithelial cell. (Courtesy, W. P. Reed and D. Selinger, Albuquerque, New Mexico; photo by J. Huser.)

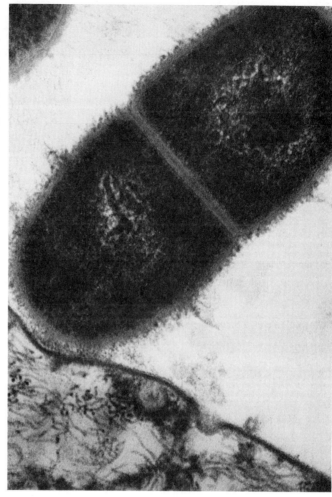

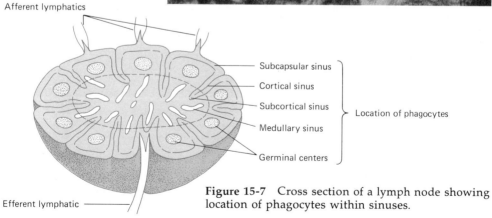

Afferent lymphatics

Subcapsular sinus
Cortical sinus
Subcortical sinus — Location of phagocytes
Medullary sinus
Germinal centers

Efferent lymphatic

Figure 15-7 Cross section of a lymph node showing location of phagocytes within sinuses.

335

Table 15-2 COMPARTMENTS OF BLOOD TRANSPORTING PARTICULAR MICROORGANISMS

| | | WHITE BLOOD CELLS | |
PLASMA	RED BLOOD CELLS	MONONUCLEAR CELLS	POLYMORPHONUCLEAR CELLS
Streptococcus pneumoniae	*Plasmodium species*	*Mycobacterium leprae*	pyogenic bacteria
Bacillus anthracis	Colorado tick fever virus	*Listeria monocytogenes*	
Borrelia recurrentis		*Brucella abortus*	
Leptospira interrogans		*Leishmania donovani*	
Trypanosoma species		*Toxoplasma gondii*	
polio virus		measles virus	
yellow fever virus		smallpox virus	
		herpes simplex virus	
		cytomegalovirus	

SOURCE: Adapted from C. A. Mims, *The Pathogenesis of Infectious Disease* (New York: Grune & Stratton, 1976).

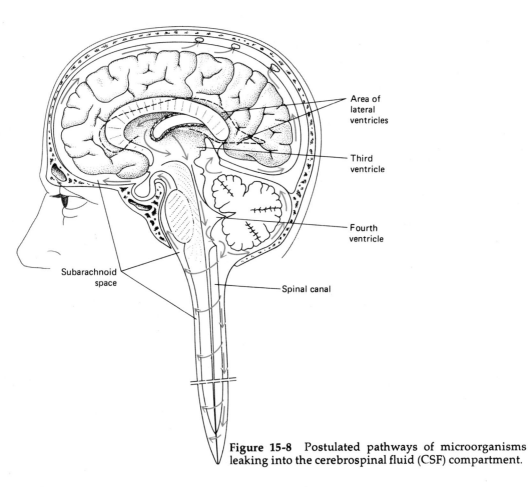

Figure 15-8 Postulated pathways of microorganisms leaking into the cerebrospinal fluid (CSF) compartment.

organisms or their products. It is, indeed, a rapid transit system which promotes microbial migration to points far removed from a lymph node or a portal of entry. Microorganisms are carried in the plasma or within red or white blood cells (Table 15-2). Some protozoa and microfilariae circulate in the plasma; protozoa, a few bacteria, and many viruses are frequently transported by lymphocytes and monocytes; malarial parasites find refuge in red blood cells. Toxins are carried by the plasma.

In addition to acting as a vehicle for transporting microorganisms or their products to distant points, blood is an excellent culture medium permitting rapid proliferation of microorganisms.

Cerebrospinal Fluid. The cerebrospinal fluid (CSF) flows slowly compared to blood. Microorganisms leaking into the CSF compartment cross into the subarachnoid space or lining of the ventricles or spinal canal with ease (Figure 15-8). CSF, like blood, is an excellent culture medium. Invasions of the brain and spinal cord are sure to follow if proliferation of microorganisms is not inhibited.

Nerve Tissue. A few microorganisms, such as the rabies virus, and some toxins of microorganisms have a predilection for nerve tissue. Peripheral nerves frequently serve as reservoirs for particular viruses or as pathways for microbial toxins. Viruses may travel from far distant points along the perineural lymphatics, through interspaces of the nerve, by sequential infection of

the Schwann cells, or by means of axons (Figure 15-9).

Toxin-producing bacteria often remain localized at the point of entry, but toxins elaborated by the organisms disseminate to far removed anatomic sites. For example, the toxoid of tetanus spreads to the anterior horns of the spinal cord. It is generally believed that the tissue spaces provide the major corridor for transporting toxins.

An alternate method for microorganisms to gain entrance to tissues of the CNS is by way of the blood. Microorganisms sometimes leave capillaries in the dorsal root ganglia. A few viruses actually travel across the blood-brain barrier. The major factor blocking the passage of most microorganisms from cerebral capillaries to brain tissue itself appears to be certain anatomic features (Figure 15-10). The endothelial cells of cerebral capillaries are so close to one another that extremely tight junctions are formed between contiguous cells. The presence of a substantial basement membrane separating capillaries from supporting tissue of the CNS (neuroglia) contributes to the barrier. Furthermore, the basement membrane is almost completely surrounded by extensive cytoplasmic processes or footplates of neuroglial cells known as *astrocytes*. Presumably, viruses travel across the blood-brain barrier with greater ease in children because the basement membrane is less well developed as capillaries are growing.

Muscle Tissue. Muscle tissue supplies conditions which attract certain protozoa and viruses. The protozoan

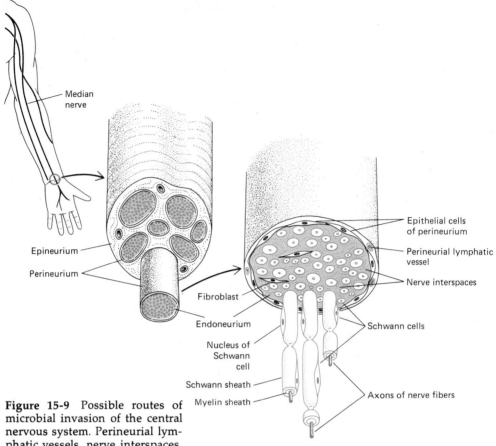

Median nerve

Epineurium

Perineurium

Fibroblast

Endoneurium

Nucleus of Schwann cell

Schwann sheath

Myelin sheath

Epithelial cells of perineurium

Perineurial lymphatic vessel

Nerve interspaces

Schwann cells

Axons of nerve fibers

Figure 15-9 Possible routes of microbial invasion of the central nervous system. Perineurial lymphatic vessels, nerve interspaces, Schwann cells, and axons of nerve fibers may facilitate dissemination.

which causes Chagas' disease migrates to cardiac, skeletal, and smooth muscle tissue. Larval forms of the nematode causing trichinosis and some arthropod-borne viruses find refuge in striated muscle tissue.

Peritoneum and Pleura. The peritoneum is the membrane lining of the abdominal cavity and covering of the abdominal organs. It extends from the diaphragm to the pelvic floor. If micro-organisms enter the peritoneal cavity, they can spread rapidly to any organ in the cavity on the moist surfaces of the lining.

The pleura is the membrane lining the chest cavity; it also encloses the lungs. Microorganisms gaining entrance to the pleural cavity can spread on the moist surfaces of the pleura.

Macrophages line both the peritoneal and pleural cavities, but an overwhelming number of microorganisms gaining

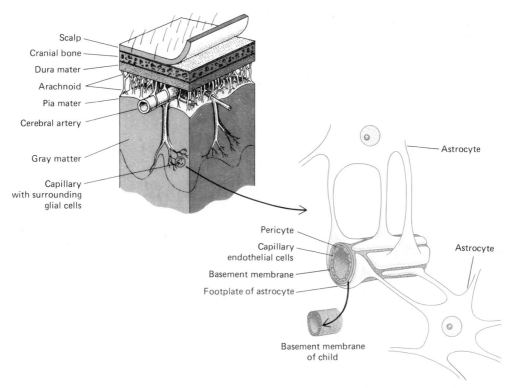

Scalp
Cranial bone
Dura mater
Arachnoid
Pia mater
Cerebral artery
Gray matter
Capillary with surrounding glial cells
Astrocyte
Astrocyte
Pericyte
Capillary endothelial cells
Basement membrane
Footplate of astrocyte
Basement membrane of child

Figure 15-10   Anatomic factors contributing to blood-brain barrier. Footplates of astrocytes almost completely surround a well-defined basement membrane and densely packed endothelial cells of cerebral capillaries.

entrance through an abdominal or chest wound readily overcome activity of macrophages.

TRANSMISSION OF INFECTIOUS DISEASE

Infectious disease may be transmitted by *direct contact* with an infected individual or a carrier of a pathogen. Sexually transmissable diseases (STD's) are usually spread by direct contact during sexual intercourse; enteric diseases are often transmitted by contaminated hands; the viruses of the upper respiratory tract infections can be spread by kissing.

Infectious disease may also be spread by *indirect contact* with an object or substance contaminated with the infectious agent. Water and food are often responsible for epidemics of diseases such as cholera, typhoid fever, or amebic dysentery. Inanimate objects responsible for the transmission of infectious disease are called *fomites*. Fomites in the

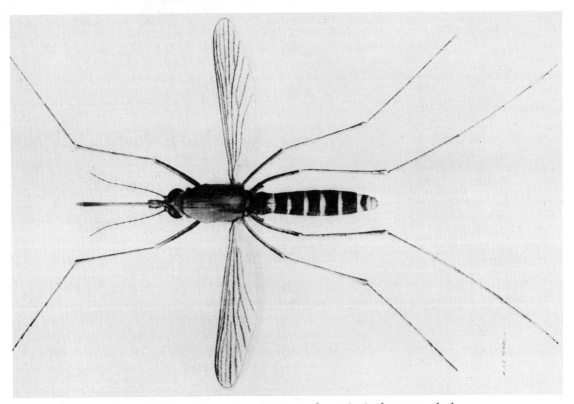

Figure 15-11 *Culex quinquefasciatus,* the principal vector of elephantiasis. The mosquito deposits larvae of a filarial worm near a
bite when feeding on the blood of humans. The larvae migrate into
the wound and travel to the lymphatic vessels. (USDA photo.)

hospital environment include utensils, bedpans, bedding, and toilet seats. Animate agents responsible for transmission of infectious disease, such as the biting or sucking arthropods, are called *vectors* (Figure 15-11).

Microorganisms are often transported by air in dried organic matter, dust, or droplets. Most organisms do not survive long in air, but humidifying devices or air-conditioning units frequently supply enough moisture to permit growth of some fungi and bacteria.

PORTALS OF ENTRY AND EXIT

Microorganisms may enter through the digestive, respiratory, or genitourinary tracts or by way of the skin or mucous membranes. Less often, organisms are introduced by the bite of an insect or arachnid or by the parenteral route through contaminated needles, syringes, or infusion sets. The most effective route for the microorganism is by direct inoculation into the blood.

Infectious agents leave the body by

way of the same systems. Waste products, such as stool, urine, sputum, saliva, pus, or secretions, provide excellent vehicles of transportation for microorganisms (Figure 15-12). Shedding of microorganisms may persist long after symptoms of disease have disappeared. Shedding has even been reported to occur following vaccination with living rubella viruses.

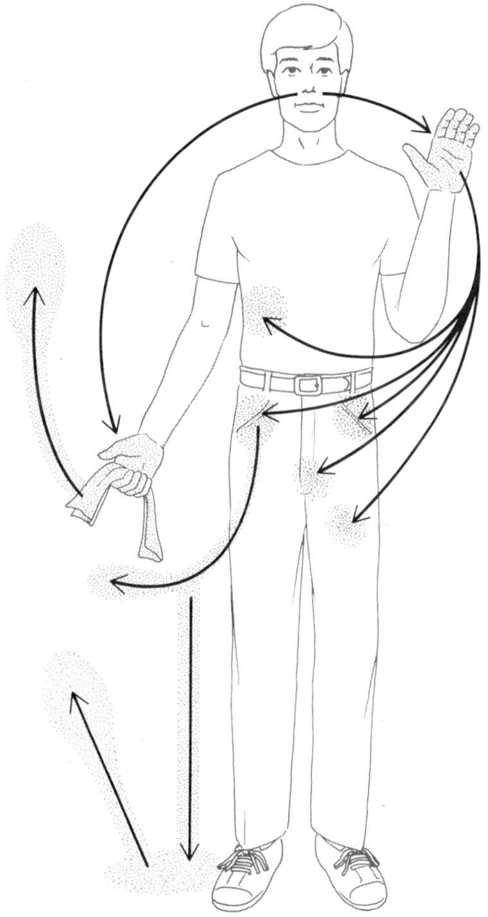

Figure 15-12 Dissemination of microorganisms by aerosols of nasal secretions. The organisms can spread from hands or tissue to clothing, the air, and the floor. The smaller aerosols may be carried in air currents for minutes or hours. The larger aerosols settle to the floor or shoes and can be transported far away from the point of origin.

SUMMARY

Pathogenicity of a microorganism is determined by both microbial and host factors. Various microbial products contribute to invasiveness and toxigenicity of an infectious agent. Exotoxins, liberated into the environment during the course of an infection, are sometimes specific in their action on particular tissues. They may cause serious and even fatal disease. Endotoxins, released only upon lysis of microbial cells, are less specific in their action, but can also produce serious disease. The anatomy and physiology of the host aid microorganisms in establishing infections. Infectious diseases are transmitted by direct or indirect contact with a diseased individual or a carrier of a pathogen.

QUESTIONS FOR STUDY

1. What is the difference between a communicable and an infectious disease?
2. Define the following types of infections and provide an example for each, other than the one described in the chapter.

   primary   superimposed
   secondary   local
   opportunistic   disseminated
   acute   specific
   chronic   nonspecific

3. Name four microbial factors which influence the ability of a microorganism to establish an infection and give an example of each.
4. Differentiate between host and microbial factors which contribute to the phenomenon of adherence.
5. Name five host factors which contribute to the dissemination of microorganisms.
6. How are infectious diseases transmitted?
7. How do infectious agents enter and leave the body?

SELECTED REFERENCES

Aly, R.; Shinefield, H. I.; Strauss, W. G.; and Maibach, H. I. Bacterial adherence to nasal mucosal cells. *Infect. Immun.* 17:546, 1977.

Brock, T. D., and Brock, K. M. *Basic Microbiology with Applications.* 2d ed. Englewood Cliffs, N.J.: Prentice-Hall, 1978.

Costerton, J. W.; Geesey, G. G.; and Cheng, K. J. How bacteria stick. *Sci. Amer.* 238:86, 1978.

Joklik, W. K., and Willett, H. P. *Zinsser Microbiology.* 16th ed. Englewood Cliffs, N.J.: Prentice-Hall, 1976.

Mims, C. A. *The Pathogenesis of Infectious Disease.* New York: Grune & Stratton, 1976.

Reed, W. P., and Williams, R. C., Jr. Bacterial adherence: First step in pathogenesis of certain infections. *J. Chron. Dis.* 31:67, 1978.

Volk, W. A., and Wheeler, M. F. *Basic Microbiology.* 4th ed. Philadelphia: Lippincott, 1980.

Willoughby, D. A.; Giroud, J. P.; and Velo, G. P. *Perspectives in Inflammation.* Baltimore: University Park Press, 1977.

Unit Four

MICROBIAL AND HELMINTHIC DISEASES OF HUMANS

Chapter 16

Bacterial and Mycotic Diseases of the Skin, Hair, and Nails

After you read this chapter, you should be able to:

1. Explain why the skin constitutes a primary line of defense against invading microorganisms.
2. Describe how microorganisms gain entrance through the skin.
3. List the lesions associated with infections of the skin.
4. Describe the most common infections of the skin caused by bacteria.
5. Discuss the transmission, laboratory diagnosis, immunity, and prevention of the common bacterial infections of skin.
6. Identify five major Lancefield groups of streptococci.
7. Classify the tineas according to site of infection.
8. List three genera to which the causative organisms of tineas belong.
9. Compare sites infected in cutaneous candidiasis, sporotrichosis, and the chromomycoses.
10. Discuss the transmission, laboratory diagnosis, immunity, and prevention of fungal infections of the skin.
11. Compare sites infected in the actinomycoses and mycetomas.
12. Discuss the transmission, laboratory diagnosis, immunity, and prevention of the funguslike infections of the skin.

The skin, hair, nails, and integumentary glands make up the covering of the body. Together they act as both a mechanical and a physiological barrier to the colonization and entry of most pathogenic microorganisms.

The basic components of this covering layer are shown in Figure 16-1. The skin is composed of a layer of closely packed epithelial cells, the *epidermis,* and a layer of dense connective tissue, the *dermis,* which contains the integumental glands, nerves, and blood vessels. The skin is continuous with the mucous membranes lining the nose, mouth, anus, vagina, and urethra.

Infections of the skin are characterized by the production of lesions. The specific terms used to identify particular types of lesions are given in Table 16-1.

BACTERIAL INFECTIONS

Bacteria are frequently associated with *suppuration* (the process of pus formation by the skin) and resulting abscesses (localized accumulations of pus surrounded by inflamed tissue). If a suppurative infection is untreated, the causative organisms can spread to subcutaneous tissues, gain entrance to the blood, and spread through the bloodstream to almost any organ of the body. Surgical intervention to permit appropriate drainage and antimicrobial therapy are frequently necessary to prevent the spread of the infection. Isolation of the patient may be required to prevent cross-infections.

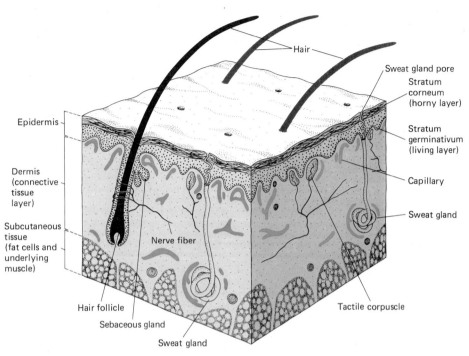

Figure 16-1 Diagrammatic representation of a section of skin and subcutaneous tissue.

Table 16-1 LESIONS COMMONLY ASSOCIATED WITH INFECTIONS OF THE SKIN

TYPE OF LESION	DESCRIPTION
Abscess	circumscribed cavity containing pus
Bulla	large blister containing serous or seropurulent fluid
Carbuncle	circumscribed multicentric abscess with a hard core
Erythema	area of diffuse redness caused by hyperemia
Furuncle (boil)	circumscribed unicentric abscess with a soft core
Macule	circumscribed, flat, red, or brown lesion
Papule (pimple)	circumscribed raised lesion without visible contents
Pustule	circumscribed raised lesion containing pus
Ulcer	open, craterlike lesion varying in size
Vesicle	small blister containing serous or seropurulent fluid
Wheal	firm, circumscribed, elevated, red lesion

STAPHYLOCOCCAL INFECTIONS

Staphylococcal infections are among the most common bacterial infections of the skin. The etiological agents are strains of *Staphylococcus aureus*. An infection may vary in severity from a simple *pimple,* which involves only superficial layers of the epidermis, to an *ulcer,* which may be extensive enough to obstruct the flow of blood in capillaries of deep tissues. An example of a severe infection is the decubitus ulcer (bedsore), a consequence of pressure exerted by body weight on the skin of immobilized patients (Figure 16-2). The increased pressure weakens the tissue and ultimately provides a portal of entry for *S. aureus.* Toxins secreted by the staphylococci and enzymes liberated by polymorphonuclear leukocytes contribute to destruction of tissue and formation of the abscess cavity. Upon healing, the resulting scar tissue often leaves permanent disfigurement.

Furuncles and carbuncles are the result of staphyloccal infections. A furuncle or boil arises from an inflammation of a hair follicle (Figure 16-3). A *stye* is an abscess formed in a hair follicle of the eyelids. A *carbuncle* is a more serious lesion because its depth and multicentric origin increase the danger of the spread of the infection to other tissues or organs should the abscesses rupture.

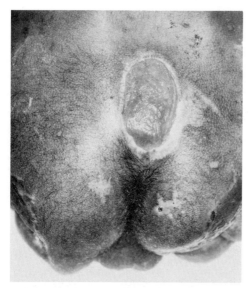

Figure 16-2 A decubitus ulcer occurring over the sacral region. This type of lesion is commonly observed in prolonged immobility. (Armed Forces Institute of Pathology Photograph, Neg. No. 68-13506.)

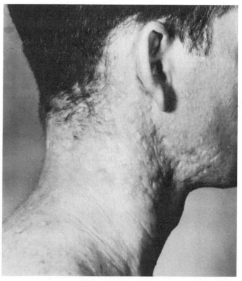

Figure 16-3 Furuncles on the face and neck. (Armed Forces Institute of Pathology Photograph, Neg. No. 55-2744-1.)

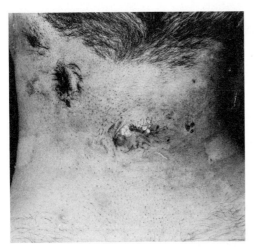

Figure 16-4 A carbuncle on the nape of the neck. (Armed Forces Institute of Pathology Photograph, Neg. No. DET B-525-B.)

It is associated with considerable discomfort (Figure 16-4). If a pathway is established for drainage of pus from a ruptured abscess, the channel is called a *sinus*.

A recently described infection, known as the *scalded-skin syndrome* (SSS), occurs mostly in small children. It is caused by a phage type II of *S. aureus*. The infection spreads rapidly and causes exfoliation of the skin. The loss of skin is attributed to production of an exfoliative toxin, coded by a plasmid, which promotes intraepidermal separation.

A highly communicable form of staphylococcal infection is *impetigo*, a disease common in infants and young children. It is sometimes complicated by the concurrent presence of streptococci. Rupture of the vesicles, induced by scratching, rapidly spreads the staphylococci or both staphylococci and streptococci contained in the serous exudate.

In recent years, colonization of prosthetic devices with *S. epidermidis*, once considered a nonpathogen, has been the source of some severe infections. It appears that distinctly invasive strains of the organism have evolved as potential hazards. Such infections present therapeutic problems because the strains of *S. epidermidis* are often resistant to the penicillins.

Transmission. Since *S. aureus* is ubiquitous in distribution, the organism causing an infection may be of endogenous or exogenous origin, and it may not always be possible to ascertain the mode of transmission or source in a particular infection. The organism may be transmitted by air, by direct contact with an infected individual, or by contact with contaminated objects.

Laboratory Diagnosis. Gram stains of smears prepared from pus reveal grampositive cocci which are approximately 1μm in diameter, frequently occurring in clusters (Figure 16-5). Pigmentation of colonies is variable ranging from white to golden yellow. On blood agar plates some strains of *S. aureus* produce beta hemolysis; others are nonhemolytic. The major characteristic used to differentiate the pathogen from the normal skin resident, *S. epidermidis*, is the ability of *S. aureus* to clot normal human or rabbit plasma after incubation for 4 to 24 hours at 35°C. Strains of *S. aureus* grow in 7.5 percent sodium chloride, ferment mannitol, produce catalase,

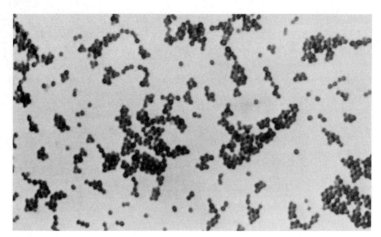

Figure 16-5 Gram-stained smear of *Staphylococcus aureus.* The cocci frequently occur in clusters. (Courtesy, Saint Joseph Medical Center, Burbank, California.)

and are often resistant to many antimicrobial agents. The mechanisms of resistance are discussed elsewhere in the text.

Immunity. Little is known about the role of specific antibodies to antigens or products of staphylococci. Acquired humoral immunity is believed to be negligible. Phagocytosis of the extracellular cocci appears to be the most significant factor in defense against disease. Active immunization procedures using an autogenous vaccine, that is, a vaccine made from the isolate of a patient, are sometimes employed for therapy. Prophylactic use of staphylococcal vaccines is not recommended because of the large number of strains of staphylococci.

Prevention. Patients debilitated by a primary disease, such as diabetes, or compromised by chemo- or radiother-

apy have lowered resistance to a number of microorganisms, including staphylococci. The large number of staphylococcal infections in compromised hosts is a result of the ubiquity of the organisms in home and hospital environments. Isolation of patients with staphylococcal infections, proper disposal of contaminated objects, and careful attention to hygienic habits can do much to prevent their spread.

STREPTOCOCCAL INFECTIONS

Most infections of the skin caused by streptococci are secondary to a primary lesion. A variety of streptococci can be involved, but the organisms are usually classified on the basis of their hemolytic and serological characteristics only.

Streptococci can be classified as members of one of three groups on the basis of their hemolytic activity on blood agar. *Alpha hemolysis* is character-ized by the appearance of green zones surrounding streptococcal colonies. Green zones are associated with incom-plete or partial hemolysis of red blood cells. *Beta hemolysis* is characterized by clear zones surrounding colonies. The clear zones indicate that complete he-molysis of red blood cells has occurred. *Gamma streptococci* produce no detecta-ble change around colonies denoting a lack of hemolytic activity.

The streptococci can be further di-vided into serological groups by a pro-cedure devised by Rebecca Lancefield. By an application of the precipitin test, Lancefield demonstrated the presence of specific antigens which she used as a basis for classifying streptococci. The group-specific substances are polysac-charides, designated as C carbohy-drates, associated with the cell wall. By the seroidentification of polysac-charides of the streptococci, the organ-isms can be classified into 13 groups. Human infections can be caused by or-ganisms belonging to most groups, but typically human pathogens belong to one of five major groups (Table 16-2). Members of Lancefield group A are the most common causes of human infec-tion.

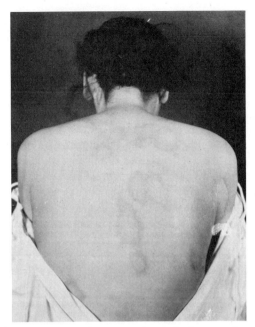

Figure 16-6 Lesions of erysipelas on the back of a patient showing dermal and sub-cutaneous inflammation. (Armed Forces In-stitute of Pathology, Neg. No. 58-6180.)

The association of streptococci with staphylococci in impetigo has already been described, but streptococci alone can cause an acute infection known as *erysipelas* (Figure 16-6). Group A strep-tococci are usually the etiological agents. The lesions may be small at

Table 16-2 HEMOLYTIC REACTIONS AND PROTOTYPE SPECIES OF FIVE MAJOR LANCEFIELD GROUPS

GROUP	HEMOLYTIC REACTION	PROTOTYPE SPECIES
A	beta	*S. pyogenes*
B	alpha, beta, none	*S. agalactiae*
C	alpha, beta	*S. dysgalactiae*
D	alpha, beta, none	*S. faecalis*
H	alpha	*S. sanguis*

first, but rapidly spread over body areas when scratched.

Scarlet fever is a streptococcal infection of the respiratory tract, with an accompanying rash. An erythrogenic toxin of a lysogenic strain of group A beta-hemolytic streptococci is responsible for the rash. If an infected area of the skin is injected with antiserum specific for the erythrogenic toxin, the rash of scarlet fever disappears; nonspecific rashes and those caused by other infectious agents are unaffected. The blanching of the scarlet fever rash is known as the *Schultz-Charlton phenomenon*.

Susceptibility to the erythrogenic toxin can be demonstrated by the *Dick test*. If a small amount of erythrogenic toxin is injected subcutaneously, localized redness around the site of injection within 24 hours indicates susceptibility; the absence of a color change indicates immunity. The reaction demonstrated by susceptible individuals constitutes a positive Dick test.

Transmission. Hemolytic streptococci of group A are not present on normal skin, so most streptococcal infections are the consequence of direct contact with infected individuals, carriers, or contaminated material. Often the infections occur as sequelae following primary lesions, burns, or wounds of traumatic or surgical origin.

Laboratory Diagnosis. Gram stains on smears of exudates reveal gram-positive cocci approximately 0.5 to 1.0 μm in diameter, occurring singly, in pairs, and frequently chains (Figure 16-7). The colonies on blood agar appear translucent to opaque, colorless or grey, and convex. Most streptococci causing infections of the skin are beta-hemolytic and do not hydrolyze hippurate or bile-esculin.

Streptococci of group A are susceptible to the antimicrobial agent bacitracin. In most laboratories, since extraction of group antigens and serological groups is time consuming, bacitracin is used for differentiating group A beta-hemolytic streptococci and from other beta-hemolytic streptococci.

Group A streptococci are uniformly susceptible to penicillin, so it is not necessary to perform antimicrobial susceptibility tests unless an alternative drug is being considered.

Immunity. Precipitating antibodies are formed against group-specific cell substances and products of streptococcal metabolism, including eryth-

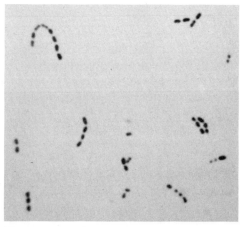

Figure 16-7 *Streptococcus pyogenes* showing typical chains. (From *Laboratory Identification of Pyogenic Cocci*, Part I, Baltimore: University Park Press, 1975.)

rogenic toxin, two streptolysins, streptokinase, and hyaluronidase. Unfortunately, antibodies formed against a single strain of streptococci afford little or no protection against infections caused by other streptococci. It is generally agreed that the number of streptococcal types is too numerous to make artificial immunization practical.

Prevention. Early diagnosis and prompt treatment of streptococcal skin diseases is essential for prevention of continued outbreaks. Prophylactic use of penicillin, in the event of possible exposure, is recommended in some circumstances. Rigorous aseptic precautions must be taken during surgery, debridement (removal of damaged tissue) of burns, and dressing of wounds.

ANTHRAX

Although anthrax is primarily a disease of cattle, goats, and sheep, it is transmissible to humans as cutaneous, pulmonary, or gastrointestinal disease. The most frequent form is a skin infection which is associated with lesions ranging from small pustules to large abscesses (Figure 16-8). The causative organism, *Bacillus anthracis*, is a gram-positive aerobic sporeformer. The spores can survive as many as 30 years in wool, yarn, hides, bristles, or soil. The disease is most prevalent in Asia, Africa, and a few countries of Europe.

Transmission. Cattle and sheep swallow spores from infected pastures or contaminated feed. The most common form of the disease in animals is therefore gastrointestinal; only occasionally do pustules develop on hides from direct contact with the organism. Humans are exposed to spores by handling animals or animal products, by inhaling the spores, or by ingestion of anthrax-infected meat. Probably humans are not involved in direct transmission of the disease.

Laboratory Diagnosis. The type of specimen required by the laboratory depends on the form of the disease. Serous fluid from lesions, sputum, or stool may be submitted for Gram staining, fluorescent antibody tests, or culturing. Gram-stained smears of clinical material reveal the presence of gram-positive bacilli measuring approximately 4.5 to 10 μm in length and 1.0 to

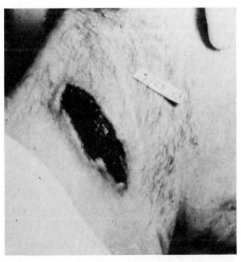

Figure 16-8 Cutaneous anthrax. The typical lesion is fully developed in 7 to 10 days after contact with the causative organism. (Armed Forces Institute of Pathology Photograph, Neg. No. 75-4203-9.)

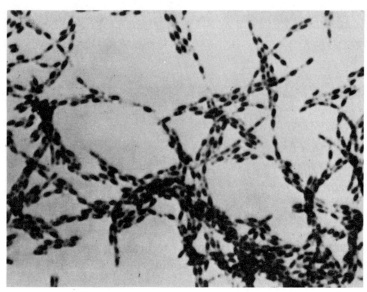

Figure 16-9 *Bacillus anthracis* showing spores and typical arrangement of bacilli in chains. (From N. Groman and V. Chambers, *Basic Laboratory Techniques for Microbiology,* © 1972, Harper & Row Publishers, Inc.)

1.25 μm in width. The cells occur singly or in long chains and are nonmotile (Figure 16-9).

B. anthracis grows on ordinary culture media and forms off-white, nonhemolytic, irregular colonies with a curled appearance very similar to those produced by the nonpathogen *B. cereus.* The colonies are tenacious, that is, tend to adhere to the agar when attempts are made to transfer them.

A battery of biochemical tests is necessary to distinguish the pathogen from *B. cereus.* An indirect hemagglutination test for detection of antibodies is available at the Center for Disease Control in Atlanta, Georgia.

Immunity. Certain species of animals are very resistant to anthrax. The resistance is believed to be related to a tissue protein. Recovery from an infection provides permanent immunity. It has never been practical to immunize humans against the anthrax organism, but two forms of immunization have been used in animals. Cattle, goats, and sheep can be immunized with a vaccine of attenuated *B. anthracis* or with a mixture of spores and antiserum. Both methods of immunization cause mild infections. Unfortunately, protection rarely lasts more than one year.

Prevention. Careful inspection of herds and removal of animals suspected of having anthrax could be important in endemic areas of Asia, Africa, and Europe. Recommended control measures are vaccination, appropriate disposal of animal carcasses, preferably by cremation, and thorough disinfection of animal products.

GAS GANGRENE

Gas gangrene is a wound infection which can be caused by a number of *Clostridium* species, but the species classically associated with it is *Clostridium perfringens*. The anaerobes of gangrenous disease establish themselves in devitalized tissue where damage to blood vessels has occurred. A particularly potent lecithinase (alpha toxin), produced by *C. perfringens*, promotes necrosis of tissues. Illness can be mild or very severe with or without production of gas in the tissues involved. Accumulation of gas interferes with the blood supply to affected areas, causing additional death of tissue. Invasion of the blood by clostridia can be life-threatening.

Transmission. The clostridia usually gain entrance through a deep puncture wound, but infections with *C. perfringens* can follow abdominal surgery or injury. A prerequisite for growth is the availability of devitalized tissue where an anaerobic atmosphere exists.

Laboratory Diagnosis. A diagnosis of gas gangrene can be made on a clinical basis, but laboratory confirmation is important. More than one clostridial organism is frequently present, and other facultative anaerobes may also contaminate wounds and contribute to the infectious process. *C. perfringens* appears on Gram-stained smears as gram-positive bacilli 1.0 to 1.5 μm wide and 4.0 to 8.0 μm long. The bacilli frequently produce a double zone of hemolysis on blood agar and promote a "stormy fermentation" of milk (see Figure 20-6).

Prevention. Gas gangrene can be prevented by prompt treatment of wounds and prophylactic immunization with a polyvalent antitoxin. A procedure known as *hyperbaric oxygen therapy* is used as treatment. The patient inhales pure oxygen in a pressurized chamber. The oxygen combines with hydrogen, the predominant gas produced by *C. perfringens*, to form hydrogen peroxide, which is detrimental to the organism.

LEPROSY

Leprosy was one of the most prevalent infectious diseases of ancient times. It still represents a major health problem in parts of Africa, Asia, the South Pacific, and some South American countries (Figure 16-10). Cases of leprosy in the United States are largely confined to Hawaii, Louisiana, Florida, Texas, and California. Under 100 new cases occur annually in the United States. The causative organism was demonstrated by Armauer Hansen to be *Mycobacterium leprae*.

The clinical entity known as leprosy or Hansen's disease has two major forms. The *lepromatous* form or progressive disease causes cutaneous lesions and frequently leads to disfigurement. Masses of granulation tissue, called *lepromas*, replace macules with time and ulceration may occur. The *tuberculoid* form involves the peripheral nerves and

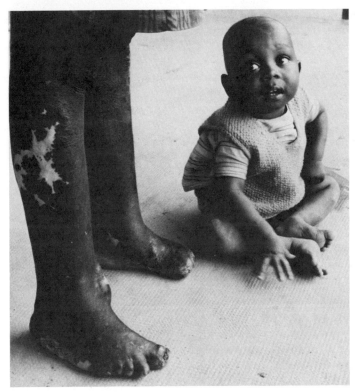

Figure 16-10 Lesions of leprosy on the feet and legs of an African mother standing beside her small boy. (Courtesy, World Health Organization, Geneva.)

causes impairment of sensory responses. Anesthesia is common and severe atrophy of muscle, skin, and bones may occur in the extremities.

Transmission. Leprosy, once feared as transmissible by even the slightest contact, is actually less communicable than most other infectious diseases. It is now known that the only reservoir is the human and that the causative organism is transmitted only upon close and prolonged contact with an infected individual. The organism is frequently contained in oral or nasal discharges of infected persons, so it is assumed that inhalation is a mode of transmission. Contaminated objects, very likely, could also be implicated in indirect contact.

Laboratory Diagnosis. Acid-fast *Mycobacterium leprae* can be demonstrated on smears of skin or nasal scrapings of leprosy patients, but clinical evidence of the disease is very important in establishing a diagnosis. An intradermal skin test using heat-treated

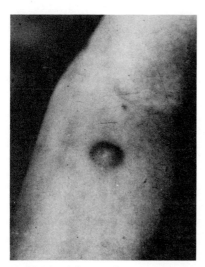

Figure 16-11 A lepromin reaction. A positive skin test is diagnostic for tuberculoid leprosy. A negative skin test is usually obtained with lepromatous leprosy. (Armed Forces Institute of Pathology Photograph, Neg. No. 55-12646.)

lepromatous material known as *lepromin* is sometimes useful in following the disease (Figure 16-11). Unlike the closely related tuberculosis organism, Hansen's bacillus does not grow on artificial culture media.

Immunity. Humans are very resistant to *M. leprae.* The organism is slow growing and probably takes years to manifest evidence of the disease. No form of artificial immunization is available. The immune response, as with tuberculosis, is believed to be largely cellular in nature.

Prevention. Prompt diagnosis and reporting of all cases of suspected leprosy are important in control of the disease.

Segregation of diagnosed lepers from infants is especially important. Hospitalization may be required in the lepromatous form of the disease. Although isolation in leprosaria, like the hospital in Carville, Louisiana, is not essential, the services that can be provided by experts is often important to future well-being. Persons working with or near individuals with possible leprosy should take care to disinfect possibly contaminated articles and take necessary precautions to avoid inhalation of aerosols arising from contaminated oral or nasal discharges.

PSEUDOMONAS INFECTIONS

The pseudomonads have become increasingly important in recent years as causes of infections in postsurgical patients and in those with extensive burns. The pathogen most frequently implicated is *Pseudomonas aeruginosa,* but other species also can invade damaged tissue. Septicemia is a common consequence of surface wound infections caused by *Pseudomonas* species.

Transmission. Soil and water are natural reservoirs for the pseudomonads. In the hospital environment most contamination has been traced to hospital water or equipment. The organisms can be recovered from the gastrointestinal and genital tracts of some healthy individuals, but these reservoirs do not appear to be related to transmission.

Laboratory Diagnosis. Gram stains on smears of exudates reveal gram-negative bacilli approximately 1.5 to 3 μm in length and 0.5 μm wide occurring singly, in pairs, or in short chains. They are not distinguishable on smears from many other gram-negative bacilli. Many species produce a soluble blue-green or yellow-green pigment which diffuses into the medium rather than coloring the colonies.

Biochemical tests and antimicrobial susceptibilities are valuable in identifying different species of the organisms.

Immunity. Resistance to *Pseudomonas* infections appears to be high in healthy individuals. The infections are most severe in the compromised host. Recovery from an infection does not seem to provide much immunity. No artificial immunization is available.

Prevention. The ubiquity of pseudomonads in the hospital environment and their ability to survive for long periods of time in moist environments present special problems. (Some of the problems caused by pseudomonads are considered in more depth in Chapter 29.) Careful monitoring of water supplies and equipment for the presence of contaminating pseudomonads can substantially reduce hospital-acquired infections caused by the organisms.

MYCOTIC INFECTIONS

Of the more than 200,000 known species of fungi, only 45 cause superficial infections of the skin, hair, and nails. However, other fungi are capable of acting as opportunists in the compromised host. Fungi which infect the skin or its keratinized tissue are called *dermatophytes*. Some fungi penetrate into subcutaneous tissues and promote chronic infections known as chromomycoses, mycetomas, or actinomycoses.

THE TINEAS

The infections caused by keratolytic fungi are called *tineas*. The causative organisms of the tineas belong to three genera: *Trichophyton, Microsporum,* and *Epidermophyton*. The great variation in superficial mycotic infections makes it necessary to have laboratory evidence to confirm a diagnosis. The many types of tineas are differentiated by the part of the body affected (Table 16-3). The term ringworm is popularly used to describe the lesions. In tinea pedis ("athlete's foot") lesions typically occur between the toes; they are associated with redness, severe cracking, and peeling (Figure 16-12). In chronic infections the lesions spread over the entire feet. Serous exudates are frequently found in acute lesions; purulent exudates are produced only in the most severe cases

Table 16-3   CLASSIFICATION OF TINEAS ACCORDING TO SITE OF INFECTION

Type of Tinea	Site of Infection
Barbae	beard
Capitis	scalp
Corporis	any skin surface
Cruris	groin, axillae, submammary, umbilical, perineal, or perianal areas
Manum	hands
Pedis	feet
Unguium	nails

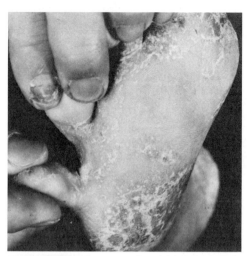

Figure 16-12 Tinea pedis showing typical lesions between the toes. (From N. F. Conant, D. T. Smith, R. D. Baker, and J. L. Callaway, *Manual of Clinical Mycology*, 3rd ed., Philadelphia, Saunders, 1971.)

or in those in which a secondary bacterial infection is superimposed.

A particularly serious and chronic form of tinea capitis (tinea of the scalp) is known as *favus*. The disease occurs in the Orient, Africa, Asia, and some parts of Europe. Mycelial elements and cellular debris cover lesions forming thick crusts. Healing is accompanied by severe scarring. Persons with favus are denied permission to enter the United States.

A more common form of tinea capitis is characterized by scaly lesions on the surface of the scalp. In one type of the infection, "black dot" ringworm, the fungus grows into the hair follicle and penetrates the hair shaft, destroying keratin. The loss of keratin makes the hair particularly susceptible to breakage. Infection within the hair shaft is called *endothrix* infection; appearance of fungi outside the hair shaft is *ectothrix* infection.

Transmission. Soil is a natural reservoir for some *Microsporum* species, most *Trichophyton* species, and *Epidermophyton floccosum*, the single species of that genus causing disease. The dermatophytes are usually transmitted, however, from person to person or from animal to person either by direct contact or by indirect contact through contaminated articles, showers, or locker rooms (Table 16-4). Those fungi associ-

Table 16-4 MAJOR SOURCES OF INFECTION FOR COMMON DERMATOPHYTES

ORGANISM	SOURCE OF INFECTION
Epidermophyton	
floccosum	humans, towels, clothing
Microsporum	
audouinii	infected hairs, epidermal scales
canis	dogs, cats
gypseum	soil
Trichophyton	
equinum	horses
mentagrophytes	epidermal scales, dogs, horses, guinea pigs
rubrum	epidermal scales
schoenleini	humans, towels, clothing
violaceum	humans, towels, clothing

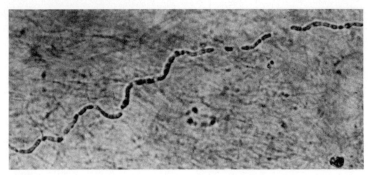

Figure 16-13 Potassium hydroxide mount of a dermatophyte showing hyphae. (Courtesy, E. W. Koneman, Denver, Colorado.)

ated with humans rather than animals are called *anthropophilic;* those having a predilection for animals are *zoophilic.*

Laboratory Diagnosis. Hyphae of typical fungi can be observed on smears of epidermal scales or nail scrapings placed in 10 percent potassium hydrox-

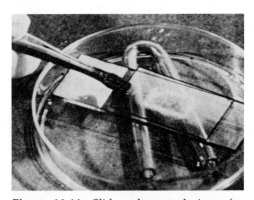

Figure 16-14 Slide culture technique for dermatophytes. Fungi are grown on a thinly sliced piece of agar on a slide and placed in a moistened Petri plate chamber. (From E. W. Koneman and S. E. Fann, *Practical Laboratory Mycology,* Part II, New York, Famous Teachings in Modern Medicine, Medcom, Inc., 1971.)

ide (KOH) and heated gently over the flame of a Bunsen burner (Figure 16-13). A periodic acid Schiff (PAS) stain can be used to stain hyphae for permanent mounts.

Infected hairs in tinea capitis or tinea barbae are examined for endothrix or ectothrix infection. A special ultraviolet light source, known as a Wood's lamp, causes fluorescence of scalp hairs if hairs are invaded by *M. audouinii,* the most common cause of tinea capitis in the United States.

Epidermal scales, nail scrapings, or hair can be cultured on a slightly acid carbohydrate-enriched medium, such as Sabouraud's dextrose agar, contained in bottles, tubes, or slide chambers (Figure 16-14).

Identification of specific organisms is made on the basis of macroscopic and microscopic morphology. Important macroscopic characteristics are colony morphology and color (Figure 16-15). The morphology of the macroconidia, when present, is helpful in assigning the organism to a particular genus (Table 16-5).

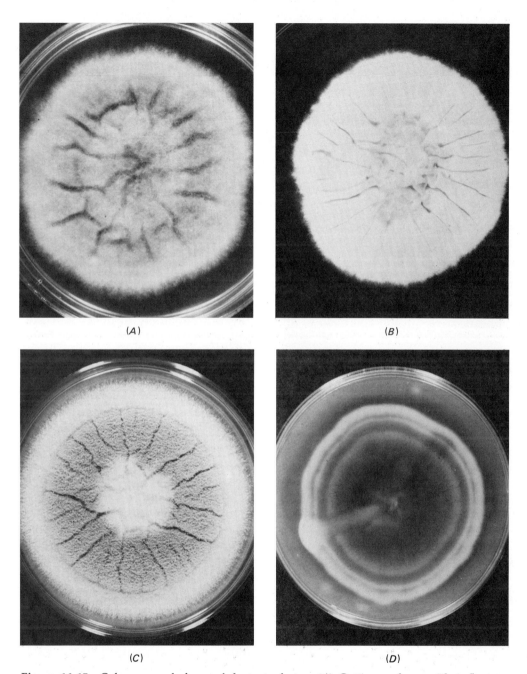

Figure 16-15 Colony morphology of dermatophytes. (*A*) Cottony colony with a floccose mycelium. (*B*) Velvety colony with a dense low mycelium. (*C*) Granular colony with a rough surface and an abundance of spores. (*D*) Glabrous or smooth colony with a waxy appearance and no mycelium. (Courtesy, E. W. Koneman, Denver, Colorado.)

Table 16-5 DIFFERENTIATION OF DERMATOPHYTES FROM APPEARANCE OF MACROCONIDIA

GENUS	FREQUENCY	SIZE (IN NM)	NUMBER OF SEPTATIONS	TYPE OF WALL
Microsporum	numerous, except *M. audouinii*	5–100 × 3–8	3–15	thick, rough, except *M. gypseum* and *M. nanum*
Trichophyton	usually rare	20–50 × 4–6	2–8	thin, smooth
Epidermophyton	numerous	20–40 × 6–8	2–4	thick, smooth

SOURCE: Adapted from U. S. Department of Health, Education, and Welfare, *CDC Laboratory Manual for Medical Mycology* (Washington, D.C.: U.S. Government Printing Office, 1963).

Immunity. The presence of circulating antibodies to the dermatophytes has not been demonstrated, but there appears to be considerable natural immunity in most individuals. No additional immunity is conferred by a superficial mycotic infection. Existing immunity is believed to be cellular in nature.

Prevention. The prevention of the tineas is somewhat dependent on the anatomic target site of the organism. Sharing of combs, hairbrushes, and caps, particularly among children, should be discouraged. Frequent disinfection of decking of public swimming pools, showers, and locker rooms, and the use of disinfectant foot baths can aid in eliminating potential infectivity of epidermal scales. Periodic inspection of pets for typical fungal lesions and subsequent treatment with a fungicide can reduce human infection with zoophilic species. In the event of tinea, disinfection of clothes, towels, and bedding can do much to prevent the spread of the infection to another member of the family or self-reinfection.

CUTANEOUS CANDIDIASIS

Yeasts, belonging to the genus *Candida,* can cause a variety of infections. *Candida albicans* is the most common cause of all candidiasis, but other species, such as *C. stellatoidea, C. parapsilosis, C. guilliermondii, C. krusei,* and *C. tropicalis* are being isolated with increasing frequency.

Generalized cutaneous candidiasis is common in diabetics or debilitated patients. It occurs occasionally in persons who have been subjected to long-term antimicrobial therapy. Chronic cutaneous candidiasis is rare, but it can cause discomfort and may even result in permanent disfigurement.

A superficial infection known as *intertriginous candidiasis* occurs in the groin, gluteal folds, umbilicus, axillae, between the toes and fingers, and under the breasts. The moisture and protection afforded by these areas often allows yeasts to produce moist, weeping vesicles or pustules.

Paronychia, an inflammation of the tissue surrounding the nail, is a more localized form of candidiasis. The in-

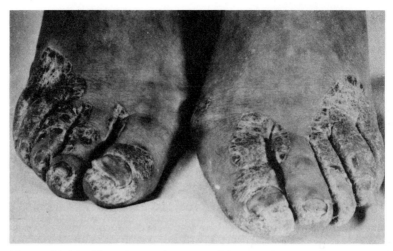

Figure 16-16 Chronic onychia caused by *Candida albicans* showing marked distortion of nails. (From N. F. Conant, D. T. Smith, R. D. Baker, and J. L. Callaway, *Manual of Clinical Mycology*, 3rd ed., Philadelphia, Saunders, 1971.)

flammation is called *onychomycosis* if it spreads to the nail (Figure 16-16).

An infection of the tongue, oral mucosa, or soft palate caused by *Candida* species is called *thrush*; it is usually a disease of the newborn.

Transmission. Many parts of the body are colonized by *Candida* species, especially *C. albicans*, so the primary source of infection is most often endogenous. The organisms are prominent in the upper respiratory tract, oral cavity, gastrointestinal tract, and vagina. The infection sometimes begins in the mucous membranes of those sites and spreads to contiguous epithelium of the skin near the nose, mouth, anus, or genitalia. Thrush is transmitted from mucous membranes of the birth canal during delivery. Exogenous sources, such as fruit or water containing the yeasts, do cause some candidiasis. Exposure to environmental organisms may be the source of infection for intertriginous candidiasis or paronychia.

Laboratory Diagnosis. *Candida* species grow well on Sabouraud's dextrose agar, but a more important diagnostic feature of the *Candida* yeasts is their ability to produce chlamydospores on corn meal agar.

C. albicans can be differentiated from other species by its ability to form short filaments, known as germ tubes, within a few hours, when the cells are placed in human serum or albumin (Figure 16-17). The oxidative and fermentative characteristics of yeasts on carbohydrates, such as glucose, maltose, sucrose, lactose, galactose, raffinose, and xylose, constitute important diagnostic aids in speciation.

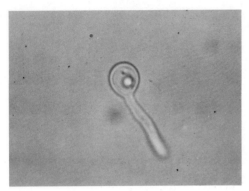

Figure 16-17 Germ tube of *Candida albicans* after incubation of the yeast cell in human serum. (From P. I. Bowman and D. G. Ahearn, *J. Clin. Microbiol.* 2:356, 1975.)

Immunity. Healthy individuals are resistant to candidiasis. Although circulating antibodies are demonstrable in persons who have recovered from candidiasis, no correlation between antibodies and immunity is apparent. The role of cellular immunity has been substantiated by successful treatment of chronic mucocandidiasis with transfer factor (Figure 16-18).

Prevention. Detection and treatment of vaginal candidiasis during the third trimester of pregnancy can prevent thrush in the newborn. Early detection of infections developing during antimicrobial therapy is important so that medication can be discontinued or supplemented with antifungal medication such as nystatin or amphotericin B.

Segregation measures and stringent attention to personal cleanliness are recommended in cutaneous candidiasis. Topical application of fungicides can sometimes prevent the spread of the infection.

In work requiring continual handling of fruit or exposure to water, wearing gloves decreases exposure to the fungus.

SPOROTRICHOSIS

Sporotrichosis is primarily an occupational disease of farmers, gardeners, and horticulturists. The causative organism is a dimorphic fungus, *Sporothrix schenckii*. The organism grows rapidly at room temperature as a mold, but converts to a yeast form on enriched media at 35°C. The disease is characterized by the formation of a nodule at the

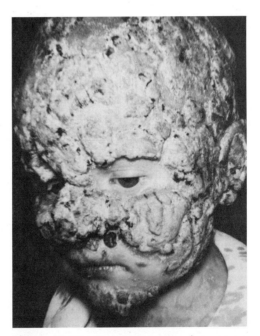

Figure 16-18 A severe case of mucocutaneous candidiasis in a child which was resolved by treatment with transfer factor. (From M. L. Schulkind, W. H. Adler III, W. A. Altemeier III, and E. M. Ayoub, *Cellular Immunol,* 3:606, 1972.)

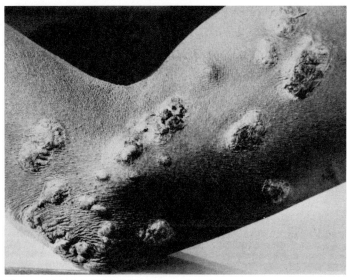

Figure 16-19 Advanced lesions of sporotrichosis on the arm and elbow. (From N. F. Conant, D. T. Smith, R. D. Baker, and J. L. Callaway, *Manual of Clinical Mycology,* 3rd ed., Philadelphia, Saunders, 1971.)

site of inoculation (Figure 16-19). Draining lymphatics can promote dissemination and formation of more nodules which sometimes ulcerate. The involvement of subcutaneous tissues allows the infection to persist for a long period, despite treatment. Arthritis, pneumonitis, and meningitis may be complications, but, fortunately, the disease is rarely fatal.

Transmission. The soil, vegetation, and wood are natural reservoirs for *S. schenckii*. Inoculation usually follows trauma from a splinter of wood or a thorn, although it is possible that organisms could have gained entry through a previously incurred wound.

Laboratory Diagnosis. The identification of *S. schenckii* is dependent on the conversion of the mycelial form to yeast cells on enriched media at 35°C. Cultures of the organism grown at room temperature are characterized by slender hyphae and conidia borne in a bouquet arrangement (Figure 16-20). With age, colonies change from white to yellow to black.

Differentiation of the pathogen from morphologically similar saprophytes can be accomplished by intraperitoneal inoculation of spores from a pure culture into mice or rats. The fungus produces an orchitis (inflammation of the testicle) in male animals.

Immunity. Little is known about immunity to sporotrichosis. Agglutinating, precipitating, and complement-fixing antibodies occur in sera of infected persons, but their significance in promoting resistance is uncertain.

Prevention. The sporadic occurrence of the disease makes it impossible to recommend universal preventative measures. Treatment of lumber with fungicides, in areas known to harbor the causative organism, could reduce exposure of individuals. Prompt treatment of small puncture wounds from splinters of wood or thorns could limit the spread of the organisms.

CHROMOMYCOSES

The chromomycoses are localized chronic infections of the skin and subcutaneous tissues. The fungi causing chromomycoses belong to three genera: *Phialophora*, *Cladosporium*, and *Fonsecaea*. The feet and legs are the most frequently affected sites. Lesions first appear as nodules, but later as verrucoid, ulcerated, or crusted lesions. The diseases are more common in tropical and subtropical climates than in temperate zones. They occur more often in males than in females, probably because of occupational exposure.

Transmission. The fungi causing chromomycoses are saprophytes commonly found in soil or on wood. The smallest cutaneous injury, even one that is virtually invisible, is sufficient for the spores to be introduced into the skin. Because of this ease of entry, individuals who lack the protection of shoes or clothes are very susceptible. The initial lesion can spread both laterally into epidermal cells and vertically into subcutaneous tissue, lymph, and even blood.

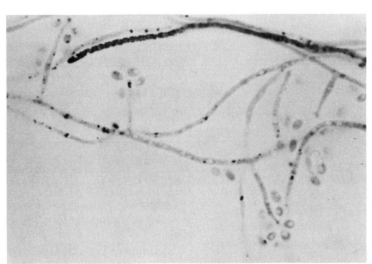

Figure 16-20 Microscopic view of conidia borne in a bouquet arrangement on slender hyphae from a culture of *Sporothrix schenckii*. (From E. W. Koneman and S. E. Fann, *Clinical Laboratory Mycology*, Part II, New York, Famous Teachings in Modern Medicine, Medcom, Inc., 1971.)

Laboratory Diagnosis. The causative organisms of the chromomycoses grow slowly and develop a smoky or dark appearance on Sabouraud's dextrose agar. The spores are borne on three types of conidiophores which are morphologically distinct one from the other. The types of sporulation are described as *acrotheca* type, *cladosporium* type, or *phialophora* type (Figure 16-21). In the acrotheca type of sporulation oval conidia occur along the sides of swollen club-shaped conidiophores. Cladosporium type of sporulation is characterized by the production of chains of oval or elliptical conidia at the ends of conidiophores which are slightly enlarged at their distal tips. In the phialophora type of sporulation oval conidia are produced in flask-shaped conidiophores (phialides). Although members of the genus *Phialophora* are typically associated with phialides and species of *Cladosporium* with the cladosporium type of sporulation, any of the three types of sporulation may be seen with species of *Fonsecaea*. Slide cultures are especially useful in demonstrating the types of sporulation.

Immunity. There is no evidence that circulating antibodies have a protective role against the chromomycoses. Like other infections caused by fungi, cellular immunity is probably more important. There is no evidence that persons who have had the disease are any less susceptible upon subsequent exposure.

Prevention. Since trauma is a prerequisite for the entrance of the causative organisms of the chromomycoses, ade-

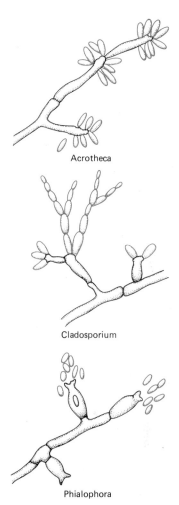

Figure 16-21 Types of conidia-bearing structures and spores found among agents of chromomycoses.

quate protection by shoes and clothes could prevent most of the infections. Since this is not possible in all parts of the world, immediate attention to puncture wounds, if evident, is important. Most cases have occurred in persons who have had little or no medical care for initial lesions and who have had less than adequate personal habits of hygiene.

FUNGUSLIKE INFECTIONS

Some moldlike bacteria produce cutaneous infections which spread by contiguity to subcutaneous tissue. The infections are usually chronic and are characterized by the formation of sinus tracts which drain suppurative lesions.

ACTINOMYCOSES

The actinomycoses are diseases of humans and cattle. Two organisms can cause the disease in cattle: *Actinomyces bovis* and *A. israelii*. *A. israelii* is the major pathogen of humans, but *A. propionicus*, *A. naeslundii*, *A. viscosus*, and *A. odontolyticus* all may be implicated in disease. All actinomycotic lesions contain other bacteria and distinct "sulfur granules," which are actually colonies of actinomyces.

The two most prominent sites for the cutaneous actinomycoses are the cervicofacial and temporofacial areas. Less frequently, thoracic or abdominal regions are involved. Primary lesions are almost always in the mandible or maxilla. The skin overlaying lesions may be discolored, but is usually devoid of identifiable lesions. The subcutaneous swelling is often considerable. An actinomycosis, known as "lumpy jaw," was once common in cattle.

Transmission. The actinomyces are ubiquitous in nature and particularly abundant in the soil. The major source in human infections is probably endogenous, however, because *A. israelii* is part of the indigenous flora of the mouth. Often lesions are extensions of periodontal abscesses or fractures of the jaw. Primary skin lesions can follow a human bite.

Laboratory Diagnosis. Sulfur granules can often be identified in specimens of pus. Gram strains of smears reveal gram-positive branching filaments of *Actinomyces* and usually other bacteria (Figure 16-22). Both *A. bovis* and *A. israelii* are anaerobic or microaerophilic and usually grow well in thioglycollate broth. Definitive speciation may require determining volatile and nonvolatile acids by gas chromatography.

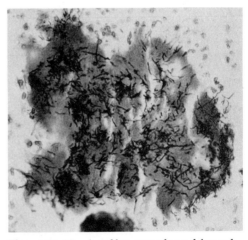

Figure 16-22 A sulfur granule and branching filaments from a case of actinomycosis. (Armed Forces Institute of Pathology Photograph, Neg. No. 59-7300.)

Immunity. Most individuals have a high level of immunity to the actinomycoses. Trauma may merely provide a portal of entry or may predispose persons to infection. Agglutinating, precipitating, and complement-fixing antibodies are produced by patients with actinomycoses, but there is no evidence that they are protective. Cellular immune mechanisms are more important.

Prevention. It is probable that the prophylactic use of antimicrobial agents in periodontal disease, fractures of the jaw, or following dental extractions can prevent the actinomycoses. Prompt diagnosis and treatment of suspected cases is important in limiting the spread of suppuration.

MYCETOMAS

The mycetomas are cutaneous lesions which extend deeply into subcutaneous tissue, including bone. The lesions usually occur on feet or hands and often exhibit considerable swelling (Figure 16-23). Madura foot is an old name for mycetoma of the foot. Multiple sinus tracts and secondary bacterial infections are common. The diseases occur in both tropical and temperate countries. They occur more frequently in rural than urban areas and are more common among males than females.

The causative organisms include the moldlike bacteria *Streptomyces, Actinomyces,* and *Nocardia,* as well as many true fungi and bacteria. The infectious agents are frequently found in

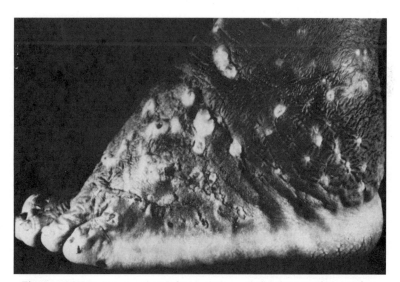

Figure 16-23 Appearance of mycetoma of the foot with tumefaction, deformity, and multiple draining fistulae. (From C. W. Emmons, C. H. Binford, and J. P. Utz, *Medical Mycology,* Philadelphia, Lea & Febiger, 1970.)

masses of organisms in the form of granules.

Transmission. The etiological agents of the mycetomas are ubiquitous, but particularly prominent in soil. Humans are infected by subcutaneous implantation through trauma, usually from a thorn or splinter.

Laboratory Diagnosis. Microscopic examination of pus reveals the presence of granules. However, biopsy material from deep tissues is preferable to pus, since contamination with secondary invaders is less frequent. The size, shape, color, and consistency of granules vary with the pathogen. The crushing of granules is necessary to observe the organisms. Most of the organisms will grow on a modified Sabouraud's agar. The necessity for additional tests depends on the nature of the isolate.

Immunity. Natural immunity is probably quite high against most of the etiological agents which have been implicated in the mycetomas. No definitive role for circulating antibodies has been established. Cellular immunity may be more important in limiting the spread of the disease.

Prevention. Prompt attention to puncture wounds and prophylactic administration of antimicrobials could prevent the colonization of pathogens following subcutaneous implantation. However, often the traumatic episode is unrecognized. The use of antimicrobials may stop dissemination of the causative agents, but amputation of an affected extremity may be necessary.

SUMMARY

The skin, hair, nails, and glands prevent the entrance of most microorganisms by providing both a mechanical and a physiological barrier. However, breaks in the skin, caused by insect bites, abrasions, lacerations, or puncture wounds, provide a portal of entry for pathogens as well as opportunistic bacteria and fungi. The invasion of cutaneous tissue by microorganisms is usually accompanied by the formation of a variety of lesions, some of which produce purulent or serous exudates. The most common bacterial infections are caused by staphylococci and streptococci. The fungi which cause infections of the skin, hair, or nails are called dermatophytes. The tineas are caused by species of *Trichophyton*, *Microsporum*, or *Epidermophyton*. Infections caused by yeast belonging to the genus *Candida* occur on the skin or mucous membranes of the body. Infections spreading to deeper tissues include sporotrichosis, the chromomycoses, actinomycoses, and mycetomas. Etiological agents of deep-tissue infections include true fungi, moldlike bacteria, and bacteria.

QUESTIONS FOR STUDY

1. Name the types of skin lesions produced by *Staphylococcus aureus*.
2. List the genera of fungi which cause tineas.
3. Name and describe two clinical types of leprosy.

4. Why should antimicrobial susceptibility tests be performed on all staphylococci isolated from infections?
5. Name five common Lancefield groups and the prototype species of each group.
6. What microbiological methods are of most value in the diagnosis of fungal infections?
7. Describe the conditions necessary for clostridia to establish infections in tissue.

SELECTED REFERENCES

Crouch, J. E. *Functional Human Anatomy.* 2d ed. Philadelphia: Lea & Febiger, 1972.

Emmons, C. W.; Binford, H. H.; and Utz, J. P. *Medical Mycology.* Philadelphia: Lea & Febiger, 1970.

Joklik, W. K., and Willett, H. P. *Zinsser Microbiology.* 16th ed. Englewood Cliffs, N.J.: Prentice-Hall, 1976.

Koneman, E. W., and Fann, S. E. *Practical Laboratory Mycology.* New York: Medcom Press, 1971.

Langley, L. L.; Telford, I. R.; and Christensen, J. B. *Dynamic Anatomy and Physiology.* 4th ed. New York: McGraw-Hill, 1974.

Lennette, E. H.; Spaulding, E. H.; and Truant, J. P. *Manual of Clinical Microbiology.* 2d ed. Washington, D.C.: American Society for Microbiology, 1974.

Wistreich, G. A., and Lechtman, M. D. *Microbiology and Human Disease.* 2d ed. Beverly Hills, Calif.: Glencoe Press, 1976.

Youmans, G. P.; Paterson, P. Y.; and Sommers, H. M. *The Biologic and Clinical Basis of Infectious Diseases.* Philadelphia: Saunders, 1975.

Chapter 17

Viral and Helminthic Diseases of the Skin

After you read this chapter, you should be able to:

1. Contrast the distribution of skin lesions in smallpox, chickenpox, and shingles.
2. Describe major skin infections caused by viruses.
3. Discuss the transmission, laboratory diagnosis, immunity, and prevention of the common viral infections of the skin.
4. Explain how it was possible to eradicate smallpox.
5. List the possible defects of congenital rubella syndrome.
6. List the helminths which have a predilection for cutaneous tissue.
7. Discuss the transmission, laboratory diagnosis, immunity, and prevention of the helminths causing cutaneous disease.

Since skin lesions frequently accompany systemic or subcutaneous diseases caused by organisms other than bacteria or fungi, it is sometimes difficult to classify some infections as to anatomic site. Although rickettsial diseases and bites of many arthropods cause lesions varying from a maculopapular rash to distinct bullae, the primary site of infection is often blood. Many viruses, such as those of smallpox, herpes, chickenpox, and measles, have a predilection for the skin. The larvae of some helminths migrate within tortuous channels in cutaneous tissue.

VIRAL INFECTIONS

The diseases of the skin caused by viruses may remain localized or spread by the bloodstream to produce systemic disease. Some viral diseases are self-limiting; others proceed from a *prodromal stage*, that is, an initial stage characterized by symptoms other than a rash, to an acute phase involving one or more organs. Unlike proliferation of bacteria in skin infections, viral replication may sometimes be diminished by natural host mechanisms before symptoms appear.

HERPES SIMPLEX INFECTIONS

The ubiquity and tendency for latency of the herpes simplex virus makes it an important opportunistic pathogen. Initial infections usually occur in children under 2 years of age and are frequently asymptomatic. If a primary disease develops, the herpetic vesicles occur on the mucous membranes of the mouth or on mucocutaneous borders. After the initial lesions have healed, the virus can persist in the ganglia of trigeminal

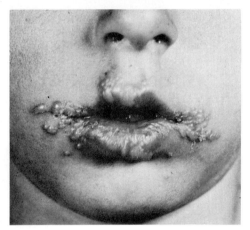

Figure 17-1 Multiple herpetic lesions on the lips. (Armed Forces Institute of Pathology Photograph, Neg. No. 55-11961.)

nerve cells. For that reason the herpes simplex virus was considered as a part of the indigenous microbiota in Chapter 11. Ultraviolet light, X ray, heat, cold, hormonal imbalance, and emotional disturbances may induce viral multiplication and recurrent disease. The virus can affect the skin on any part of the body, but most often manifests itself as a lesion on the lips (Figure 17-1). A disseminated form of herpetic infection may occur in children suffering from malnutrition, patients receiving immunosuppressive drugs, or individuals with defects in cell-mediated immunity.

Transmission. The initial infection usually occurs subsequent to a break in the skin or mucous membranes by direct contact with a herpetic lesion. The virus is often transmitted by kissing or sexual intercourse. For that reason some epidemiologists have termed the herpes simplex virus the "virus of love." Recurrent infections may be endogenous or exogenous in origin. A form of infection called herpes gladiatorum is believed to be transmitted by the close body contact provided by the sport of wrestling.

Laboratory Diagnosis. Herpes simplex infections are usually diagnosed without the aid of the laboratory. However, if confirmatory evidence is needed to supplement a clinical diagnosis, scrapings from the base of lesions can be submitted for histopathological studies. Multinuclear giant cells with intranuclear eosinophilic inclusion bodies are characteristic of cells infected with the virus (Figure 17-2). Vesicle fluid from lesions may

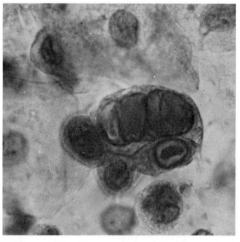

Figure 17-2 Group of multinuclear giant cells with intranuclear eosinophilic inclusion bodies from a case of herpetic esophagitis. (From S. M. Shah, R. F. Schaefer, and E. Araoz, *Acta Cytologica* 21:109-111, copyright © 1977 by International Academy of Cytology.)

be used to inoculate laboratory animals, chick embryos, or human embryonic lung fibroblasts for demonstration of inclusion bodies after an appropriate incubation period at 35°C. Specific antigens may be detected in smears of vesicle fluid by an immunofluorescent technique using fluorescein-tagged antibodies.

Immunity. It is uncertain if circulating antibodies to type 1 or 2 herpes simplex virus afford much protection against the virus infections. Since persons with impaired cell-mediated immunity, such as those with Wiskott-Aldrich syndrome or Hodgkin's disease, are very susceptible to infection by the virus, it is generally assumed that cellular mechanisms are more important than humoral response.

Prevention. The large number of asymptomatic infections and the latency potential of the virus make control difficult. Isolation of all cases with suspected herpetic infections is important to prevent the spread of the disease, particularly in susceptible hospital populations, that is, in those having impaired cellular immunity caused by disease or immunosuppressive therapy. It has been proposed that herpetic infections in infants could be prevented by performing cesarean sections in women having genital lesions caused by herpes simplex at term.

VARICELLA-HERPES ZOSTER INFECTIONS

The etiologic agents of varicella (chickenpox) and herpes zoster (shingles) are physically and immunologically identical. Both are caused by the varicella-zoster virus (V-Z). Chickenpox is the primary disease, whereas shingles is the recurrent form of the disease. The lesions of both diseases are similar. In both they start with macules, proceed to papules, and terminate in vesicles and also occur in crops so that all three types may be observed simultaneously. However, the distribution of lesions varies in the two diseases. The rash occurs typically on the trunk and face in chickenpox, whereas vesicles erupt along the distribution of a single sensory nerve in shingles (Figure 17-3). An intercostal

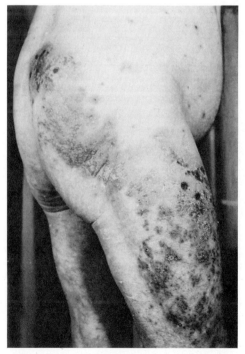

Figure 17-3 Distribution of lesions in shingles. (Armed Forces Institute of Pathology Photograph, Neg. No. ACC 219482-16013.)

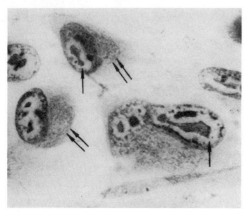

Figure 17-4 Intranuclear eosinophilic inclusion bodies in human embryonic cells infected with varicella-herpes zoster virus (single arrows). Eosinophilic bodies in the paranuclear area (double arrows). (From T. H. Weller et al., *J. Exp. Med.* 108:843, 1958.)

nerve is frequently involved. The infection is accompanied by inflammation and severe neuralgia.

Transmission. Chickenpox is transmitted primarily by direct contact with an infected person or with droplets from secretions of the respiratory tract of an infected person. It may also be transmitted indirectly by articles freshly contaminated with nasal or vesicle discharges. The scabs are not infective. The period of communicability is probably limited to the first week following primary eruption of vesicles. Shingles is usually of endogenous origin, but the virus can be transmitted by direct contact producing chickenpox in the susceptible host.

Laboratory Diagnosis. It is usually not necessary to use laboratory tests to diagnose chickenpox or shingles, but

infection with the V-Z virus can be confirmed by a complement-fixation (CF) or fluorescent antibody (FA) technique on paired sera. Antigens of the virus may be demonstrated in smears taken from epithelial cells underlying vesicles by using fluorescein-tagged antibodies. The virus can be grown in a variety of human and monkey cells. Eosinophilic inclusions and chromosomal aberrations occur in infected cells (Figure 17-4).

Immunity. Recovery from chickenpox almost always produces permanent immunity to that form of the disease, but predisposes the individual to shingles in later life.

Prevention. Children with chickenpox should avoid contact with susceptible adults and children and should not attend school for at least a week after vesicle eruption. The disease can be modified by the administration of pooled immunoglobulins, but this treatment is not recommended for general use.

POXVIRUS INFECTIONS

A number of poxviruses cause infections in animals, but those important to humans are the viruses of smallpox, vaccinia, and molluscum contagiosum. The history of smallpox dates back to antiquity and the attempts to eradicate the disease, beginning with Jenner's prophylactic technique, represent the most dramatic success story known in the prevention of infectious diseases. The vaccinia virus is also an important

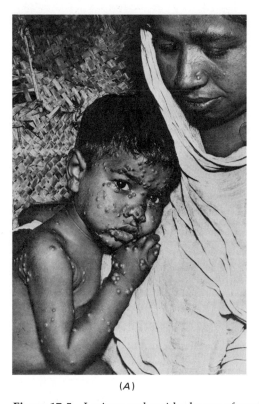

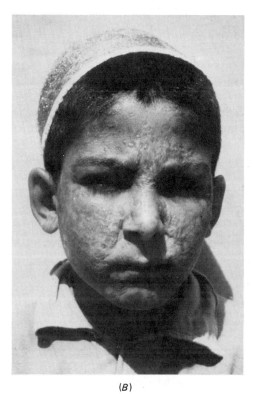

(A)

(B)

Figure 17-5 Lesions and residual scars of smallpox. (*A*) Typical pustules of a young victim — a sight the world hopes never to see again. The lesions dry up on the eleventh or twelfth day after eruption, leaving scars. (*B*) Scars which another victim will carry for a lifetime. (Courtesy, World Health Organization, Geneva.)

virus historically, for the agent, indigenous to cattle, is indistinguishable from the smallpox virus. Worldwide deliberate inoculation with the vaccinia virus has eliminated smallpox as a major public health problem.

Smallpox is a systemic disease characterized by fever, malaise, headache, and skin lesions which pass through macular, papular, vesicular, and pustular stages and terminate in scab and scar formation (Figure 17-5). The lesions do not occur in crops as in chick-

enpox, but are at any one time essentially all at the same stage of development. They display a centrifugal pattern of distribution and are more abundant on the face and extremities than on the trunk. Two types of smallpox have occurred: *variola major*, the classical disease, and *variola minor* or alastrim. Skin lesions are similar in both, but milder systemic symptoms are manifested in variola minor. Fatality rates up to 50 percent or greater have been reported for variola major; fatality rates for variola minor rarely exceed 2 percent.

The virus of molluscum contagiosum causes wartlike lesions of the skin which are usually devoid of an inflammatory response. The disease is found more frequently in children and participants of contact sports. Lesions occur most frequently on the hands or face and only rarely on the lower extremities. The lesions can be removed effectively by curettage or electrodesiccation.

Transmission. Both smallpox and molluscum contagiosum are spread by direct contact with an infected patient or by indirect contact with material from lesions. Viruses of smallpox may be acquired by inhalation. The organisms invade the respiratory mucosa and spread to the regional lymph nodes and bloodstream. Transmission of smallpox to laundry workers by bedding has been documented. Both smallpox and molluscum contagiosum are communicable for the duration of lesions.

Laboratory Diagnosis. A diagnosis of smallpox can usually be made without the aid of the laboratory by its sudden onset and distribution of lesions, if it can be established that the patient has not been vaccinated and has a history of possible exposure. The smallpox virus can be isolated from vesicular and pustular fluid or crusts in embryonated eggs or tissue cultures. It produces typical pocks on chorioallantoic membranes of chick embryos (see Figure 4-12).

Early lesions of molluscum contagiosum may resemble warts, but scrapings from the lesion, when placed in 10 percent potassium hydroxide (KOH), reveal intracytoplasmic inclusion bodies.

Immunity. Recovery from either form of smallpox produces permanent immunity. It is doubtful that the person with molluscum contagiosum develops any protection against subsequent attacks. There appears to be little or no natural immunity to either disease.

Prevention. In the event of a smallpox outbreak isolation, quarantine, appropriate disinfection of contaminated materials, immunization of contacts, and investigation of possible sources of infections are all important control measures. Widespread vaccination with vaccinia virus has proved to be the most important prophylactic measure in the eradication of the once dreaded disease.

Since man is the only source of infection for molluscum contagiosum, it is important to identify the source of the virus, to remove any lesions, and to reexamine the patient several times in order to detect any further eruptions of lesions.

PAPOVAVIRUS INFECTIONS

Although viruses belonging to the papovavirus group produce benign tumors which may undergo malignant changes in a number of animals, the only virus of this group known to cause disease in humans is the human-wart virus. Warts frequently occur on the backs of hands, wrists, fingers, or around nailbeds (Figure 17-6).

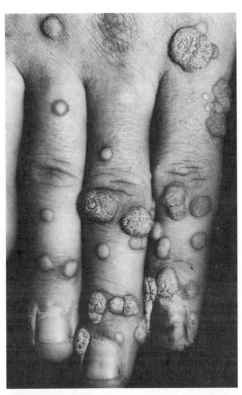

Figure 17-6 Common warts on the hand and fingers. Proliferation of epithelial cells infected with a papovavirus and progressive keratinization cause the solid growths. (Courtesy, G. W. Korting, Mainz, Germany.)

Transmission. Transmission of the human-wart virus is by direct contact with an infected person. No cases of indirect contact have been documented.

Laboratory Diagnosis. Warts can usually be recognized easily, but if doubt exists regarding the etiology, the excised lesion can be sent to the laboratory for histologic examination. Eosinophilic or basophilic inclusion bodies, representative of abnormal keratinization, indicate a viral etiology for the proliferative disease.

Immunity. There is no evidence that having had a wart affords any protection against subsequent invasion of epidermal cells by the human-wart virus.

Prevention. Treatment of warts by excision or chemicals, such as trichloroacetic acid, is important in preventing the spread of the infectious disease to other members of the family or to those having close contact with the patient. Complete control may necessitate examination of other members of the family in an attempt to discover a reservoir.

RUBEOLA-RUBELLA INFECTIONS

It is unfortunate that for many years rubeola and rubella infections have both been designated as measles, because the infections differ in severity, duration of symptoms, and possible complications. Rubeola, sometimes called the 14-day measles, is an acute, highly communicable disease characterized by maculopapular lesions (Figure 17-7). It occurs almost always in children and is caused by a paramyxovirus. A prodromal period in which the patient exhibits fever, conjunctivitis, coryza, and cough lasts for three or four days. Koplik's spots on the buccal mocosa are diagnostically important.

Rubella, often called German or three-day measles, has an insidious onset, that is, it develops so gradually that it is well established before symptoms are apparent, but it is only moderately contagious. It is caused by a togavirus but, unlike other members of that group, is not arthropod-borne. The disease is mild in both children and adults,

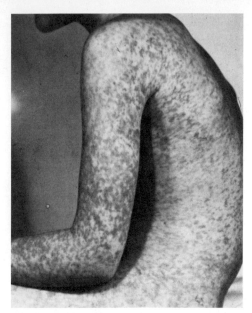

Figure 17-7 Rash of rubeola showing extent of lesions at the peak of skin involvement. (Courtesy, D. H. Koobs and Department of Pediatrics, Loma Linda School of Medicine, Loma Linda, California.)

but if acquired during pregnancy, it can produce *congenital rubella syndrome*, a group of defects present at birth in the infant. Purpura, heart disease, encephalitis, blindness, deafness, and mental retardation are but a few of the possible complications.

Transmission. Both rubeola and rubella are transmitted by direct contact with an infected individual or by indirect contact through materials contaminated with nasopharyngeal secretions, blood, urine, or feces of infected persons. Individuals with rubeola excrete large amounts of the virus in nasal secretions during the prodromal period. The virus may be shed in the urine up to four days after the rash appears. The virus of rubella is shed from the naso-

pharynx for seven to ten days before clinical signs of disease are present and up to a week thereafter. Infants with congenital rubella syndrome may shed virus for months after birth. Some individuals vaccinated with attenuated strains of the rubella virus have also been shown to shed virus, but it is unlikely that it is an important mode of transmission.

Laboratory Diagnosis. The rubeola or rubella virus can be detected by hemagglutination-inhibition (HI), complement-fixation (CF), or immunofluorescent antibody (FA) techniques. The HI antibody appears soon after onset of disease whereas CF antibody appears later. A four-fold or greater rise in titer on paired sera is diagnostic for the diseases. The diagnosis of rubella in pregnant women should be confirmed by isolation of the virus from the throat in tissue cultures. The presence of IgM antibodies in early infancy is diagnostic for congenital rubella infection, since the IgM molecules cannot cross the placental barrier.

Immunity. Immunity after an attack of rubeola is permanent; no recurrence has ever been documented. Infection with rubella was once thought to confer lifelong immunity, but recent reports of reinfection have cast some doubt on longevity of the immune state following infection. Congenital immunity to rubella lasts 6 to 12 months if the mother is immune to the disease.

Prevention. Mass immunization for rubeola and rubella has caused substantial declines in both diseases in the last five years. However, the lasting quality of immunity from vaccination with attenuated measles viruses is in some doubt; evidence suggests that there may be a need for booster immunization in the future. The incidence of congenital rubella syndrome has decreased, but the need still exists to identify and immunize susceptible women of child-bearing age.

HELMINTHIC INFECTIONS

The larva of certain parasitic nematodes invade the skin, subcutaneous tissues, and occasionally the viscera of vertebrate hosts, including humans. The dermatitis is called cutaneous larva migrans or creeping eruption. Creeping eruption is more common in tropical and subtropical climates than in temperate zones; in the United States it occurs mainly along the Gulf of Mexico and in the southern Atlantic states. Three filarial worms or their larvae can invade cutaneous and subcutaneous tissues producing rashes, nodules, or ulcers. Cutaneous filariasis is common in the tropics.

CUTANEOUS LARVA MIGRANS

Ancylostoma braziliense, the most common etiological agent of cutaneous larva migrans, is a frequent intestinal inhabitant of dogs and cats. Feces from man's favorite pets pollute beaches, backyards, and parks. Developing larvae penetrate the skin of barefoot chil-

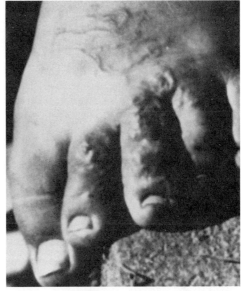

Figure 17-8 Lesions of cutaneous larva migrans (creeping eruption) on the foot. (From J. W. Smith et al., *Diagnostic Medical Parasitology: Intestinal Helminths*, Chicago: American Society of Clinical Pathologists, © 1976. Used by permission.)

dren or adults and make intracutaneous tunnels beneath the surface of the skin (Figure 17-8). At the point if invasion, a papule develops; vesicles form along the course of tunnels.

Transmission. The disease is transmitted only by contact with soil containing larvae excreted by infected dogs or cats.

Laboratory Diagnosis. There is usually no need for laboratory tests since diagnosis can be made in endemic areas by evidence of tunneling in the skin and by the presence of subcutaneous nodules. There is a marked eosinophilia. Biopsy material is necessary for species identification of larval forms.

381

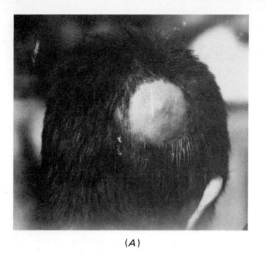
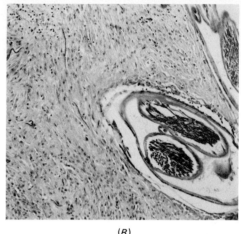

(A)　　　　　　　　　　　　　　　　　(B)

Figure 17-9 Onchocerciasis. (A) Scalp nodule containing masses of adult worms. (B) Microscopic view of a nodule section showing microfilariae in adult worms. (Armed Forces Institute of Pathology Photograph, Neg. Nos. N-79133 and N-80606.)

Immunity. All individuals are uniformly susceptible if exposed to soil contaminated with feces from infected dogs or cats. Little or no protection from subsequent infection is obtained by an initial contact with causative agents of cutaneous larva migrans.

Prevention. Creeping eruption of hookworm origin can be prevented by controlling infections in household pets and protecting children from stray dogs and cats. For example, covering children's sandboxes, when not in use, can sometimes prevent contamination of sand with dog or cat feces.

CUTANEOUS FILARIASIS

The three major forms of cutaneous filariasis are onchocerciasis (river blindness), loaiasis (eye worm infection), and dracontiasis (guinea worm infection). All are caused by filarial nematodes with a propensity for cutaneous tissues.

Adult worms of *Onchocerca volvulus*, the etiological agent of onchocerciasis, can be found in masses within cutaneous or subcutaneous nodules (Figure 17-9). The nodules constitute the eventual graveyards for the adult forms, for in time they degenerate and die there. Microfilariae, released by the mature females, migrate into subcutaneous tissues and sometimes to the eye, where they cause blindness. The disease occurs only in Africa and some parts of Central and South America.

The etiological agent of loaiasis, *Loa loa*, is known for its continuous migratory excursions in subcutaneous tissue. The typical Calabar lesion is named for an area in which the disease is endemic. Calabar lesions consist of transient red swollen areas usually on the upper extremities or the eye caused by the extensive migratory action of the parasite (Figure 17-10). Larvae mature

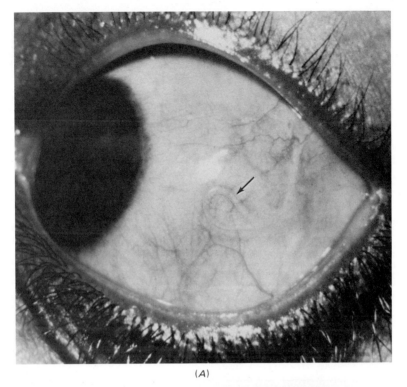

(A)

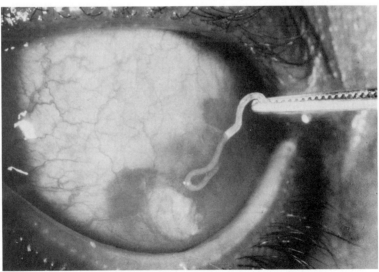

(B)

Figure 17-10 *Loa loa* in the eye. (*A*) Wandering adult worm. (*B*) Removal of adult worm from the eye. (From P. Fenton, *Arch. Ophthalmol.* 76(December):867, 1966. Copyright 1966 by American Medical Association.)

in the subcutaneous and muscular tissue in about one year. Damage is minimal despite the extensive migrations undertaken by microfilariae when released by mature female worms. The sheathed microfilariae appear in blood with a diurnal periodicity, that is, always in the daytime. Loaiasis is endemic in tropical West Africa.

Dracontiasis differs from other forms of cutaneous filariasis in that the initial contact with the causative agent, *Dracunculus medinensis,* is by ingestion of larval forms of the worm. Larvae, freed during digestion, migrate into connective tissue and mature in about 10 weeks. Upon maturation the adult female parasite produces a blister. Later, a vesicle occurs on the skin as the worm surfaces to discharge microfilariae. Rupture of the vesicle produces a small opening into which a probe can be inserted to extract the worm (Figure 17-11). It has been estimated that over 48 million persons in Africa, South America, and Southwestern Asia are infected with the guinea worm.

Transmission. The three forms of cutaneous filariasis are transmitted to the human host by intermediate hosts. The initial traumatic event in onchocerciasis is the bite of a fly belonging to the genus *Simulium,* which harbors the larvae of *O. volvulus* (Figure 17-12). The larvae penetrate the wound when the fly bites the human host. Infection with *L. loa* is spread by species of the deerfly, *Chrysops.* Infection of humans with *D. medinensis* follows the drinking of water infested with the parasite's intermediate host, the crustacean *Cyclops.*

Laboratory Diagnosis. The presence of cutaneous filariasis can be suspected in the presence of typical lesions in endemic areas. Definitive identification of *O. volvulus* or *L. loa* depends on finding

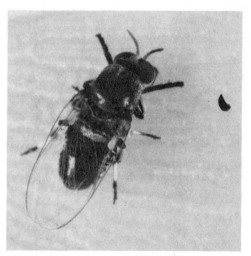

Figure 17-12   Dorsal view of the black fly *Simulium damnosum,* magnifiied 13 times. The fly is the intermediate host for the filarial nematode *Onchocerca volvulus.* (Photograph by D. H. Connor, Armed Forces Institute of Pathology Photograph, Neg. No. 72-4519-B.)

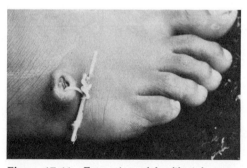

Figure 17-11   Extraction of the filarial worm *Dracunculus medinensis* from a ruptured vesicle on the surface of the skin. (Courtesy, P. E. C. Manson-Bahr, London.)

Table 17-1 CHARACTERISTICS OF *ONCHOCERCA VOLVULUS* AND *LOA LOA*

CHARACTERISTIC	*O. VOLVULUS*	*L. Loa*
Length (in μm)	150–185 or 285–370	250–300
Appearance (in stained smears	smooth, sweeping coils	irregular, kinky coil
Sheath	absent	present
Stylets	none	1
Nuclei in tail	do not extend to tip	extend to tip

microfilariae in slices of skin or blood. Repeated examinations may be necessary. Microfilariae of *O. volvulus* or *L. loa* can be differentiated by their appearance on stained smears or sections (Table 17-1). Sometimes *D. medinensis* can be palpated, detected by reflected light, or suspected by the pattern of erythema. Upon extraction, the adult female filarial worm measures 3 feet or more in length. Eosinophilia is always present in cutaneous filariasis. Complement-fixation tests for the agents of cutaneous filariasis are available and may be of some value.

Immunity. Persons living in endemic areas are universally susceptible. One infection provides little or no protection against a second attack.

Prevention. Destruction of vectors with insecticides and protection of skin with appropriate clothing and repellents could do much to eliminate onchocerciasis and loaiasis. Surgical removal of adult worms may be somewhat effective in controlling onchocerciasis. Chlorination, filtering, or boiling of water to be used for drinking could help eliminate the intermediate hosts of dracontiasis and, therefore, prevent human infections.

SUMMARY

The skin lesions caused by most viruses and helminths are similar to those of bacterial infections. Among those producing distinctly different lesions are the human-wart virus, the virus of molluscum contagiosum, and the filarial worm *Loa loa*. Few diseases of viruses have definitive pathognomonic signs, but the distribution and eruption times of lesions may be important in differential diagnosis. Effective vaccination programs have eradicated smallpox and reduced the incidence of rubeola, rubella, and congenital rubella syndrome.

QUESTIONS FOR STUDY

1. Why is the herpes simplex virus called the "virus of love"?
2. Identify the following characteristics as being associated with rubeola or rubella.

   insidious onset   cough
   conjunctivitis   coryza
   congenital defects
   highly contagious

3. How have mass immunization measures affected the incidence of smallpox, rubeola, and rubella?
4. Name the etiological agents of the following helminthic infections.
   river blindness
   eye worm infection
   guinea worm infection
   cutaneous larva migrans
5. Identify the type of cutaneous filariasis spread by the following arthropod vectors.
   Simulium
   Chrysops
   Cyclops

SELECTED REFERENCES

Brown, H. W. *Basic Clinical Parasitology*. 4th ed. Englewood Cliffs, N.J.: Prentice-Hall, 1975.

Davis, B. D.; Dulbecco, R.; Eisen, H. N.; Ginsberg, H. S.; and Wood, W. B., Jr. *Microbiology*. 2d ed. New York: Harper & Row, 1973.

Hoeprich, P. D. *Infectious Diseases*. 2d ed. New York: Harper & Row, 1977.

Koneman, E. W.; Richie, L. E.; and Tiemann, C. *Practical Laboratory Parasitology*. New York: Medcom, 1974.

Kortin, G. W. *Diseases of the Skin in Children and Adolescents*. Philadelphia: Saunders, 1970.

Markell, E. K., and Voge, M. *Medical Parasitology*. 4th ed. Philadelphia: Saunders, 1976.

Rothschild, H.; Allison, F., Jr.; and Howe, C. *Human Diseases Caused By Viruses*. New York: Oxford, 1978.

Chapter 18

Bacterial, Mycotic, and Protozoal Diseases of the Respiratory Tract

After you read this chapter, you should be able to:

1. Explain how the respiratory tract is adapted to resist infections.
2. Differentiate between upper and lower respiratory tract infections.
3. Describe the most common bacterial infections of the lungs.
4. Discuss the transmission, laboratory diagnosis, immunity, and prevention of the common bacterial infections of the lungs.
5. List factors which predispose individuals to infections caused by *Streptococcus pneumoniae*.
6. List the major serological groups of commonly isolated streptococci.
7. Explain the role of animal inoculation in the diagnosis of bacterial and fungal diseases of the respiratory tract.
8. Discuss the transmission, laboratory diagnosis, immunity, and prevention of the three major deep mycoses.
9. Discuss the transmission, laboratory diagnosis, immunity, and prevention of actinomycosis, nocardiosis, and aspergillosis.
10. Describe the circumstances which permit *Pneumocystis carinii* to establish an infection in the lung.

The respiratory tract consists of the nose, pharynx, larynx, trachea, bronchi, and lungs (Figure 18-1). With the aid of a number of accessory organs, including the diaphragm and intercostal muscles, the organs provide a passageway for the transportation and exchange of the gases of respiration. The procurement of oxygen and elimination of water and carbon dioxide are necessary to sustain life.

The exposure of the respiratory tract to microbial contaminants in the atmosphere is unavoidable. Microorganisms of varying sizes become airborne as solid or liquid particles known as *aerosols*. The particle size and moisture content influence the deposition of aerosols following inhalation. Most particles larger than 6 μm in diameter are trapped in the nose. Of those under 6 μm, hygroscopic particles, that is, those with the capacity to absorb moisture readily, are deposited with greater frequency than nonhygroscopic particles of the same size (Table 18-1). The

Table 18-1 DEPOSITION OF SMALL HYGROSCOPIC PARTICLES (UNDER 6 μM DIAMETER)

ANATOMIC SITE	PERCENT OF DEPOSITION
Nose	36
Pharynx, secondary bronchi	1
Tertiary bronchi, bronchioles	25
Alveolar ducts	21
Total retained	83

SOURCE: Adapted from V. Knight, *Viral and Mycoplasmal Infections of the Respiratory Tract* (Philadelphia: Lea & Febiger, 1973).

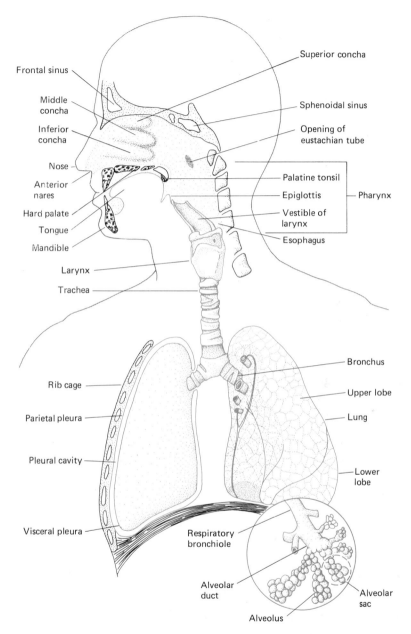

Figure 18-1   The upper and lower respiratory tract, pleura, and diaphragm.

continuity of the mucous membrane lining of the respiratory tract provides the means for infectious aerosols to spread throughout the air passageways and even into the auditory tubes or paranasal sinuses.

Infections of the respiratory tract are classified as upper respiratory infections (URI) if the nose, paranasal sinuses, middle ear, pharynx, or tonsils are involved. The nose, pharynx, and tonsils are the most frequently affected sites. Infection of the airway can be specified by use of such terms as rhinitis, sinusitis, or pharyngitis, but more often the term URI is used since frequently multiple sites are involved. Lower respiratory infections involve the trachea, bronchi, alveolar spaces, or supporting interstitial tissue of the lungs. In infections of the lower respiratory tract, it is more common to differentiate the specific anatomic site of the infection.

BACTERIAL INFECTIONS

The bacteria causing upper or lower respiratory tract disease are derived from indigenous flora of the oropharynx or nasal cavities or from aerosols in coughs or sneezes of carriers or infected persons. Bacteria are small enough to gain access to alveoli, but defense mechanisms prevent their implantation and colonization in healthy individuals. However, inhalation of large numbers of bacteria or an immunosuppressed state provides favorable conditions for proliferation and possible invasion.

STAPHYLOCOCCAL INFECTIONS

Staphylococci rarely cause disease of the respiratory tract in the healthy adult, but are common opportunists in the host compromised by surgical intervention or antimicrobial therapy. Staphylococcal pneumonia, does not generally occur in the absence of a predisposing virus infection except in children under the age of 2 years. Infants become colonized with staphylococci shortly after birth. The typical etiological agent is *Staphylococcus aureus*, but coagulase-negative strains of staphylococci have also been implicated. The inflammatory reaction may be absent or edema and abscess formation may be so severe as to cause death within a few hours (Figure 18-2).

Transmission. *S. aureus* may be of endogenous or exogenous origin in staphylococcal pneumonia. Floors, bedding, laundries, and infected patients represent hospital reservoirs for the organism. Healthy carriers of *S. aureus*, harboring the organism in the nose or throat, constitute special hazards.

Laboratory Diagnosis. Gram stains of sputum show numerous polymorphonuclear leukocytes and gram-positive cocci, which may not be distinguishable from streptococci (Figure 18-3). Pure cultures of *S. aureus* are frequently grown on blood plates inoculated with sputum of patients with

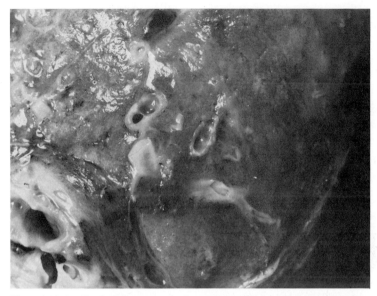

Figure 18-2 Typical lesions of a lung in staphylococcal pneumonia. (Armed Forces Institute of Pathology Photograph, Neg. No. 55-6150.)

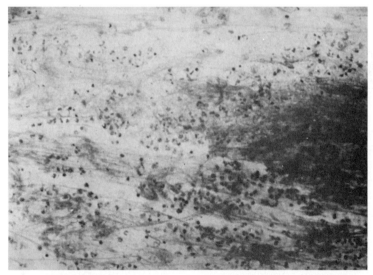

Figure 18-3 Sputum with an abundance of neutrophils and absence of squamous epithelial cells. (Courtesy, American Society for Microbiology, Washington, D.C.)

staphylococcal pneumonia. A positive coagulase reaction is a better index of pathogenicity than either pigmentation or hemolysis.

Immunity. Healthy adults appear to have substantial natural immunity to staphylococcal pneumonia. Only young infants and immunosuppressed patients lack the ability to mobilize defense mechanisms against *S. aureus* in the lower respiratory tract.

Prevention. The numbers of cases of staphylococcal pneumonia can be reduced by surveillance of patients recovering from viral infections and those compromised by age, therapy, or underlying disease. In addition, hospital-acquired staphylococcal pneumonias can be prevented by instituting rigorous environmental controls.

STREPTOCOCCAL INFECTIONS

So-called "strep throat," caused by group A streptococci, is one of the most common infectious diseases. Streptococci belonging to serological groups other than group A are rarely isolated from patients with pharyngitis or tonsillitis. The "strep throat" can occur as a localized infection or as a part of disseminated streptococcal infection of contiguous membranes of the upper or lower respiratory tract. Most usually, the posterior pharyngeal mucous membranes and tonsils are involved, but organisms can invade the middle ear, sinuses, bloodstream, joints, or heart.

Streptococcus pneumoniae probably causes few cases of acute bacterial pharyngitis, but is the primary cause of lobar pneumonia. Sometimes a single lobe is involved; other times all the lobes of one lung or one lobe of both lungs are infected. There are 83 documented capsular types of *S. pneumoniae*, but only 14 cause serious disease. Pneumococcal disease is a problem in closed populations, such as military recruits, and in the elderly. It has been estimated that the fatality rate for pneumococcal pneumonia approximates 5 to 10 percent.

Scarlet fever is a disease of the upper respiratory system caused by an erythrogenic toxin-producing strain of group A beta-hemolytic streptococci. The distinguishing characteristic of the disease is a fine rash appearing on the chest, neck, groin, and thighs. Typically, a desquamation of skin from the fingers, toes, palms of hands, and soles of feet occurs during convalescence.

Transmission. Streptococci usually are spread by aerosols from a cough or a sneeze of an infected individual or a carrier; only rarely are they transmitted by indirect contact with contaminated objects. Healthy carriers constitute the primary reservoir of *S. pneumoniae*. Predisposing factors to infection include age, debilitating disease, and immunosuppression. Alcoholics and persons who have had splenectomies are particularly susceptible to *S. pneumoniae*. The reason for the increased susceptibility is not well understood.

Laboratory Diagnosis. Gram stains of smears from throat swabs or sputum reveal gram-positive cocci in pairs or

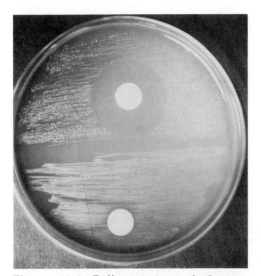

Figure 18-4 Differentiation of *Strepto-coccus pneumoniae* and alpha-hemolytic streptococci on a blood agar plate. The upper half of the plate demonstrates suscep-tibility of *S. pneumoniae* to optochin. The lower half of the plate demonstrates resis-tance of alpha-hemolytic streptococci to op-tochin. (Courtesy, Saint Joseph Medical Center Laboratories, Burbank, California.)

short chains. Group A streptococci pro-duce beta hemolysis; *S. pneumoniae* produces alpha hemolysis. Hemolytic characteristics of other Lancefield groups of streptococci may be variable. *S. pneumoniae* is soluble in bile and sus-ceptible to the chemical optochin. If an optochin-impregnated disc is placed on a blood agar plate inoculated with the organism, growth is inhibited (Figure 18-4). Group A beta-hemolytic strepto-cocci are susceptible to small amounts of bacitracin, but not to optochin.

Immunity. In the absence of previous contact with a particular strain suscep-tibility to streptococcal infection is gen-eral. Immunity against type-specific erythrogenic toxin following scarlet fever is permanent, but second attacks of scarlet fever can occur since there are three immunologic types of erythro-toxin. Passive immunity explains pro-tection afforded to newborns from streptococcal infections. Although the means exists to provide prophylactic immunization against streptococci, the large number of strains makes the pro-cedure impractical.

Prevention. To control contact with infected persons, isolation of cases, and the reduction of crowding in institu-tions are important. It is virtually im-possible to control healthy carriers of beta-hemolytic streptococci.

A polyvalent polysaccharide vaccine against 14 capsular types of *S. pneumo-niae* has now been licensed for use in the United States. It is recommended for high-risk populations. It appears that particularly the elderly and chil-dren over 2 years of age with chronic diseases or splenic impairment may benefit from the polyvalent polysac-charide vaccine. The duration of immu-nity provided by the vaccine is not yet known.

KLEBSIELLA INFECTIONS

Klebsiella pneumoniae, or Friedlander's bacillus, has long been recognized as a cause of lobar pneumonia in males over 40 years of age and in chronic alcoholics of both sexes. Patients with Fried-lander's pneumonia almost always enter the hospital with the disease.

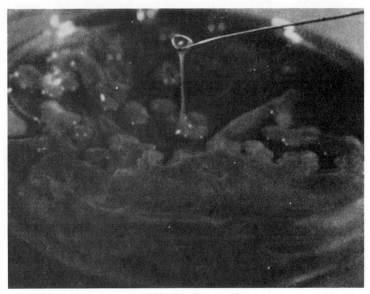

Figure 18-5 Mucoid growth of *Klebsiella pneumoniae* on Endo agar. (Courtesy, Abbott Laboratories, *Atlas of Diagnostic Microbiology*, p. 19, July, 1974.)

More recently, *K. ozaenae, K. oxytoca,* and *K. rhinoscleromatis* have been recognized as opportunistic pathogens of both the lower and upper respiratory tracts. The opportunists cause degenerative changes in the nasal and pharyngeal mucosa.

Transmission. *Klebsiella* species are spread directly by aerosols or indirectly by contact with freshly soiled discharges of infected persons. Nasal carriers with no symptoms of disease may be the primary reservoirs of the organism.

Laboratory Diagnosis. Bacilli belonging to the genus *Klebsiella* resemble the enteric organism *Enterobacter aerogenes,* but they have large amounts of capsular material, are nonmotile, and have a mucoid appearance on the surface of agar (Figure 18-5). Klebsiella species are not fastidious in their growth requirements; they are easily isolated on MacConkey's agar, blood, or eosin methylene blue (EMB) agar.

Of the klebsiellae, *K. pneumoniae* of capsular types 1 and 2 cause the most serious lung disease.

Immunity. Resistance to *Klebsiella* organisms is usually high except in alcoholics and debilitated persons. Limited immunity to a serological type of *K. pneumoniae* probably occurs after an attack.

Prevention. Friedlander's pneumonia and other upper respiratory infections caused by *Klebsiella* species can be reduced by isolation of infected individuals and avoidance of crowding in institutions.

HAEMOPHILUS INFECTIONS

Haemophilus influenzae is a common cause of acute bronchiolitis in infants and young children and of chronic bronchitis in adults. The name *influenzae* has no etiological significance today, but the organism was once believed to be the cause of the 1918–1919 pandemic of influenza. In 1933 the influenza virus A was unequivocally shown to be the cause of epidemic influenza. The bacterial pathogen had assumed the role of a secondary invader. Today, pneumonia caused by *H. influenzae* accounts for almost all bacterial pneumonias not caused by pneumococcus *(S. pneumoniae)* or *Klebsiella* species. *H. influenzae* and *S. pneumoniae* are sometimes isolated from the same individual. *H. influenzae*, type B, is the primary serological type promoting infections in children.

Transmission. Like other etiological agents of pneumonia, most *H. influenzae* is spread by aerosols or by articles freshly contaminated with nasal or pharyngeal discharges from infected individuals or carriers. The organism is quite susceptible to cold so does not survive for long periods of time after expectoration.

Laboratory Diagnosis. *H. influenzae* is one of the smallest gram-negative bacilli, typically measuring approximately 1.5 μm in length by 0.3 μm in width. Some strains are highly pleomorphic and occur as long filaments. The coccobacilli are sometimes encapsulated; the filamentous forms never have capsules. *H. influenzae* requires two growth factors: an X factor or hemoglobin component and a V factor which has been identified as the coenzyme nicotinamide adenine dinucleotide (NAD). Although both substances are present in blood agar, the V factor tends to be sequestered in the red blood cells. Best results are obtained when red cells are lysed by heating blood agar to 80° to 90°C to make a preparation called chocolate agar.

H. influenzae produces a phenomenon called *satellism* on blood agar inoculated with *S. aureus*. The colonies of *H. influenzae* grow abundantly surrounding a colony of the gram-positive coccus which supplies V factor to the fastidious *Haemophilus* organisms (Figure 18-6). Precipitin or quellung reaction tests can be used to differentiate the six serological types, designated as a through f.

Immunity. Healthy adults appear to have a high degree of resistance to *H. influenzae*. Immunity after an attack may be limited. Immunization with capsular polysaccharides, while effective, has been used very little to date.

Prevention. Whenever practical, crowding in institutions should be minimized. Prompt institution of antimicrobial therapy can effectively decrease the period of communicability in infectious states.

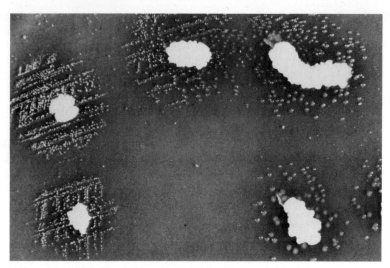

Figure 18-6   Satellism demonstrated by *Haemophilus influenzae* surrounding colonies of staphylococci on blood agar. (Courtesy, Abbott Laboratories, *Atlas of Diagnostic Microbiology*, p. 25, July, 1974.)

BORDETELLA INFECTIONS

Several *Bordetella* species have been incriminated in cases of acute bronchiolitis in both young children and adults, but the primary pathogen of the genus is *B. pertussis*, the cause of whooping cough, or pertussis, by far the most serious disease caused by the genus. Other *Bordetella* species cause at least a small proportion of the cases. Whooping cough is characterized by three distinct phases. During the *catarrhal* phase, which lasts approximately two weeks, the cough is usually nonproductive and nocturnal, a rhinorrhea and low-grade fever persists, and a leukemoid reaction (an increase in leukocytes, predominantly lymphocytes) is pathognomonic. The *paroxysmal* phase, which lasts two to four weeks, is associated with paroxysms of coughing. Unlike the cough of the catarrhal phase, the paroxysmal spasms enable the patient to bring up thick mucus. An actual whoop may or may not be present. During the *convalescent* phase, another two weeks or longer, the cough subsides.

Transmission. *B. pertussis* is spread directly by contact with laryngeal or bronchial discharges or indirectly by articles contaminated with the discharges. The disease is most communicable during the catarrhal stage.

Laboratory Diagnosis. The specimen of choice for the isolation of *B. pertussis* is the nasopharyngeal swab. If the swab is taken during the catarrhal stage, it is estimated that there is a 95 percent chance for recovery of the organism.

The organism is very sensitive and swabs should be streaked immediately on Bordet-Gengou agar, a medium enriched with glycerol, potato, and blood. Gram stains of smears or colonies from Bordet-Gengou reveal gram-negative bacilli measuring 1.0 μm by 0.3 to 0.5 μm in size. Some pleomorphism may be observed, particularly in old cultures, where filamentous forms may actually predominate. The organism is hemolytic, but somewhat inert biochemically. Slide agglutination tests using specific antiserum can be helpful in confirming a diagnosis. A fluorescent antibody procedure can be applied to smears of exudate in lieu of culturing the organism. Complement-fixation and agglutination tests on paired sera may show rising titers if sampling for the second specimen is done late in convalescence.

Immunity. Recovery from whooping cough is generally associated with permanent immunity to recurrent attacks. Development of demonstrable antibodies is notably slow in whooping cough.

Prevention. In the United States vigorous adherence to the immunization of preschool children has substantially reduced the threat of whooping cough as a major public health problem. Pertussis vaccine is combined with diphtheria and tetanus toxoids (DPT) for simultaneous immunization against the three diseases. The initial immunization procedure consists of three injections four to eight weeks apart. The first injection can be given as early as 2 months of age. Boosters are recommended one year after the third injection and before the child enters school.

CORYNEBACTERIUM INFECTIONS

The most important pathogen of organisms belonging to the genus *Corynebacterium* is *C. diphtheriae*. It can cause disease of any part of the upper respiratory tract, but is most often the etiological agent of a type of pharyngitis known as diphtheria. *C. diphtheriae* can be a part of the resident population of the upper respiratory tract in healthy individuals and cause no discernible harm. However, if an individual is susceptible to the exotoxin of the organism, a severe pharyngitis occurs which is often complicated by a myocarditis and mild to complete paralysis.

Transmission. *C. diphtheriae* is transmitted by direct contact with aerosols composed of nasal or pharyngeal discharges of infected persons or carriers; only rarely is it transmitted indirectly by contaminated fomites. Since the organism can cause skin lesions, contact with such lesions cannot be ruled out as a source of the pharyngeal organism.

Laboratory Diagnosis. Smears made from nasopharyngeal swabs and stained with methylene blue reveal the presence of pleomorphic bacilli ranging from 1 to 6 μm in length and 0.3 to 0.8 μm in width. Club-shaped and branching forms are common; irregular staining caused by an abundance of granules is characteristic (Figure 18-7).

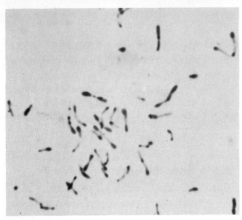

Figure 18-7 Irregular staining of *C. diphtheriae* demonstrated with methylene blue. (Courtesy, Center for Disease Control, Atlanta, Georgia.)

Loeffler's medium, which contains coagulated beef serum and nutrient broth, is frequently used for primary isolation of the organism. A virulence test must be performed for confirmation of toxigenicity of isolated strains of *C. diphtheriae*. Guinea pigs or the Elek *in vitro* procedure described in Chapter 14 may be used to demonstrate virulence.

Immunity. Susceptibility to diphtheria is low until the age of 6 months, increases in unvaccinated children until the age of 4 or 5, and then gradually declines. The use of toxoid in DPT preparations has eliminated diphtheria as a major disease in the United States. The *Schick* skin test is useful in determining susceptibility to diphtheria. The test employs an intradermal injection into the forearm of a small amount of diphtheria toxin.

Prevention. Active immunization with diphtheria toxoid is the most effective measure for preventing diphtheria. Following primary immunization, in which three intramuscular injections of DPT are given, booster doses should be given one year after the third injection and when a child starts school.

PULMONARY ANTHRAX

Pulmonary anthrax is not a common disease. It has occurred only sporadically in the last 50 years. It follows a somewhat different course than the other bacterial pneumonias. The inhaled spores of *Bacillus anthracis* lodge in the pulmonary parenchyma, where they are phagocytized by macrophages. The spores germinate following transportation of macrophages to lymph nodes. The organisms spread to the lungs via the bloodstream. The widening congestion and consolidation caused by the infection almost invariably culminate in death.

Transmission. Pulmonary anthrax does not require direct contact with contaminated wool or hides. Air containing spores of *B. anthracis* can be the source of the infection. No evidence exists that the disease can be transmitted from one individual to another.

Laboratory Diagnosis. Gram-stained smears of sputum reveal gram-positive bacilli occurring in chains. *B. anthracis* grows on ordinary culture media; its similarity to *B. cereus* was described in Chapter 16.

Immunity. Although some animals are immune to anthrax, humans appear to be universally susceptible. No second attacks have been documented, since pulmonary anthrax is usually fatal. Although vaccination is available for animals, it has never been deemed practical to immunize people.

Prevention. Despite lack of evidence for person-to-person transmission, cases of pulmonary anthrax should be isolated promptly to avoid exposure to other individuals. Disinfection of wool, hair, hides, or other animal products from endemic areas is recommended to prevent dissemination of anthrax spores into other countries.

PNEUMONIC PLAGUE

Pneumonic plague can occur as a secondary infection to the bubonic form of the disease or can be present as a primary infection. It is usually fatal. The causative organism, *Yersinia pestis*, is highly communicable and has been responsible for many devastating epidemics throughout the years.

Transmission. Pneumonic plague is transmitted by aerosols. The disease is highly communicable. The epizootic disease, also known as *sylvatic plague*, can be transmitted to man by the bite of infected rat fleas (*Xenopsylla cheopis*).

Laboratory Diagnosis. Gram stains of sputum in pneumonic plague reveal the presence of gram-negative cocco-bacillary forms measuring 1.0 to 2.0 μm in length and 0.5 to 1.0 μm in width. The organism grows readily on ordinary media and resembles some coliforms. *Y. pestis* is nonmotile and differs from two related species, *Y. enterocolitica* and *Y. pseudotuberculosis*, in that it is urease negative. Agglutination tests or animal inoculations may be undertaken to confirm an identification.

Immunity. There appears to be uniform susceptibility to pneumonic plague. Even after recovery from the bubonic form of the disease, immunity is often only temporary. During World War II the United States Army used killed bacilli to immunize soldiers. The successful control of rodent and flea populations has obviated the necessity of using the vaccine as a prophylactic measure.

Prevention. No country currently has laws making vaccination for plague mandatory prior to entry. However, during an epidemic of pulmonary plague an individual can be required to be placed in isolation for a minimum of six days before leaving a country or disembarking from a ship. Single doses of attenuated *Y. pestis* organisms are used by some countries in endemic areas. Two or three doses of a vaccine containing killed cells of *Y. pestis* are recommended for high-risk populations. It is wise to avoid contact with wild rodents of any kind whether or not plague has been reported in animal populations.

MYCOBACTERIUM INFECTIONS

The major pathogen in the pulmonary disease known as tuberculosis is *Mycobacterium tuberculosis*, but other

Mycobacterium species, sometimes described as atypical acid-fast bacilli, cause pulmonary disease which is indistinguishable from tuberculosis. Tuberculosis was the leading cause of death in the United States at the beginning of the twentieth century. With the advent of chemotherapy there has been a substantial decrease in mortality rate and a reduction in hospitalization times for most patients.

Transmission. *Mycobacterium tuberculosis* is spread directly by aerosols from a person with active pulmonary disease to a susceptible individual. It is probably only rarely transmitted by contaminated materials from a patient. In the United States *M. bovis*, a pathogen of cows, has been almost eliminated as an etiological agent of human tuberculosis by pasteurization of milk.

Laboratory Diagnosis. Chest X rays are of importance in screening large numbers of persons in high-incidence populations for pulmonary tuberculosis. Positive findings on X rays, seen as shadows on posteroanterior or lateral chest films, constitute only presumptive evidence for presence of the disease. The confirmatory diagnosis of pulmonary tuberculosis requires additional tests and the isolation and identification of the etiological agent from sputum or gastric washings.

Individuals infected with tubercle bacilli demonstrate a cell-mediated type of hypersensitivity to a purified protein derivative (PPD) of tuberculin or old tuberculin (OT). The Mantoux procedure and Tine modification were described in Chapter 13.

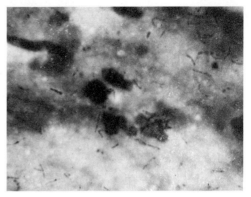

Figure 18-8 A microscopic field showing numerous acid-fast bacilli stained by the Ziehl-Neelsen method. With the technique the bacilli can be observed as brilliant red rods against a blue background. (From G. D. Roberts, *J. Clin. Microbiol.* 2:261, 1975.)

The presence of acid-fast bacilli, measuring 0.2 to 0.6 μm in width by 1.0 to 10 μm in length, on smears supports a presumptive diagnosis of mycobacterial pulmonary disease (Figure 18-8). Mycobacteria can also be demonstrated by fluorescent microscopy using auramine. With appropriate filters the organisms appear yellow against a dark background.

The guinea pig is susceptible to small numbers of *M. tuberculosis* and *M. bovis*. For that reason and because the guinea pig can tolerate contaminating organisms rather well, it is the animal of choice to document a diagnosis of tuberculosis. Upon death or sacrifice of an inoculated guinea pig, typical lesions of tuberculosis (tubercles) can be found on various organs if the isolate is an acid-fast pathogen. Although the validity of negative tests is questionable, guinea pigs are still used on a limited basis in the diagnosis of tuberculosis.

Immunity. Susceptibility to tuberculosis is general, but approximately one-third of the reported new cases in the United States occur in persons between the ages of 45 and 64. Most active cases in adults occur as reinfections from an exogenous or endogenous source. An endogenous reinfection arises from the breakdown of inactive lesions from a primary, often unrecognized, infection. Tuberculosis differs from other pulmonary infections in that the disease process is merely arrested by treatment and persons with residual lesions remain reservoirs of potential infectivity.

Prevention. The vaccine BCG (Bacille Calmette-Guérin), developed by the French scientists Calmette and Guérin early in the twentieth century, has been employed successfully in many parts of the world to prevent tuberculosis. The vaccine, which contains an attenuated bovine strain of the tubercle bacillus, has not been used on a large scale in the United States. The tuberculin sensitivity resulting from use of the vaccine negates the usefulness of diagnostic skin tests. BCG is recommended for household contacts of tuberculous individuals.

An alternate preventative measure, in the event of high risk because of age, underlying disease, or prolonged immunosuppressive therapy, is the administration of isoniazid. Isoniazid is particularly effective in preventing relapse in arrested cases of tuberculosis. This form of chemoprophylaxis is, however, too expensive for entire communities. Correction of overcrowding and poverty, routine chest X rays, and periodic tuberculin skin tests are essential in the prevention of tuberculosis as long as reservoirs exist in persons with present or past infections.

MYCOPLASMA INFECTIONS

Mycoplasmas have been known for many years to be important pathogens of animals, but *Mycoplasma pneumoniae* is the only member of the wall-deficient organisms causing respiratory disease in humans. Although the lung is the primary site of infection, the nasopharynx, larynx, trachea, and bronchi may be involved. Mycoplasmal pneumonia is sporadic and affects primarily older children and young adults. The pneumonia caused by the mycoplasmal organism is described as primary atypical pneumonia.

Transmission. It appears that *M. pneumoniae* is not highly communicable for it takes weeks for it to spread even among members of the same family. The risk of infection is greater in congested areas. Outbreaks in military recruits and college populations suggest that repeated contact with respiratory secretions may be necessary for transmission to occur.

Laboratory Diagnosis. No rapid test exists for the diagnosis of primary atypical pneumonia caused by *M. pneumoniae*. The organism can be isolated from sputum on media enriched with yeast extract and horse serum, but grows slowly. Colonies of *M. pneumoniae*, with their typical "fried-egg" appearance, can be observed in one to three weeks on solid media after incubation at 35°C (Figure 18-9). Specific serologi-

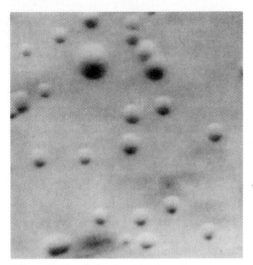

Figure 18-9 Colonies of *Mycoplasma pneumoniae* grown on PPLO agar. (From C. Liu in P. D. Hoeprich, *Infectious Diseases*, 2d ed., New York, Harper & Row, 1977.)

cal tests, including complement-fixation, indirect hemagglutination, and metabolic inhibition tests, are infrequently used outside of the research laboratory. Streptococcus MG and cold agglutinins are present in the blood of some patients with primary atypical pneumonia caused by *M. pneumoniae* one to four weeks after the onset of the disease, but the agglutination tests are nonspecific.

Immunity. The susceptibility of young people to mycoplasmal pneumonia is not well understood. However, the production of specific antibodies to the organism in response to an infection either prevents or modifies a subsequent infection. Both inactivated or attenuated vaccines and the use of tem-

perature-sensitive mutants of *M. pneumoniae* show promise for the eventual development of a vaccine.

Prevention. The avoidance of crowding, particularly among military recruits and college populations, can substantially reduce respiratory infections caused by *M. pneumoniae*. Intrafamilial transmission can sometimes be prevented by the prophylactic use of antimicrobial agents.

MELIOIDOSIS

Melioidosis is a pulmonary disease which is endemic in southeast Asia. The disease can manifest itself as a chronic lung infection similar to tuberculosis. However, the course of the infection is sometimes characterized by a latency period during which no symptoms are evident. When the latent infection is reactivated, an acute septicemia, which usually terminates in death, can occur. The suddenness with which the highly fatal form of melioidosis appears has caused it to be known as the "Vietnamese time bomb." During the Vietnam war a significant number of cases of melioidosis occurred in American soldiers.

The causative organism, *Pseudomonas pseudomallei*, a gram-negative bacillus, is a soil inhabitant in southeast Asia and can be isolated from surface waters as well. The organism gains entrance to the body by inhalation or through a break in the skin. Prompt recognition and treatment are important in reducing fatalities. No form of immunization is available.

LEGIONNAIRES' DISEASE

Legionnaires' disease is a serious infection of the lung with a mortality rate of approximately 20 percent. It was thought to have made its first appearance as an outbreak of a febrile respiratory illness in Philadelphia in the summer of 1976 and was given its name because individuals affected were attending a state American Legion convention. It now appears that the pulmonary infection is widespread and had occurred as early as 1947.

The etiological agent is a small pleomorphic gram-negative bacillus which has been named *Legionella pneumophila*. The organisms are difficult to recover by conventional culturing techniques. Charcoal yeast extract agar, egg yolk sacs, and intraperitoneal inoculation of guinea pigs have been used successfully to isolate the bacilli from pleural fluid or transtracheal aspirates (Figure 18-10). Direct and indirect fluorescent antibody tests are also proving useful for the diagnosis of Legionnaires' disease. The natural habitat of *L. pneumophila* has not yet been defined, but it has been found in surface water, mud, and water in air-conditioner cooling towers. No forms of immunization have been developed.

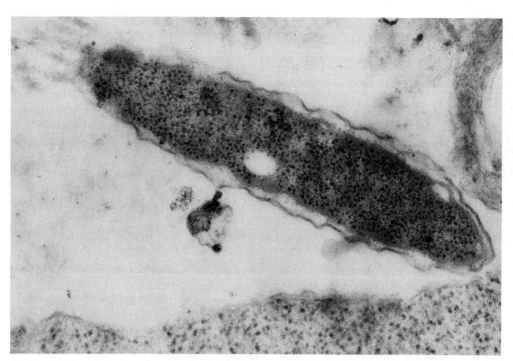

Figure 18-10   Electron micrograph of a thin section of *Legionella pneumophila* in the yolk sac of an embryonated hen's egg. (Courtesy, Center for Disease Control, Atlanta, Georgia.)

FUNGAL INFECTIONS

Other than the skin, hair, and nails, the most common primary sites of fungal infections are the lungs. The fungi which infect deeper tissues and internal organs are distinct from those which cause superficial infections. The diseases which they cause are called *deep mycoses*. The major deep mycoses are histoplasmosis, coccidioidomycosis, and blastomycosis.

HISTOPLASMOSIS

Acute pulmonary infections caused by *Histoplasma capsulatum* occur in all age groups of both sexes but are more frequent in adult males, probably because of greater exposure. The chronic form of the disease simulates tuberculosis on chest X rays. Its clinical course also resembles tuberculosis. The progressive systemic form of the disease is most often observed in the very young, the aged, or those with immunologic deficiencies. Again like tuberculosis, primary histoplasmosis may be asymptomatic. It differs from tuberculosis in that favorable resolution of the infection is more frequent.

Transmission. *H. capsulatum* is transmitted by inhalation of airborne spores of the fungus. Soil around old chicken houses, starling roosts, and caves harboring the common brown bat serve as reservoirs for the organism. The disease is contracted mostly by persons in rural communities. In the United States it is especially prevalent in the Mississippi and Ohio river valleys.

Laboratory Diagnosis. Wet mounts or Wright-stained smears of sputum, gastric washings, pleural fluid, excised pulmonary lesions, and occasionally blood or bone marrow reveal the presence of typical organisms in the yeast phase. The yeasts measure 3.0 μm by 4.0 to 5.0 μm in size.

Definitive morphology of the mycelial phase is obtained when the organism is isolated on Sabouraud's dextrose agar at 30°C (Figure 18-11). A white aerial mycelium, which turns brown with age, is characteristic of the mycelial phase. Large round tuberculate macroconidia, approximately 7.5 μm in diameter, are important in the identification of the histoplasmosis organism.

A number of serological tests are useful, but the most reliable is the complement-fixation test using antigens of either the yeast or mycelial phase. Yeast-phase antibodies are common in acute histoplasmosis, whereas mycelial-phase antibodies are usually present in chronic forms of the disease. Animal inoculation and skin tests with histoplasmin, a protein analogous to tuberculin, may also be employed in the diagnosis of histoplasmosis.

Immunity. Susceptibility to a primary infection of *H. capsulatum* is general, but middle aged and older men appear to be more susceptible to the disseminated and chronic forms of the disease. Endogenous reactivation of

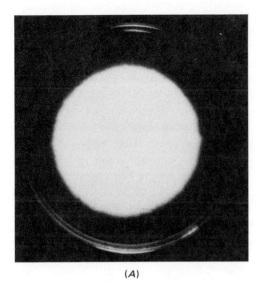
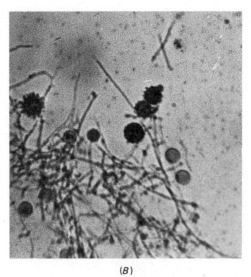

(A)

(B)

Figure 18-11 *Histoplasma capsulatum.* (A) Macroscopic view of mycelial phase showing a white aerial mycelium. (B) Microscopic view showing tuberculate macroconidia. (Courtesy, H. Larsh, Norman, Oklahoma.)

histoplasmosis similar to that found in tuberculosis can occur. No vaccine for histoplasmosis is available.

Prevention. Decontamination of soil harboring *H. capsulatum* spores is not practical for very large areas, but attempts to minimize exposure to soil containing fowl or bat excreta can reduce cases of the disease. No effective vaccine is available.

COCCIDIOIDOMYCOSIS

San Joaquin Valley fever or coccidioidomycosis is endemic in the southwestern part of the United States. Its causative organism, *Coccidioides immitis*, grows well in soil as a mold, reproducing asexually by arthrospores.

The organism infects cattle, dogs, sheep, burros, pigs, rodents, and humans. Only a few people who have contact with the arthrospores develop symptoms of respiratory disease. In most people the disease is self-limiting and no treatment is necessary for mild to moderate primary coccidioidomycosis. The disseminated form of the disease, which occurs more frequently in dark-skinned individuals, can be fatal.

Transmission. *C. immitis* is transmitted by inhalation of arthrospores from soil, dust, or plants from arid areas. It is also readily transmitted from cultures in the laboratory. The white cottony mycelium on laboratory cultures bears abundant infectious spores and should

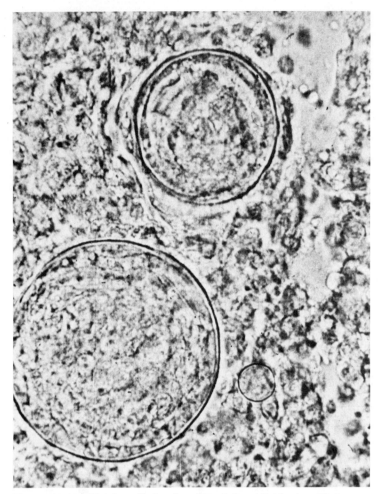

Figure 18-12 Thick-walled spherules of *Coccidioides immitis* in unstained wet mount of sputum. (From H. W. Larsh and N. L. Goodman, in E. H. Lennette et al., *Manual of Clinical Microbiology*, 2d ed., Washington, D.C., American Society for Microbiology, 1974.)

only be handled by experienced personnel. There is no evidence that the organism is transmitted by an infected individual to a susceptible person.

Laboratory Diagnosis. Direct examination of sputum may reveal thick-walled spherules, measuring 30 to 60 μm in diameter, which contain numerous endospores (Figure 18-12). Definitive diagnosis requires culturing the organism on Sabouraud's dextrose agar at 30°C. The arthrospores are readily demonstrated by a lactophenol cotton

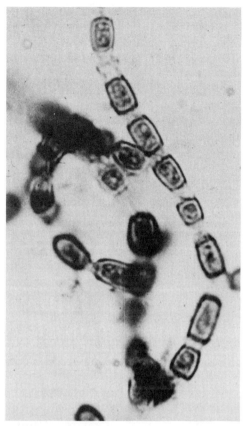

Figure 18-13 Arthrospores of *Coccidioides immitis* stained with lactophenol cotton blue in a wet mount. (From H. W. Larsh and N. L. Goodman, in E. H. Lennette et al., *Manual of Clinical Microbiology*, 2d ed., Washington, D.C., American Society for Microbiology, 1974.)

blue stain in a wet mount. The arthrospores are barrel-shaped and alternate with empty cells (Figure 18-13). Confirmation of *C. immitis* is obtained by intratesticular injection of guinea pigs with a suspension of spores. Severe orchitis (inflammation of the testitle) occurs in 7 to 10 days.

Precipitating antibodies against *C. immitis* are produced early in the disease, but complement-fixing antibodies are not present until four to eight weeks following onset. Intracutaneous administration of coccidioidin, prepared in a similar fashion to tuberculin, produces 5 mm or more of induration in pulmonary infections and a weak or no reaction in disseminated infections.

Immunity. Susceptibility to a primary infection of *C. immitis* is general. Recovery is followed by permanent immunity. No vaccine for coccidioidomycosis is available.

Prevention. Since disinfection of soil is virtually impossible, persons in endemic areas are bound to be exposed to *C. immitis*. Oiling of dirt roads and planting of grass does limit dissemination of arthrospores by wind. Recruitment of road or farm workers from nonendemic areas should probably be discouraged.

BLASTOMYCOSIS

Blastomycosis is an acute or chronic disease of the lungs or skin caused by the dimorphic fungus *Blastomyces dermatitidis*. The pulmonary form of the disease is generally mild and is often unrecognized. The cutaneous form of the disease usually follows systemic involvement. Blastomycosis occurs most frequently in the central and southeastern parts of the United States. It is sometimes called North American blastomycosis to differentiate it from a similar clinical entity found in Central and

South America caused by *Paracoccidioides brasiliensis.*

Transmission. The conidiospores of the mycelial phase of *B. dermatitidis* from soil reservoirs are probably inhaled in spore-laden dust, although the organism has not been isolated from soil in endemic areas with any regularity. There is no evidence that blastomycosis is transmitted directly from person to person.

Laboratory Diagnosis. Smears of sputum, pleural fluid, exudates, or biopsy

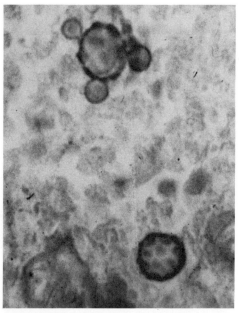

Figure 18-14 Spherical, thick-walled yeast-like cells of *Blastomyces dermatitidis* stained with lactophenol cotton blue in a wet mount. (From H. W. Larsh and N. L. Goodman, in E. H. Lennette et al., *Manual of Clinical Microbiology,* 2d ed., Washington, D.C., American Society for Microbiology, 1974.)

material, stained with lactophenol cotton blue or hematoxylin and eosin, reveal large, spherical, thick-walled yeastlike cells 8 to 15 μm in diameter (Figure 18-14).

No culture should be identified as the etiological agent of North or South American blastomycosis without demonstration of yeast forms. Intratesticular or intraperitoneal inoculation of hamsters may be required to convert mycelial growth to the yeast phase. Cells of *B. dermatitidis* produce single buds with broad bases in contrast to the multiple buds on narrow bases formed by *P. brasiliensis.* The appearance of the large, spherical cells of *P. brasiliensis,* which reach diameters of 30 μm or more, and their daughter cells has been likened to the wheel of a ship; the buds are often variable in size (Figure 18-15). The yeast phase of both *B. dermatitidis* and *P. brasiliensis* can be obtained on blood agar at 35°C.

Mycelial phases of the organisms grow on Sabouraud's dextrose agar at 30°C and produce lateral or terminal conidia. The mycelia are initially white, but may turn tan or brown with age.

Both precipitating and complement-fixing antibodies are produced in North American blastomycosis, but the tests have limited value because of cross-reactions encountered in cases of histoplasmosis and coccidioidomycosis. Blastomycin skin tests are of little help in diagnosing blastomycosis.

Immunity. There is no definitive information about susceptibility of populations to *B. dermatitidis* or *P. brasiliensis* or any about possible immunity derived from exposure to the fungi.

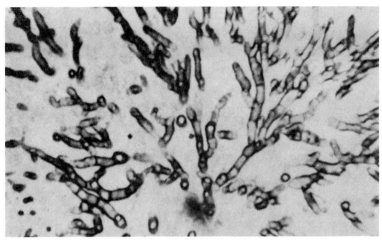

Figure 18-17 Human lung tissue showing short fragments of hyphae of *Aspergillus fumigatus*. (From E. L. Hazen, M. A. Gordon, and F. C. Reed, *Laboratory Identification of Pathogenic Fungi Simplified*, 3rd ed., 1970. Courtesy, Charles C Thomas, Publisher, Springfield, Illinois.)

Immunity. Resistance to pulmonary nocardiosis is high in general populations. The increased susceptibility in the compromised host is caused by a depression of cellular immune mechanisms. It is unknown if immunity follows an attack of nocardiosis.

Prevention. The ubiquity of *N. asteroides* in soil precludes effective control methods. Aggressive surveillance of patients on long-term glucocorticoids and prompt administration of an antimicrobial regimen in the event of lung infection could prevent chronic pulmonary disease and dissemination to other organs.

PULMONARY ASPERGILLOSIS

Pulmonary aspergillosis is caused by one or more species of *Aspergillus*, a mold found in decaying plants, stored hay, and cereal grains. The most important human pathogen is *A. fumigatus*, but other species are occasionally isolated from the lung. There are four major forms of pulmonary disease designated as aspergillosis: (1) primary acute pneumonia, (2) formation of a "fungus ball" within a previously existing cavity, (3) allergic bronchopulmonary aspergillosis, and (4) secondary pulmonary aspergillosis, occurring as an opportunistic infection.

Transmission. Aspergillus species are transmitted by inhalation of the spores. There is no evidence of person-to-person transmission.

Laboratory Diagnosis. *A. fumigatus*, which causes approximately 90 percent of aspergillosis, can often be observed in wet mounts of sputum after digestion with 10 percent potassium hydroxide. In biopsy material only short fragments of hyphae are usually visible when sections are stained with hematoxylin and eosin (Figure 18-17). The or-

411

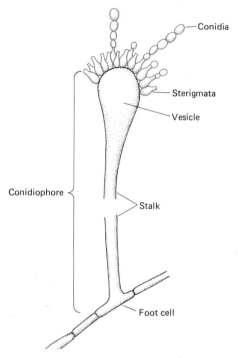

Figure 18-18 Flask-shaped vesicle of *Aspergillus fumigatus* showing conidiophore, a single row of sterigmata, and conidia.

ganism grows rapidly on Sabouraud's dextrose agar as a dark blue or green mold. It produces flask-shaped vesicles, a single row of sterigmata, and conidia (Figure 18-18).

Biochemical tests, serological techniques, and animal inoculations have little application. Skin tests may aid in screening patients suspected of allergic bronchopulmonary aspergillosis.

Immunity. Resistance to *A. fumigatus* is high in general populations. Underlying disease processes, especially those providing cavities in the lungs, predispose some individuals to infec-tion. Long-term chemotherapy or ad-ministration of glucocorticoids predis-poses other persons to opportunistic infection with *Aspergillus* species.

Prevention. There are no recom-mended control methods for aspergil-losis. Aggressive surveillance of pa-tients with weakened cellular defense mechanisms is necessary to permit early diagnosis and prompt treatment.

PROTOZOAL INFECTIONS

The lung can become involved as a sec-ondary site of infection caused by some protozoa as well as a few helminths. There is, however, one extracellular protozoan which occurs as a primary invader in premature and debilitated infants and more rarely in im-munosuppressed adults. The organism, *Pneumocystis carinii*, causes interstitial plasma cell pneumonia, a disease char-acterized by thickened alveolar septa infiltrated with plasma cells (cells derived from B-cell lymphocytes). The alveoli become filled with fat-laden cells, exudate, and the parasites, occur-ring as sporelike bodies in clusters en-closed within a thin membrane (Figure 18-19).

The mode of transmission for *Pneumocystis carinii* has not been defi-nitely established, but the protozoan appears to be widespread in nature. It is likely that the organism is airborne and that it can reside in the naso-pharynx of asymptomatic individuals. Like other opportunistic microorga-nisms, the ubiquity of the parasites makes control measures difficult.

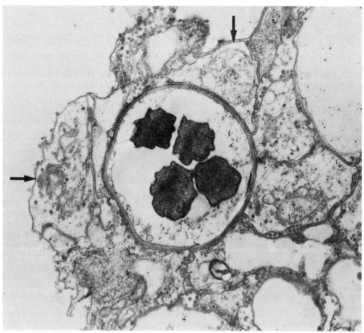

Figure 18-19 Electron micrograph of a thick-walled cyst of *Pneumocystis carinii* containing sporelike bodies. The surrounding thin-walled cysts (indicated by arrows) display marked variation in configuration suggestive of a pliable outer limiting membrane. (Courtesy, H. Sepp, Toronto.)

SUMMARY

The constant exposure of the respiratory tract to atmospheric air makes it impossible to protect the respiratory organs from environmental contaminants. The site of microbial deposition is a function of particle size and moisture content, but the invasive characteristics of the microorganisms and host susceptibility determine the nature and extent of the infection. In most bacterial diseases resolution is accompanied by destruction of invading microorganisms; in tuberculosis and some fungal diseases organisms can remain viable in walled-off cavities. Artificial immunization and chemotherapy have eliminated whooping cough, diphtheria, and tuberculosis as major public health problems, but "strep throat" remains as one of the most common infectious diseases. There is no substitute for early diagnosis and prompt institution of antimicrobial therapy in preventing dissemination of the respiratory pathogens within an infected individual or a susceptible population.

QUESTIONS FOR STUDY

1. Why are the lungs so vital for sustaining life?
2. How does particle size and moisture content influence the deposition of microorganism-laden aerosols?
3. What bacterium produces a "satellite phenomenon" in the presence of *Staphylococcus aureus?*
4. Describe the role of skin tests in the diagnosis of bacterial and fungal infections.
5. Describe three phases of whooping cough.
6. Differentiate between pneumonic and sylvatic plague.
7. What specimens are required to culture the tubercle bacilli from a pulmonary infection?
8. List the differential morphological characteristics of the fungi which cause histoplasmosis, coccidioidomycosis, and blastomycosis.

SELECTED REFERENCES

Baum, G. L. *Textbook of Pulmonary Diseases.* 2d ed. Boston: Little, Brown, 1971.

California State Department of Public Health. *A Manual for the Control of Communicable Diseases in California.* Berkeley: 1971.

Crouch, J. E. *Functional Human Anatomy.* 2d ed. Philadelphia: Lea & Febiger, 1972.

Emmons, C. W.; Binford, C. H.; and Utz, J. P. *Medical Mycology.* Philadelphia: Lea & Febiger, 1970.

Joklik, W. K., and Willett, H. P. *Zinsser Microbiology.* 16th ed. Englewood Cliffs, N.J.: Prentice-Hall, 1976.

Kirby, B. D.; Snyder, K. M.; Meyer, R. D.; and Finegold, S. M. Legionnaires' disease—a cluster of cases. *Clinical Research* 26:399A, 1978.

Knight, V. *Viral and Mycoplasmal Infections of the Respiratory Tract.* Philadelphia: Lea & Febiger, 1973.

Prier, J. E., and Friedman, H. *Opportunistic Pathogens.* Baltimore: University Park Press, 1974.

U.S. Department of Health, Education, and Welfare, Public Health Service. Pneumococcal polysaccharide vaccine. *CDC Morbidity and Mortality Weekly Report* 27:25, 1978.

Chapter 19

Viral, Rickettsial, and Chlamydial Diseases of the Respiratory Tract

After you read this chapter, you should be able to:

1. Identify five groups of viruses associated with respiratory disease.
2. Discuss the transmission, laboratory diagnosis, immunity, and prevention of the chief respiratory diseases caused by viruses, rickettsiae, and chlamydiae.
3. Describe a pulmonary infection caused by a rickettsia.
4. Explain how the transmission of Q fever differs from the transmission of other rickettsial diseases.
5. Describe a pulmonary infection caused by a chlamydia.
6. Explain the role of IgA antibodies in resistance to infections of the respiratory tract.
7. Explain why etiological agents of most common colds remain undiagnosed.

It has been estimated that at least 90 percent of acute upper respiratory infections and nearly 50 percent of lower respiratory infections are caused by viruses. The respiratory infections of rickettsial and chlamydial origin are small in number, but important because they may simulate viral, bacterial, or fungal diseases of the lung.

The devastating pandemic of influenza virus pneumonia in 1918–1919 attacked 20 million persons throughout the world and killed 850,000 in the United States alone, but the etiological agent went unrecognized until 1933 when influenza A virus was isolated from humans. Since 1933 a large number of additional viruses belonging to five groups have been isolated from human respiratory tract disease (Table 19-1). Influenza viruses continue to be uncontrolled despite the availability of vaccines. Most viral infections do not respond well to chemotherapy and do, therefore, have life-threatening potential.

VIRAL INFECTIONS

The multiplicity of viral agents involved in acute respiratory illnesses, along with the varying symptoms produced in humans, complicates the identification of specific etiological agents. However, at least 13 viruses are now known to cause serious lower respiratory tract disease: influenza A and B, respiratory syncytial virus, parainfluenza virus types 1, 2, 3, and 4, and adenovirus types 1, 2, 3, 4, 5, and 7. The 90 serotypes of rhinoviruses and several strains of coronaviruses colonize in cells of the upper airways.

Table 19-1 MAJOR GROUPS AND SEROTYPES OF RESPIRATORY VIRUSES

VIRUS	SEROTYPES	MAJOR DISEASE
Orthomyxovirus		
influenza	A, B	influenza
Paramyxovirus		
respiratory syncytial (RS)	1	bronchiolitis
parainfluenza	1, 2, 3, 4	croup
Adenovirus	1, 2, 3, 4, 5, 6, 7, 14, and 21	acute respiratory disease
Picornavirus		
rhinovirus	1–90	common cold
coxsackievirus	A2, A4, A5, A6, A7, A12, and A21; B2, B3, and B5	pharyngitis
Coronavirus	B814, 229E, and OC43	common cold

SOURCE: Adapted from R. M. Chanock, Control of Acute Mycoplasmal and Virus Disease, *Science* 169:248, 1970.

INFLUENZA VIRUS INFECTIONS

There is no doubt that influenza viruses A and B rank as primary causes of epidemics or pandemics of respiratory tract infection. Type C influenza virus almost never causes recognizab e disease. Influenza has an incubation time of only one to three days and is most often characterized by an abrupt onset of fever, chills, headache, and muscle aches.

Transmission. There is little information available on the natural transmission of influenza, but the infectious particles are believed to have their origin in aerosols of respiratory secretions from coughs or sneezes of infected persons. The viruses can remain viable in the aerosols for at least an hour. Small aerosols travel relatively large distances within a single hour.

Laboratory Diagnosis. Specific diagnosis of influenza depends on isolation of the virus from nasal washings or demonstration of at least a four-fold rise in antibody titer in convalescent sera when compared with sera obtained during the acute phase of the disease. Type A viruses grow well in embryonated chick eggs; type B viruses can be recovered in primary Rhesus monkey cells. Influenza viruses agglutinate red blood cells of some animals, including humans (Figure 19-1). Antibodies to the influenza viruses can be identified using a hemagglutination inhibition test or a neutralization technique.

Immunity. Resistance to influenza after an attack or following vaccination is limited because new antigenic variants emerge with such frequency. There probably are a finite number of antigenic subtypes, some of which are dormant for long periods of time.

Prevention. Vaccination with subtypes of influenza A and B viruses is the only means available for control of in-

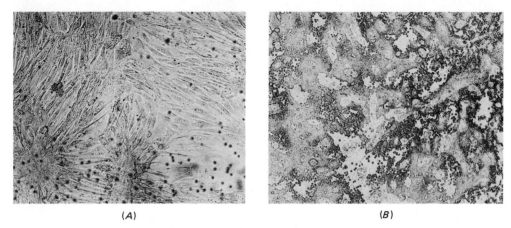

(A)   (B)

Figure 19-1   A comparison of negative and positive hemadsorption. (A) Uninfected Rhesus monkey kidney cells showing no hemadsorption. (B) Rhesus monkey kidney cells containing type A influenza virus showing guinea pig red blood cells adhering to the surfaces. (From V. Knight and J. A. Kasel, in *Viral and Mycoplasmal Infections of the Respiratory Tract*, Lea & Febiger, Philadelphia, 1973.)

fluenza. Mass production of vaccine presents some problems, however. Newly isolated viruses need to be adapted for production of high yields under laboratory conditions.

RESPIRATORY SYNCYTIAL VIRUS INFECTIONS

The respiratory syncytial (RS) virus is a member of the paramyxovirus group to which parainfluenza, mumps, and rubeola viruses belong. The RS virus is an important respiratory pathogen of children under 6 months of age and of elderly persons with underlying pulmonary disease. The infection is rarely fatal in infants unless severe pneumonia occurs. The role of RS virus as a forerunner to bacterial infections may be a more important consequence than symptoms resulting from viral in-

vasion. Most often, presence of the RS virus goes unrecognized.

Transmission. RS virus infections are generally transmitted by the aerosol route, but direct contact with nasal secretions may take place in young children. It is not known if RS virus is shed after the acute illness disappears.

Laboratory Diagnosis. The correlation between RS virus isolations and serological evidence for RS viral antibodies has been disappointing. The virus grows in human HeLa cells, human embryo fibroblasts, and primary monkey kidney cells, but has not been isolated from all cases shown to have RS viral infection by other methods. Infected cells are characterized by the presence of eosinophilic cytoplasmic inclusions and formation of

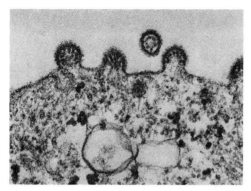

Figure 19-2 The process of budding whereby viruses are released in a green monkey kidney cell infected with a respiratory syncytial (RS) virus. (From E. Norrby, H. Marusyk, and C. Örvell, *J. of Virol.* 6:240, 1970.)

syncytia, that is, fused masses of cells. RS viruses are released from cells by a budding process on the surface (Figure 19-2). Both complement-fixing and neutralizing antibodies can be demonstrated in adults with RS viral infections, but very young infants may not produce antibodies in sufficient amounts to be detected.

Immunity. Susceptibility to the RS virus appears to be particularly high in infants during the first six months of life, but no active immunization against RS virus is available. During an early investigation of vaccine feasibility inoculation with inactivated viral vaccines caused severe illnesses in children exposed subsequently to RS virus. The adverse effect was attributed to a possible Arthus reaction, with antigen-antibody complexes or hypersensitivity induced by administration of the vaccine.

Prevention. Care should be taken with the very young and the very old to prevent exposure to possible RS viral infection. The use of masks during close contact with infants or the elderly is of some value in preventing spread of nasopharyngeal aerosols.

PARAINFLUENZA VIRUS INFECTIONS

Serotypes 1, 2, 3, 4A, and 4B of the parainfluenza viruses cause natural infection in animals, but are also human pathogens (Table 19-2). Viruses belong-

Table 19-2 HUMAN SEROTYPES AND ANIMAL DESIGNATIONS OF PARAINFLUENZA VIRUSES

SEROTYPE	ANIMAL INFECTED	ANIMAL DESIGNATION
1	mice	Sendai agent
2	monkeys	simian virus 5
		simian virus 41
3	cattle	SF4
4A	—	—
4B	—	—

SOURCE: Adapted from V. Knight, *Viral and Mycoplasmal Infections of the Respiratory Tract* (Philadelphia: Lea & Febiger, 1973).

ing to serotype 4 are less frequently isolated in human disease. Parainfluenza viruses cause less than 10 percent of respiratory infections in hospitalized children, but are responsible for approximately one-third of the cases diagnosed as croup. Serotypes 1 and 2 are the most common etiological agents in URI's in both children and adults. Serotype 3 is more commonly isolated from lower respiratory disease in infants.

Transmission. Parainfluenza viruses are transmitted by aerosols of nasopharyngeal secretions from infected persons. The virus is spread most rapidly in institutions and among members of the same family.

Laboratory Diagnosis. The diagnosis of parainfluenza virus infections depends on isolation of the virus in tissue culture, immunofluorescent demonstration of the virus in nasopharyngeal cells, or rises in complement-fixing, neutralizing, or hemagglutination-inhibiting antibody titers. The parainfluenza viruses grow well on primary Rhesus monkey kidney cells and some human cell lines, but cytopathic effects may not be detectable for at least two weeks.

Immunity. Neutralizing antibodies of the IgA type in nasal secretions have been shown to be better deterrents to infection with parainfluenza viruses than serum antibodies. The stability of such antibodies may, however, be limited, so that recurrent infections upon exposure are inevitable.

Prevention. The parenteral administration of attenuated or inactivated parainfluenza virus has not been effective in preventing infections. Administration of inactivated parainfluenza virus in the form of an aerosol to stimulate IgA antibody production by mucosa of the respiratory tract may hold promise in the future.

ADENOVIRUS INFECTION

Although there are at least 33 serotypes of human adenovirus, serotypes 1, 2, 3, 4, 5, and 7 cause the most serious infections. Serotypes 1 and 2 cause about 60 percent of all adenovirus infections, but the adenoviruses cause less than 10 percent of all nonbacterial respiratory tract infections in civilians. Serotypes 4 and 7 have been responsible for the high incidence of acute respiratory disease in military recruits. Serotype 7 has been incriminated in fatal cases of pneumonia in children.

Transmission. The adenoviruses are spread by aerosols of nasopharyngeal secretions from infected persons. It is uncertain if a focus of gastrointestinal infection could represent a reservoir from which the viruses can spread by the fecal-oral route. It is known that fecal shedding of adenoviruses occurs, but the role of feces in transmission of the viruses is unknown.

Laboratory Diagnosis. Isolation of adenoviruses from clinical material is the preferred diagnostic method. They can be isolated from throat, conjunctival swabs, and stool specimens. The adenoviruses grow in primary human embryonic kidney cells or continuous human cell lines. In addition, useful serological methods include tests for complement-fixing, neutralizing, and hemagglutination-inhibiting antibodies.

Immunity. Resistance to a specific serotype of adenovirus is not long lasting after an infection, despite the prevalence of antibodies in general populations. Inactivated whole adenoviruses, live viruses, and capsid antigen preparations have been used to immunize military recruits.

Prevention. The ubiquity of adenoviruses in respiratory tracts of apparently healthy individuals makes it impossible to avoid exposure. No vaccines are in general use, except for military recruits.

RHINOVIRUS INFECTIONS

The rhinoviruses are the most frequent cause of the common cold. At least 90 serotypes have been identified to date throughout the world. Although colds caused by rhinoviruses occur at any time during the year, an increased incidence is usually observable in the fall and late spring.

Transmission. The method of transmission for rhinoviruses has not been clearly defined, but aerosols from an infected person are suspected as the vehicles for transport. Rhinovirus infections are known to spread within 24 hours in family groups.

Laboratory Diagnosis. Because of the mild nature and short duration of rhinovirus infections, specific etiological agents are rarely identified. Although rhinoviruses may be isolated from nasopharyngeal washings, nasal swabs, or throat swabs, detection of neutralizing antibodies in paired sera is the preferred diagnostic procedure. Individuals with rhinovirus infection usually develop a four-fold or greater increase in neutralizing antibody titer.

Immunity. Type-specific secretory IgA antibodies against rhinoviruses are more important than serum antibodies in protecting persons from rhinovirus infections. An infection appears to provide at least temporary resistance to reinfection with one or more serological types of rhinovirus.

Prevention. The large number of antigenic types of rhinovirus negates the practicality of using vaccines for general populations. The mild nature of rhinovirus disease makes it impossible to avoid exposure, since individuals are often unaware of infections. It would appear that, for now, the common cold caused by rhinoviruses is but one of the inconveniences that humans must endure.

COXSACKIEVIRUS INFECTION

A limited number of coxsackieviruses cause acute respiratory disease; most of them cause more serious disease such as pericarditis, meningitis, myocarditis, pleurodynia, or paralysis. Coxsackieviruses A21 and B3 are the only

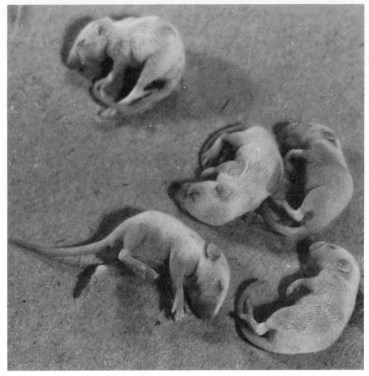

Figure 19-3 Four-day-old suckling mice inoculated intraperitoneally with a group A coxsackie virus. Severe myositis causes paralysis and death. (From A. Levensohn, *Postgrad. Med.* 10:448, 1951.)

ones consistently isolated from cases of respiratory illness, but more aggressive searches for coxsackieviruses would probably implicate others in pharyngitis. Coxsackievirus A21 infection occurs in epidemic proportions mainly in military personnel in late summer or early fall.

Transmission. Coxsackieviruses are spread almost exclusively by virus-laden aerosols. The virus is shed in feces, but evidence for a fecal-oral route for transmission is obscure.

Laboratory Diagnosis. Although coxsackieviruses grow in human diploid and primary monkey renal cell cultures, isolation of the viruses from nasal washings or feces does not necessarily confirm an etiological role for the viruses in respiratory illness. Other viruses are almost always present. Suckling mice can be inoculated intraperitoneally to differentiate the A and B varieties of coxsackievirus (Figure 19-3). The group A viruses, including A21, produce a myositis which can be identified in tissue sections; the group B viruses not only produce myositis, but also necrosis of fat pads and inflammatory reactions in the pancreas, liver, cerebral cortex, and meninges. Type-specific identification can be

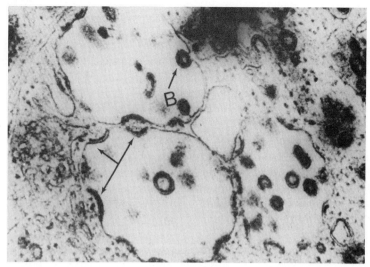

Figure 19-4 Appearance of coronavirus in a human diploid cell. Several mature particles are present within vacuoles. A particle (B) budding into a vacuole is also seen. (From B. D. Davis et al., *Microbiology*, 2d ed., New York, Harper & Row, 1973.)

made by performing neutralizing antibody tests on acute and convalescent sera.

Immunity. Susceptibility to coxsackievirus infection is probably general. Little information is available on immunity resulting from a respiratory infection, but type-specific resistance is presumed to be present for at least a limited period.

Prevention. The ubiquity of coxsackieviruses precludes prevention of exposure. At the present time development of vaccines does not appear practical.

CORONAVIRUS INFECTION

The coronaviruses are the latest major group of viruses found to cause upper respiratory tract infections. The viruses cause symptoms resembling those of the common cold in humans, but dis-

seminate in both chickens and mice, causing bronchitis or hepatitis. With time more information on this latest addition to respiratory viruses will be available.

Transmission. From studies on the mode of transmission of other respiratory viruses, it is likely that coronaviruses are aerosol-borne. The tendency of the viruses to disseminate, at least in animals, makes other routes of transmission possible. More studies will be necessary to assess possible alternate modes of transmission.

Laboratory Diagnosis. No vigorous attempts have been made to isolate the coronaviruses from individuals with symptoms of a common cold, so their frequency as a cause of upper respiratory infection is unknown. The viruses grow only in human embryotracheal organ cultures and primary monkey kidney cells (Figure 19-4). The availability of antigens for serological studies is therefore limited. Both complement-fixing and neutralizing antibodies are produced by persons with coronavirus infection.

Immunity. The protective effect of coronavirus antibodies has not been studied sufficiently to provide any definitive information. Based on antigens recovered from tissue and organ cultures, it is known that there are at least two groups.

Prevention. There are no vaccines available for human coronavirus infections. Both live and inactivated vaccines for avian coronavirus disease have been effective in controlling the disease in chickens. The probable ubiquity of coronaviruses and the benign nature of the common cold make it impossible to avoid exposure.

RICKETTSIAL INFECTIONS

Most rickettsial diseases follow the bite of an infected arthropod which permits entry of the rickettsial organisms into the bloodstream. The rickettsiae invade endothelial cells lining the blood vessels causing widespread peripheral vasculitis. With the exception of the respiratory disease known as Q fever, headache, rash, and fever are common symptoms. The causative organism of Q fever can be transmitted in aerosol form as well as by arthropod bite. Inhalation of the airborne rickettsiae causes a pulmonary infection which resembles viral or fungal disease of the lungs.

Q FEVER

Q fever is an acute febrile disease caused by *Coxiella burnetii*. It simulates many other respiratory infections. The disease is characterized by pulmonary lesions with little or no involvement of the upper respiratory tract. Q fever is endemic in California, but has also been reported in other states and in countries all over the world.

Transmission. Q fever is transmitted by aerosols containing excreta of infected animals. Cattle, sheep, goats, ticks, and some wild animals are natural reservoirs of *C. burnetii*. Raw milk has long been suspected as a mode of transmission for the rickettsial agent. Infected ticks pass the organism to offspring transovarially and to humans by a bite, but transmission from person to person is rare.

Laboratory Diagnosis. The diagnostic procedure of choice for Q fever is a complement-fixation test on sera obtained during the acute and convalescent stages. Microagglutination tests may also be performed on paired sera in capillary tubes, slides, or wells of microtiter equipment.

Immunity. Susceptibility to Q fever is general, but recovery following a bout of the disease renders an individual immune for life. No vaccination procedures have been widely employed, but a vaccine of inactivated organisms prepared from *C. burnetii* grown in egg yolk sacs can be used for workers in occupations involving constant exposure.

Prevention. Adherence to strict cleaning procedures in barns can prevent the exposure of barnyard personnel to *C. burnetii*—laden aerosols. Appropriate disposal of animal placentas and pasteurization of milk can also reduce the risk of infection. Boiling of raw milk will kill the rickettsiae.

CHLAMYDIAL INFECTIONS

The chlamydiae are included in a single genus *Chlamydia* which was once known as *Bedsonia*. Along with the rickettsiae and mycoplasmas, they were once thought to be viruses. The chlamydiae reproduce only within host cells and are considered true energy parasites since they depend on host cells for adenosine triphosphate (ATP). The chlamydiae appear to have a predilection for particular types of tissue.

PSITTACOSIS

Psittacosis or ornithosis was at one time thought to be limited to members of the parrot family, but many kinds of birds can harbor the causative organism. Many of the infections in birds remain latent, surfacing only under conditions of stress. In humans psittacosis may be a relatively mild disease, a severe pulmonary infection, or a septicemia. The etiological agent, *Chlamydia psittaci*, is the only known chlamydial respiratory pathogen of man.

Transmission. Psittacosis is spread from bird to bird and bird to human by aerosols or by contact with discharges from infected birds. In some birds *C. psittaci* is transmitted vertically from parents to offspring in sex cells. The disease is not generally transmitted from human to human.

Laboratory Diagnosis. The clinical picture of psittacosis is not definitive. Diagnosis must be made, therefore, by demonstrating a rising titer of complement-fixing antibodies in paired sera. *C. psittaci* usually cannot be observed on stained smears of sputum or lung tissue. The organisms will grow in embryonated eggs, mice, and irradiated cell monolayers, but successful recovery of the chlamydiae from clinical specimens is difficult if antimicrobial therapy has been instituted prior to specimen collection.

Immunity. Susceptibility to psittacosis is general, but the most severe cases occur in older adults. One attack of the disease confers limited immunity, and resistance can be overcome by a massive challenge of the chlamydial agent. Evidence of delayed hypersensitivity is often present during the course of an infection.

Prevention. Regulation of bird traffic, as well as surveillance of pet shops and aviaries, can prevent the sale of infected birds. In California birds are banded to identify breeders in the event of a psittacosis outbreak. Aviary workers attending sick birds or nurses taking care of patients with diagnosed psittacosis should wear masks to reduce the risk of exposure to the chlamydial agent.

SUMMARY

Over the past several decades an increasing number of microbial agents, including viruses, rickettsiae, and chlamydiae, have been discovered to cause acute disease of the respiratory tract. The viruses constitute the largest group of microorganisms associated with respiratory tract infections. The infections range from the common cold to severe pneumonia. Protection against viral infections is complicated by the large number of etiological agents, the antigenic instability of some viruses, the transient nature of immunity, and variation in host response. Submission of paired serum specimens to the laboratory is necessary for definitive diagnosis of viral, rickettsial, and chlamydial diseases. The development of vaccines against only the major respiratory pathogens is practical. Evidence suggests that serum antibodies are not the most important mediators of immunity in some localized respiratory infections, but that antibodies of the IgA class of immunoglobulins present in respiratory tract secretions have a major role in resistance.

QUESTIONS FOR STUDY

1. Why is it difficult to control influenza outbreaks by vaccination?
2. What is the major mode of transmission for virus infections of the respiratory tract?
3. Why are chlamydiae described as energy parasites?
4. What is the primary microbial method used in the diagnosis of viral, rickettsial, and chlamydial diseases of the respiratory tract?
5. Why does the common cold persist as an important infectious disease?

SELECTED REFERENCES

Baum, G. L. *Textbook of Pulmonary Diseases.* 2d ed. Boston: Little, Brown, 1974.

California State Department of Public Health. *A Manual for the Control of Communicable Diseases in California.* Berkeley: 1971.

Chanock, R. M. Control of acute mycoplasmal and viral respiratory tract disease. *Science* 169:248, 1970.

Davis, B. D.; Dulbecco, R.; Eisen, H.; Ginsberg, H. S.; and Wood, W. B., Jr. *Microbiology.* 2d ed. New York: Harper & Row, 1973.

Knight, V. *Viral and Mycoplasmal Infections of the Respiratory Tract.* Philadelphia: Lea & Febiger, 1973.

Swain, R. H. A., and Dodds, T. C. *Clinical Virology.* Baltimore: Williams & Wilkins, 1967.

Youmans, G. P.; Paterson, P. Y.; and Sommers, H. M. *The Biologic and Clinical Basis of Infectious Diseases.* Philadelphia: Saunders, 1975.

Chapter 20

Bacterial, Viral, and Toxin-Associated Diseases of the Gastrointestinal Tract

After you read this chapter, you should be able to:

1. Differentiate between a food poisoning and a food infection.
2. Explain how microorganisms or toxins entering the intestine are sometimes transported to distant sites.
3. Discuss the transmission, laboratory diagnosis, immunity, and prevention of the common bacterial infections of the gastrointestinal tract.
4. Compare the symptoms and time of onset of four types of bacterial food poisoning.
5. Discuss the transmission, laboratory diagnosis, immunity, and prevention of bacterial food poisoning.
6. List the major virus groups causing infections of the gastrointestinal tract.
7. Compare the incubation time and mode of transmission for hepatitis A and hepatitis B.
8. Explain the significance of the presence of an antigen designated as HB_sAg in blood.
9. Contrast the nature of the health hazard to humans of paralytic shellfish and aflatoxin poisoning.

The gastrointestinal tract, or alimentary canal, is a continuous tube which begins with the mouth, includes part of the pharynx, the esophagus, the stomach, the small intestine, and large intestine, and ends with the anus. The accessory organs are the teeth, tongue, salivary glands, liver, gallbladder, and pancreas (Figure 20-1).

The gastrointestinal tract and its accessory organs are responsible for the processes of digestion of food, absorption of nutrients, and elimination of undigested food. The organs that lie outside the alimentary canal contribute to the processes by secretion or storage of digestive juices.

The terms *enteric infection, enteritis,* or *gastroenteritis* are often used interchangeably to describe inflammation of the intestinal tract of microbial origin. However, gastroenteritis is usually accompanied by the presence of gastric symptoms which may include nausea and vomiting. Enteric infections are characterized by the rapid secretion of fluid from mucosa of the small intestine or by an acute inflammatory response. The watery discharge causes the clinical syndrome known as *diarrhea;* the inflammatory response, characterized by the presence of blood and pus in the stool, is more appropriately called *dysentery.* If a fever is produced as a result of the infectious process, the disease may appropriately be called an *enteric fever.* If microorganisms enter the bloodstream a *septicemia* is produced. Septicemias produced by bacteria are known as *bacteremias* whereas those caused by viruses are called *viremias.*

BACTERIAL DISEASES

Diarrheal disease caused by bacteria is still a major cause of illness and death, particularly in developing countries. Several geographic and socioeconomic

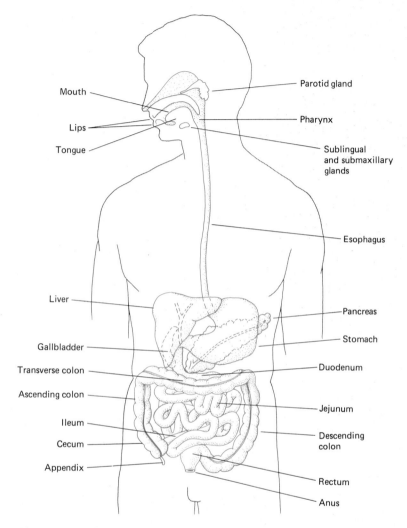

Mouth

Lips

Tongue

Parotid gland

Pharynx

Sublingual
and submaxillary
glands

Esophagus

Liver

Gallbladder

Transverse colon

Ascending colon

Ileum

Cecum

Appendix

Pancreas

Stomach

Duodenum

Jejunum

Descending
colon

Rectum

Anus

Figure 20-1 Organs comprising the gastrointestinal tract and accessory organs of digestion.

factors play roles as determinants of types of gastroenteric disease prevalent in particular populations. The prevalence of certain parasitic diseases in some areas causes persons in those areas to be more susceptible to bacteria as secondary invaders. The incidence of enteric disease caused by bacterial pathogens tends to be higher in tropical than in temperate climates, but just as people travel with greater ease than a few decades ago, so do the bacteria that colonize humans. And, whatever the geographic factors, the availability of clean water, adequate sewage disposal, and a balanced diet influence the incidence of enteric disease in a particular location more than the climate.

SALMONELLA INFECTIONS

The widespread dissemination of salmonellae makes them among the most prominent of the enteric pathogens. Domestic fowl constitute the largest single reservoir of salmonellae, but other domestic and wild animals also harbor the organisms. Human *Salmonella* infections, or salmonelloses, produce three forms of disease: enteric fever, gastroenteritis, and a septicemia. It has recently become accepted protocol to consider three species of *Salmonella* as the etiological agents: *S. typhi*, the cause of the enteric fever known as typhoid; *S. cholerae-suis* and *S. enteritidis*, both of which cause gastroenteritis. Septicemia is observed with both *S. typhi* and *S. cholerae-suis*. The multiple serotypes of salmonellae are considered to be antigenic varia-

tions of *S. enteritidis*. Although approximately 1800 serotypes of *S. enteritidis* have been identified, most human disease in the United States is caused by 8 serotypes (Table 20-1).

Transmission. The salmonellae are transmitted indirectly by contaminated poultry, eggs, meat, and water or directly by the fecal-oral route. Domestic pets, including cats, birds, dogs, and even turtles, host a wide variety of salmonellae. Undetected carriers of typhoid may unknowingly spread the disease. The familiar term "typhoid Mary" is derived from stories about a real or fictional carrier who reportedly worked in several restaurants before public health authorities identified her as a source of *S. typhi*.

Laboratory Diagnosis. A diagnosis of salmonellosis can be made by isolating the organism from stool or blood during the acute stage of the disease. The gram-negative bacilli may appear in the bloodstream in septicemias and enteric

Table 20-1 COMMON ETIOLOGICAL AGENTS OF SALMONELLOSIS IN HUMANS

ORGANISM	REPRESENTATIVE SEROTYPE	MAJOR HUMAN DISEASE
Salmonella cholerae-suis		septicemia
Salmonella typhi		typhoid fever
Salmonella enteritidis	*paratyphi A.*	
	schottmuelleri	
	dublin	
	typhimurium	gastroenteritis
	derby	
	enteritidis	
	heidelberg	
	newport	

SOURCE: Adapted from G. P. Youmans, P. Y. Paterson, and H. M. Sommers, *The Biologic and Clinical Basis of Infectious Diseases* (Philadelphia: Saunders, 1975).

fevers during the first two weeks of illness. *S. typhi* can sometimes be isolated from urine during peak periods of bacteremia. Direct microscopic examination is of no value because the gram-negative bacilli are indistinguishable in size or shape from nonpathogenic enteric flora.

The salmonellae grow on differential and moderately selective media, such as deoxycholate-citrate, Hektoen enteric, or Salmonella-Shigella (SS) agar. Biochemical properties are used to separate *Salmonella* species, but serologic confirmation is required (Table 20-2). The Widal test for detecting agglutinins in patients' sera to O or somatic antigens of the typhoid organism can be employed in suspected cases of typhoid fever.

Immunity. Antibodies of the anti-O and anti-Vi variety both play a role in immunity to infections caused by *S. typhi*. The amount of resistance derived from a naturally acquired infection is dependent on the amount of the challenging dose or course of the disease. Although somatic antigens are shared by some salmonellae, individual variation is great enough to minimize cross-immunizing protective effects.

Prevention. Of primary importance in preventing salmonelloses are adequate sewage disposal, a safe supply of drinking water, pasteurization of milk, thorough cooking of meat, poultry, and eggs, and exclusion of convalescent or chronic carriers as food handlers. A convalescent carrier of typhoid fever is defined as an individual who harbors salmonellae for three months following onset of the disease. A chronic carrier may excrete salmonellae for a year or more after recovery from the illness.

Table 20-2   DIFFERENTIATION OF THREE MAJOR *SALMONELLA* SPECIES

TEST OR SUBSTRATE	S. CHOLERAE-SUIS	S. TYPHI	S. ENTERITIDIS
Hydrogen sulfide (TSI)	+/−	+	+
Citrate (Simmons)	+	−	+
Ornithine	+	−	+
Gas from glucose	+	−	+
Dulcitol	+/−	+/−	+
Inositol	−	−	+/−
Trehalose	−	+	+
Arabinose	−	−	+
Rhamnose	+	−	+
Cellobiose	−	+/−	+
Erythritol	+/−	−	−
Sodium acetate	+/−	−	+
Mucate	−	−	+/−
Stern's glycerol fuchsin	−	−	+

SOURCE: Adapted from E. H. Lennette, E. H. Spaulding, J. P. Truant, *Manual of Clinical Microbiology*, 2d ed. (Washington, D.C.: American Society for Microbiology, 1974).

Administration of killed typhoid bacilli of high antigenicity in two doses confers protection for up to three years if the Vi antigen is not destroyed. Routine typhoid immunization is not recommended in the United States except for household contacts of known carriers or in the event of an outbreak of the disease in a community. However, travelers to endemic areas should avail themselves of typhoid vaccine. Vaccines for other salmonellae have not proved to be effective in prevention of gastroenteritis or septicemia.

SHIGELLA INFECTIONS

The shigellae, unlike the salmonellae, are found only in humans. Bacillary dysentery, or shigellosis, is characterized by an onset of abdominal cramps, fever, and diarrhea one to four days after ingestion of the organisms. Although all shigellae produce a common endotoxin, a potent neurotoxin is elaborated by *Shigella dysenteriae*, type 1, as an exotoxin. *S. sonnei* is the most prevalent cause of bacillary dysentery in the United States.

Transmission. Most bacillary dysentery is transmitted by contaminated water, milk, and food. Both flies and food handlers have been incriminated in the spread of the disease. However, documented cases of venereal transmission are increasing in incidence among homosexual men. More aggressive searches for means of enteric-disease transmission may reveal that other enteric infections can spread by the venereal route.

Laboratory Diagnosis. The shigellae can be isolated from stool specimens during the acute phase of the disease. Unlike the salmonellae, they cannot be isolated from blood or urine. Direct microscopic examination is not useful as the shigellae, like the salmonellae, are indistinguishable from other gram-negative bacilli. Deoxycholate citrate, Hektoen enteric, or Salmonella-Shigella (SS) agar are of value for isolation of *Shigella* from stool specimens or rectal swabs. The shigellae are nonmotile in contrast to the motility exhibited by most salmonellae. Isolates of shigellae may be classified on the basis of mannitol fermentation, ornithine decarboxylase activity, and serological group (Table 20-3). The presence of significant titers of antibodies to *Shigella* organisms is an unpredictable indicator of infection.

Immunity. Circulating antibodies to shigellae from either an apparent or

Table 20-3 DIFFERENTIATION OF FOUR *SHIGELLA* SPECIES

ORGANISM	SEROLOGICAL GROUP	MANNITOL	ORNITHINE DECARBOXYLASE
S. dysenteriae	A	−	−
S. flexneri	B	+	−
S. boydii	C	+	+/−
S. sonnei	D	+	+

SOURCE: Adapted from D. B. Davis, et al., *Microbiology*, 2d ed. (New York: Harper & Row, 1973).

inapparent infection are not particularly protective against subsequent attacks of bacillary dysentery. Local immune factors may be of more importance in protecting the intestinal tract from invasion.

Prevention. The most important prophylactic measures for preventing shigellosis include control of food handlers, control of flies, and provision for adequate disposal of human wastes. Since humans are the only natural host, prevention of shigellosis should be simpler than for the salmonelloses. However, the inordinate number of undiagnosed mild infections makes the elimination of person-to-person transmission difficult. No vaccine is available since the efficacy of circulating antibodies is doubtful.

ENTERIC DISEASE ASSOCIATED WITH *ESCHERICHIA COLI*

For decades it has been known that particular serotypes of *Escherichia coli* cause severe diarrhea in newborn infants. The serotypes associated with epidemics of the disease are described as enteropathogenic *E. coli* (EEC). The number and severity of infant cases of diarrhea attributable to EEC have decreased substantially in recent years.

More recently, enterotoxin-producing or enteroinvasive strains of *E. coli* have been associated with diarrheal disease of both adults and infants. The enteric disease, well known to travelers, is characterized by a precipitous onset of watery stools. The loss of fluid has been attributed to either a heat-labile (LT) or a heat-stable (ST) enterotoxin.

Transmission. Enterotoxin-producing and enteroinvasive strains of *E. coli* are spread by contaminated water or food and from person to person by the fecal-oral route. Transmission in nurseries can result from not washing hands before feeding infants or following diaper changes. Spread of the organisms by aerosols, dust, or flies cannot be discounted in epidemics.

Laboratory Diagnosis. The disease-producing strains of *E. coli* are indistinguishable from *E. coli* comprising the normal intestinal flora in direct microscopic examination and when grown on typical selective media, such as eosin methylene blue (EMB) or MacConkey's agar. Identification of genus and species can be made biochemically using a series of carbohydrates, amino acids, and other organic substrates (Table 20-4). Enterotoxin production can be demonstrated by inoculating rabbit ileal loops with suspected enterotoxin producers. Enterotoxin-producing strains of *E. coli* cause fluid accumulation and distension of ileal loops. Differentiation of LT and ST requires the inoculation of suckling mice with supernatants from both cultures. The ST promotes loss of intestinal fluid.

Demonstration of invasive properties of strains of *E. coli* requires a guinea pig model or the human neoplastic cells He La. Enteroinvasive strains produce a keratoconjunctivitis (inflammation of the cornea and mucous membranes of the eye) in guinea pigs and death of He La cells. Procedures for demonstrating enterotoxin production or enteroinvasiveness are cumbersome and not yet practical for the clinical laboratory.

Table 20-4 SELECTED BIOCHEMICAL REACTIONS OF *ESCHERICHIA COLI*

TEST OR SUBSTRATE	TYPICAL REACTION
Dextrose	+
Citrate	−
Gelatin (22°C)	−
Hydrogen sulfide	−
Indole	+
Lysine decarboxylase	−
Methyl red	+
O-nitrophenyl 1-β-D-glactoside (ONPG)	+
Ornithine decarboxylase	+/−
Phenylalanine deaminase	−
Urease	−
Voges Proskauer	−

Thirteen serotypes of *E. coli* caused about 75 percent of infantile diarrheal disease in the past. However, serotyping of isolates of *E. coli* from infants with diarrhea is no longer recommended as a routine procedure.

Immunity. It is not known if significant immunity follows enteric disease caused by *E. coli*. The severe nature of the symptoms caused by the enteric pathogens in infants and in some adults may be attributable to lack of previous exposure to the organisms. The presence of local or humoral immune factors from prior contact with the enterotoxins may explain mild symptoms occurring in other adults.

Prevention. Treatment of water to be used for drinking or cooking with a dilute solution of chlorine or tincture of iodine while traveling in countries with less than adequate sanitation can prevent some forms of enteric disease (Table 20-5). In areas where chlorinated

Table 20-5 TREATMENT OF WATER WITH CHLORINE OR TINCTURE OF IODINE

	DROPS TO BE ADDED PER QUART OR LITER	
	CLEAR WATER	CLOUDY WATER
Chlorine solution*		
1%	10	20
4–6%	2	4
7–10%	1	2
unknown	10	20
Tincture of		
iodine, 2%	5	10

*Most chlorine bleach solutions have 4 to 6 percent available chlorine. Water treated with chlorine or iodine should be allowed to stand for 30 minutes before using.
SOURCE: Adapted from *Health Information for International Travel 1977*, HEW Publication No. (CDC) 77-8280 (Washington, D. C.: U.S. Government Printing Office, 1977).

water is not available, only tea and coffee made with boiled water, canned or bottled carbonated beverages, beer, or wine may be safe to drink. Wet cans or bottles should always be dried before opening and wiped clean with chemically treated water, if possible. Food should be selected with a good deal of care. Only pasteurized milk and milk products should be consumed. It is also prudent to eat only fruit or vegetables that can be peeled or freshly cooked hot food.

Special attention to hand washing and disinfection can reduce disease associated with *E. coli* in hospital nurseries. Isolation of infants with suspected enteric disease can help prevent spread of the disease to healthy newborns.

ENTERIC DISEASE ASSOCIATED WITH OTHER GRAM-NEGATIVE BACILLI

The isolation of a number of seemingly atypical bacteria from individuals with diarrhea and extraintestinal infections has led to the recognition of other gram-negative bacilli as opportunistic pathogens. Bacteria belonging to the genera *Edwardsiella*, *Arizona*, *Citrobacter*, *Enterobacter*, *Hafnia*, *Proteus*, *Morganella*, *Providencia*, and *Serratia* must be differentiated from *Salmonella*, *Shigella*, or *Escherichia* species.

A variety of substrates are required to differentiate the genera from one another and to speciate the organisms within a single genus. Figure 20.2 shows a commercially prepackaged

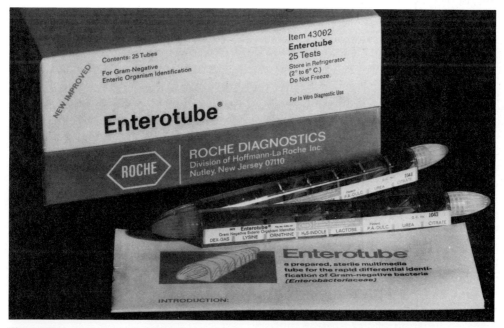

Figure 20-2 An example of a self-contained system for the rapid identification of enteric organisms. (Courtesy, Roche Diagnostics, Division of Hoffmann-La Roche, Nutley, New Jersey.)

testing system valuable for rapid identification if speciation is required.

The ubiquitous nature of gram-negative bacilli provides ample opportunity for the spread of the organisms in hospital populations. Surveillance of hospital-acquired infections and strict adherence to guidelines for disinfection can do much to prevent disease associated with these opportunistic bacilli.

CHOLERA

Cholera, like shigellosis, has been described in humans only. It is endemic in Asia and India, but also occurs sporadically in other parts of the world. The causative organism, *Vibrio cholerae*, multiplies rapidly in the intestinal tract and ruptures, releasing a potent enterotoxin and an enzyme, neuraminidase. The two substances act on the intestinal mucosa causing an exceptional loss of fluid. In severe cases as much as 15 percent of the body weight can be lost in just a few hours.

Transmission. The vibrios of cholera are spread by the fecal-oral route, which most often includes contaminated water as the vehicle of transmission. An English physician, John Snow, first recognized the role of "spoiled water" in 1854 as the mode of transmission for cholera. He succeeded in controlling the spread of the disease by removing the handle of London's Broad Street pump. Air travel and population shifts in some parts of the world have made elimination of the disease more complex in the twentieth century.

Laboratory Diagnosis. Direct microscopic examination of a stool under dark-field microscopy reveals the vibrios of cholera. The organisms grow in alkaline peptone broth (pH 8.5), which is inhibitory to other enteric pathogens and coliforms. Growth of the vibrios is sparse on most enteric media with the exception of MacConkey's agar. Tellurite-taurocholate gelatin agar (TTGA) and thiosulfate citrate bile salts (TCBS) agar are both useful for the primary isolation of *V. cholerae*. Vibrios from pure cultures can be subjected to fluorescein-labeled specific antisera for confirmation or can be used for inoculation of differential media (Figure 20-3). A particularly virulent and persistent biotype of *V. cholerae*, known as El Tor, can be identified by phage typing.

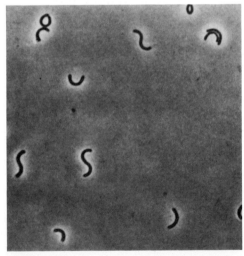

Figure 20-3 Appearance of *Vibrio cholerae* observed under dark field. (From N. Groman and V. Chambers, *Basic Laboratory Techniques for Microbiology*, © Copyright Harper & Row Publishers, Inc., 1972.)

Immunity. Susceptibility to cholera is not well understood. Only a small percentage of individuals are affected even when the disease occurs in epidemic form. Strain-specific antitoxins and vibriocidal antibodies can be demonstrated in serum and feces after recovery from cholera, but resistance to the cholera vibrios is probably more dependent on the nutritional status of the host. Malnutrition is a predisposing factor in many parts of the world where cholera is endemic.

Prevention. A vaccine, consisting of heat-killed vibrios, administered in two doses, provides temporary immunity. Booster doses can be given every six months as necessary. Vaccination is recommended for persons traveling to areas in which cholera is endemic. Elimination of carriers, purification of water, adequate disposal of sewage, and attention to habits of personal hygiene can all be effective control measures.

BRUCELLOSIS

Brucellosis (undulant fever) is one of the oldest infections of animals. The disease has been endemic for years in Mediterranean countries, but the incidence of brucellosis has been markedly reduced in the United States by pasteurization of milk. Three common species of *Brucella* organisms are recognized: *B. melitensis* from goats, *B. abortus* from cattle, and *B. suis* from pigs. During the past decade most cases of human brucellosis in the United States have been caused by *B. suis*. A fourth species, *B. canis*, causes disease in dog colonies and therefore constitutes a health hazard to animal attendants and laboratory workers.

Transmission. Human brucellosis is transmitted by ingestion of contaminated meat or dairy products or by contact with infected animal fetuses, placentas, waste products, or carcasses. The infectious agents can gain entrance through the skin or mucous membranes. Furthermore, aerosols containing brucellae can be inhaled by farmers, rendering plant workers, or animal handlers. Person-to-person transmission is probably almost nonexistent.

Laboratory Diagnosis. Brucellae may be isolated from blood and bone marrow. Growth of the gram-negative coccobacilli, which seldom measure more than 0.4 to 1.5 μm in length, is dependent on, or enhanced by, 10 percent CO_2 in the atmosphere. The inhibitory action of basic fuchsin and thionin, production of H_2S, and urease activity can be used to speciate *Brucella* (Table 20-6). Antisera to the three major species of brucellae can be employed to confirm results of biochemical tests. High or rising titers indicate infections, but negative results do not exclude the possibility of the disease.

Skin tests using antigens of brucellae are of limited value in the diagnosis of brucellosis. If present, the cell-mediated response to *Brucella* antigens can be a diagnostic aid. However, lack of a delayed hypersensitivity reaction does not exclude the possibility of infection.

Table 20-6   DIFFERENTIATION OF THREE MAJOR *BRUCELLA* SPECIES

TEST OR SUBSTRATE	B. ABORTUS	B. MELITENSIS	B. SUIS
CO_2 requirement	+/−	−	−
H_2S production	+/−	−	+/−
Basic fuchsin, 1:100,000 inhibition, 1:100,000	−	−	+
Thionin inhibition	+	−	−
Urease activity	+	+	+++

Immunity. There is no indication that resistance follows human brucellosis. To the contrary, exposure to the brucellae may increase susceptibility of an individual to the etiological agents.

Prevention. Prevention of brucellosis in humans depends on the control of the infection in animals. A vaccine which provides permanent immunity is available for cattle, sheep, and goats. A testing program for swine herds, combined with an effective vaccination procedure, is needed to eliminate pigs as potential sources of the infection.

YERSINIOSIS

Enteric infections caused by *Yersinia enterocolitica* and *Y. pseudotuberculosis* have been increasingly reported from all parts of the world. A majority of cases have occurred in western Europe. Fewer isolates have been obtained in the United States, but sources of isolates have varied. The yersiniae have been recovered from stool, blood, sputum, abscesses, and wounds.

Transmission. The mode of transmission for *Y. enterocolitica* or *Y. pseudotuberculosis* is unknown. It is assumed that the fecal-oral route has validity in the spread of enteric infections, but the nature and source of other types of infections are unclear. Since the yersiniae occur in a variety of wild and domestic animals, direct contamination of food or water from infected animals probably does occur. Apparently, healthy humans can also carry the disease-producing yersiniae.

Laboratory Diagnosis. *Y. enterocolitica* is a gram-negative coccobacillus measuring 0.8 to 3.0 μm long by 0.8 μm wide; *Y. pseudotuberculosis* is sometimes larger and pleomorphic (Figure 20-4). Both organisms grow readily on blood agar and most media selective for gram-negative bacilli. The species can be differentiated by biochemical tests. Antisera are not available commercially for serological confirmation.

Immunity. Little or no information is available on resistance conferred by an attack of yersiniae-caused enteric infection. Serological evidence points to a significant drop in antibody titers within two months following an infection.

Prevention. Purification of drinking water and pasteurization of milk appear important deterrents to enteric disease caused by yersiniae. Adherence to strict habits of personal hygiene could prevent spread of the disease from non-suspected carriers of *Y. enterocolitica*.

LEPTOSPIROSIS

Leptospirosis was first described more than 100 years ago as an icteric (relating to jaundice) syndrome called Weil's disease. The causative organism, a tightly wound motile spirochete, is acquired by contact with water contaminated with waste products of rats. In humans

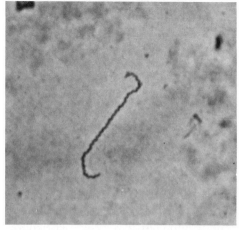

Figure 20-5 A phase-contrast photomicrograph of *Leptospira interrogans*, serotype icterohaemorrhagiae, the causative agent of human leptospirosis. (Courtesy, D. A. Kuhn, Northridge, California.)

the most serious disease is caused by *Leptospira interrogans*, serotype icterohaemorrhagiae (Figure 20-5). In recent years other leptospires have been isolated from dogs, cattle, and swine.

Transmission. Leptospires are spread by water contaminated with urine of infected animals or by direct contact with animals having leptospirosis. The organisms can enter the body by ingestion or through cuts and abrasions on the skin. Infections are common in farmers working in rice paddies or sugarcane fields.

Laboratory Diagnosis. Leptospires are difficult to demonstrate by direct microscopic examination, but may be observed by dark-field examination if they are present in large numbers. The cells are typically helical and range in

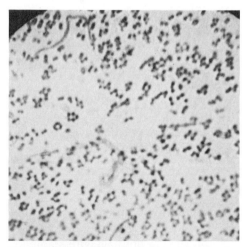

Figure 20-4 Gram stain of *Yersinia pseudotuberculosis* isolated from fluid aspirated from a pericardial cavity.

size from 6 to 20 μm in length and 0.1 μm in diameter. One or both ends may be bent or hooked. The organisms can be isolated from blood during the first week of the disease and from urine for several months. Most strains of leptospires will grow in media enriched with rabbit serum at 30°C. An occasional isolate may require several weeks for evidence of growth. Weanling hamsters or young guinea pigs may be inoculated as an alternate to culturing. Leptospires isolated in cultures or animals in clinical laboratories are sent to leptospirosis reference laboratories for serotyping.

Agglutinins against leptospiral antigens are detectable within two weeks after onset of illness as a rule. Titers reach a maximum in three to four weeks.

Immunity. The amount of resistance conferred by an attack of leptospirosis remains largely speculative. Only if titers of antibodies remain high can it be assumed that an individual has some immunity to a particular serotype. More than 100 serotypes have been identified from sources all over the world. It is doubtful that mild forms of the disease afford any subsequent protection.

Prevention. Protective clothing, such as gloves and boots, may protect farm workers from exposure to leptospires. Disinfection of barns, pigsties, pastures, and ponds can be accomplished with chlorine or creosols. Killed leptospires have been used on a limited scale for vaccination of certain occupational groups in a few countries. Animal vaccination programs may prove effective for future control of leptospirosis.

STAPHYLOCOCCAL FOOD POISONING

It is important to differentiate between staphylococcal enteritis and staphylococcal food poisoning. The cocci are found in limited numbers in the gastrointestinal tract of healthy individuals. In the absence of effective competition by other indigenous flora, the staphylococci proliferate and produce sufficient enterotoxin to cause enteritis.

Staphylococcal food poisoning occurs after ingestion of a sufficient amount of preformed enterotoxin to cause nausea, vomiting, and diarrhea. The symptoms usually occur two to six hours after eating contaminated food, but do not last longer than a day or two. Food poisoning was at one time referred to as *ptomaine poisoning.* Ptomaine is a nitrogenous product derived from putrefactive action of bacteria. The enterotoxin elaborated by certain strains of *Staphylococcus aureus* is not a product of putrefaction, nor are other enterotoxins derived from bacterial metabolism. True ptomaine poisoning is probably rare since evidence of putrefaction is usually recognizable by distinctly unpleasant odor or taste.

Transmission. Enterotoxin-producing staphylococci gain entrance to food from persons or animals with staphylococcal disease or from carriers of *S. aureus.* The cocci grow especially well in dairy products, cream-filled pastries, custards, ham, sausage, and mayonnaise-containing salads or sandwich spreads. After contamination, food must stand at room temperature for several hours to permit sufficient growth of *S. aureus* for enterotoxin production.

Laboratory Diagnosis. Samples of food, vomitus, or stool in a suspected staphylococcal food poisoning outbreak can be cultured on blood agar or on selective media. Selective media, such as mannitol-salt agar (MSA) or *Staphylococcus* medium no. 110 (SM110), containing 7.5 to 10 percent sodium chloride, inhibit the growth of most other bacteria, but permit staphylococci to grow. The microscopic appearance of staphylococci has been described in an earlier chapter. Strongly positive coagulase-producing staphylococci will cause normal plasma to clot within four hours. All coagulase-positive staphylococci do not produce enterotoxin, however. In order to incriminate staphylococci as etiological agents in cases of food poisoning, enterotoxins must be recovered from broth or food and typed serologically as A, B, C, D, or E.

Immunity. Detection of antibodies to the various types of staphylococcal enterotoxin has been hampered by difficulty in obtaining purified preparations of toxin. Both precipitating and hemagglutinating antibodies against highly purified enterotoxin B (SEB) have been demonstrated in human sera. All precipitating antibodies in one study were shown to be associated with the IgG class of immunoglobulins. Limited studies indicate that humoral antibodies to SEB offer resistance to a parenteral, but not an alimentary challenge.

Prevention. All food processors should be adequately informed on proper food storage. No food should be stored for prolonged periods at room temperature. Individuals with suspected or diagnosed staphylococcal lesions should refrain from active involvement in preparing or serving food.

BOTULISM

Like staphylococcal food poisoning, botulism is not classified as an infection, but rather as an intoxication from a potent exotoxin of *Clostridium botulinum*. The effect of the toxin is not limited to the gastrointestinal tract, but botulism is included here because of the toxin's portal of entry. When the neurotoxin is ingested, it is absorbed by the stomach and small intestine. The toxin disseminates 18 to 36 hours after ingestion and blocks release of acetylcholine by nerve fibers. Symptoms include facial paralysis, difficulty in speaking, muscle weakness, vertigo, double vision, nausea, vomiting, and respiratory failure. The high fatality rate for botulism, which approximates 20 to 30 percent in the United States, is related to the irreversible "fixing" of toxin to efferent nerve endings.

Botulism has recently been reported as a "new disease" in infants with profound muscle weakness. The disease appears to be the result of intraintestinal production of toxin by *C. botulinum*. In most cases the source of the organisms remains a mystery. To date, all recognized cases of infant botulism have recovered without neurological complications.

A clinical entity called "wound botulism" has also been described in recent years in the United States. The spores of *C. botulinum*, abundant in soil, presumably gain entrance through a deep puncture wound. Neurological effects are evident only after sufficient time has elapsed to permit multiplication of the organisms. After 4 to 14 days, sufficient exotoxin may be produced to cause sensory disturbances in an affected extremity.

Transmission. Most food-borne botulism outbreaks in the United States have been traced to home-processed foods in which heating has been inadequate to kill *C. botulinum* cells or to inactivate preformed botulinal toxin. A temperature of 100°C for 10 minutes is sufficient to destroy the toxin. Home-canned lamprey, beans, mushrooms, fermented salmon eggs, and smoked fish, and commercially processed tunafish and beef stew have been incriminated as sources for the neurotoxin in outbreaks of botulism. Honey has been implicated as a source for botulinal organisms in infant botulism.

Laboratory Diagnosis. Botulism is usually diagnosed clinically on the basis of symptoms and recent history of consuming suspected food within the past several days. If samples of the suspected foods are available, they can be homogenized to extract possible toxin. Supernatants, or serum or gastric contents from a patient, can be injected intraperitoneally into mice; the mice often exhibit neurological symptoms and die within several hours.

Food samples may also be cultured in cooked-meat medium. Organisms can be subcultured in prereduced trypticase-peptone glucose (TPG) broth in order to obtain sufficient toxin for inoculation purposes. Gram stains made directly on food samples are of no value, because merely finding the gram-positive bacilli, which measure 1.0 to 1.5 μm by 4.0 to 8.0 μm in size, does not provide proof that the food contained a toxin.

Immunity. Recovery from botulism offers little resistance upon subsequent exposure to botulinal toxin. Antibody response appears minimal and too late to provide protection within the time required for toxin to act.

Prevention. Prophylactic measures, including education on appropriate food-preserving methods, could minimize the number of cases of botulism. Toxoids are recommended for cattle in endemic areas. Vaccination programs for humans do not appear warranted except for specific laboratory personnel. A pentavalent toxoid is available on a limited basis to high-risk employees.

PERFRINGENS POISONING

Perfringens poisoning ranks second as a cause of food poisoning in the United States. Only *S. aureus* is responsible for more outbreaks of food poisoning than *Clostridium perfringens.* Abdominal pain, diarrhea, and nausea usually occur within 12 hours after ingestion of contaminated food. Five distinct biotypes of the organism, based on toxin production, have been identified. An alpha toxin, identified as lecithinase, is produced by all biotypes of C. *perfringens.* Other toxins include both hemolytic and necrotizing substances.

Transmission. C. *perfringens* is a part of the normal intestinal flora of humans and animals. If meat or poultry is insufficiently cooked, the organism is transmitted on ingestion. Lack of attention to personal hygiene habits contributes to the spread of the organism from human sources.

Laboratory Diagnosis. Gram stains of smears prepared from food samples containing C. *perfringens* reveal the presence of gram-positive bacilli 1.0 to 1.5 μm wide by 4.0 to 8.0 μm long. Endospores may or may not be present. Suspected food or stool samples can be cultured on tryptose-sulfite-cycloserine (TSC) agar under anaerobic conditions. Lecithinase-producing colonies, which appear black on TSC agar, can be used to subculture isolates in thioglycolate broth. C. *perfringens* is nonmotile, reduces nitrate, and produces "stormy fermentation" of milk. The evolved gas is readily visible in the curd (Figure 20-6).

Immunity. There is general susceptibility to perfringens poisoning. Recovery from the effects of the toxin is generally so rapid that antibody response is negligible.

Prevention. Precaution in food handling and strict adherence to personal

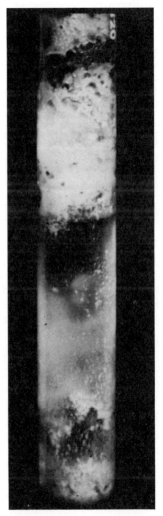

Figure 20-6 "Stormy fermentation" produced by *Clostridium perfringens* in milk. (Courtesy, Center for Disease Control, Atlanta, Georgia.)

hygiene can prevent contamination of food with the intestinal organism. Thorough cooking of foods containing meat or poultry and immediate refrigeration of cooked foods can reduce the risk of perfringens poisoning. If food is kept at room temperature for long periods of time, spores of *C. perfringens* which survive an inadequate heating process can germinate, multiply, and elaborate sufficient enterotoxin to cause perfringens poisoning within a few hours.

HALOPHILIC VIBRIO POISONING

Facultative halophilic (salt-loving) vibrios have been associated with a type of food poisoning in both Japan and the United States. At least three biotypes of the organism, based on biochemical and antimicrobial susceptibility characteristics, have been recognized. The marine vibrio, *Vibrio parahaemolyticus*, is responsible for over 50 percent of diarrhea occurring during the summer months in Japan. The onset of symptoms may be rapid or delayed as long as 8 to 10 days after ingestion of contaminated seafood. All cases, except one in the United States, have originated in an ocean-bound state.

Transmission. In the United States halophilic vibrio poisoning is transmitted by ingestion of raw oysters or improperly cooked crab, shrimp, or clams. In Japan sushi, a vinegar-treated rice-ball topped with fish, is frequently associated with outbreaks of the poisoning.

Laboratory Diagnosis. Direct microscopic examination of stool specimens in suspected cases of halophilic vibrio poisoning is not recommended. Rectal swabs or suspected food samples can be streaked on bromthymol blue "teepol" (TBT teepol) or thiosulfate citrate bile salts sucrose (TCBS) agar or placed in alkaline peptone broth (pH 8.5) supplemented with 3.5 percent NaCl. A complete battery of biochemical tests is necessary to differentiate vibrios causing food poisoning. The taxonomic status of marine vibrios has not been clearly defined.

Immunity. Susceptibility to halophilic vibrio poisoning is probably general. There is no evidence that exposure to contaminated seafoods provides protection in the event of subsequent ingestion of the vibrios or their products.

Prevention. Control measures are aimed at keeping the numbers of marine vibrios or their products below the minimal infective dose in seafoods. Since it is impossible to rid the oceans of *V. parahaemolyticus* or related vibrios, eating raw fish should be avoided. Special care should be taken not to allow seafoods to stand at room temperature for long periods of time.

CAMPYLOBACTER GASTROENTERITIS

A gram-negative vibrio, *Campylobacter fetus*, may be associated with a variety of infections, but probably most commonly causes gastroenteritis. The gastrointestinal disease is usually short in duration, but may be accompanied by bloody stools. Chickens have been incriminated as a source of the organism. Immunocompromised hosts are particularly susceptible to *Campylobacter* infections. The organism grows well at 45°C under reduced oxygen tension on a selective medium containing vancomycin, polymyxin, and trimethoprim. Distinctive characteristics of the vibrio include the inability to ferment carbohydrates, motility by a single polar flagellum at one or both ends of the cell, and production of both oxidase and catalase.

PSEUDOMEMBRANOUS COLITIS

Pseudomembranous colitis is a complication of antimicrobial therapy associated with toxin-producing strains of *Clostridium difficile*. The anaerobe is widespread in nature and can be isolated in small numbers from intestinal contents of healthy individuals. The competition from other indigenous organisms keeps the numbers low in the absence of antimicrobial agents. Presence in a Gram stain of a stool of both large numbers of white blood cells and gram-positive bacilli with or without subterminal spores suggests the possibility of the antimicrobial agent–associated disease. Confirmation of the presence of toxin-producing strains of *C. difficile* requires demonstration of toxin in stool and isolation of the anaerobe from stool on an enriched egg yolk agar containing cycloserine and cefoxitin. The toxin is cytotoxic for human amnion cells.

VIRAL INFECTIONS

There is no doubt that the digestive system provides a major portal of entry for viruses. Some that invade the body through the gastrointestinal tract affect organs outside the alimentary canal, while others produce distinct gastrointestinal disease. Symptoms resulting from viral invasion of the gastrointestinal tract may resemble those arising from bacterial invasion or toxigenicity. In the absence of a specific bacterial etiological agent, a virus is usually assumed to be the agent of disease. If symptoms are mild and recovery is rapid, the specific virus is usually not identified. However, it is important to recognize that gastrointestinal symptoms may indicate the entry of a virus which can cause more serious diseases of the respiratory and central nervous systems (Table 20-7).

PICORNAVIRUS INFECTIONS

The picornaviruses are small RNA-containing viruses. A large number of them enter the human host by means of the oral route. They include the echoviruses, coxsackieviruses, and polioviruses. The 31 echoviruses are probably the major enteric pathogens, but they can also cause fever, rash, and central nervous system (CNS) disease. All of the echoviruses, even those that do not have a predilection for alimentary tract tissue, find easy access to the human host by way of the oral route. The en-

Table 20-7 MAJOR GROUPS AND SEROTYPES OF GASTROINTESTINAL VIRUSES

VIRUS	SEROTYPES	MAJOR DISEASE
Picornavirus		
echovirus	1–31	enteritis, epidemic diarrhea
coxsackievirus	A1–23, B1–6	undifferentiated febrile disease
poliovirus	1–3	poliomyelitis
Herpesvirus		
cytomegalovirus	1, 2	cytomegalovirus inclusion disease, inapparent infection
Unclassified		
hepatitis, type A (HAV)	MS-1	hepatitis A
hepatitis, type B (HBV)	MS-2	hepatitis B
hepatitis, non-A, non-B (NANB)	Unknown	non-A, non-B hepatitis
Reovirus	1–3	inapparent infection

teritis and diarrheal syndrome, following ingestion of echoviruses, are manifestations of localized invasion.

Coxsackieviruses may cause undifferentiated febrile disease, but more often are respiratory pathogens. Polioviruses, while entering by the oral route, manifest themselves primarily as pathogens of the CNS and are discussed in Chapter 23.

Transmission. The echoviruses are transmitted by contaminated food, water, and aerosols. The severity of enteric disease appears to be related to the number of the viruses ingested.

Laboratory Diagnosis. Echoviruses can be grown in monkey kidney cells from throat washings, nasal secretions, or stool samples (Figure 20-7). Hemagglutinating, hemagglutination-inhibiting, and neutralizing antibodies can be detected serologically in convalescent sera of infected patients. In most cases the echovirus remains unidentified be-

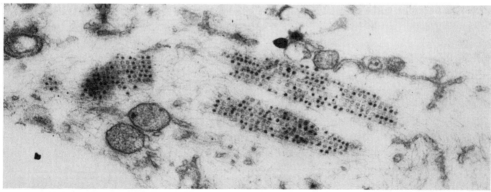

Figure 20-7 Assembly of echovirus, type 9, in cytoplasm of infected cells. (Courtesy, G. C. Godman, New York.)

cause laboratory procedures required for diagnosis are too time-consuming and expensive for general use.

Immunity. It is doubtful that significant permanent immunity is a consequence of any echovirus infection. The large number of viruses belonging to this group precludes resistance other than to a specific agent and that resistance may be short in duration.

Prevention. There are no effective control measures for prevention of echovirus infections. Artificial immunization is not recommended because of the large number of echoviruses implicated in gastrointestinal infections.

HERPESVIRUS INFECTIONS

The cytomegalovirus causes a severe and sometimes fatal illness in newborns known as cytomegalovirus inclusion disease. The virus causes increases in cell size of the invaded tissue. It has a predilection for salivary glands and may disseminate from the glands to produce cytopathology of the brain, kidneys, liver, spleen, or lungs. Motor aberrations, mental retardation, and loss of sight are common sequelae in surviving infants.

Transmission. Cytomegalovirus usually is transmitted by parenteral routes (introduced other than by way of the intestines). Transmission across the placenta from a mother with an inapparent infection is the usual means of entry in newborns. Blood transfusion is the most likely route in adults, although in disseminated disease the virus is shed in aerosols and urine. The fact that the virus has been recovered from both semen and cervical secretions suggests that venereal transmission is also possible.

Laboratory Diagnosis. The presence of cytomegalovirus can be established by culturing saliva, urinary sediment, sputum, or gastric washings on human embryonic fibroblasts. The intranuclear eosinophilic inclusion bodies are pathognomonic for the disease (Figure 20-8). The cytoplasm of infected cells may be vacuolated and frequently contains numerous basophilic bodies rich in DNA. Hemagglutinating and complement-fixing antibodies can be detected in sera of children and adults with clinical evidence of disease, but also in more than half of the population between 18 and 25 years of age in the United States.

Immunity. Although host response to cytomegalovirus infection is consistent, the antibodies do not seem to alter the course of the disease. Persons with natural or acquired immunological deficiencies are particularly prone to active infections. It is likely that cellular immune mechanisms play a larger role than does humoral immunity.

Prevention. The large number of asymptomatic infections makes it impossible to detect carriers or to ascertain if the source of the virus is exogenous or endogenous in actual disease. Effective measures for prevention of congenital or acquired illness caused by cytomegalovirus can be developed only when more is known about its transmission.

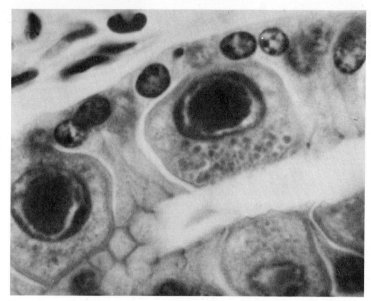

Figure 20-8 Intranuclear and intracytoplasmic inclusions in an epithelial cell of a salivary gland duct infected with cytomegalovirus. (Courtesy, J. S. Nelson, St. Louis.)

HEPATITIS VIRUS INFECTIONS

Information on the exact nature of the hepatitis viruses is somewhat limited, since the organisms multiply only in humans, although the infectious nature of the disease they cause has been long recognized.

The two viruses responsible for most cases of hepatitis (inflammation of the liver) are type A (HAV) and type B (HBV). The disease caused by HAV was formerly known as infectious hepatitis and by HBV as serum hepatitis. Although the two types are clearly distinct from one another, the diseases they cause have several characteristics in common (Table 20-8). The effect of invasion by either virus varies from an inapparent infection to severe liver necrosis and death. The classical clinical feature of both is jaundice, which may be minimal and of short duration or quite severe over a prolonged period of time. Fatality rates for reported cases range from 10 to 50 percent for hepatitis B and about 1 percent for hepatitis A.

A third type of viral hepatitis has recently been described. It is caused by an agent designated as a non-A, non-B (NANB) particle.

Transmission. The most common mode of transmission for hepatitis A is the fecal-oral route through contaminated food or water. The parenteral route, principally through blood, accounts for much disease caused by the

Table 20-8 SOME CHARACTERISTICS OF HEPATITIS A AND HEPATITIS B INFECTIONS

CHARACTERISTIC	HEPATITIS A	HEPATITIS B
Communicability	highly contagious	mildly contagious
Incidence	autumn and winter	year round
Incubation period	15–40 days	60–160 days
Onset	abrupt	insidious
Target organ	liver	liver
Clinical hallmark	jaundice	jaundice
Fever	present	usually absent
Severity	mild to moderately severe	frequently severe
Serum transaminases	elevated	elevated
HB_sAg in serum	absent	present
HB_cAg in serum	absent	present
Prophylactic immune serum globulin (ISG)	80–90% effective	40–70% effective

type B hepatitis virus and for infections caused by the NANB particle. Infections may be transmitted through blood transfusions, contaminated hypodermic needles, and contaminated instruments such as razors or tattoo needles. Parenteral transmission of HAV is rare. The virus of hepatitis B can also spread from person to person in intensive care, pediatric, surgical, oncology, and hemodialysis units by means of infective secretions. Recently oral, venereal, and neonatal transmission for the type B particle have been established.

Laboratory Diagnosis. The clinical course of both types of hepatitis may mimic other viral or toxic liver diseases. Tests of liver function do not differentiate the causative agents, but provide information only on the extent of hepatocellular injury. Elevated glutamic oxaloacetic (SGOT) and glutamic pyruvic (SGPT) transaminases are common in both hepatitis A and B.

Type B can be differentiated from type A by the presence of the hepatitis B surface antigen (HB_sAg) in the blood of patients with the type B virus. The surface antigen is present during the prodromal stage of the disease; it persists during early phases of illness in all patients and for months or even years in 5 to 10 percent of them. The most sensitive technique for identifying HB_sAg is a radioimmunoassay.

The core antigen HB_cAg appears to be present during acute phases of hepatitis B. It can be detected by radioimmunoassay, complement-fixation, and fluorescent antibody techniques, or electron microscopy. Anti-HB_cAg activity is high in sera obtained from patients with acute or chronic progressive hepatitis. Antibodies to HB_sAg tend to be abundant in blood donors and patients who have received multiple blood transfusions.

Serum antibody against HAV can be demonstrated by complement-fixation immune adherence hemagglutination, and radioimmunoassay. The HAV antibodies remain detectable in serum for many years after an initial infection.

Immunity. Antibodies to HB_sAg provide partial or complete immunity to hepatitis B. The role of antibodies against the core antigen is less clear. Anti-HAV antibodies confer lifelong immunity. The serum of over half of the adults in the United States contains antibodies affording protection from type A hepatitis virus. For the most part contact with HAV produces no overt symptoms of disease.

Prevention. The dissemination of hepatitis viruses can be minimized by strict adherence to personal hygiene, testing of transfusion blood for HB_sAg, careful surveillance by public health agencies, and broad educational programs. Eliminating commercialism in obtaining donor blood is a goal of federal public health agencies in the United States. Blood from paid donors carries a higher risk for potentiating hepatitis than blood from volunteers.

Immune serum globulin (ISG) can be used to reduce the severity of hepatitis A or hepatitis B. A dose of 0.02 ml per kilogram of body weight is recommended immediately upon possible exposure to HAV. Passive immunization with 0.05 to 0.07 ml of ISG per kilogram of body weight is recommended in the event of accidental exposure to a large inoculum of HBV or in certain endemic settings.

REOVIRUS INFECTIONS

The role of reoviruses in gastrointestinal disease has been in doubt because the viruses can be isolated from the stool of asymptomatic individuals. Recent reports from such widely separated countries as the United States, Guatemala, and Bangladesh, however, have implicated members of the reovirus group, known as rotaviruses, as causes of gastroenteritis in infants and young children. Rotavirus infections also occur in a variety of animals, including calves, piglets, and lambs. A recently developed enzyme-linked immunosorbent assay (ELISA) may make it possible to identify human rotavirus serotypes in the future. The reason for the propensity of rotaviruses for intestinal tissue of young children or animals and the possible role of animals as reservoirs in human disease are not understood.

ALGAL AND FUNGAL TOXIN-ASSOCIATED DISEASE

Despite the ubiquity of both algae and fungi in the human environment, toxigenic algae and fungi have not been studied as much as toxigenic bacteria. Evidence has accummulated during recent years, however, which incriminates cyanobacteria (blue-green algae), eucaryotic algae, and a variety of fungi in animal and some human toxin-associated diseases. Blooms of cyanobacteria belonging to the genus *Anabaena*, for example, have been responsible for some serious wildlife and livestock poisonings. Another cyanobacterium, *Lyngbya majuscula*, is associated with a type of human dermatitis known as Hawaiian swimmer's itch. Moldy grains have long been associated with toxicosis in domestic birds, sheep, and cattle. The role of mycotoxins is less well established in human disease. At least two types of poisoning associated with algal and fungal toxins constitute major health hazards, paralytic shellfish poisoning, and aflatoxin poisoning.

PARALYTIC SHELLFISH POISONING

Paralytic shellfish poisoning is a particularly dramatic type of intoxication resulting from eating shellfish, such as mussels, clams, cockles, oysters, or periwinkles, infested with the dinoflagellate *Gonyaulax catenella*. The marine alga produces a potent alkaloid neurotoxin. Symptoms of shellfish poisoning occur almost immediately after ingestion of shellfish muscle or viscera. Tingling followed by numbness in the lips, tongue, and fingers usually precedes vertigo, double vision, dryness of the throat, muscular incoordination, and respiratory paralysis.

Transmission. The transmission of the neurotoxin of the microscopic alga *G. catenella* to a cold-blooded animal and ultimately to a human is a form of "food-chain" transmission. The unicellular photosynthetic alga is found in abundance as a part of plankton along the Pacific coast from May through October. Presence of the alga in large amounts sometimes causes the so-called red tide phenomenon, that is, a reddening of coastal waters. Lack of red water, however, does not preclude the presence of the poisonous dinoflagellates. *G. catenella* and other organisms comprising the Pacific plankton are consumed by shellfish. The poison, which is nontoxic to shellfish, is stored in their muscle tissue or digestive glands. Mussels and clams represent the most frequently incriminated seafoods causing the neurological poisoning.

Laboratory Diagnosis. The diagnosis of paralytic shellfish poisoning presents few problems because of the dramatic symptoms occurring soon after ingestion of shellfish. Unfortunately, toxic shellfish do not look or taste different from harmless ones. For confirmation of a diagnosis mice may be given an intraperitoneal inoculation of extracts of gastric contents or suspected seafood; the inoculation is lethal within 15 minutes.

Immunity. Susceptibility to paralytic shellfish poisoning is general. There is no evidence that previous exposure to small amounts of the neurotoxin is beneficial as a deterrent to the disease.

Prevention. Both educational and legislative measures have been employed to prevent paralytic shellfish poisoning. For example, mussels are quarantined in California during periods when *G. catenella* is abundant in coastal waters. Highway signs are posted along beaches in summer months to warn seafood enthusiasts. Contrary to popular belief among some coastal residents, oil spills are not associated with shellfish poisoning. The microbial etiology of the disease needs greater publicity to correct misunderstandings and to reduce numbers of cases.

AFLATOXIN POISONING

There has been a great deal of recent interest in metabolic products of the fungi *Aspergillus flavus*, *A. parasiticus*, and *Penicillium notatum*, all of which frequently contaminate animal feed. The products of the contaminating fungi, called *aflatoxins*, cause severe poisoning with liver damage in many species of animals. It is likely that ingestion of aflatoxins in moldy grain, nuts, or milk is the cause of human hepatic disease in some parts of the world. At least six aflatoxins, B_1, B_2m, B_{2a}, G_1, G_2, and G_{2a}, have been characterized. All are tumorigenic for rats, but the role of aflatoxins in human tumorigenesis remains to be elucidated.

SUMMARY

Bacterial pathogens or their toxins can gain entrance to the gastrointestinal tract through contaminated food or water, or by means of the fecal-oral route. Preformed toxins may directly affect the alimentary canal or be absorbed and carried by blood to target organs other than the gastrointestinal tract. Bacteria may colonize within the intestines, or even invade deeper tissues, and produce enterotoxins with a primary affinity for the alimentary canal. The enteric viruses gain entrance by the oral route as a rule and may cause intestinal disturbances, affect accessory digestive organs, or disseminate to distant body parts. Despite the ubiquity of toxigenic algae and fungi, only two types of poisoning constitute major health hazards. Much bacterial, viral, or toxin-associated disease of the gastrointestinal tract can be prevented by understanding the etiology of the diseases, providing for adequate surveillance, educating the general public, and applying special precautions for high-risk populations.

QUESTIONS FOR STUDY

1. Classify each disease as a food poisoning or food infection.
   salmonellosis   cholera
   botulism   brucellosis
   bacillary dysentery leptospirosis
2. Distinguish between the terms diarrhea and dysentery.
3. Compare the time required for the onset of symptoms in staphylococcal food poisoning, botulism, perfringens poisoning, halophilic vibrio poisoning, and paralytic shellfish poisoning.
4. What accounts for the pathogenicity of some strains of *Escherichia coli?*
5. What advice can you give travelers to countries with less than adequate sanitation to prevent "travelers' diarrhea"?
6. What steps can be taken to prevent hepatitis?

SELECTED REFERENCES

Bader, M.; Pedersen, A. H. B.; Williams, R.; Spearman, J; and Anderson, H. Venereal transmission of shigellosis in Seattle-King County. *Sexually Transmitted Diseases* 4:89, 1977.

Benner, D. J.; Farmer, J. G., III; Hickman, F. W.; Asbury, M. A.; and Steigerwalt, A. G. Taxonomic and nomenclature changes in *Enterobacteriaceae.* HEW Publication No. (CDC) 78-8356. Atlanta, Ga.: Center for Disease Control, 1977.

Burrows, W.; Lewert, R. M.; and Rippon, J. W. *Textbook of Microbiology.* 19th ed. Philadelphia: Saunders, 1963.

California State Department of Public Health. *A Manual for Control of Communicable Diseases in California.* Berkeley: 1971.

Davis, B. D.; Dulbecco, R.; Eisen, H. N.; Ginsberg, H. A.; and Wood, W. B., Jr. *Microbiology.* 2d ed. New York: Harper & Row, 1973.

Edmonds, P. *Microbiology: An Environmental Perspective.* New York: Macmillan, 1978.

Housaini, A. A. Selected topics in immunology: infectious mononucleosis and Australia antigen. *Prog. in Clin. Path.* 4:211, 1972.

Joklik, W. K., and Willett, H. P. *Zinsser Microbiology.* 16th ed. Englewood Cliffs, N.J.: Prentice-Hall, 1976.

Lennette, E. H.; Spaulding, E. H.; and Truant, J. P. *Manual of Clinical Microbiology.* 2d ed. Washington, D.C.: American Society for Microbiology, 1974.

Lorian, V. *Significance of Medical Microbiology in the Care of Patients.* Baltimore: Williams & Wilkins, 1977.

MacFaddin, J. F. *Biochemical Tests for Identification of Medical Bacteria.* Baltimore: Williams & Wilkins, 1976.

McGann, V. G.; Rollins, J. B.; and Mason, D. W. Evaluation of resistance to staphylococcal enterotoxin: naturally acquired antibodies of man and monkey. *J. of Inf. Dis.* 124:206, 1971.

Peery, T. M., and Miller, F. N. *Pathology: A Dynamic Introduction to Medicine and Surgery.* 2d ed. Boston: Little, Brown, 1971.

Silver, S. Progress in hepatitis research. *Amer. J. Med. Tech.* 41:154, 1975.

Steele, J. H. The zoonoses: an epidemiologist's viewpoint. *Prog. in Clin. Path.* 5:239, 1973.

U.S. Department of Health, Education, and Welfare. Perspectives on the control of viral hepatitis, type B. *CDC Morbidity and Mortality Weekly Report Supplement* 25:3, 1976.

U.S. Department of Health, Education, and Welfare. Immune globulins for protection against viral hepatitis. *CDC Morbidity and Mortality Weekly Report* 26:425, 1977.

U.S. Department of Health, Education, and Welfare. Follow-up on infant botulism—United States. *CDC Morbidity and Mortality Weekly Report* 27:17, 1978.

Wade, N. New vaccine may bring man and chimpanzee into tragic conflict. *Science* 200:1027, 1978.

Youmans, G. P.; Paterson, P. Y.; and Sommers, H. M. *The Biologic and Clinical Basis of Infectious Diseases.* Philadelphia: Saunders, 1975.

Chapter 21

Protozoal and Helminthic Diseases of the Gastrointestinal Tract

After you read this chapter, you should be able to:

1. Describe the primary features of three protozoal infections of the gastrointestinal tract.
2. List the major protozoa and the infective stages which cause gastrointestinal disease.
3. Differentiate between trophozoites and cysts of the major intestinal protozoal parasites.
4. Describe the major helminthic infections of the gastrointestinal tract.
5. List the major helminths and the infective stages which cause gastrointestinal disease.
6. Describe the life cycles of the major helminths causing gastrointestinal disease.
7. Describe two tapeworm infections caused by larval forms.
8. Identify the helminthic diseases that are the most common in children.
9. Explain the role of the snail in the life cycle of flukes.
10. Compare methods required to prevent protozoal and helminthic gastrointestinal disease in the United States with methods required where the diseases are endemic.

The host-parasite relationships between humans and protozoa or helminths that cause enteric disease are often more complex than those involving bacteria or viruses. In the course of their life cycle the intestinal protozoa or helminths establish a parasitic relationship within the alimentary tract. The parasites live in a protected environment within the host and benefit from the more than adequate source of nutrition to support growth and multiplication. The host, however, is injured in the relationship, if harmful effects are substantial enough, disease or death ensues. Death is a catastrophe for both the host and the parasites.

PROTOZOAL INFECTIONS

Pathogenic protozoa have probably been significant causes of diarrheal disease and dysentery throughout the history of the world. Although it is not possible to incriminate any one protozoan, it is likely that protozoa were among the etiological agents of the epidemic diarrheal diseases that decimated Napoleon's troops during the Russian campaign and severely hampered efforts of the British soldiers in India at one time.

AMEBIC INFECTIONS

The pathogenicity of *Entamoeba histolytica* for humans was established early in the twentieth century. At one time *E. histolytica* was believed to be the sole etiological agent of amebic dysentery, but other amebas, including *Entamoeba coli, Endolimax nana, Iodamoeba bütschlii,* and *Dientamoeba fragilis,* are also associated with the disease. The true incidence of amebiasis is difficult to establish because symptoms of disease may be absent. It has been estimated that the worldwide incidence is close to

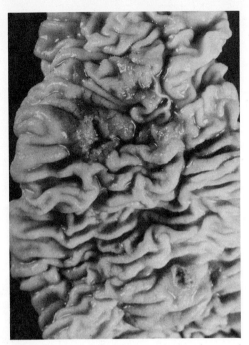

Figure 21-1 Typical buttonhole ulcers of the large intestine showing irregular margins. (From H. Brandt, in R. A. Marcial-Rojas, ed., *Pathology of Protozoal and Helminthic Diseases with Clinical Correlation,* Baltimore, William & Wilkins, 1971.)

10 percent. Entamebic dysentery can mimic a variety of intestinal disorders, but ulceration is the rule (Figure 21-1).

Life Cycle. Humans are the principal host for *E. histolytica* (Figure 21-2). Under most conditions the cyst is the infective stage. Ingested cysts are resistant to the highly acid gastric juice, but their walls are ultimately digested by the action of intestinal enzymes. The entamoebic parasite multiples within the cyst, so that on excystation the immature amebas are liberated. The trophozoites migrate to the large intestine

where stasis contributes to their ability to colonize effectively. The trophozoites have a predilection for the cecum, but also penetrate blood vessels and can be transported to other organs such as the brain, liver, or lungs. Trophozoites ultimately cease moving, become round, and secrete wall-forming cysts. A stage intermediate between the trophozoite and cyst stages, when cytoplasm is undergoing reorganization and movement is sluggish, is called the precystic stage. Trophozoites and precystic amebas may be found in liquid stools, but the lack of cytoplasmic organization makes the precystic stages of doubtful diagnostic value. Cysts are eliminated in formed stools. If trophozoites are eliminated in stools, they undergo the metamorphosis from trophozoites to cysts outside the host.

Transmission. Most amebic dysentery is transmitted by ingestion of food or water containing cysts of *E. histolytica*. However, flies have been shown to have significant roles as vectors in outbreaks of amebiasis in military or civilian camps. The cysts can also be transmitted directly from person to person by the fecal-oral route.

Laboratory Diagnosis. Diagnosis of amebic dysentery is made by demonstrating trophozoites or cysts in wet mounts or permanent mounts prepared from fresh stool (Figure 21-3). The trophozoites of *E. histolytica* range in size from 10 to 60 μm and often contain red blood cells in otherwise clear refractile cytoplasm. The cysts are variable in size, measuring 5.0 to 20 μm and may

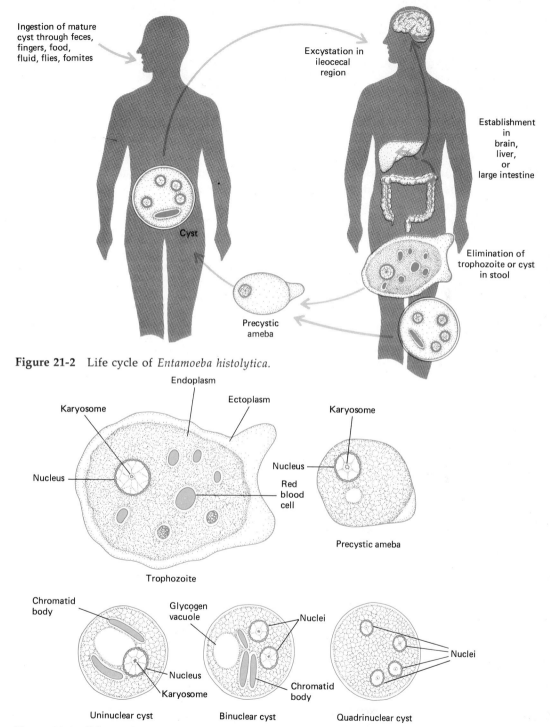

Figure 21-2 Life cycle of *Entamoeba histolytica.*

Figure 21-3 Schematic representation of stages of development of *Entamoeba histolytica.*

457

contain glycogen vacuoles and dark-staining cigar-shaped chromatoidal bodies. The cysts rarely have more than four nuclei bounded by chromatin on the inner nuclear membranes. Small central karyosomes are sometimes observed within nuclei. Serological tests are usually reserved for extraintestinal amebiasis. Complement-fixing (CF), indirect hemagglutinating (IH), and precipitating antibodies are elevated when the parasite migrates to extraintestinal sites.

Immunity. Very little is known about the protection afforded by antibodies produced in amebiasis. However, in countries in which amebic dysentery is endemic, residents have less severe symptoms than do visitors exposed to *E. histolytica.*

Prevention. Amebic dysentry can be prevented by purification of drinking water, provision for adequate disposal of sewage, detection of carriers, elimination of insects, effective treatment of infections, and warnings to travelers in endemic areas. If purity of water is questionable, water should be boiled or treated with dilute chlorine or tincture of iodine (see Table 20-5). In no instance should a person with a diagnosed amebic infection or a carrier state be allowed to handle food intended for human consumption.

GIARDIASIS

Giardiasis is an infection of the duodenum or jejunum of humans caused by the flagellate *Giardia lamblia.* The cyst constitutes the infective stage almost without exception. Many people harbor the protozoan in a commensal relationship, that is, a symbiotic relationship in which the parasite is provided with protection and nourishment without apparent harm to the host. For other individuals the intestinal invasion causes chronic diarrhea, sometimes accompanied by impaired absorption of fat and vitamin A.

Life Cycle. Humans are the major host for *G. lamblia,* but some rodents may be accidentally infected. After ingestion the cysts undergo excystation in the duodenum. The young trophozoites colonize in the duodenum or jejunum and only rarely migrate to the liver, bile ducts, or gallbladder. Both trophozoites and cysts may be found in unformed stool; only cysts occur in formed stool.

Transmission. Giardiasis is transmitted by food or water contaminated with cysts of *G. lamblia* or directly by the fecal-oral route. Flies and other insects can transmit the cysts after feeding or landing on contaminated material.

Laboratory Diagnosis. Diagnosis of giardiasis is made by demonstrating the cysts or trophozoites in stained wet or permanent mounts made from stool or duodenal contents. The trophozoite is bilaterally symmetrical, measures 12 to 15 μm in length, is pear-shaped with a rounded anterior and tapered posterior, has four pairs of flagella, and has two prominent nuclei (Figure 21-4). The cyst is ellipsoidal, measures approxi-

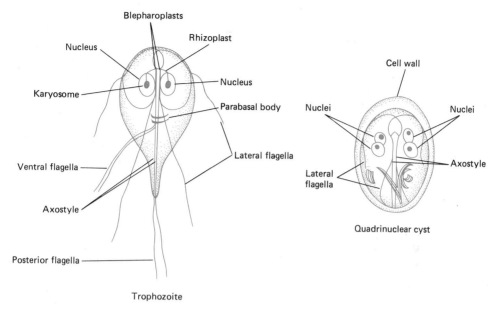

Figure 21-4 Schematic representation of trophozoite and quadrinuclear cyst of *Giardia lamblia.*

mately 9 to 12 μm, has a smooth, readily visible wall, and has two to four nuclei. No serological tests are of value in establishing a diagnosis of giardiasis.

Immunity. *G. lamblia* infections are more common and tend to be more severe in children than adults. It is not known if prior exposure to small doses of the flagellate can establish partial immunity to the parasite or if nonspecific immune factors account for the differences in susceptibility.

Prevention. Measures used to prevent amebic dysentery can also be used to control giardiasis. Recognition of *G. lamblia* as a true pathogen has emphasized the need to treat carriers of the intestinal flagellate. Addition of cysticidal iodine compounds to drinking water is recommended for travelers in endemic areas.

BALANTIDIASIS

Balantidiasis is a rare cause of dysentery in humans, but of considerable interest, because it is caused by the only pathogenic ciliate and the largest protozoan to infect humans. Cysts are the infective forms of the ciliate, *Balantidium coli,* but the trophozoite lives mainly in the lumen of the ileum or cecum of the host and is able to penetrate the intestinal mucosa with apparent ease. Penetration may be minimal with hyperemia the only effect, or it may be deep enough to cause marked ulceration. The ciliate rarely invades the liver or appendix, but secondary bacterial invasion is common.

Life Cycle. The life cycle of *B. coli* mimics that of *E. histolytica* but the ciliate does not multiply within cysts as is characteristic of the entamoebic parasite. The trophozoite divides by transverse binary fission. Invasion of intestinal mucosa follows liberation of trophozoites from cysts.

Transmission. Pigs are the most important source of *B. coli*, even though all herds of swine are not uniformly susceptible to infection. Asymptomatic rats and humans may also harbor the parasites. Only about half of the patients with balantidial infections have a history of exposure to pigs, and only

rarely has poorly cooked pork been implicated in the disease. Contaminated food or water and direct person-to-person transmission are important in the dissemination of balantidiasis.

Laboratory Diagnosis. Definitive diagnosis of balantidiasis can be made only by finding trophozoites or cysts in stained wet or permanent mounts prepared from stool or from scrapings obtained during sigmoidoscopy. Trophozoites are more commonly observed and are unmistakable because of their large size. The trophozoites average 60 by 45 μm and are shaped much like a sac (Figure 21-5). A mouth and gullet are frequently visible at the anterior end, and a less distinct excretory opening may be seen at the posterior end.

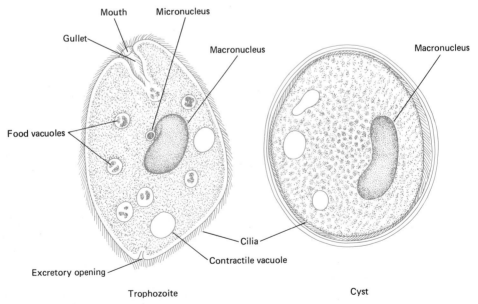

Figure 21-5 Schematic representation of trophozoite and cyst of *Balantidium coli*.

Both a micro- and a macronucleus are usually discernible. The cilia may be more difficult to see. The cysts, if present, are round or oval and average 52 to 55 μm in size. The cilia of cysts are retracted and a distinct cyst wall is visible.

Immunity. Healthy individuals probably have a high degree of resistance to *B. coli*. Nutritional deficiencies or the presence of other underlying disease probably increase susceptibility to the ciliate.

Prevention. Balantidiasis can be prevented by attention to the same prophylactic measures recommended for amebic dysentery and giardiasis. In addition, because of the suspected role of pigs in the transmission of the disease, swine herders should take extra sanitary precautions.

ROUNDWORM INFECTIONS

The parasitic nematodes can invade many parts of the body as immature forms (larvae) or as adults, but the intestines provide one of the most favorable environments for their development. Most nematodes have a single definitive host; a few species have arthropods as intermediate hosts; one roundworm requires a crustacean to complete its life cycle. In most instances embryonated ova, unembryonated ova, or larvae are excreted in feces. Embryonated ova are immediately infec-

tive for the same or another host. Unembryonated eggs must be incubated in the soil for 10 to 40 days before becoming infective. Larvae may be excreted in the noninfective, feeding rhabditiform stage or develop directly into the nonfeeding, infective filariform stage.

PINWORM INFECTION

Enterobiasis has the widest geographic distribution of any helminthic disease. The pinworm *Enterobius vermicularis* reportedly affects an estimated 208.8 million persons in the world and 18 million individuals in Canada and the United States. The disease is particularly common in children. The worms rarely cause serious lesions, but poor appetite, insomnia, and irritability caused by migratory habits of the female worm are common.

Life Cycle. Humans are the only natural host for *E. vermicularis*. Ingested ova hatch in the duodenum, but adult worms colonize and multiply in the ileum, cecum, or appendix (Figure 21-6). Gravid females, containing up to 11,000 ova, deposit their eggs in the perianal and perineal regions four to six weeks after ingestion of ova. Only rarely do female worms migrate to the vagina or urinary bladder. Female worms usually die after ovideposition. The cycle is completed only if embryonated ova are ingested by the same or another individual.

Transmission. The infective embryonated ova are usually transmitted

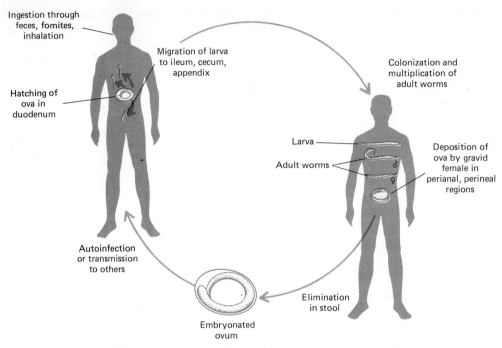

Figure 21-6   Life cycle of the pinworm *Enterobius vermicularis.*

by the fecal-oral route, by contaminated fomites, or by inhalation of ova-laden dust. Household pets do not harbor pinworms, but their fur can become a reservoir for eggs. Bedding, bath tubs, and toilet seats are common sources of contamination. In many communities *E. vermicularis* is best known as the "seatworm."

Laboratory Diagnosis. Diagnosis of pinworm infection is often made by finding the adult worms in stool or in the perianal region. The female worm is 6 to 12 μm long and 0.3 and 0.55 μm wide. The male worm is smaller and seldom seen. Because ova are rarely found in stool specimens, swabs of the perianal region, made with Scotch adhesive tape, are usually submitted to the laboratory for diagnostic purposes. Ova measure 50 to 60 μm in length and 20 to 30 μm in width. Shells of the ova are smooth, thick, and bilayered. Embryos may have a tadpole- or larvalike appearance (Figure 21-7)

Immunity. Susceptibility to pinworm infection is general. Even multiple infections produce no apparent resistance to a subsequent attack. Differences in intensity of the infection are related to numbers of ova encountered during exposure. The disease is self-limiting in two to eight weeks if reinfection does not occur.

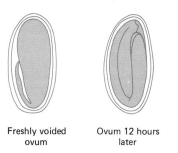

Freshly voided
ovum

Ovum 12 hours
later

Figure 21-7 Ova of *Enterobius vermicularis,* showing appearance of embryos within a freshly voided ovum and an ovum 12 hours later.

Prevention. Enterobiasis has proved to be difficult to control. A strict regimen of personal hygiene which includes proper washing of hands, frequent bathing, regular changes of bedding, underclothing, and night clothes, elimination of nail-biting, and relief from itching of the perianal region is important in preventing the spread of ova. Ova on discarded linen can be killed by exposure to 55°C for a few seconds. Toilet seats should be cleaned daily with disinfectants to prevent exposure of uninfected members of a family or an institution. Sunlight or ultraviolet lamp radiation readily destroy ova in the environment.

HOOKWORM INFECTION

Hookworm infection is most commonly caused by the presence of the adult nematode *Ancylostoma duodenale* or *Necator americanus* in the small intestine. *A. duodenale* is most often described as the Old World hookworm. *N. americanus* was so named because at one time it was believed to be a parasite of the New World, but study has shown that the parasite was transported to the United States with the importation of slaves from West Africa. The worldwide incidence of hookworm disease is surpassed only by malaria. At least 700 million people are believed to be victims of hookworm disease. In the United States most cases have occurred in rural areas of the southern states where moist, warm climates favor development of larvae. Alternating episodes of diarrhea and constipation, irritability, and tenderness of the abdomen may occur, but blood loss from the intestinal wall is the most serious consequence of hookworm infection.

Life Cycle. Humans are the usual host for *A. duodenale* and *N. americanus*. The hookworms attach themselves to the intestinal mucosa by cutting plates or teeth and feed on blood of the host (Figure 21-8). Embryonated eggs, which are produced at rates of more than 10,000 per day by a single worm, are excreted in feces and form rhabditiform larvae within one or two days in suit-

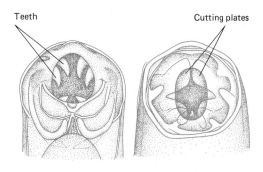

Teeth

Cutting plates

Ancylostoma duodenale

Necator americanus

Figure 21-8 Mouth parts of hookworms.

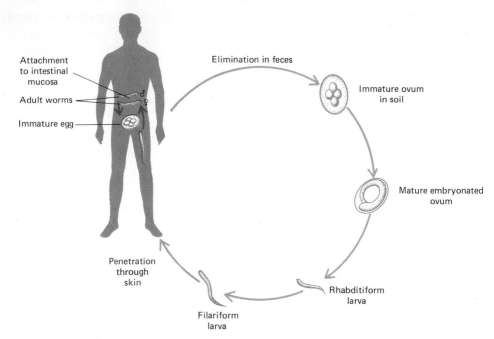

Attachment
to intestinal
mucosa

Adult worms

Immature egg

Elimination in feces

Immature ovum
in soil

Mature embryonated
ovum

Rhabditiform
larva

Filariform
larva

Penetration
through
skin

Figure 21-9   Life cycle of the hookworms *Ancylostoma duodenale*
and *Necator americanus.*

able soil. Feeding on organic material
and bacteria, they mature into the filariform stage within a week. The filariform larvae penetrate the skin of the
human host and begin the week-long
journey to the small intestine (Figure
21-9). Eggs do not appear in feces for a
month or two after initial exposure to
the hookworm larvae. If filariform larvae do not find a host, they die in about
six weeks when their endogenous food
supplies have been exhausted.

Transmission. Infective larvae usually penetrate the skin of bare feet exposed to soil contaminated with *A. duodenale* or *N. americanus.* Water or food is
rarely a source of the filariform larvae,

but asymptomatic individuals may constitute a reservoir for both hookworms.
Countries using human wastes for fertilization of crops provide exceptional
opportunity for dissemination of embryonated eggs into permissive soils.

Laboratory Diagnosis. Diagnosis of
hookworm infection is made by finding
the ova in stained wet or permanent
mounts made from stool. The eggs of *A.
duodenale* and *N. americanus* are virtually identical except for size. The eggs
of *Ancylostoma* are 56 to 60 μm long and
36 to 40 μm wide; the *Necator* eggs are
similar in width, but may be as long as
76 μm. A hyaline shell and a definitive
number of cells can be discerned in

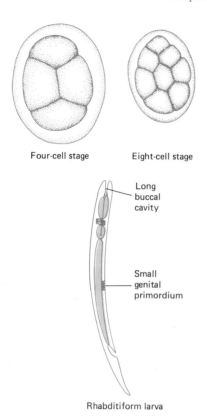

Four-cell stage   Eight-cell stage

Long
buccal
cavity

Small
genital
primordium

Rhabditiform larva

Figure 21-10 Developmental stages of hookworm ova and a rhabditiform larva.

early developmental stages of the ova of both parasites (Figure 21-10). Rhabditiform larvae of *A. duodenale* or *N. americanus* must be carefully distinguished from those of *Strongyloides* (see Figure 21-12).

Immunity. Susceptibility to hookworm infection is general, but some immunity, directed against larvae, follows an infection.

Prevention. It is important to treat all diagnosed cases of hookworm disease

to prevent spread of the infection. Safe disposal of human waste is an important deterrent to the spread of embryonated ova from unsuspected carriers. The simple practice of wearing shoes in rural areas and discouraging promiscuous defecation could do much to eliminate hookworm disease.

STRONGYLOIDIASIS

Strongyloidiasis was originally described in 1876 as "Cochin China" diarrhea in French soldiers returning from China. The causative agent, *Strongyloides stercoralis*, is widespread in distribution, but is particularly prevalent in warm, humid climates. Larvae of *Strongyloides*, much like those of the hookworm, can migrate to other organs.

Life Cycle. The life cycle of *S. stercoralis* may take one of three forms: a direct life cycle involving humans and soil, an indirect life cycle in which the larvae develop into sexually mature forms in the soil, or an endogenous life cycle which is completed within the human host (Figure 21-11).

In the direct life cycle infective filariform larvae penetrate the skin of man, and are carried by the venous and pulmonary circulation to the heart and lungs, respectively. The young parasites migrate to the bronchi, trachea, and pharynx, where the act of swallowing propels them into the digestive system. Larvae may also migrate to other organs during their developmental stages. Mature females deposit ova in the intestinal mucosa about 21 days after ingestion of filariform larvae.

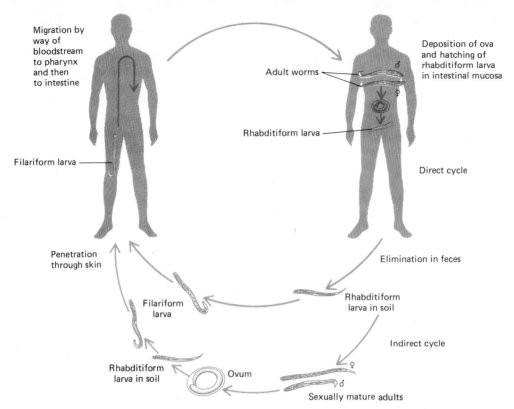

Figure 21-11 Direct and indirect life cycles of *Strongyloides stercoralis*.

Rhabditiform larvae are hatched in the mucosa and, after gaining access to appropriate soil, mature into the infective filariform forms in two or three days.

The indirect, or free-living, cycle is more common in tropical and subtropical climates. Under optimal conditions in soil or within the host, the life cycle may be completed in a single environment. The successful establishment of a life cycle within a host is responsible for recurrent autoinfections.

Transmission. Infective larvae penetrate the skin of bare feet exposed to soils contaminated with feces or de-velop within a previously infected host. Contaminated food or water is not a usual source of infection, but both can serve as vehicles for transmission of strongyloidiasis.

Laboratory Diagnosis. A diagnosis of strongyloidiasis is made by demonstrating rhabditiform larvae in stained wet or permanent mounts prepared from stool or duodenal drainage. Several specimens may be required to find larvae since the larvae are expelled intermittently. The larvae are present in sputum only if pulmonary disease is severe. The rhabditiform larvae are 200 to 300 μm long and 14 to 16 μm wide.

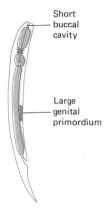

Figure 21-12 labels:
- Short buccal cavity
- Large genital primordium

Figure 21-12 A rhabditiform larva of *Strongyloides stercoralis*.

Their tails are short and bluntly pointed (Figure 21-12). The buccal cavity of *S. stercoralis* is shorter than those of *A. duodenale* or *N. americanus*. Ova are rarely present in feces.

Immunity. Susceptibility to strongyloidiasis is general. Definitive immune responses to invasion by the parasite have not been demonstrated in humans, but repeated infections with *S. stercoralis* promote partial immunity in experimental animals.

Prevention. The adaptation of the intestinal parasite to a single environment of the host provides a highly effective method for self-perpetuation. Autoinfection can be prevented only by aggressive search techniques and treatment in endemic areas. Exposure to the infective larvae can be reduced by protective shoes and clothes, elimination of the use of human wastes as fertilizer, strict adherence to personal hygiene, and installation of sanitary privies in rural areas.

ASCARIS INFECTION

Ascaris infection, or ascariasis, was probably the first parasitic infection to be recorded. Reference is made to its etiological agent, *Ascaris lumbricoides*, in books from China, Mesopotamia, Greece, and Rome. The large nematode is cosmopolitan in its distribution, affecting millions in Asia, Europe, Central and South America, and Africa. Ascaris infection is particularly prevalent in China. In the United States the incidence is high in southern rural areas. Children are more commonly infected than adults.

Larval migration typically produces an allergic response in the host with an accompanying eosinophilia. Adult ascarids can make their way through the intestinal wall into the peritoneal cavity, or migrate to the common bile duct, pancreas, or liver. Larvae can enter the circulatory system and be carried to the lung. It is not unusual for a child to pass worms through the umbilicus (Figure 21-13). A cough, fever, difficulty in

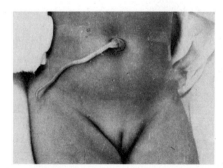

Figure 21-13 A 4-year-old girl passing an *Ascaris* through the umbilicus. (Courtesy, H. Schenone, Santiago, Chile. From J. M. Ausin et al., *Boletin Chileno de Parasitologia* 21:88, 1966.)

breathing, and hemorrhaging may occur in lung infections. The presence of adult worms in the intestine has an adverse effect on the host's nutritional status and may even cause an obstruction.

Life Cycle. Ascarids, residing in the lumen of the small intestine, can produce as many as 200,000 ova daily. Fertilized eggs are passed in the feces and develop into infective larvae in approximately three weeks in well-aerated soil at 25°C. If fertilized eggs are ingested by man, rhabditiform larvae hatch in the intestine. The hatched larvae penetrate the intestinal mucosa and begin their migration to distant parts, most commonly to the lungs. From the lungs larvae travel by way of bronchi, trachea, pharynx, esophagus, and stomach to the small intestine where they mature into adult parasites capable of mating.

Transmission. Ascaris infections are usually transmitted by ingestion of fertilized ova from contaminated soil or fomites, most often toys. In countries using human wastes as fertilizer raw vegetables are common vehicles of transmission. Other foods and drinking water are not common sources of the ascarid eggs.

Laboratory Diagnosis. The diagnosis of ascariasis is made by finding the ova in stained wet or permanent mounts prepared from stool or by identifying adult worms passed spontaneously through the anus, mouth, nose, or umbilicus. The fertilized ova are 45 to 75 μm long and 35 to 50 μm wide, are un-

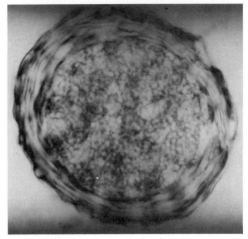

Figure 21-14 A fertilized ovum of *Ascaris lumbricoides*. (Courtesy, Abbott Laboratories, *Atlas of Diagnostic Microbiology*, p. 55, July, 1974.)

segmented, and demonstrate well-defined, clear spaces at the end of each pole. They are most often corticated, that is, with shells; the thick shells are coarsely mammillated (having many small projections) (Figure 21-14). Decorticated eggs (without shells) may be confused with hookworm eggs. In unisexual infections unfertilized ova may be found. Unfertilized eggs are longer, narrower, and tend to be decorticated. The adult female of *A. lumbricoides* ranges from 20 to 35 cm in length; adult males range from 15 to 31 cm. The worms are white to pink in color with blunt anterior and pointed posterior ends.

Immunity. Susceptibility to ascaris infection is general. Exposure to the parasite promotes an antibody response, but the role of antibodies in development of resistance is poorly understood. Hypersensitivity reactions, common during larval migration, are believed to be cell-mediated responses to larvae-associated metabolites.

Prevention. Ascaris infections can be prevented by appropriate disposal of feces, elimination of the practice of using human wastes as fertilizer, and strict adherence to personal hygiene. Antihelminthic treatment, without attention to personal hygiene and sanitation, is of little value in endemic areas.

WHIPWORM INFECTION

Whipworm infection, or trichuriasis, has probably been around for a long time. *Trichuris trichiura*, the causative agent, is the most common parasite of humans in some parts of the world. It is particularly prevalent in tropical countries where as many as 80 percent of persons may be infected. More children than adults harbor the parasite. The climate in the southern part of the United States meets the needs of *T. trichiura* for the extracorporal part of its life cycle.

Anemia is almost always present in severe infections, and eosinophilia is characteristic of acute infections.

Life Cycle. As many as 3,000 to 10,000 ova are produced by a female worm. Fertilization occurs within the intestines, but embryonic development takes place in warm, shaded, moist soil. The eggs become infective in about three weeks. Embryonated eggs, in-gested by humans, release larvae in the small intestine. The larvae reach maturity about three months after migrating to the cecum. The anterior ends of the mature parasites burrow into the intestinal mucosa where they can survive, if uninterrupted, for several years.

Transmission. Infective ova are transmitted by the fecal-oral route or by contaminated toys, food, or water. Reinfections are common.

Laboratory Diagnosis. The diagnosis of whipworm infection is made by finding the ova in stained wet or permanent mounts prepared from stool. The eggs are barrel-shaped and have a mucous plug at each end (Figure 21-15). The ova have thick shells and measure 50 to 54 μm long and 22 to 23 μm wide. The adult worms can be demonstrated in stool following treatment. They measure 3.5 to 5.0 cm in length and have slender, whiplike anterior ends. The blunt, thicker posterior ends are typically coiled in males (Figure 21-16).

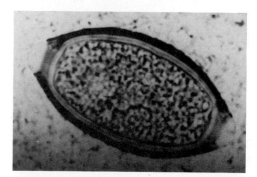

Figure 21-15 A fertilized ovum of *Trichuris trichiura*. (Courtesy, Abbott Laboratories, *Atlas of Diagnostic Microbiology*, p. 67, July, 1974.)

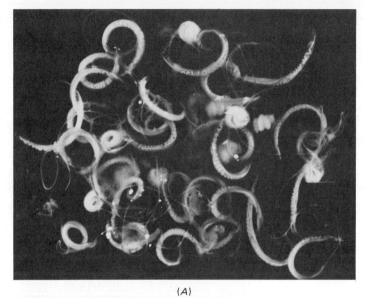

(A)

(B)

Figure 21-16 *Trichuris trichiura.* (*A*) Adult worms passed by a child after treatment with mebendazole. The worms were still moving within a mucoid mass when passed. (*B*) Adult pair. The threadlike esophagus followed by a thick body simulates a whip and handle, thus the common name whipworm. Coiled posterior end with protruding spicule identifies the male. (Courtesy, J. F. Maldonado-Mall, San Juan.)

Immunity. Susceptibility to whipworm infection is general. Since reinfection is common, trichuriasis probably does not establish any significant degree of immunity.

Prevention. Treatment of all infected individuals is essential in halting the spread of whipworm infections. Appropriate disposal of human waste, hand washing, and thorough washing of raw vegetables are especially important in eliminating the disease. As with other parasitic infections, more aggressive attempts to educate individuals, particularly children, could eradicate trichuriasis as a major enteric disease.

TRICHINOSIS

The Biblical recommendation against the eating of pork is believed by some to be the first recognition of the hazard of ingesting viable cysts of *Trichinella spiralis*, but the larval forms of the parasite were not described until 1835. The disease caused by the encysted larvae is called trichinosis. It is worldwide in distribution, but incidence varies with eating habits. Migration of larvae to muscles produces fever, headache, myalgia, muscle spasm, and frequently periorbital edema (Figure 21-17). Larvae can migrate to the myocardium, brain, or meninges causing symptoms which resemble those of severe bacterial or viral infections. Trichinosis can be fatal.

Life Cycle. Within a few hours after encysted larvae are ingested, capsules are digested in the small intestine. The freed larvae penetrate the intestinal mucosa and attain sexual maturity within a day. The female produces ova which are hatched *in vivo*. Embryos are

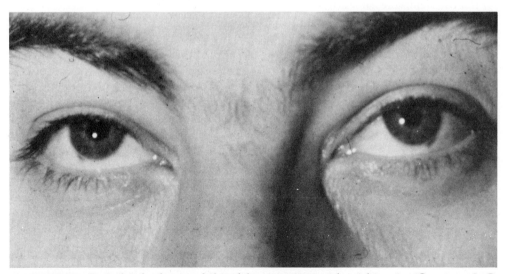

Figure 21-17 Periorbital edema exhibited by a patient with trichinosis. (Courtesy, I. G. Kagan, Center for Disease Control, Atlanta, Georgia.)

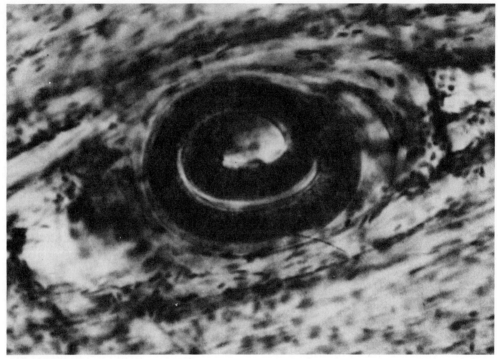

Figure 21-18 Encysted larva of *Trichinella spiralis* in muscle. (Courtesy, I. G. Kagan, Center for Disease Control, Atlanta, Georgia.)

discharged at a rate of about one every one-half hour during the usual life span of five weeks. The male adult parasite usually is excreted in feces shortly after fertilization occurs. Larvae penetrate the lymphatic spaces and are carried to the bloodstream. The migrating larvae have a predilection for striated muscle where they encyst about three weeks after reaching the target tissue (Figure 21-18). Humans are accidental hosts and do not contribute to the life cycle. The life cycle is maintained when pigs eat garbage containing improperly cooked pork, harboring the encysted larval forms.

Transmission. Humans become infected by eating insufficiently cooked pork, pork products, adulterated beef, or meat from wild animals. Both walrus and bear meat have been responsible for human trichinosis. Beef may be adulterated purposely by adding pork scraps to ground beef or inadvertently through use of a common grinder. Animal hosts can contain larvae in muscle tissue for several months. Person-to-person transmission does not occur.

Laboratory Diagnosis. Trichinosis is sometimes difficult to diagnose despite the availability of a skin test as well as tests for detecting complement-fixing and precipitating antibodies. All three tests may be negative early in the disease. Eosinophilia in trichinosis is marked and persists for several months unless a secondary bacterial infection occurs. Definitive diagnosis requires demonstration of living larvae in a biopsy of muscle tissue.

Immunity. Susceptibility to trichinosis is general and protection against reinfection from a single attack is of very limited duration. Second infections do occur in groups who regularly consume pork or pork products.

Prevention. Inspection of pork for evidence of trichinosis is considered to be too costly as a preventative measure against trichinosis. The macroscopic inspection of pork is not a reliable way to detect the presence of encysted larvae. However, the now mandatory requirement for sterilizing garbage before feeding it to hogs has successfully interrupted the life cycle of *T. spiralis*. The need to cook pork, pork products, and game meat so that all parts reach a minimal temperature of 65.5°C (150°F) or until meat turns from pink to distinct gray should be emphasized in educational campaigns.

TAPEWORM INFECTIONS

Most parasitic cestodes invade the intestinal tract of humans as adults and spend their adolescence as larvae in tissues of other vertebrates or invertebrates. The long, flat, ribbonlike adult worms are divided into segments called *proglottids*. The anterior ends or *scolices* contain specialized organs, the suckers and hooks, which attach to the mucosa of the ileum. Most flatworms, when mature, are hermaphroditic, that is, contain both male and female reproductive organs. Each proglottid having dual reproductive systems provides overwhelming potential for ova production.

A few of the cestodes have a larval form which invades humans. These larvae, called *cysticerci*, have two forms: the *cysticercus larva*, sometimes called a bladder larva because it has a fluid-containing bladder, and a *cysticercoid* or solid larva which has a tail (Figure 21-19). The reason for the well-developed migratory capacity of the larval forms is not known.

TAENIASIS AND CYSTICERCOSIS

Taeniasis and cysticercosis are cosmopolitan in distribution, but particularly prevalent in Africa, Central and South

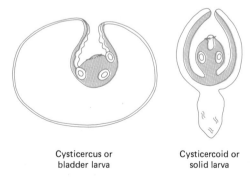

Cysticercus or bladder larva   Cysticercoid or solid larva

Figure 21-19 Two immature stages of human tapeworms.

America, Europe, and some parts of South Asia. Taeniasis is an infection of humans caused by the adult beef tapeworm, *Taenia saginata*, or the adult pork tapeworm, *T. solium*. Cysticercosis is an infection caused by cysticerci. Cysticerci of the beef tapeworm, *Cysticercus*

bovis, cause disease primarily in their herbivorous hosts. Cysticercosis in humans is usually caused by cysticerci of the pork tapeworm, *C. cellulosae*. The infection is rare in the United States. Humans are the only definitive hosts for both the adult beef and pork tape-

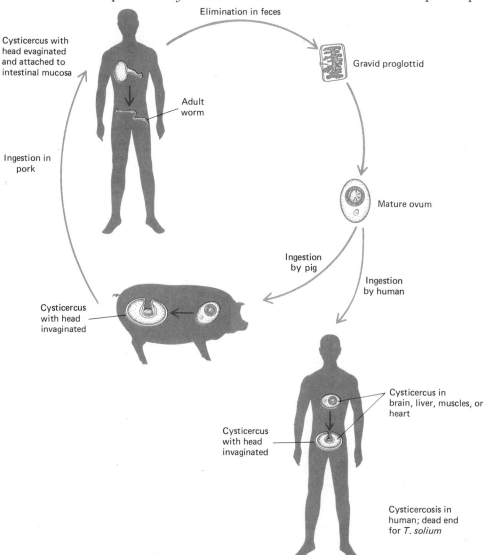

Figure 21-20   Life cycle of *Taenia solium*.

worms. The cysticerci of *T. saginata* rarely migrate in their herbivorous hosts, but the cysticerci of *T. solium* can cause lesions of the brain, meninges, eyes, heart, skin, or skeletal muscles in humans. They may remain in the human host for several years. Generally only one tapeworm is present.

Life Cycle. When ova of *T. saginata* or *T. solium* are swallowed by cattle or pigs, their shells are destroyed by pancreatin and bile salts (Figure 21-20). Liberated embryos penetrate the intestinal mucosa where they encyst and form cysticerci. The cysts are eaten by humans in raw or insufficiently cooked beef or pork. The scolex of the larvae evaginate and attach to the intestinal mucosa where adult parasites develop. Proglottids are shed in the stool with regularity. Ova are released when the proglottids rupture or expel egg-laden fluid. A single proglottid may consti-

tute a reservoir for as many as 100,000 eggs. The infective ova are ingested in food or water by cattle or pigs to complete the life cycles.

Transmission. Either cysticerci or ova constitute infective stages of *T. solium*. The ova of *T. saginata* are not infective for humans. Cysticerci are transmitted by consuming inadequately cooked beef or pork; the ova of *T. solium* are transmitted by the fecal-oral route or by ingesting contaminated food or water.

Laboratory Diagnosis. Taeniasis can be diagnosed by finding either proglottids in stool or ova in stained wet or permanent mounts prepared from stool. The spherical eggs of the taenias are morphologically indistinguishable. They measure 30 to 40 μm, radial striations in the shell are distinct, and hooklets may be faintly visible in the embryo (Figure 21-21).

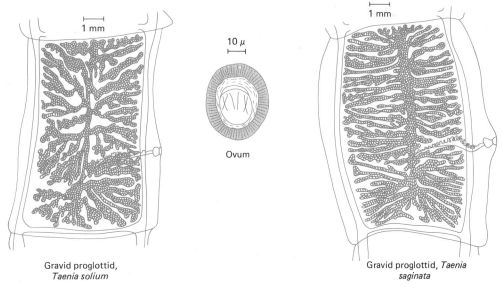

Gravid proglottid,
Taenia solium

Ovum

Gravid proglottid, *Taenia
saginata*

Figure 21-21   *Taenia* ovum and proglottids.

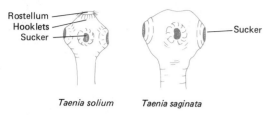

Figure 21-22 Scolices of *Taenia solium* and *Taenia saginata*.

A differential diagnosis is made by observing proglottids expelled in feces or scolices after treatment. Gravid proglottids of *T. solium* are smaller and have only 7 to 12 lateral uterine branches. The mature worms of *T. saginata* have 1000 to 2000 proglottids and reach 4 to 10 meters in size. Gravid proglottids of *T. saginata* have 15 to 20 lateral uterine branches. Adult parasites of *T. solium* contain 800 to 1000 proglottids and attain lengths of 2 to 4 meters. The scolices of the two tapeworms are quite different. The scolex of *T. saginata* has 4 suckers, and no well-developed rostellum or hooks. The scolex of *T. solium* has 4 suckers, and a rostellum armed with 25 to 30 hooks (Figure 21-22).

Immunity. Susceptibility to taeniasis and cysticercosis is general. Adult *Taenia* worms probably stimulate little antibody response because of their sequestered existence in the intestines. Cysticerci of *T. solium* may induce slightly more, but still limited, immunological responses, since their distribution is more widespread in the human host.

Prevention. The prevention of human cysticercosis is dependent on immedi-

ate treatment of individuals with intestinal taeniasis caused by *T. solium*. Taeniasis of cattle or swine origin can be controlled by thorough cooking of beef and pork, elimination of the use of sewage effluent for fertilization or irrigation, and strict adherence to personal hygiene. Governmental inspection of packing houses can be effective in eliminating sale of infected meat. Refrigeration of pork or beef at −10°C for at least five days kills cysticerci.

DIPHYLLOBOTHRIASIS AND SPARGANOSIS

Diphyllobothriasis, sometimes called broad fish tapeworm infection, is especially prevalent in countries bordered by the Baltic Sea. Norwegians, Swedes, Finns, and Russians, who consume freshwater fish with regularity, have high rates of infection. The fish of the Great Lakes in the United States are sporadically infected with the causative agent, *Diphyllobothrium latum*. Sparganosis is an infection caused by larvae (spargana) of worms related to *D. latum*. The symptoms of diphyllobothriasis range from vague abdominal distress to nausea, vomiting, and anemia. The worm competes effectively with the host for vitamin B_{12} when it is attached in the upper portion of the small intestine. One type of anemia in humans is caused by a Vitamin B_{12} deficiency. *Spirometra mansonoides* is the cause of most sparganosis in the United States.

Life Cycle. Immature ova of *D. latum*, or related parasites, are discharged at a rate of several million per day by the adult female worm. Development of the

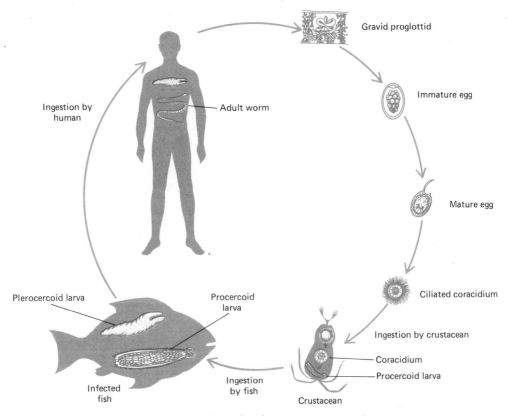

Figure 21-23 Life cycle of *Diphyllobothrium latam.*

embryos is dependent on a suitable freshwater environment (Figure 21-23). Ciliated coracidia emerge from ova in 10 days to several weeks, but survive only for a day or two unless they are ingested by a freshwater crustacean. Both *Diaptomus* and *Cyclops* species make suitable primary intermediate hosts. The developing parasites are eaten by a freshwater fish as procercoid larvae and undergo continuing metamorphosis into plerocercoid larvae. Ingestion of plerocercoid forms in inadequately cooked fish provides a mode of entry for the parasite in man. The intestine provides a suitable environment for larvae to reach maturity in three to five weeks.

Transmission. The plerocercoid larvae are ingested in raw or improperly cooked fish. Procercoid larvae are usually transmitted by water contaminated with infected *Cyclops* or by eating frogs or snakes harboring the parasites. There is no person-to-person transmission of diphyllobothriasis or sparganosis.

Laboratory Diagnosis. A diagnosis of diphyllobothriasis is made by finding proglottids of *D. latum* in stool or by finding the ova in stained wet or permanent mounts prepared from stool. The gravid proglottids are 2 to 4 mm long and 10 to 12 mm wide; they contain long, coiled uterine canals. The ova are approximately 70 μm long and 45 μm wide and frequently have recognizable opercula (Figure 21-24). The scolex, which appears in stool only after successful dislodgement by treatment, is almond-shaped with dorsal and ventral suckers.

Sparganosis can be diagnosed only by demonstrating larvae in tissue.

Immunity. Individuals are universally susceptible to infective larvae of *D. latum* or related species. There is no evidence that one infection provides immunity in the event of a subsequent exposure to the parasites.

Prevention. Diphyllobothriasis and sparganosis can best be controlled by prohibiting the disposal of untreated sewage into bodies of fresh water. However, since the source of freshwater fish may be lakes or ponds in which control measures are not operative, other steps need to be taken to kill infective larvae. Freezing freshwater fish for a day or more at −10°C or cooking for at least 10 minutes at 50°C (120°F) destroys infective larvae of *D. latum*. In endemic areas boiling of water may be necessary to destroy intermediate hosts of the parasites.

DWARF TAPEWORM INFECTION

The so-called dwarf tapeworm infection is a relatively mild disease caused by *Hymenolepis nana*. It is estimated that over 20 million individuals in the world, mostly children, are infected with the parasite. Hundreds of adult worms may parasitize a single host. Light infections in children may be asymptomatic. Heavy infections may produce an inflammatory response with accompanying abdominal pain, nausea, vomiting, and sometimes diarrhea.

Life Cycle. Definitive hosts for *H. nana* are humans, mice, and rats. Although no intermediate host is required for completion of its life cycle, one marine variety is associated with

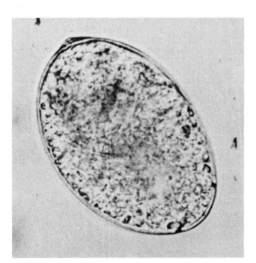

Figure 21-24 Ovum of *Diphyllobothrium latum*. (From J. W. Smith, ed., et al., *Diagnostic Medical Parasitology: Intestinal Helminths,* Chicago, American Society of Clinical Pathologists, © 1976. Used by permission.)

fleas and beetles as intermediate hosts. Ingested ova hatch within 4 days in the intestine, penetrate villi, and develop into adult worms in 10 to 12 days. Ova may be eliminated in the stool or hatch in the intestine.

Transmission. The human is the primary source for dwarf tapeworm infection although mice and rats harbor the parasite. *H. nana* can be transmitted by the fecal-oral route and less frequently by contaminated water or food since the ova are quite fragile. Autoinfection can occur by the fecal-oral route or by endogenous hatching of eggs in the intestine.

Laboratory Diagnosis. A diagnosis of dwarf tapeworm infection is dependent on finding the infective ova in stained wet or permanent mounts prepared from stool. The eggs are nearly spherical, range from 30 to 47 μm in diameter, and contain 4 to 8 polar filaments (Figure 21-25). Proglottids are broad and the uterus is saclike. The scolex, if obtainable, is almost round and has 4 suckers and a rostellum containing a single row of 24 to 30 hooks.

Immunity. Unlike most parasitic diseases, recovery from an infection of *H. nana* confers some resistance on the host. It is not known if that immunity is transient, or endures over a period of years.

Prevention. Prevention of dwarf tapeworm infection is dependent on understanding the need for personal hygiene. All infected persons should be treated. Proper disposal of sewage and effective control of rodent and flea populations are also of paramount importance.

ECHINOCOCCOSIS OR HYDATID DISEASE

Echinococcosis has been known since the earliest days of medicine. It is prevalent in Europe and the southernmost countries of South America. The disease is also an important debilitating disease in parts of Africa. Echinococcosis is caused by a hydatid cyst, a larval form of the dog tapeworm *Echinococcus granulosis*. Localization of the larval stage occurs when embryos are trapped in hepatic veins, pulmo-

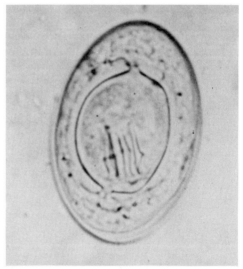

Figure 21-25 Ovum of *Hymenolepis nana* showing polar filaments. (From J. W. Smith, ed., et al., *Diagnostic Medical Parasitology: Intestinal Helminths*, Chicago, American Society of Clinical Pathologists, © 1976. Used by permission.)

nary capillaries, or arterial vessels of other organs. More than half of the reported cases of hydatid disease involve the liver. The cysts grow slowly, but ultimately give rise to considerable discomfort. Symptoms in humans depend on the location of cysts, but are usually the result of pressure. Pressure on bile ducts or ureters may cause obstructions. In the brain cysts may promote epileptic seizures. Pulmonary cysts are often associated with difficulty in breathing. Abdominal cysts may cause only minor discomfort. The disease is asymptomatic in the canine host.

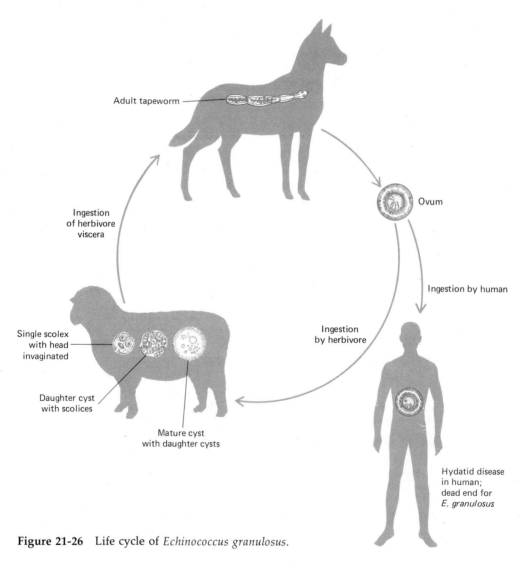

Figure 21-26   Life cycle of *Echinococcus granulosus.*

Life Cycle. Infective eggs are swallowed by accident, most frequently by animals other than humans. Shells of ova are digested in the duodenum, and liberated embryos are transported to the liver or other body organs in the bloodstream. The bladderlike cysts develop about a month after implantation. If mature cysts rupture, metastasis occurs, and protoscolices, sometimes called *hydatid sand,* are carried by the bloodstream to other anatomic sites. The life cycle of the tapeworm ends if humans are the hosts; the life cycle is maintained if fertile cysts containing protoscolices are eaten by dogs (Figure 21-26). Adult worms develop in the canine intestine to start the cycle again.

Transmission. Echinococcosis is transmitted to humans directly from infected dogs by contact with fur or feces and from contaminated soil, water, or food. The ova can remain viable for months in moist soils. Water and vegetables are then easily contaminated. Toys shared by children and dogs are frequently the source of infective eggs of the parasite.

Laboratory Diagnosis. A diagnosis of echinococcosis is sometimes difficult to establish. Symptoms may not differ from tumors, but the patient's history always reveals a close association with dogs. X rays are sometimes of value, but definitive diagnosis depends on finding protoscolices, capsules, or cysts in tissue after surgical intervention. Indirect hemagglutination, bentonite flocculation, and skin tests are not always dependable. Rupture of cysts some-

times releases hydatid fragments in sputum or urine, but considerable skill may be required to identify specific hydatid forms.

Immunity. There is general susceptibility to infection with the larval form of *E. granulosus.* Although humoral antibodies are demonstrable in some cases, the amount of protection afforded by them is probably negligible.

Prevention. If dogs had no access to raw viscera of domestic or wild animals, the life cycle of *E. granulosis* could be effectively interrupted. Discouragement of home slaughter, incineration of carcasses, thorough cooking of meat and vegetables, boiling of water, and prophylactic treatment of dogs are recommended for areas in which echinococcosis is endemic. Children and adults should be warned that the affectionate, but unhygienic, habit of kissing dogs can be hazardous.

DIPYLIDIASIS

Dipylidiasis, or dog tapeworm infection, is primarily a disease of dogs, cats, and wild animals, but humans can be infected accidentally with the etioligical agent *Dipylidium caninum.* The adult worm favors the small intestine of the host as a habitat, but usually does not cause much distress.

Life Cycle. Food, fleas, or lice containing the infective cysticercoid larvae of *D. caninum* are swallowed by the animal host. Liberated larvae penetrate the intestinal mucosa and reach maturity in about 20 days. Embryonated eggs are deposited in the anal area and become enmeshed in animal fur. The ova are, in turn, ingested by immature fleas or lice where the infective cysticercoid larvae develop.

Transmission. Dog tapeworm infection is transmitted indirectly by immature fleas or lice which infest the fur of dogs or other animals or directly by the fecal-oral route. Food or toys are frequent vehicles of transportation for embryonated ova. Swallowing infected fleas enables the cysticercoid larvae to gain access to the small intestine of the host. The disease occurs most often in infants, under 6 months of age, who have close contact with household pets.

Laboratory Diagnosis. Dipylidiasis is diagnosed by finding proglottids in stool or ova in stained wet or permanent mounts prepared from stool. The gravid proglottids demonstrate motility and contain an abundance of capsules with 15 to 25 eggs each. The ova, which measure 36 to 60 μm in diameter, typically occur in clusters.

Prevention. Control of flea and lice populations that infest cats and dogs could do much to eliminate dog tapeworm infections. Dogs and cats not only cannot resist scratching arthropod-infested skin or fur, but frequently zero in on the ectoparasites with well-aimed bites. Household pets should be treated periodically for helminths, fleas, and lice to interrupt the life cycle of *D. caninum.*

FLUKE INFECTIONS

The life cycle of all flukes, including those which infect the intestinal tract or liver, is complex. Completion of the cycle often requires one or more intermediate hosts, and the primary intermediate host is always a snail. Some ova need considerable time in fresh water to develop into larvae which are infective for a secondary intermediate host or for humans, who serve as definitive hosts.

Relatively few species of snails are adapted to serve as suitable intermediate hosts for trematodes. Humans become infected by consuming aquatic plants, water, or inadequately cooked freshwater fish which contain encysted larval stages known as *metacercariae.* Encysted metacercariae attach themselves to the intestinal mucosa of the duodenum or ileum, or establish residence in bile ducts. The intestinal flukes are hermaphroditic, but self-fertilization occurs more frequently than cross-fertilization. Adult parasites occasionally migrate to other organs producing *ectopic* (displaced) disease. Prognosis is good except in heavy infections involving liver damage.

FASCIOLOPSIASIS

Fasciolopsiasis is an infection caused by one of the largest flukes, *Fasciolopsis buski.* It is particularly prevalent in southeast Asia and has occurred in some American military personnel stationed in that part of the world. The adult fluke usually resides in the duodenum or jejunum, but may inhabit the stomach or colon. It has a short, but productive life, liberating around 25,000 eggs a day. Abdominal pain, nausea, and diarrhea are common complaints in fasciolopsiasis. Abscesses sometimes occur at points of attachment. Symptoms appear to be most severe in early morning hours before ingestion of food.

Life Cycle. *F. buski*, inhabiting the intestine of humans, pigs, and sometimes dogs, liberate undeveloped ova. If the ova are deposited in stagnant fresh water and a temperature of 27° to 32°C is maintained, the eggs hatch into free-living miracidia in three to seven weeks (Figure 21-27). To continue the life cycle, the free-living miracidia must find a suitable snail within a couple of days. Planorbid snails of the genera *Segmentina*, *Hippeutis*, and *Gyraulus* are common primary intermediate hosts.

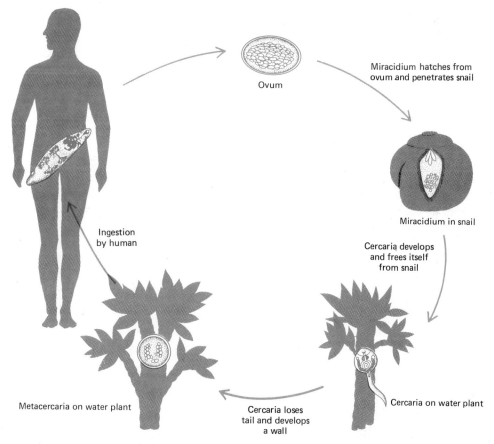

Ovum

Miracidium hatches from ovum and penetrates snail

Miracidium in snail

Cercaria develops and frees itself from snail

Ingestion by human

Metacercaria on water plant

Cercaria loses tail and develops a wall

Cercaria on water plant

Figure 21-27   Life cycle of *Fasciolopsis buski*.

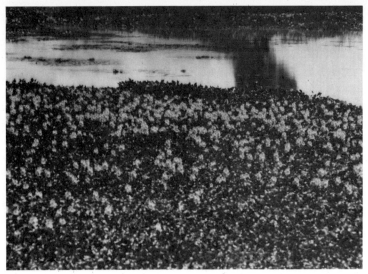

Figure 21-28 Water hyacinths. Such aquatic plants provide ample surface for encystment of cercariae and maturation of metacercariae of *Fasciolopsis buski*. (Courtesy, A. Villa, Van Nuys, California.)

During the intramolluscan phase sporocysts, first and second generation rediae, and ultimately cercariae are produced; the process usually takes four to seven weeks. The emerging cercariae find refuge on water plants, such as the water caltrop, hyacinth, chestnut, or bamboo, where they encyst and mature into metacercariae in another three to four weeks (Figure 21-28). The most common vehicle whereby the encysted metacercariae gain entrance to the human host is the water caltrop. The metacercariae excyst in the intestine and reach maturity in approximately three months.

Transmission. Metacercariae of *F. buski* are ingested with raw pods of water caltrop and bulbs of the water chestnut, which are frequently peeled with the teeth. Dipping leafy plants in water to retain freshness probably contributes to the viability of metacercariae

and the spread of fasciolopsiasis in some parts of the world.

Laboratory Diagnosis. A diagnosis of fasciolopsiasis is made by finding ova in stained wet or permanent mounts prepared from stool. The unembryonated ova are shaped like hens' eggs, have opercula, and measure 130 to 140 μm by 80 to 85 μm. The adult flukes, which are fleshy by comparison with other flukes, are 2 to 7 cm long, 0.5 to 3.0 mm thick, and about 2.0 cm wide. Mature flukes are occasionally found in feces or vomitus.

Immunity. Susceptibility to fasciolopsiasis is general. There is no evidence that an infection produces any protective immune response.

Prevention. Metacercariae of *F. buski* are susceptible to both drying and heat. Allowing suspected plants to dry or

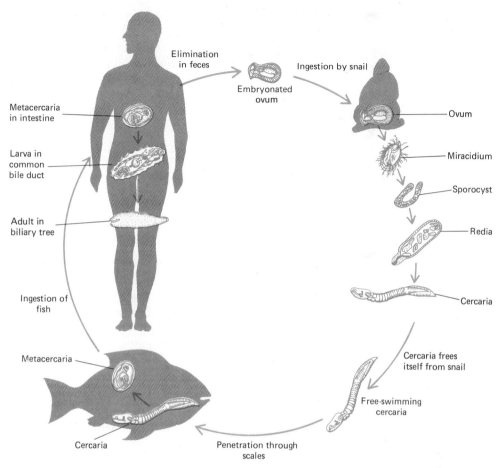

Figure 21-29 Life cycle of *Clonorchis sinensis.*

dipping them into boiling water for several seconds will kill metacercariae. Treatment of infested soil with unslaked lime destroys ova. Education of persons living in endemic areas on the disease-producing capacity of the fluke could reduce the incidence of parasitism.

CLONORCHIASIS

Clonorchiasis is an important parasitic liver infection in certain populous areas of the Far East, such as China, Korea, Hong Kong, and Taiwan. It is caused by the Oriental liver fluke, *Clonorchis sinensis.* Adult flukes typically reside in bile ducts causing, at the least, mechanical irritation. In severe infections the liver may become enlarged and functionally impaired. The lowered resistance resulting from sometimes thousands of worms makes individuals susceptible to other infections.

Life Cycle. Mature ova of *C. sinensis* are excreted in feces of an infected host (Figure 21-29). The miracidia are hatched only when an appropriate snail ingests the eggs from water polluted with ova-laden feces. Species of *Bulimus* and *Parafossarulus* are particularly suitable primary intermediate hosts. The miracidia undergo metamorphosis in the snail's digestive tract, producing sporocysts, rediae, and finally cercariae, which are released into water. The free-swimming forms die within 48 hours unless they can make contact with fish. A wide variety of fish can serve as secondary intermediate hosts. The cercariae penetrate scales and encyst as metacercariae in muscle or subcutaneous tissue. The life cycle is completed when a person ingests encysted parasites. The metacercariae excyst in the intestine, and the liberated larvae migrate to the common bile duct. From the common bile duct the larvae move progressively higher into the biliary tree. The larvae mature into egg-laying adult flukes in three or four weeks. The embryonated ova pass with bile into the intestine and are evacuated with feces.

Transmission. The encysted metacercariae of *C. sinensis* are consumed in raw, pickled, salted, or insufficiently cooked freshwater fish. The infective metacercariae may be present in drinking water. Heavy infections are almost always the result of regular ingestion of uncooked fish or water contaminated with the liver fluke.

Laboratory Diagnosis. Clonorchiasis is diagnosed by finding ova in stained wet or permanent mounts prepared from stool or biliary drainage. The eggs are bulb-shaped, are distinctly opercu-

late, and average 29 by 16 μm in size. They are often difficult to distinguish from ova of *Heterophyes* or *Metagonimus*. Antibodies cross-react with other trematodes, so serological tests have had limited diagnostic use.

Immunity. Susceptibility to clonorchiasis is universal, but the disease does provoke an immune response. Precipitating and hemagglutinating antibodies have been described. However, the protective abilities of the antibodies are unknown.

Prevention. There is no substitute for thorough cooking of freshwater fish in preventing clonorchiasis, but dietary habits are difficult to change. Control of contamination of fish ponds by eliminating pond-side privies is also sometimes difficult to enforce (Figure 21-30). The life cycle can be most easily interrupted at the stage of the primary intermediate host. The snail population, being susceptible to the action of chemicals, can be best controlled on land upon which fresh water drains. The addition of chemicals to ponds is not feasible since fish and aquatic plants may also be destroyed. Simply cutting back of aquatic plants during snail-breeding periods reduces the opportunity for fish to consume *C. sinensis*-laden snails.

FASCIOLIASIS

Fascioliasis is chiefly a disease of herbivorous animals caused by the trematode *Fasciola hepatica*, but it can cause a parasitosis in humans. The disease is

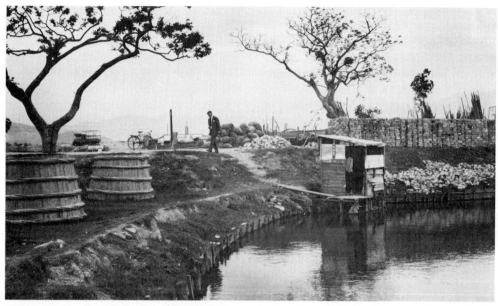

Figure 21-30 Location of privies on fish ponds, like the one pictured, contributes to the spread of clonorchiasis when raw fish is eaten. (From T. Sun and J. B. Gibson, *International Path.* 6:95, 1965.)

widespread. The incidence of fascioliasis in humans is directly related to the incidence of infection in animals. In France 100 percent of the sheep and 20 percent of the cattle harbor the parasite. *F. hepatica* resides in the bile ducts of its hosts causing enlargement of the liver, fever, and abdominal pain.

Life Cycle. Immature ova of *F. hepatica* are discharged from the host in the feces, but require an aquatic environment for maturation. Temperatures of 22° to 25°C cause the miracidia to hatch in 10 to 15 days. In order to survive the free-swimming forms must penetrate the soft tissue of a snail within a few hours. At least 21 species of the genus *Lymnaea* can serve as primary interme-

diate hosts. In the snail metamorphosis proceeds to the sporocyst stage, through first and second generation rediae, to the cercariae in about four weeks. The mature cercariae become attached to aquatic plants, shed their tails, and eventually encyst as metacercariae. Infective metacercariae are ingested by animals or humans, lodge in the stomach or duodenum, escape into the peritoneal cavity, and enter the liver capsule, where they mature in about 12 weeks. The ova, deposited by the adult trematodes in bile ducts, are transported with bile into the intestine. They gain access to the external environment in the feces and are ready to begin the life cycle again if circumstances permit.

Transmission. *F. hepatica* is usually transmitted by the ingestion of fresh watercress or other aquatic plants, but it can also spread by drinking water containing the infective metacercariae.

Laboratory Diagnosis. Diagnosis of fascioliasis may be difficult since symptoms do not differ from those of other types of liver disease. A definitive diagnosis requires finding operculate ova of the fluke in stained wet or permanent mounts prepared from stool or biliary drainage. The eggs are 130 to 150 μm long and 63 to 90 μm wide. However, since the eggs, which are noninfective, can be ingested with raw liver, a history of dietary habits is important in establishing the significance of ova in feces. Intracutaneous and complement-fixation (CF) tests, using *Fasciola* antigens, are of some value in ectopic infections.

Immunity. The antibodies produced in response to an infection with *F. hepatica* appear to be of little or no value in protecting the vertebrate host against repeated infections with the fluke.

Prevention. It is difficult to eradicate any parasite with widespread distribution in herbivorous animals and, likewise, difficult to eliminate snail populations. Infection in humans can be prevented by sufficient warning of the hazards of eating watercress or drinking unboiled water in areas where fascioliasis is endemic.

PARAGONIMIASIS

Paragonimiasis is primarily an infection of the lung found in the Far East, including Japan, South Korea, China, and the Philippines. It is caused by the fluke, *Paragonimus westermani*, which has a considerable migratory capacity. If the flukes are confined to the lung, the disease is characterized by a fever, cough, and blood-tinged sputum. The abdominal wall, abdominal cavity, mesenteric lymph nodes, and intestinal wall are frequent extrapulmonary sites. Abdominal infection causes pain, rigidity, and diarrhea.

Life Cycle. Two intermediate hosts, a snail and either a freshwater crab or crayfish, are required to complete the life cycle of *P. westermani* (Figure 21-31). Undeveloped eggs escape the definitive host, which can be humans or a variety of both wild and domestic animals, in sputum or stool. Miracidia in sputum or stool develop in approximately three weeks at temperatures of 27°C. The free-swimming miracidia must find a suitable snail to penetrate in order to continue the life cycle. Snails belonging to the genera *Hua, Semisulcospira, Syncera,* and others can be primary intermediate hosts. Cercariae emerge from infected snails in about 13 weeks. If cercariae find an appropriate crustacean host, they encyst in gills, legs, muscles, or viscera and develop into metacercariae. Crustaceans can also become infected by ingesting snails. Without refuge supplied by crustacean hosts cercariae die within 48 hours. A variety of crabs and crayfish can be involved. When the definitive host ingests crustaceans containing metacercariae, the excysted metacercariae pass through the intestinal wall into the abdominal cavity to begin their migration upward.

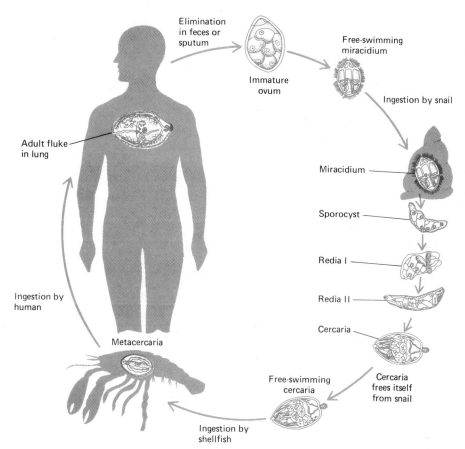

Figure 21-31 Life cycle of *Paragonimus westermani*.

The young flukes burrow through the diaphragm reaching the lungs in about 20 days. Some excysted metacercariae may take alternate routes to other organs. The worms reach maturity in five or six weeks. The cycle is repeated if eggs are released in sputum or stool and find suitable intermediate hosts.

Transmission. Paragonimiasis is transmitted by the ingestion of metacercariae in raw or improperly cooked freshwater crabs or crayfish. It may also be transmitted in shellfish freshly pickled in vinegar or wine, because the metacercariae can survive for at least several hours in the pickling solution. Inadequately treated drinking water can also be a source of infection in endemic areas.

Laboratory Diagnosis. A diagnosis of paragonimiasis is made by finding ova in stained wet or permanent mounts prepared from stool, sputum, or pleural effusions. The ova are oval, yellow-

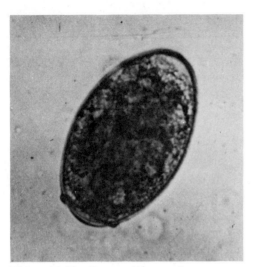

Figure 21-32 Ovum of *Paragonimus westermani*. (From J. W. Smith et al., *Diagnostic Medical Parasitology III: Intestinal Helminths,* Chicago, American Society of Clinical Pathologists, © 1976. Used by permission.)

brown, and thick-shelled and measure at least 80 by 55 μm. The operculum and well-defined shoulders are apparent (Figure 21-32). Repeated samplings of sputum or stool are often necessary to establish a diagnosis. X rays of lungs are of limited value since cavities produced by invasion of the flukes are indistinguishable from those of tuberculosis.

Immunity. Susceptibility to paragonimiasis is general. Complement-fixing antibodies can be demonstrated in some infections, but the amount of immunity afforded by their presence may be negligible.

Prevention. Paragonimiasis can be prevented by not eating raw, freshly pickled, or improperly cooked freshwater crustaceans and by drinking only filtered or boiled water in endemic areas. It is not practical or possible to attempt the elimination of either the snail or the crustacean intermediate hosts.

SUMMARY

Most of the enteric protozoal and helminthic infections are cosmopolitan in distribution. The numbers of individuals infected in any one part of the world depend on diet, method of sewage disposal, availability of intermediate hosts, soil conditions, water temperature, and personal habits of hygiene. The diagnosis of most protozoal and helminthic infections requires identification of the parasites in stool. For the most part little or no immunity follows a parasitic infection. Control of protozoal and helminthic diseases requires a knowledge of life cycles, reservoirs, vectors, and both definitive and intermediate hosts of individual parasites. Prevention of parasitic disease may also require changes in dietary and personal hygiene habits. Thorough cooking of all foods, boiling of water, and adequate hand washing are important deterrents to the spread of parasitic disease in endemic areas.

QUESTIONS FOR STUDY

1. Name the disease caused by each parasite.
   Trichinella spiralis
   Balantidium coli
   Enterobius vermicularis
   Diphyllobothrium latum
   Hymenolepis nana
   Taenia saginata

Trichuris trichiura
Ascaris lumbricoides
Necator americanus
Strongyloides stercoralis

2. Name the infective stage for each parasite.
   Entamoeba histolytica
   Giardia lamblia
   Balantidium coli
   Trichinella spiralis
   Taenia solium
   Paragonimus westermani
   Fasciola hepatica
   Clonorchis sinensis
   Dipyltidium caninum
   Echinococcus granulosis

3. What is the role of arthropods in transmission of helminthic infections?

4. How can washing of fresh vegetables and hands prevent protozoal and helminthic infections?

5. Identify the target organ or organs for each parasite.
   Fasciola hepatica
   Clonorchis sinensis
   Echinococcus granulosis
   Paragonimus westermani
   Enterobius vermicularis
   Necator americanus
   Trichinella spiralis
   Trichuris trichiura
   Giardia lamblia
   Entamoeba histolytica
   Ascaris lumbricoides
   Fasciolopsis buski

SELECTED REFERENCES

Beck, J. W., and Davies, J. E. *Medical Parasitology.* 2d ed. St. Louis: Mosby, 1976.

Brown, H. W. *Basic Clinical Parasitology.* 4th ed. Englewood Cliffs, N.J.: Prentice-Hall, 1975.

California State Department of Public Health. *A Manual for the Control of Communicable Diseases in California.* Berkeley: 1971.

Davidsohn, I., and Henry, J. B. *Todd-Sanford Clinical Diagnosis by Laboratory Methods.* 14th ed. Philadelphia: Saunders, 1969.

Koneman, E. W.; Richie, L. E.; and Tiemann, C. *Practical Laboratory Parasitology.* New York: Medcom Press, 1974.

Lennette, E. H.; Spaulding, E. H.; and Truant, J. P. *Manual of Clinical Microbiology.* 2d ed. Washington, D.C.: American Society for Microbiology, 1974.

Marcial-Rojas, R. A. *Pathology of Protozoal and Helminthic Diseases with Clinical Correlation.* Baltimore: Williams & Wilkins, 1971.

Markell, E. K., and Voge, M. *Medical Parasitology.* 4th ed. Philadelphia: Saunders, 1976.

U.S. Naval Medical School, National Naval Medical Center. *Medical Protozoology and Helminthology.* Washington, D.C.: U.S. Government Printing Office, 1965.

Chapter 22

Microbial Diseases of the Genitourinary Tract

After you read this chapter, you should be able to:

1. Explain why urinary tract infections are more common in women than in men.
2. List the major sites for inflammatory lesions of the male and female genital tracts.
3. Name the most common isolates of urinary tract infections.
4. Name several common anaerobic organisms associated with pelvic inflammatory disease (PID).
5. Discuss measures which can be employed to prevent postpartum and postabortal sepsis.
6. Explain the significance of penicillinase-producing *Neisseria gonorrhoeae* (PPNG) as a cause of sexually transmissible disease (STD).
7. Compare clinical manifestations of infections caused by *Neisseria gonorrhoeae* and *Treponema pallidum*.
8. List three common nontreponemal screening tests used in the diagnosis of syphilis.
9. Explain why treponemal confirmatory tests may be necessary in the diagnosis of syphilis.
10. Compare the etiological agents and symptoms of chancroid, lymphogranuloma venereum, and granuloma inguinale.
11. Name one fungus and one protozoan which are common causes of vaginal or urethral infections.

Although the genital (reproductive) and urinary systems perform different functions, the anatomic proximity of the organs and their environment provide ample opportunities for microorganisms to invade one or both systems and to be transmitted easily from one to another. For this reason we can conveniently combine the study of infections of both systems as diseases of the genitourinary tract.

The urinary system in both sexes consists of the kidneys, ureters, urinary bladder, and urethra (Figure 22-1). The Skene's glands consist of two tubular glands near the orifice of the female urethra. The genital organs of the male include the scrotum, testes, seminal vesicles, prostate gland, and the paired Cowper's glands which are located anteriorly to the prostate gland (Figure 22-2); those of the female include the ovaries, fallopian tubes, uterus, vagina, vulva, clitoris, and Bartholin's glands which are the counterparts of the male Cowper's glands (Figure 22-3).

The area bounded by the buttocks and thighs in both sexes is called the *perineum*. It can be divided into a *urogenital triangle*, which contains the external genitals, urethral orifice, and surrounding tissue, and an *anal triangle*, which contains the anus and surrounding tissue (Figure 22-4).

In men the perineum is contaminated with indigenous organisms of the intestinal tract and lower portion of the urethra. Microorganisms of the intestines, lower urethra, and vagina colonize the perineum of women. The warm, moist, and protected environment supplied by the perineum provides especially favorable conditions for colonization by bacteria.

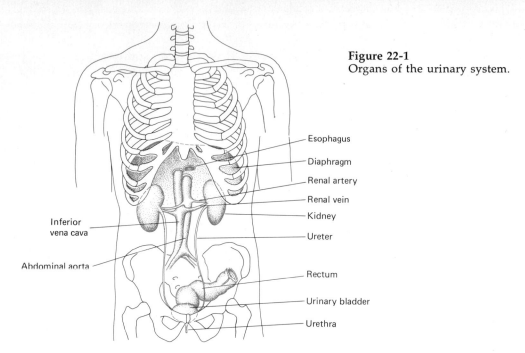

Figure 22-1
Organs of the urinary system.

Esophagus

Diaphragm

Renal artery

Renal vein

Kidney

Inferior
vena cava

Ureter

Abdominal aorta

Rectum

Urinary bladder

Urethra

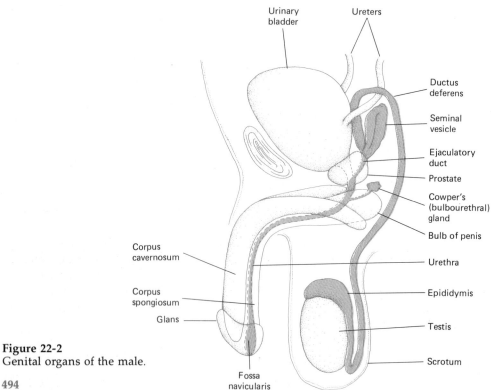

Urinary
bladder

Ureters

Ductus
deferens

Seminal
vesicle

Ejaculatory
duct

Prostate

Cowper's
(bulbourethral)
gland

Bulb of penis

Corpus
cavernosum

Urethra

Epididymis

Corpus
spongiosum

Glans

Testis

Scrotum

Figure 22-2
Genital organs of the male.

Fossa
navicularis

BACTERIAL INFECTIONS

Urinary tract infection can affect men and women at any age. The number of urinary tract infections in women is about 30 times greater than the number reported in men. Incidence of bacteriuria is as high as 10 percent in the elderly. The relatively short female urethra which averages 4 cm and warm moist area under the labia minora, where it ends, provides favorable conditions for colonization of microorganisms. Sexual intercourse may injure the short urethra and provide a means for bacteria of the perineum to gain entrance. Following invasion of the bladder mucosa, microorganisms can multiply in bladder urine. Bacteria or their endotoxins can interfere with peristaltic action and permit reflux of urine into ureters. In this manner organisms or their products can migrate against the pressure gradient to the kidneys.

Venereal diseases, or, as they are now often called, sexually transmissible diseases (STD's), constitute the most

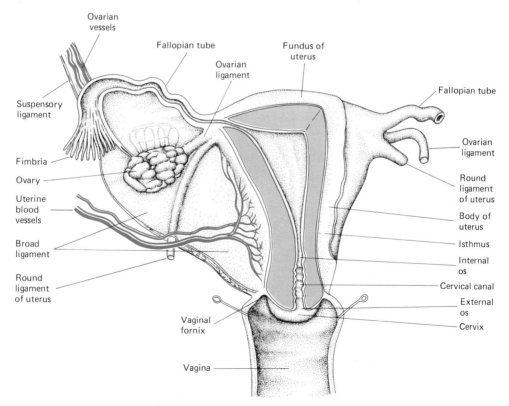

Figure 22-3 Genital organs of the female.

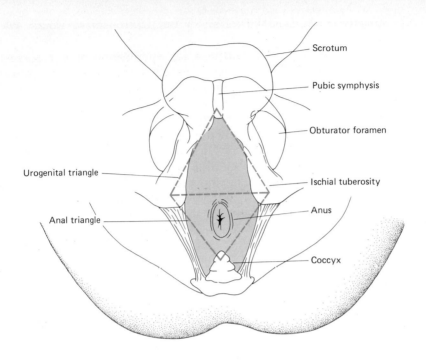

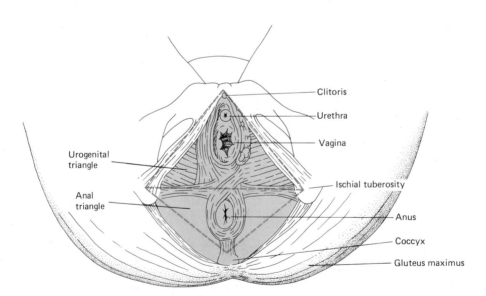

Figure 22-4 External genitalia of male and female (vulva) showing urogenital and anal triangles of the perineum in both sexes.

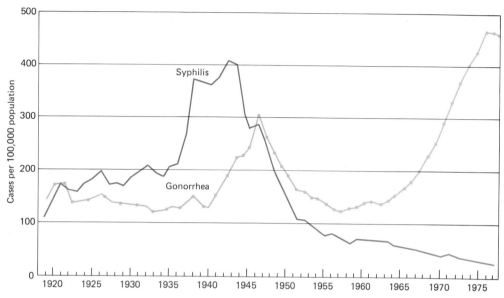

Figure 22-5 Reported cases of gonorrhea and syphilis (all stages) in the United States. Figures for 1914–1940 are based on the fiscal year, for 1941–1977 on the calendar year; military cases are included for 1919–1940 and excluded from 1941 on; all states are included from 1939 on. (From *Reported Morbidity and Mortality in the United States, Annual Summary, 1977,* Atlanta, Ga.: Center for Disease Control, 1977.)

serious infectious diseases of the genital tract. If untreated, the invading microorganisms can cause severe disease and even death. During the years 1960 to 1975 the number of cases of gonorrhea increased precipitously in the United States (Figure 22-5). Fewer cases of syphilis were reported in the same time period, but until recently an increase in the number of total early syphilis cases was evident. More liberal attitudes about sex in the past decade have allowed greater promiscuity in choice of sexual partners and encouraged sexual activity at earlier ages. Unfortunately, venereal disease educational programs and governmental surveillance measures have not kept pace with changes in sexual behavior.

NONSPECIFIC URETHRITIS (NSU)

Nonspecific urethritis (NSU) refers to an infection of the urethra caused by a microbial agent other than the gonorrheal organism. Bacterial agents include staphylococci, streptococci, mycoplasmas, chlamydiae, gram-negative cocci, and gram-negative bacilli. The mycoplasmas causing urethritis are *Mycoplasma hominis* and *Ureaplasma urealyticum* (human T mycoplasmas) (Figure 22-6). Symptoms of nonspecific urethritis include discomfort, pain, and burning on urination as well as frequency of urination. The urethra may be inflamed.

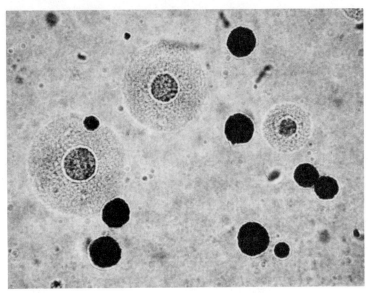

Figure 22-6 A mixture of colonies of *Mycoplasma hominis* and *Ureaplasma urealyticum* on a differential agar medium. The deep colored colonies of *U. urealyticum* can easily be differentiated from the colorless colonies of *M. hominis*. (Courtesy, M. C. Shepard, Camp Lejeune, North Carolina.)

Transmission. The major means of transmission for nonspecific urethritis is sexual intercourse.

Laboratory Diagnosis. Microscopic examination of Gram-stained smears of urethral discharge reveals the morphology and gram reaction of bacteria, other than mycoplasmas or chlamydiae, if they are present in sufficient numbers. Blood agar, eosin methylene blue (EMB) agar, and phenylethyl alcohol blood (PEA) agar can be used for primary plating or for subculturing organisms isolated in an enriched broth. Appropriate media and biochemical tests can be employed to identify gram-positive or gram-negative isolates. Mycoplas-mas can be grown on enriched media, but isolation of chlamydiae requires embryonated eggs, special cell lines, or laboratory animals. The time and expense involved preclude most laboratories from attempting to isolate mycoplasmas or chlamydiae from cases of nonspecific urethritis.

Immunity. It is unlikely that superficial infection of the urethra generates antibody activity. Recurrent nonspecific urethritis is relatively common.

Prevention. A complete regimen of appropriate antimicrobial treatment is important in preventing ascending urinary tract infection and persistence or recurrence of an existing infection. The vulnerability to subsequent infection cannot be obviated, however, in sexually active individuals.

CYSTITIS AND PYELONEPHRITIS

Cystitis (inflammation of the urinary bladder) and pyelonephritis (inflammation of the kidney and its pelvis) are usually caused by gram-negative bacilli of intestinal origin. *Escherichia coli* is the most frequently isolated organism, but *Proteus, Enterobacter, Citrobacter, Klebsiella,* and *Pseudomonas* species are also isolated with regularity. Staphylococci and streptococci are isolated less frequently. Anaerobic streptococci, *Bacteroides* species, and *Clostridium* species are rarely isolated, but when present, the anaerobes may act synergistically with other bacteria to produce necrosis. Cystitis causes suprapubic pain and tenderness. Frequency and burning on urination may be present. Renal infections may be associated with loin pain. Unfortunately, both cystitis and pyelonephritis may be asymptomatic.

Transmission. Cystitis and pyelonephritis are usually ascending infections caused by bacteria with access to the urethra. In women even slight trauma to the urethra, which can occur during intercourse, is believed to be sufficient to attract bacterial migrations. Bacteria in the blood rarely invade healthy kidneys or the bladder. When they do, the organs have generally sustained significant damage from previous exposure to bacteria or their endotoxins.

Laboratory Diagnosis. The bacteria causing cystitis or pyelonephritis can be isolated from catheterized, clean voided, midstream urine or urine obtained by cystoscopy or suprapubic aspiration. Urethral catheterization solely for culture purposes cannot be justified. Contamination of urine by the indigenous organisms of the distal urethra can be prevented by suprapubic aspiration. Cystoscopic specimens, obtained from the bladder and each ureter, are of value in determining locations of infections.

Clean voided, midstream urines are obtained after thorough cleansing of the labia and periurethral region in women or the penis in men. It is important in obtaining specimens that no part of the perineum touch the containers. As a rule, urines are submitted to the laboratory for both qualitative and quantitative analysis. Urine that cannot be cultured within an hour after delivery to the laboratory can be stored for 24 hours at refrigerated temperatures and will still give satisfactory results.

If a calibrated loop, designed to deliver 0.01 ml, is used for inoculating well-mixed, clean voided urine on plates of EMB and blood agars, a colony count of more than 100,000 or 10^5 is considered significant bacteriuria, that is, indicative of urinary tract infection. In drug-induced diuresis colony counts below 10^5 may still indicate an infective state. Most urinary tract infections are caused by a single bacterial species. Isolates can be identified using standard cultural and biochemical tests.

Immunity. The sequestering of bacteria in uncomplicated cystitis or pyelonephritis prevents formation of antibodies. Some patients with pyelonephritis develop high antibody titers against the infecting organism, while others show little or no antibody activity. The protection afforded by even limited antibody production is probably more than offset by vulnerability to subsequent infection afforded by trauma to the urinary tract.

Prevention. The anatomic proximity of urogenital orifices makes it difficult to prevent contamination of the distal urethra with coliforms or intestinal anaerobes. In women fecal flora colonize in the vaginal vestibule or periurethral area before ascending into the urinary tract. Prompt and complete treatment for cystitis and pyelitis is an important deterrent in preventing recurrent infections or pyelonephritis.

PROSTATITIS

Acute prostatitis can be caused by a variety of bacteria including *Neisseria gonorrhoeae, E. coli, Proteus vulgaris, Pseudomonas aeruginosa,* staphylococci, and streptococci. Mixed infections are common. Single or multiple abscesses lead to swelling of the gland, a urethral discharge, and interference with micturition. Chronic prostatitis may follow an acute infection. A postinflammatory fibrosis, occurring after long-standing prostatitis, causes hardening of the prostate gland.

Transmission. In most instances the prostate becomes infected following a urethral or bladder infection. In patients with no history of urethritis or cystitis microorganisms which gain entrance to the bloodstream in some unrelated manner account for spontaneous prostatitis. Any manipulative or surgical procedure can initiate the infection.

Laboratory Diagnosis. Gram stains of urethral smears may reveal the morphology and gram reaction of causative organisms, but culturing on selective media is necessary to isolate the organisms. Depending on the types of bacteria which grow, appropriate biochemical tests can be applied for species identification.

Immunity. It is doubtful that any immunity follows prostatitis. In fact, the trauma caused by invading bacteria may predispose an individual to subsequent infections.

Prevention. Prompt diagnosis and treatment of urethritis or cystitis can prevent some ascending tract infections. Administration of prophylactic antimicrobial agents when instrumentation or surgery is necessary is sometimes recommended.

ACUTE GLOMERULONEPHRITIS

The etiology of acute glomerulonephritis, following streptococcal pharyngitis as an autoimmune phenomenon, was discussed in Chapter 13. Acute glomerulonephritis can occur, however, during the course of or following other bacterial or viral infections. In addition, circulating host antigens or immune complexes may lodge in glomeruli. In all instances the offending agent is a humoral antibody. In most cases of suspected immune complex nephritis, the nature of the offending antigen remains an enigma.

PELVIC INFLAMMATORY DISEASE (PID)

Pelvic inflammatory disease (PID) occurs almost without exception in sexually active women of child-bearing age. In most instances the cervix, uterus, fallopian tubes, ovaries, or perineum are infected with anaerobic cocci or bacilli (Table 22-1). *Bacteroides fragilis* is the most commonly recovered anaerobe, but mixed infections are not infrequent. Symptoms of PID include fever, chills, malaise, and lower abdominal pain. A purulent discharge may be present. In severe infections scar tissue may block the lumen of the fallopian tubes. Repeated infections may lead to the chronic state as well as irreparable damage to reproductive organs.

Transmission. Pelvic inflammatory disease is frequently a complication of a primary ascending genitourinary tract infection, but may spread by means of lymphatic vessels. The attraction of anaerobes may be enhanced by trauma caused by injury or a primary infective agent. Peritonitis may ensue if pus spills into the peritoneal cavity.

Laboratory Diagnosis. Gram stains of smears made from purulent discharges may reveal a mixture of gram-negative and gram-positive bacteria. More fastidious anaerobes will grow in thioglycollate broth, supplemented with Vitamin K and hemin. Specific identification often requires time-consuming procedures.

Immunity. The frequency of reinfection in pelvic inflammatory disease suggests that few, if any, protective antibodies are formed.

Prevention. Prompt diagnosis of mild cervicitis or endometritis is an important deterrent to serious pelvic inflammatory disease. The complications of infectious pelvic disease, including infertility, can likewise be prevented by prompt diagnosis and by appropriate and persistent antimicrobial treatment.

Table 22-1 COMMON ANAEROBIC ISOLATES FROM PELVIC INFLAMMATORY DISEASE

Gram-negative cocci
  Veillonella
	Gram-positive cocci
	  Peptococcus
	  Peptostreptococcus

Gram-negative bacilli
  Bacteroides fragilis
  Bacteroides melaninogenicus
  Bacteriodes oralis
  Fusobacterium nucleatum
  Fusobacterium necrophorum
	Gram-positive bacilli
	  Clostridium perfringens
	  Clostridium tetani
	  Clostridium novyi
	  Bifidobacterium
	  Propionibacterium

3

CHORIOAMNIONITIS

Chorioamnionitis is an inflammation of the fetal membranes. It occurs as a sequela to premature rupture of the membranes or as a complication of amniocentesis. *E. coli,* coagulase-negative staphylococci, diphtheroids, and the yeast *Candida* are frequent isolates. Infection in the fetus is the most significant hazard of chorioamnionitis, but the infection, depending on its severity, may be fatal to both the infant and the mother. Expediting delivery after membranes are ruptured and the discontinuation of other than necessary amniocentesis can substantially reduce the incidence of chorioamnionitis.

POSTPARTUM (PUERPERAL) AND POSTABORTAL SEPSIS

Postpartum or postabortal sepsis begins with an infection of the uterus following delivery or abortion. Spread of the infection to the blood or other organs by means of the lymphatic system causes serious disease and even death. A century ago epidemics of puerperal sepsis (childbirth fever) were leading causes of maternal morbidity and mortality. Today postpartum sepsis is rare, and when it does occur, it is not usually a catastrophic illness. Postabortal sepsis was much more common in the United States before abortion was legalized.

The organisms causing either postpartum or postabortal sepsis are usually indigenous flora of the vagina or colon: they include anaerobic streptococci, clostridia, staphylococci, coliforms, and *Bacteroides* species. Contaminated hands and instruments are the primary means by which the microorganisms are spread. Fever, abdominal rigidity, and hypotension are common symptoms in postpartum or postabortal infection. Aseptic postpartum or postabortal care of the perineum is a significant deterrent to the spread of indigenous flora to traumatized tissue. The use of aseptic techniques and antimicrobial agents have made childbirth and abortion relatively safe events.

GONORRHEA

Gonorrhea is the most prevalent STD; it is worldwide in distribution. Its incidence has reached epidemic proportions in the United States, where approximately 1 million new cases are reported annually. The etiological agent, *Neisseria gonorrhoeae,* invades epithelial tissue of the urogenital tract in adults and the conjunctiva of both adults and neonates.

In men acute gonorrhea may involve the urethra, testes, prostate gland, or rectum. Invasion of the urogenital tissue causes pain on urination, inflammation of the urethra, and a purulent discharge. Accumulations of scar tissue from untreated or repeated infections can lead to urethral stricture and make urination difficult. Sterility is a complication if the vas deferens is affected.

In women gonococci may colonize the urethra, cervix, Skene's glands, Bartholin's glands, rectum, or throat; the vagina is affected only in prepubescent girls. In contrast to the disease in men, approximately 75 to 90 percent of infected women have no symptoms. In symptomatic cases women are likely to have a purulent discharge from the urethra, cervix, or rectum and possibly painful urination or defecation. An ascending infection may involve the uterus, fallopian tubes, ovary, and abdominal tissues. Formation of scar tissue in the fallopian tubes may result in ectopic pregnancy or sterility; acute peritonitis may be fatal.

Gonococcal arthritis can occur in men or women as a consequence of urogenital infection. The inflammatory process is particularly debilitating if large joints are affected.

Ophthalmia neonatorum is a conjunctivitis of the newborn caused by contact with *N. gonorrhoeae* during delivery. If untreated, corneal ulcers or blindness may occur.

Public health authorities are concerned about the emergence of strains of gonococci which produce beta-lactamase (penicillinase). The penicillinase-producing *N. gonorrhoeae* (PPNG) has been identified in at least 11 countries and is being reported from an increasing number of states in the United States. The Center for Disease Control (CDC) recommends that patients with persistent gonococcal infection be screened for PPNG.

Transmission. *N. gonorrhoeae* is almost universally transmitted by sexual intercourse in the adult or during delivery in the newborn. Involvement of the throat may follow oral intercourse; rectal involvement may follow anal intercourse or self-infection from contact with cervical or urethral discharges.

Transmission by toilet seats, bath towels, sheets, chairs, or drinking glasses is almost negligible. The organism is very susceptible to drying and survives only a short period of time in the external environment.

Laboratory Diagnosis. Gram stains of urethral or cervical exudates reveal the presence of polymorphonuclear neutrophils containing gram-negative diplococci, particularly in the male. In early or very late stages of gonorrhea the organisms can be observed extracellularly. The gonococcus is 0.6 to 1.0 μm in diameter and has flattened adjacent sides like "coffee beans" (Figure 22-7). The organism grows well in an atmosphere of 5 to 10 percent CO_2 on Thayer-Martin agar, an enriched medium containing vancomycin, colistin, and nystatin. The antibiotics inhibit the

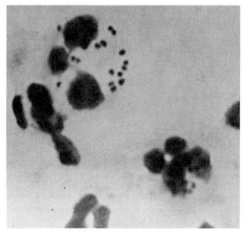

Figure 22-7 Intracellular *Neisseeria gonorrhoeae* in a gram-stained smear of urethral pus. (Courtesy, Abbott Laboratories, *Atlas of Diagnostic Microbiology*, p. 27, July, 1974.)

growth of saprophytic *Neisseria* species and other contaminants from genital organs. *N. gonorrhoeae* produces the enzyme oxidase and degrades glucose.

Immunity. Susceptibility to gonorrhea is general. No protection follows an infection.

Prevention. There is no substitute for prompt diagnosis and treatment of gonorrhea in limiting its spread in sexually active individuals. Aggressive tracing and treatment of sexual contacts can control, but not eradicate the disease. There is a need for continuing mass public educational programs. The mandatory practice in most states of applying a 1 percent solution of silver nitrate to the eyes of a newborn has been effective against ophthalmia neonatorum. There is no vaccine available for gonococcal infections, although recent success in producing a meningococcal vaccine has provided hope that a similar approach can be used to make a gonococcal vaccine.

SYPHILIS

Syphilis is an acute or chronic infection caused by the spirochete *Treponema pallidum*. The disease was once believed to have been introduced in Europe upon the return of Columbus and his crew in 1493. There is, however, much evidence that the disease existed in epidemic proportions during earlier times. The particularly virulent form of syphilis which spread during the century that followed the discovery of America was probably caused by a new strain, which could well have originated in the New World.

Syphilis occurs in four stages. *Primary syphilis* is characterized by a hard ulcer known as a *chancre*, occurring on the genitals 10 to 90 days after exposure. In men the chancre usually develops on the tip of the penis and less frequently on the scrotum. In women the primary lesion may remain undetected if it develops on the inner surface of the genital organs. The chancre heals in one to five weeks with or without treatment. *Secondary syphilis* develops six to eight weeks after the appearance of the primary chancre and manifests itself as a skin rash (Figure 22-8). The lesions of secondary syphilis are commonly present on the palms of the hands and soles of the feet, differing in that respect from other infectious skin rashes, which rarely affect the palmar or plantar surfaces. *Tertiary syphilis* may not become apparent for ten or twenty years following the secondary stage. The period during which there are no apparent signs of the infection, even though the infection may be spreading to inner organs is called *latent syphilis*. Late latent syphilis is thought to be noninfectious except in pregnant women who can transmit the disease to a fetus. The effects of the infection, which finally become apparent in the tertiary stage, are lesions of the cardiovascular, central nervous, or musculoskeletal systems. The soft tumorlike lesions of the tertiary stage are called *gummas*.

Tertiary syphilis is disabling and the outcome is always fatal if undiagnosed before symptoms appear. Any organ

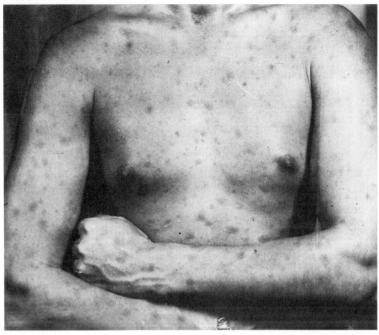

Figure 22-8 Lesions of secondary syphilis. (Armed Forces Institute of Pathology Photograph, Neg. No. 78-1413.)

can be invaded by spirochetes, but the aorta, spinal cord, brain, and long bones are more commonly affected. Manifestations of aortitis include progressive aortic regurgitation, enlargement of the left ventricle, and congestive heart failure. Changes in reflexes, coordination, speech, emotions, and memory are common in neurosyphilis. The most serious cases of tertiary syphilis exhibit such severe delusions of grandeur and paranoia that confinement in an institution is required.

Congenital syphilis occurs when the spirochetes penetrate the placental barrier and infect the fetus *in utero*. Primary or secondary maternal syphilis almost invariably causes miscarriage, stillbirth, neonatal death, or serious developmental abnormalities in the fetus

(Figure 22-9). Bullae (blisters) are present in the infant with congenital syphilis in contrast to the maculopapular or papular lesions seen in adults with secondary syphilis.

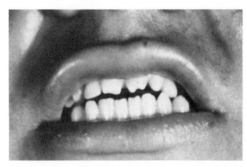

Figure 22-9 Notched teeth, known as Hutchinson's teeth, resulting from congenital syphilis. (Armed Forces Institute of Pathology Photograph, Neg. No. 53-19638.)

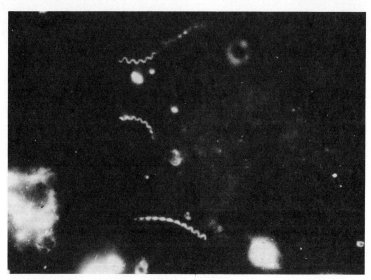

Figure 22-10 *Treponema pallidum* as observed in a dark-field preparation of fluid from a chancre. (Courtesy, Center for Disease Control, Atlanta, Georgia.)

Venereal disease in homosexuals poses serious problems for public health authorities. Not only do homosexual populations tend to underutilize available health services, but the frequency of activity with numerous, anonymous partners makes it nearly impossible to interrupt spread of disease. A few large cities have organized venereal disease clinics staffed by homosexual health professionals in an attempt to increase utilization of health services by homosexuals.

Transmission. Approximately 95 percent of all syphilis is transmitted by direct contact with exudates or lesions of infected individuals through sexual intercourse. The rest are transmitted by kissing, placental transfer, or rarely blood transfusions. The laboratory worker can contract *T. pallidum* through accidental exposure to blood or exudates containing the treponeme. Fortunately, such accidents are rare.

Laboratory Diagnosis. The bacteriological diagnosis of syphilis by darkfield microscopy depends on finding helical forms of *T. pallidum* in fluid collected from a chancre (Figure 22-10). The spirochetes measure 5.0 to 20.0 μm in length and 0.09 to 0.18 μm in width. The organisms move slowly with flexuous movements in a liquid environment. *T. pallidum* does not grow *in vitro*, but can be grown by scarification of hamster or rabbit skin and in rabbit testes.

Several serological tests for detection of treponemal antibodies are available, but the tests will not distinguish an-

Table 22-2 SEROLOGICAL TESTS FOR DIAGNOSIS OF SYPHILIS

TEST	TYPE OF REACTION
Nontreponemal screening tests	
Venereal Disease Research Laboratory (VDRL)	flocculation
Automated Reagin Test (ART)	flocculation
Rapid Plasma Reagin (RPR)	agglutination
Treponemal confirmatory tests	
Fluorescent Treponemal Antibody Absorption (FTA-ABS)	immunofluorescence
Fluorescent Treponemal Antibody Absorption Immunoglobulin M (FTA-ABS-IgM)	immunofluorescence
Fluorescent Treponemal Antibody Cerebrospinal Fluid (FTA-CSF)	immunofluorescence
Treponema pallidum Immobilization Test (TPI)	immobilization
Microhemagglutination-Treponemal Antibody Test (MHA-TP)	agglutination

tibodies for *T. pallidum* from antibodies for other treponemes (Table 22-2). Treponemes cause a number of diseases other than syphilis so clinical input is required to establish a diagnosis of syphilis. Fortunately, other treponemal infections, like yaws and pinta, are not usually found in the United States. More than a single serum sample should always be submitted for the serodiagnosis of treponemal diseases.

Immunity. Susceptibility to syphilis is general. Some resistance develops following an infection caused by *T. pallidum*, but that immunity is limited.

Prevention. It is important that individuals with gonorrhea have blood tests for syphilis two to four weeks after treatment and periodically up to three months afterwards. Gonorrhea and syphilis are not mutually exclusive diseases. Follow-up of sexual contacts and mass public educational programs can do much to control syphilis. Premarital

and prenatal testing of blood for treponemal antibodies is especially important in reducing the incidence of the venereal disease. To date, attempts to develop a vaccine for syphilis have not been successful.

NONSYPHILITIC TREPONEMAL DISEASE

Nonsyphilitic treponemal disease is more common in tropical countries and includes nonvenereal infections such as yaws, pinta, and endemic syphilis. Those diseases are transmitted by direct contact and possibly by flies. The nonsyphilitic treponemal diseases are characterized by skin lesions and may involve both the cardiovascular and central nervous systems.

CHANCROID

Chancroid is an acute, self-limiting venereal disease in which the primary lesion is an ulcer known as a soft

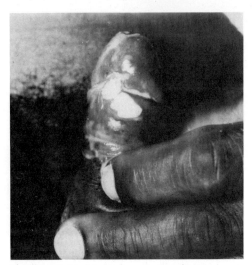

Figure 22-11 Lesions of chancroid on a penis. (Armed Forces Institute of Pathology Photograph, Neg. No. 78-1412.)

chancre (Figure 22-11). It is caused by the small, gram-negative bacillus *Haemophilus ducreyi*. The infection is frequently associated with pain and suppuration of regional lymph nodes. Chancroid is transmitted by sexual intercourse. Only rarely have dressings, instruments, or contaminated hands of attending medical personnel been implicated as a means for spreading chancroid.

The infection can sometimes be diagnosed clinically, but the gram-negative bacilli usually can be demonstrated in smears prepared from ulcers or from growth obtained on blood agar containing a meat infusion.

No immunity follows infection. All individuals with suspected or diagnosed chancroid should have blood tests for syphilis, as mixed infections do occur.

LYMPHOGRANULOMA VENEREUM

Lymphogranuloma venereum is a chlamydial disease which is worldwide in distribution, but more common in tropical and subtropical countries. The etiological agent, *Chlamydia trachomatis*, causes other urogenital and ocular diseases, including urethritis, proctitis, trachoma, and inclusion conjunctivitis. The initial lesion is a genital papule. Healing of the lesion is followed by enlargement of the inguinal or perirectal lymph nodes (buboes). The disease is transmitted by sexual intercourse or by contact with articles contaminated with material from active lesions.

Diagnosis is generally made by detecting complement-fixing antibodies in the patient's serum, since *C. trachomatis* can be grown only with some difficulty in embryonated eggs or in mice. A delayed skin reaction, known as the Frei test, can also be useful in establishing a diagnosis of the chlamydial disease.

An infection with *C. trachomatis* does not produce resistance to a subsequent venereal or ocular infection with the same organism.

GRANULOMA INGUINALE

Granuloma inguinale is an ulcerative disease caused by the pleomorphic, encapsulated, gram-negative bacillus *Calymmatobacterium granulomatis*. The initial lesion is a painless nodule, but it soon degenerates into an ulcer and causes progressive ulceration of the genitals. The lesions become infiltrated with neutrophils and monocytes. Granuloma inguinale is transmitted by sexual intercourse, but does not appear to be highly communicable. Diagnosis is made by demonstrating small pleomorphic rods, sometimes called Donovan bodies, in fresh egg-yolk medium.

Susceptibility to the venereal disease is variable, but differences in susceptibility do not appear to be caused by specific protective antibodies. The spread of granuloma inguinale can be prevented by prompt diagnosis and treatment. Eradication of the disease, like other STD's, must await the development of a suitable vaccine.

MYCOTIC INFECTIONS

Except for vulvovaginal candidiasis (sometimes called moniliasis), infections of the genitourinary tract caused by fungi are rare. However, indwelling catheters may become contaminated with *Candida albicans* and ultimately cause systemic infection. Conversely, yeast in urine may be the manifestation of disseminated mycotic disease.

VULVOVAGINAL CANDIDIASIS

Vulvovaginal candidiasis consists of an inflammation of the vulva and vagina; it can be caused by a variety of *Candida* species, but it is most frequently caused by *C. albicans*. Vulvovaginitis is common in diabetics. The high estrogen levels accompanying pregnancy, use of oral contraceptives, or administration

of corticosteroids also predispose individuals to the infection. The yeast can cause inflammatory lesions on the penis. Candidiasis can spread readily to the perineum or perianal regions.

Susceptibility is general and no immunity follows an infection. Abstinence from or protection during intercourse may be necessary to prevent reinfections. Both sex partners may require treatment.

PROTOZOAL INFECTIONS

Most pathogenic protozoa have a predilection for the intestine or blood, where access is provided through the gastrointestinal tract or by capillary invasion following the bite of an arthropod. An exception is the flagellate *Trichomonas vaginalis*, which resides in the vagina of approximately 25 percent of American women. The parasite can invade the Bartholin's or Skene's glands, but more frequently causes urethritis or cystitis.

TRICHOMONIASIS

Trichomoniasis may occur as a single infection or may coexist with candidiasis in the inflamed vagina. Sometimes there is an accompanying urethritis or cervicitis caused by gonococcal infection. Vaginal trichomoniasis causes itching, burning, and a frothy creamy yellow discharge. It is doubtful that extrasexual transmission of *T. vaginalis* occurs with any regularity.

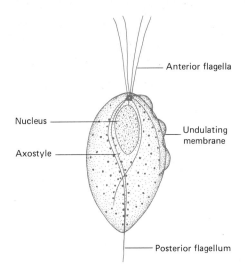

Figure 22-12   Diagrammatic representation of *Trichomonas vaginalis.*

The flagellated organisms from a discharge are readily observed when a small amount of the discharge is placed in a drop of saline on a slide and viewed with the bright-field microscope under high power (Figure 22-12).

No immunity follows the superficial infection. Abstinence from or protection during sexual intercourse may be necessary to prevent reinfections. It is important that both sex partners receive treatment.

VIRAL INFECTIONS

Both the male and female genital tracts may be sites of primary and recurrent disease caused by herpes simplex virus, type 2. The infection is transmitted by sexual intercourse. Lesions, which often are painful, may occur on the vulva, vagina, cervix, or perineum in the female and on the glans, prepuce, or shaft of the penis in the male. Like the type 1 herpes simplex virus, type 2 appears to have the potential for latency.

For many years attempts have been made to link type 2 herpes simplex virus with cancer of the cervix. Approximately 80 percent of women in the United States with cancer of the cervix have antibodies against the genital virus. The incidence of cervical cancer is high among women who have had sexual experiences early in life and who have progressed to multiple sex partners. However, the relationship between cervical cancer and herpes simplex virus, type 2, remains unclear. Greater sexual promiscuity may merely provide more opportunities for exposure to the virus. The laboratory diagnosis and prevention of herpesvirus infections were discussed in Chapter 17.

SUMMARY

The microbial diseases of the genitourinary tract comprise a heterogeneous group of infections with local manifestations which, if untreated, spread to adjacent organs causing irreparable damage. The microorganisms causing urinary tract infections are frequently a part of the indigenous intestinal flora. The infectious agents of the venereal diseases are transmitted by sexual contact with an infected individual. Gonorrhea and syphilis occur in epidemic proportions in many countries, including the United States. The increasing social acceptance of multiple sex partners provides a means for widespread dissemination of the diseases. Since vaccines are not available for the STD's, prompt diagnosis, treatment, and case-contact tracing remain the only ways to control syphilis and gonorrhea. Greater sexual promiscuity and use of oral contraceptives or corticosteroids are also providing greater opportunity for colonization by indigenous vaginal microorganisms and exposure to type 2 herpes simplex virus. The genital virus is of interest because of its potential for latency and possible association with cancer of the cervix.

QUESTIONS FOR STUDY

1. Name three factors which predispose women to urinary tract infections.
2. What is the significance of positive cultures from catheterized urine?
3. What role does trauma play in the establishment of infections of the urogenital tract?
4. Identify each lesion with a venereal disease.

   papule   bulla
   chancre   nodule
   gumma   bubo
5. What means are available to control epidemics of gonorrhea and syphilis?

SELECTED REFERENCES

California State Department of Public Health. *A Manual for the Control of Communicable Diseases in California.* Berkeley: 1971.

Charles, D., and Finland, M. *Obstetric and Perinatal Infections.* Philadelphia: Lea & Febiger, 1973.

Davidsohn, I., and Henry, J. B. *Todd-Sanford Clinical Diagnosis by Laboratory Methods.* 14th ed. Philadelphia: Saunders, 1969.

Davis, R. D.; Dulbecco, R.; Eisen, H. N.; Ginsberg, H. S.; and Wood, W. B., Jr. *Microbiology.* 2d ed. New York: Harper & Row, 1973.

Good, R. A., and Fisher, D. W. *Immunobiology.* Stamford, Conn.: Sinauer, 1971.

Judson, F. N. Sexually transmitted disease in gay men. *Sexually Transmitted Diseases* 4:76, 1977.

Langley, L.L.; Telford, I. R.; and Christensen, J. B. *Dynamic Anatomy and Physiology.* 4th ed. New York: McGraw-Hill, 1974.

Lee, Y. H.; McCormack, W. M.; Marcy, S. M.; and Klein, J. O. The genital mycoplasmas — their role in disorders of reproduction and in pediatric infections. *Ped. Clin. of No. Amer.* 21:457, 1974.

Lennette, E. H.; Spaulding, E. H.; and Truant, J. P. *Manual of Clinical Microbiology.* 2d ed. Washington, D.C.: American Society for Microbiology, 1974.

Montgomery, G. L. *Textbook of Pathology.* Vol. 1. Baltimore: Williams & Wilkins, 1965.

Peery, T. M., and Miller, F. N. *Pathology: A Dynamic Introduction to Medicine and Surgery.* 2d ed. Boston: Little, Brown, 1971.

Shepard, M. C., and Howard, D. R. Identification of "T" strain mycoplasmas in primary agar cultures by means of a direct test for urease. *Ann. N.Y. Acad. Sci.* 174:809, 1970.

Tortora, G. J., and Anagnostakos, N. P. *Principles of Anatomy and Physiology.* San Francisco: Harper & Row (Canfield Press), 1975.

Wallace, A. L., and Norins, L. C. Syphilis serology today. *Prog. in Clin. Path.* 2:198, 1969.

Youmans, G. P.; Paterson, P. Y.; and Sommers, H. M. *The Biologic and Clinical Basis of Infectious Diseases.* Philadelphia: Saunders, 1975.

Chapter 23

Microbial Diseases of the Central Nervous System

After you read this chapter, you should be able to:

1. List the bacterial organisms which commonly cause meningitis.
2. List the bacterial organisms which commonly cause brain abscess.
3. Discuss the transmission, laboratory diagnosis, immunity, and prevention of bacterial diseases of the central nervous system.
4. Identify the major viruses causing diseases of the central nervous system.
5. Discuss the transmission, laboratory diagnosis, immunity, and prevention of viral diseases of the central nervous system.
6. Explain how poliomyelitis differs from aseptic meningitis.
7. Describe a possible role for the subviral particles in disease.
8. Compare the etiological agent, reservoir of the organisms, and target organs in cryptococcosis and the phycomycoses.
9. List three genera of free-living amebas that can cause meningoencephalitis.

The central nervous system (CNS) consists of the brain and spinal cord (Figure 23-1). The brain is contained within a vault of bone known as the *cranium;* the spinal cord is encased in a tunnel of bones known as the *vertebrae.* The spinal cord passes through the *foramen magnum,* an opening in the skull, and expands into the *medulla oblongata* or brain stem.

The brain and spinal column are covered by three membranes, called meninges. The *dura mater* is the strong outermost covering; the *pia mater* is a thin membrane adjacent to the brain and spinal cord. The *arachnoid* is the delicate middle membrane separated from the dura mater by the subdural space and from the pia mater by the subarachnoid space (Figure 23-2).

The hollow central canal of the spinal cord and cavities of the brain, called *ventricles,* contain the *cerebrospinal fluid* (CSF). The same fluid circulates in the subarachnoid space and also flows a short distance along sheaths of the cranial and spinal nerves.

BACTERIAL INFECTIONS

Bacterial infections of the CNS may occur as primary infections or may be extensions of infection in other parts of the body. The bacteria can gain access to neural tissue through the bloodstream, by direct continuity from a nearby bone infection, or by penetrating wounds. (Some diseases which eventually affect neural tissue are discussed in the chapter concerned with the portal of entry or site of primary infection. For example, botulism is discussed with diseases of the gastrointestinal tract and syphilis with urogenital diseases.)

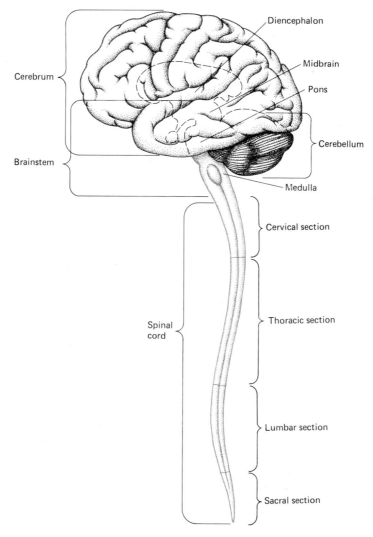

Figure 23-1   Lateral view showing major parts of the central nervous system.

MENINGOCOCCAL MENINGITIS

Meningococcal meningitis is caused by *Neisseria meningitidis.* The disease is characterized by an abrupt onset of headache, fever, and nausea. Sometimes vomiting, stiff neck, and petechiae (small hemorrhagic spots on the skin) also occur. At one time fatality rates from meningococcemia were as high as 50 percent.

Transmission. Meningococcal meningitis is transmitted by direct contact with an infected person or a carrier. It is the only type of meningitis which oc-

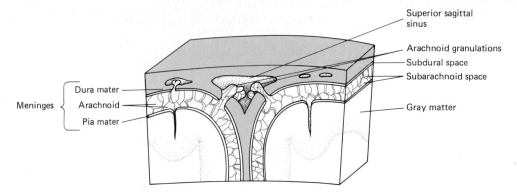

Portion of cortex, vertical section

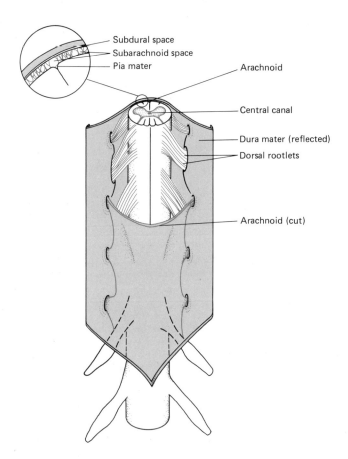

Portion of spinal cord, posterior view

Figure 23-2 The meninges of the brain and the spinal cord.

curs in epidemic form. The carrier rate is higher than the frequency of the disease. Carriers are usually free of any symptoms, but if the bacteria colonize the nasopharynx of a susceptible individual and gain entrance to the bloodstream, the bacteremia inevitably leads to invasion of the meninges.

Laboratory Diagnosis. Gram stains of sediment from CSF reveal the presence of intracellular or extracellular gram-negative diplococci approximately 1.0 μm in diameter. The organism grows on Thayer-Martin medium in an atmosphere of 10 percent CO_2. Like *N. gonorrhoeae*, colonies of meningococci exhibit a positive oxidase reaction, but *N. meningitidis* degrades both glucose and maltose. Fluorescent antibody techniques are of value in establishing the presence of a *Neisseria* species, but will not differentiate meningococci from gonococci, because the organisms possess similar antigens (Figure 23-3). Meningococci may be typed by a quellung reaction in the presence of type-specific antisera. Two serotypes, A and C, are responsible for most meningococcal meningitis.

Immunity. Children are particularly susceptible to meningococcal meningitis. Most adults, except under unusual circumstances, have sufficient humoral antibody activity to afford protection against the meningococci. Within a week even the carrier state induces the synthesis of protective antibodies against the serotype colonizing the nasopharynx.

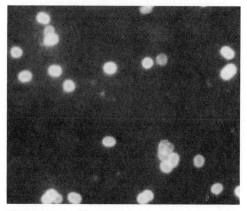

Figure 23-3 *Neisseria meningitidis,* group C, as observed in cerebrospinal fluid using a fluorescent antibody stain. (Courtesy, Center for Disease Control, Atlanta, Georgia.)

Prevention. Monovalent vaccines of purified cell wall polysaccharides against serotypes A and C and a bivalent A-C vaccine are available for selective use. Serotype C vaccine has been given to military recruits in the United States since 1971. Routine vaccination for civilians is not recommended, but it should be considered for travelers to African countries, particularly Egypt, as an adjunct to antimicrobial prophylaxis.

TUBERCULOUS MENINGITIS

Tuberculous meningitis is a possible consequence of disseminated tuberculosis, especially in children. Typical tubercles occur as small yellow lesions on the arachnoid membrane primarily at the base of the brain. The causative organism, *Mycobacterium tuberculosis,* is spread by the bloodstream or lymphatic vessels from primary lesions occurring elsewhere in the body.

Acid-fast bacilli are recoverable from CSF samples, but the low numbers present may require animal inoculation for definitive diagnoses.

Recovery from tuberculous meningitis was once unknown. However, the variety of antimicrobial agents available today has greatly improved chances for recovery. Brain damage, unfortunately, is an almost inevitable sequela to tuberculous meningitis.

NONMENINGOCOCCAL-NONTUBERCULOUS BACTERIAL MENINGITIS

Meningitis caused by organisms other than the meningococcus or *M. tuberculosis* may follow a skull fracture or may be an extension of a primary infection. Both *Streptococcus pneumoniae* and *Haemophilus influenzae* are frequent invaders of the meninges. *H. influenzae* is the most common cause of meningitis in children under 6 years of age. Other gram-negative bacilli, staphylococci, *Listeria monocytogenes,* and group B streptococci are occasional isolates. Many newborns appear to acquire group B streptococci or *L. monocytogenes* from the maternal genital tract during delivery. Diagnosis and proper treatment is dependent on rapid identification and susceptibility testing of the causative organism. Mortality rates vary from 20 percent with *S. pneumoniae* to 70 to 80 percent with *L. monocytogenes.* The use of prophylactic antibiotics may be indicated in skull or spinal column injuries, but most diagnoses must await symptoms of meningeal involvement.

BRAIN ABSCESS

A brain abscess consists of a pyogenic local infection in the brain. It commonly occurs in the cerebrum or cerebellum as a result of trauma or as an extension of a primary infection site (Figure 23-4). Bacteria commonly isolated from CSF of patients with post-trauma brain abscesses include staphylococci, streptococci, and coliforms. Most abscesses occurring as an extension of a primary infection are caused by anaerobes. Severe headache is almost always an early symptom. Nausea, vomiting, drowsiness, confusion, and loss of consciousness may occur as the disease progresses. Surgical intervention is often necessary to drain or excise an abscess.

Transmission. Both aerobes and anaerobes are prevalent throughout the body as a part of the indigenous flora. If given the opportunity, particularly in the presence of traumatized tissue, they can cause infections of the urogenital tract, pleuropulmonary regions, intra-abdominal areas, ears, and teeth. The organisms reach the brain by direct extension through bones, nerves, or the bloodstream.

Laboratory Diagnosis. Exudates or sediments from CSF are examined initially by dark-field microscopy and the light microscope after Gram staining. Some anaerobes stain faintly, have tapered ends, or are spheroidal in shape; others form distinct endospores (Table 23-1). Depending on results of the Gram stain, appropriate media are chosen for the selective cultivation of organisms observed.

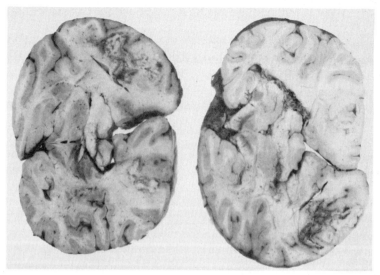

Figure 23-4 Brain abscesses in nocardiosis. (Armed Forces Institute of Pathology Photograph, Neg. No. N-33470.)

Table 23-1 COLONY AND MICROSCOPIC MORPHOLOGY OF ANAEROBES ISOLATED FROM BRAIN ABSCESSES

ORGANISM	COLONY MORPHOLOGY ON BLOOD AGAR	MICROSCOPIC MORPHOLOGY
Actinomyces sp.	convex, rough or smooth, white	long, filamentous gram-positive bacilli with branching; no spores
Bacteroides fragilis	convex, white to gray, translucent, glistening	gram-negative bacilli with rounded ends; may be pleomorphic
Clostridium perfringens	low, convex, slightly opaque	large gram-positive bacilli with blunt ends; rare, oval subterminal spores
Fusobacterium nucleatum	convex, rough or smooth, white	slender gram-negative bacilli with tapered ends
Peptococcus sp.	convex, gray to white, opaque, shiny and dull	gram-positive cocci occurring singly or in pairs, chains, or clumps
Peptostreptococcus sp.	convex, gray to white, opaque shiny or dull	gram-positive cocci occurring singly or in pairs or chains
Propionibacterium	convex, white to pink, shiny, opaque	pleomorphic, club-shaped gram-positive bacilli
Veillonella sp.	convex, translucent, glistening	gram-negative cocci in pairs, short chains, and irregular clumps

SOURCE: Adapted from V. L. Sutter, and S. M. Finegold, *Prog. in Clin. Path.* 5:219, 1973.

Immunity. Since bacteria causing brain abscesses are often sequestered in the cranial vault, it is unlikely that sufficient immune responses can be invoked to provide any substantive immunity.

Prevention. Prompt diagnosis and treatment of ear or periodontal infections can be a deterrent to dissemination of microorganisms to the brain. The administration of antimicrobial agents following injury or surgery can sometimes prevent microbial colonization of traumatized tissue.

TETANUS

Tetanus is one of the most serious bacterial diseases affecting the CNS. The causative organism, *Clostridium tetani*, is an anaerobe which produces a potent neurotoxin. The symptoms of disease occur only after the exotoxin spreads by way of retrograde axonal transport from an initial site of infection to the CNS. Early symptoms may include irritability, headache, and low-grade fever. The toxin, tetanospasmin, causes contractions of muscles which are often followed by respiratory paralysis and death. The jaw muscles are frequently affected. *Tetanus neonatorum* is a form of the disease which occurs when the umbilical cord of a newborn is infected.

Transmission. *C. tetani* is part of the indigenous intestinal flora of herbivorous animals. The organism is also widely distributed in the soil, growing readily on dead organic matter. Devitalized human tissue favors growth of the organism. The bacteria gain entrance to the body through deep puncture wounds, severe lacerations, or gunshot wounds. *Tetanus neonatorum* is caused by cutting the umbilical cord with an instrument contaminated with spores.

Laboratory Diagnosis. The isolation of *C. tetani* from a wound is not a prerequisite for diagnosing tetanus. The symptoms, if associated with a history of exposure, are so dramatic that symptoms alone can establish the diagnosis. However, the organism does grow as a thin-surface film on anaerobic blood agar plates. *C. tetani* is a gram-positive bacillus measuring 2.0 to 5.0 μm in length and 0.3 to 0.8 μm in width. The terminal swollen spores of *C. tetani* have a typical drumstick appearance (Figure 23-5). Proof of isolation of toxin-producing *C. tetani* requires demonstration of the toxic effects in mice and

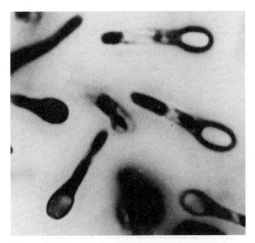

Figure 23-5 Endospores of a clostridial organism in a stained, wet-mount preparation. (From B. D. Davis et al., *Microbiology*, 2d ed., New York, Harper & Row, 1973.)

neutralization of the toxin in mice previously inoculated with antitoxin.

Immunity. Recovery from tetanus does not guarantee immunity to the disease. There have been many documented cases of tetanus occurring in individuals who have had previous exposure to the tetanus toxin.

Prevention. Tetanus can be prevented by immunization with tetanus toxoid. The toxoid is given in a series of three injections during the first year of life. For maximum protection, initial injections are followed by boosters one year later, when the child enters school, and at five-year intervals thereafter.

If a full series of tetanus toxoid injections has not been given to an individual having a deep wound, it may be necessary to supplement cleansing and debriding the wound with an additional injection of toxoid. Tetanus immune globulin (TIG) is recommended for individuals who have an uncertain or incomplete history of tetanus immunization (Table 23-2). The human product provides longer protection than does antitoxin of animal origin.

Moreover, TIG is associated with fewer allergic reactions than the animal product.

VIRAL INFECTIONS

Certain viruses have an affinity for tissue of the CNS; they are often called neurotropic viruses (Table 23-3). Most other viruses do not invade the CNS except under unusual circumstances. An exception would be dissemination of the measles or mumps viruses to the CNS during convalescence from those diseases.

The permissive role of some peripheral nerves in housing the herpes simplex and zoster viruses during long periods of dormancy is not well understood. The nerves appear unaffected by the presence of those viruses.

ASEPTIC MENINGITIS

Aseptic meningitis is an inflammation of the meninges not caused by bacteria and assumed in most cases to be caused

Table 23-2 GUIDE TO TETANUS PROPHYLAXIS IN WOUND MANAGEMENT

DOSES OF TETANUS TOXOID PREVIOUSLY ADMINISTERED	CLEAN, MINOR WOUNDS	ALL OTHER WOUNDS
Uncertain	toxoid	toxoid and TIG
0–1	toxoid	toxoid and TIG
2	toxoid	toxoid*
3	none†	none‡

*Unless wound is more than 24 hours old.
†Unless more than 10 years has elapsed since last dose.
‡Unless more than 5 years has elapsed since last dose.
SOURCE: Adapted from *CDC Morbidity and Mortality Weekly Report* 26:407, 1977.

Table 23-3 MAJOR GROUPS AND SEROTYPES OF VIRUSES CAUSING DISEASES OF THE CENTRAL NERVOUS SYSTEM

Virus	Serotypes	Major Disease
Picornavirus		
poliovirus	1, 2, 3	poliomyelitis
coxsackievirus A	1, 2, 4-11, 16-18, 22-24	aseptic meningitis
coxsackievirus B	1-6	aseptic meningitis
echovirus	1-9, 11-25, 30, 31	aseptic meningitis
Togavirus		
eastern equine virus (EEE)*		encephalitis
western equine virus (WEE)		encephalitis
Venezuelan equine virus (VEE)		encephalitis
Paramyxovirus		
mumps virus		aseptic meningitis
rubella virus		encephalitis
Herpesvirus		
herpes simplex virus	1	encephalitis
herpes simplex virus	2	aseptic meningitis
varicella-zoster virus		encephalitis
Epstein-Barr virus		aseptic meningitis
Rhabdovirus		
rabies virus		encephalitis

*No designation for serotype means that a single antigenic type has been identified.

by a virus. A variety of viruses have been implicated, but enteroviruses are considered to be the most common cause of aseptic meningitis. In a majority of cases, however, causative organisms are unknown. The disease has a sudden onset with an intense headache being a primary symptom. A fever, nausea, vomiting, stiff neck, sore throat, and drowsiness also occur with some regularity.

Transmission. The viruses causing meningitis are most probably disseminated by the bloodstream during a period of viremia. The viruses do not appear to spread easily to other patients, family members, or hospital personnel.

Laboratory Diagnosis. CSF, stool, rectal swabs, or paired sera may be sub-

mitted to a virology laboratory. Complement-fixation (CF) tests are available for mumps, herpes simplex, polio- and adenoviruses. Serological tests for cox-sackie- or echoviruses are not feasible; diagnosis of diseases caused by these viruses is dependent on recovery of the viruses from rectal swabs, stool, or CSF.

Immunity. Resistance to particular viruses, following aseptic meningitis, varies with the infectious agent. Any protective antibodies would offer limited immunity because of the large number of possible etiological agents.

Prevention. Prompt diagnosis, treatment, and surveillance of infections caused by viruses is important in controlling aseptic meningitis. Strict adherence to personal hygiene constitutes a deterrent to the spread of viral infections. Isolation of patients with aseptic meningitis may be recommended as a precautionary measure.

POLIOMYELITIS

Poliomyelitis (infantile paralysis) consists of an acute inflammation of the spinal cord and brain stem. It affects chiefly the anterior horns of the lumbar sections of the spinal cord (Figure 23-6). The paralysis which develops in some patients distinguishes the disease from aseptic meningitis. Muscle involvement is frequently unilateral, but the site of paralysis depends on the location of the nerves invaded by the virus. There are three antigenic types of poliovirus designated as 1, 2, and 3. Type 1 is the cause of most paralytic illness.

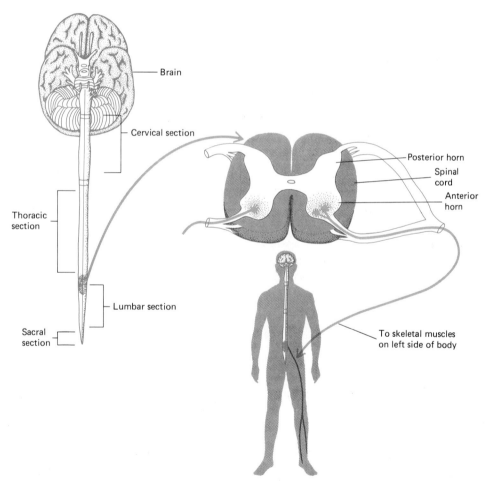

Figure 23-6 Invasion of anterior horns of lumbar section of spinal cord by poliovirus. Destruction of nerve cells frequently causes a unilateral paralysis of muscles.

Transmission. Polioviruses are spread by direct contact with pharyngeal secretions or feces of an infected person. Water, milk, and occasionally flies have been incriminated in outbreaks of the disease. A viremia is established before invasion of the CNS. From the blood, viruses may penetrate the blood-brain barrier or travel along peripheral nerve fibers to the CNS.

Laboratory Diagnosis. Poliomyelitis can be diagnosed by isolation of the virus from pharyngeal secretions early in the disease and later from stool or rectal swabs. The viruses grow readily in monkey kidney cells, producing rounding of cells, inclusion bodies, ballooning, and ultimately death of cells (Figure 23-7). Serodiagnosis can often be made on paired sera using complement-fixation or neutralization techniques.

Immunity. As with some other viral diseases, age influences host reaction to polioviruses. Susceptibility is greatest in early childhood, but paralysis is a more frequent consequence of poliomyelitis in adults. Lifelong, type-specific resistance follows apparent or sometimes inapparent infection.

Prevention. Poliomyelitis can be controlled effectively by active immunization with trivalent attenuated viruses or inactivated viruses. The live attenuated virus, or Sabin vaccine, is more easily administered and is relatively inexpensive. Booster vaccines of live or killed virus vaccines are no longer believed to be necessary.

ENCEPHALITIS

Encephalitis is an inflammation of the brain characterized by altered cerebral function, including loss of consciousness. It can be caused by a number of viruses and other etiological agents including fungi, rickettsiae, protozoa, and *Trichinella spiralis*. Fatality rates vary from 5 to 60 percent, depending on the infectious agent. Eastern equine (EEE), western equine (WEE), and Venezuela equine (VEE) encephalitis are among the most important types of arthropod-borne encephalitis.

Transmission. WEE is transmitted by the mosquito, *Culex tarsalis*. Birds, rodents, and other mammals may be significant reservoirs for WEE, but both horses and humans are dead-end hosts (Figure 23-8). The specific vectors for

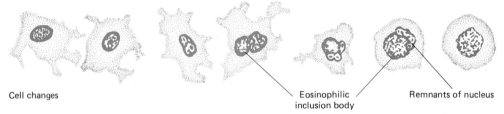

Cell changes   Eosinophilic   Remnants of nucleus
                                                                 inclusion body

Figure 23-7   Diagrammatic representation of the effect of poliovirus on an infected cell. As numbers of viruses reach a maximum, an inclusion body is produced, causing ultimate cell death.

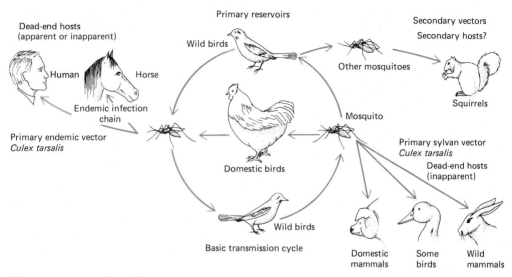

Figure 23-8 Epidemiology of WEE virus infections. (From A. D. Hess and P. Holden, *Ann. N.Y. Acad. Sci.* 70:294, 1958.)

EEE and VEE are not known. Encephalitis is not transmitted from person to person.

Laboratory Diagnosis. Serological diagnosis can be made on paired sera from persons suspected of having encephalitis caused by EEE, WEE, or VEE agents. Complement-fixation techniques are most satisfactory for early diagnosis, but complement-fixing antibodies do not persist as long as neutralizing or hemagglutination-inhibiting antibodies. The viruses can be isolated from extracts of brain and spinal cord specimens obtained at autopsy and only rarely from blood or cerebrospinal fluid.

Immunity. Susceptibility varies with the infectious agent. As a rule, children and the elderly are the most susceptible. Inapparent infection probably is

responsible for synthesis of some protective antibodies. Recovery from encephalitis is associated with immunity to the particular causative virus.

Prevention. Destruction of mosquito larvae and breeding places for mosquitoes is important in the control of arthropod-borne encephalitis. The use of insect repellents and apparel to cover exposed surfaces of the skin may be indicated in endemic areas. Immunization with formalin-inactivated viruses is an important deterrent to infection in certain high-risk groups.

RABIES

Rabies is a type of encephalitis caused by a virus occurring mainly in infected dogs, cats, cattle, skunks, bats, and squirrels. It is considered a fatal disease in humans, with only one reported case of survival in this century. Symptoms occur at variable periods after invasion by the virus. The virus migrates to the CNS by way of peripheral nerves, so the shorter the pathway from the site of a bite the shorter the incubation time for the disease. Onset of rabies is heralded by apprehension, irritability, fever, malaise, and difficulty in swallowing. Often the mere sight or thought of water induces spasmodic contractions of the muscles of deglutition. For that reason, the name hydrophobia (fear of water) was once used to describe the illness.

Transmission. Rabies is transmitted most often by a bite inflicted by a rabid animal, but it may also be transmitted by inhalation of virus-laden aerosols. Viruses are airborne in caves harboring the infected bats. Dog-to-dog transmission is rare, but an exception occurred in the sporadic outbreak of rabies in Laredo, Texas, in 1976–1977 in which more than 20 dogs were affected. Rabies occurs naturally in wild animals such as skunks, squirrels, weasels, and ferrets. Presumably it is transmitted by bites or scratches from animal to animal. Transmission from person to person has not been demonstrated.

Laboratory Diagnosis. The rabies virus can sometimes be recovered from saliva, throat washings, CSF, urine, or nasal secretions of humans. Serological techniques on patient sera are of limited value early in human rabies, since antibodies develop slowly. Definitive diagnosis in humans depends on identifying the virus in brain-impression smears from the animal that inflicted the wound, demonstrating Negri-type inclusion bodies in brain tissue, or isolating the virus from brain-tissue extracts or saliva (Figure 23-9). White laboratory mice are the animals of choice for isolation and identification of the rabies virus. A fluorescent antibody technique applied to brain impression smears from mice has largely replaced other methods of diagnosis.

Immunity. Susceptibility to rabies is general, but development of symptoms may depend on both the virulence and number of rabies viruses gaining entrance.

Prevention. The effective control of rabies requires compulsory vaccination of dogs and cats, registration of all dogs,

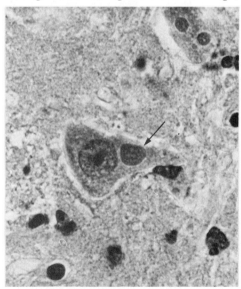

Figure 23-9 Negri inclusion body in human brain cell. (Courtesy, P. Atansiu and J. Sisman, Pasteur Institute, Paris.)

destruction of stray dogs, quarantine, and careful observation of animals inflicting wounds on humans. Prompt and vigorous cleansing and flushing of wounds can significantly reduce numbers of viruses and reduce the risk of rabies.

In the event of possible exposure to the rabies virus, prophylactic immunization should be undertaken only if deemed necessary and with a full understanding of the risks involved. The chances of vaccine-induced demyelinating encephalitis from phenolized rabbit-brain vaccine may be greater than the chance of acquiring rabies. A vaccine made from duck eggs inoculated with the rabies virus is associated with fewer side effects but it may not be as effective in confining the virus to superficial tissues. Only high-risk animal workers should consider prophylactic immunization with the avian product.

An unusual, but somewhat controversial, approach to controlling rabies in red foxes is being tested in Switzerland. Attenuated rabies virus is being spread in fox dens to stimulate the animals to produce antibodies. Since the attenuated virus is contagious, although it does not produce rabies, it is hoped that it will be spread in the same manner as the rabies-producing virus.

SUBVIRAL PARTICLE DISEASES

Diseases caused by subviral particles include a group of infections characterized by a period of latency lasting for months or years. Ultimately, the viruses produce serious or fatal illness. The first subviral particle infections described were chronic diseases of Icelandic sheep, two of which affect the CNS.

Several subviral particles cause diseases of the CNS in humans. *Subacute sclerosing panencephalitis* (SSPE) is believed to be a delayed reaction to infection with the measles virus. Infections with measles before the age of 2 is a predisposing factor in SSPE. *Kuru*, a degenerative disease of the cerebellum, has been observed in cannibals in New Guinea. The disease produces alterations in balance which cause difficulty in walking, then tremors, and eventual death (Figure 23-10). The infectious agent is believed to be a subviral particle, but has not yet been described. *Creutzfeldt—Jakob disease* (CJD) and *progressive multifocal leukoencephalopathy* (PMC) are rare human diseases associated with mental deterioration and lack of muscle coordination. The viral agents are currently being studied.

Subviral particles are the suspected etiological agents of *multiple sclerosis* (MS), a neurological disorder in which the myelin sheath surrounding nerves is destroyed. The disease affects 500,000 individuals in the United States. Several findings suggest that the paralysis, numbness, loss of coordination, tremors, and interference with balance may be caused by an autoimmune response resulting from viral infection. Epidemiological studies suggest that a measles (rubeola) or a similar virus is the primary suspect. If the measles virus is in fact involved, the widescale immunization with measles vaccines employed since 1965 should affect the incidence of MS by 1980.

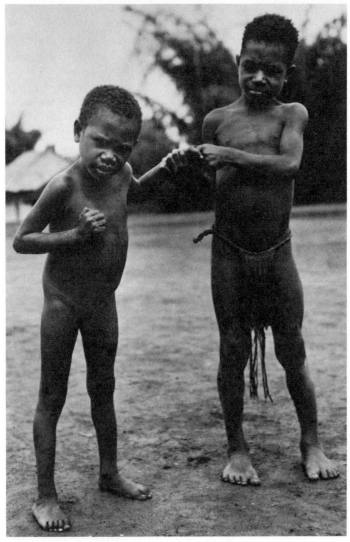

Figure 23-10   A young patient (on left) with kuru. He died at 5 years of age, several years before his mother developed kuru. (Courtesy, D. C. Gajdusek, Bethesda, Maryland.)

FUNGAL INFECTIONS

Infections of the CNS caused by fungi typically occur in the compromised host. The infections are almost universally fatal, and diagnosis is most often made at autopsy. The presence of underlying degenerative diseases predisposes some individuals to brain and spinal cord infections caused by fungi.

CRYPTOCOCCOSIS

Cyrptococcosis is a worldwide disease caused by the yeast *Cryptococcus neoformans*. The primary site of infection is the lung, and when confined to the lung, the illness is usually of a transient and uncomplicated nature. Extension of the infection to the meninges of the brain and spinal cord causes a chronic meningitis. Chronic cryptococcosis of the CNS may be present over a period of 10 to 20 years, but is more often a rapid, fulminating disease.

Transmission. Exposure to pigeon droppings is the most important factor in transmission of cryptococcosis. The yeast cells are abundant in aerosols surrounding pigeon coops. There is no evidence that the disease can be transmitted from person to person.

Laboratory Diagnosis. A diagnosis of meningeal cryptococcosis can be made by direct examination of sediment from CSF using India ink (Figure 23-11). The yeasts can be recognized by the large capsules which surround the organisms. *C. neoformans* grows readily on carbohydrate-enriched media. Ability to grow *in vitro* at 35°C, pathogenicity for mice, and hydrolysis of urea are useful identifying characteristics. The serodiagnosis of cryptococcosis is usually not practical because of cross-reactions occurring with other antibodies.

Immunity. The fact that the incidence of pulmonary and meningeal cryptococcosis is low despite the frequency of *C. neoformans* in the environment seems to indicate that natural resistance to the fungus is high. Patients with multiple myeloma, Hodgkin's disease, or those on corticosteroids appear to be especially susceptible to the disseminated form of the disease.

Prevention. Protection during exposure to pigeon dung could be a significant deterrent to inhalation of *C. neoformans*. Monitoring of particularly vulnerable patients during immunosuppressive therapy could detect pulmonary infections prior to dissemination. Amphotericin B, a polyene antimicrobial agent, is particularly effective in preventing the spread of primary infections.

PHYCOMYCOSES

The phycomycoses of the CNS include infections caused by *Absidia, Mucor,*

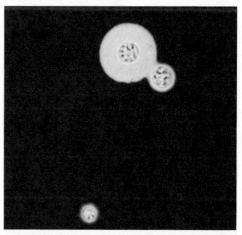

Figure 23-11 *Cryptococcus neoformans* in an India ink wet-mount preparation (Courtesy, L. Ajello, Center for Disease Control, Atlanta, Georgia.)

Rhizopus, and *Mortierella* sp. Diabetic acidosis appears to be an important factor predisposing individuals to CNS involvement. A phycomycosis of the sinuses, ocular orbits, or meninges has a grave prognosis. The infection may reach the terminal stage in 2 to 10 days.

Transmission. The etiological agents of the phycomycoses are common in the environment. They are found in old bread, decaying fruit, and animal dung. Spores may be inhaled quite accidentally.

Laboratory Diagnosis. Cultures alone are not diagnostic for the phycomycoses as *Absidia, Mucor, Rhizopus,* and *Mortierella* are common contaminants. Diagnosis must be confirmed by the demonstration of nonseptate hyphae in biopsy material and culture of tissue obtained by biopsy or at autopsy. There are no satisfactory serological tests.

Immunity. The low incidence of phycomycoses indicates that humans are resistant to the invading fungi except under unusual circumstances caused by diabetic acidosis or by drugs which suppress immune responses.

Prevention. It may be impossible to prevent phycomycoses in the compromised host, but more aggressive monitoring of such patients could be effective in diagnosing invasion by the fungi before widespread dissemination has occurred.

PROTOZOAL INFECTIONS

The migration of protozoa from intestinal or extraintestinal sites to the CNS is relatively rare. However, some trypanosomes, toxoplasmas, and amebas can gain entrance to the brain by penetrating the cribiform plate (a thin, perforated part of a skull bone) or can infect the meninges. The protozoa are frequently scattered throughout the brain substance. African trypanosomiasis (sleeping sickness) is discussed in Chapter 25 because of the blood and lymph node involvement accompanying the disease. Toxoplasmosis is presented in Chapter 24 as a cause of retinochoroiditis. CNS involvement occurs in chronic stages of African trypanosomiasis or as a result of disseminated-toxoplasmosis. In congenital trypanosomiasis and toxoplasmosis, granulomatous lesions containing extracellular parasites can be found in the brain or on the meninges.

Other protozoal parasites, namely, *Plasmodium falciparum* and more rarely *P. vivax,* cause brain damage in quite a different manner. Red blood cells infected with the malarial organisms tend to agglutinate in cerebral capillaries, causing occlusions. The surrounding tissue becomes necrotic, and hemorrhaging frequently occurs around the occluded vessels. The net effect of the blood vessel damage is to produce cerebral edema and subsequent irreversible brain damage.

There are authentic records of abscesses of the brain caused by *Entamoeba histolytica*, but they are extremely rare. However, at least one type of amebic infection is deserving of additional comment.

AMEBIC MENINGOENCEPHALITIS

Since 1965 at least 60 cases of amebic meningoencephalitis have been reported in the United States. Free-living amebas, species of *Naegleria*, *Hartmanella*, and *Acanthamoeba*, have been isolated from spinal fluid, purulent exudates, or brain tissue. The protozoa are believed to gain entrance to the brain by penetrating the cribiform plate after entering the nasal mucosa from contaminated water. Victims of the soil-water amebas had all been swimming in lakes, ponds, or bays. The mortality rate in amebic meningoencephalitis is very high since most forms of treatment have been ineffective.

SUMMARY

Infections of the central nervous system can be caused by a variety of microbial agents, including bacteria, viruses, fungi, and protozoa. Bacteria, fungi, and protozoa invade the meninges primarily. Viruses invade tissue of the brain and spinal cord and also sometimes migrate to peripheral nerve fibers. A few viruses have long incubation periods before onset of progressive degenerative disease. Viral agents are suspect as participants in a number of neurological disorders, including the debilitating multiple sclerosis. The success of the poliovirus vaccines in eliminating paralytic poliomyelitis provides hope that one day similar approaches can be used to control other microbial infections of the CNS.

QUESTIONS FOR STUDY

1. How does injury predispose an individual to infections of the central nervous system?
2. List five complications of infections of the central nervous system.
3. What are the major differences between *Neisseria gonorrhoeae* and *Neisseria meningitidis*?
4. Name the major viruses which have an affinity for tissue of the central nervous system.
5. Identify a microorganism and a disease of the central nervous system associated with each reservoir.

   pigeon droppings   stray dogs
   Culex mosquito   animal dung
   carrier state   ponds

SELECTED REFERENCES

Brown, H. W. *Basic Clinical Parasitology.* 4th ed. Englewood Cliffs, N.J.: Prentice-Hall, 1975.

Burrows, W.; Lewert, R. M.; and Rippon, J. W. *Textbook of Microbiology — The Pathogenic Microorganisms.* Philadelphia: Saunders, 1968.

California State Department of Public Health. *A Manual for the Control of Communicable Diseases in California.* Berkeley: 1971.

Davidsohn, I., and Henry, J. B. *Todd-Sanford Clinical Diagnosis by Laboratory Methods.* 14th ed. Philadelphia: Saunders, 1969.

Davis, B. D.; Dulbecco, R.; Eisen, H. N.; Ginsberg, H. S.; and Wood, B. W., Jr. *Microbiology.* 2d ed. New York: Harper & Row, 1973.

Emmons, C. W.; Binford, C. H.; and Utz, J. P. *Medical Mycology.* Philadelphia: Lea & Febiger, 1970.

Fenner, F.; McAuslan, B. R.; Mims, C. A.; Sambrook, J.; and White, D. O. *The Biology of Animal Viruses.* New York: Academic Press, 1974.

Langley, L. L.; Telford, I. R.; and Christensen, J. B. *Dynamic Anatomy and Physiology.* New York: McGraw-Hill, 1974.

Lennette, E. H.; Spaulding, E. H.; and Truant, J. P. *Manual of Clinical Microbiology.* 2d ed. Washington, D.C.: American Society for Microbiology, 1974.

Maugh, T. H., II. Multiple sclerosis: genetic link, viruses suspected. *Science* 195:667, 1976.

Peery, T. M., and Miller, F. N. *Pathology: A Dynamic Approach to Medicine and Surgery.* 2d ed. Boston: Little, Brown, 1971.

Rosenthal, M. S. Viral infections of the central nervous system. *Med. Clin. of No. Amer.* 58:593, 1974.

Salk, J., and Sack, D. Control of influenza and poliomyelitis with killed virus vaccines. *Science* 195:834, 1976.

Tortora, G. J., and Anagnostakos, N. P. *Principles of Anatomy and Physiology.* San Francisco: Harper & Row (Canfield Press), 1975.

Youmans, G. P.; Paterson, P. Y.; and Sommers, H. M. *The Biologic and Clinical Basis of Infectious Diseases.* Philadelphia: Saunders, 1975.

Chapter 24

Microbial Diseases of the Eye and Ear

After you read this chapter, you should be able to:

1. Describe anatomic structures and products of the eye and ear which act as natural barriers to pathogenic or opportunistic microorganisms.
2. Explain under what conditions microorganisms gain entrance to the eye and ear.
3. List the major microbial diseases of the eye.
4. Discuss the transmission, laboratory diagnosis, immunity, and prevention of the major microbial diseases of the eye.
5. List the factors which predispose individuals to orbital cellulitis and endophthalmitis.
6. List possible consequences of congenital toxoplasmosis.
7. Describe the symptoms and possible etiological agents of otitis media.
8. Discuss the transmission, laboratory diagnosis, immunity, and prevention of otitis media.

The eyes and ears are specialized organs which receive and convert light and sound waves into impulses which enable us to be aware of and respond to the external environment. Communication of the optic and aural receptors with specific areas of the cerebral cortex permits the interpretation of the impulses as meaningful images and sounds; communication with motor pathways of the brain and spinal cord allows us to react to changes in the environment. The ear also contains receptors for equilibrium which allow humans to maintain an upright position and to initiate directed movements.

The eyes are located within sockets known as *orbital cavities* which are formed by bones of the skull. Each orbital cavity also contains a fibrous membrane known as *fascia*. The fascia supports the blood vessels, nerves, extrinsic eye muscles, and a *lacrimal ap-* *paratus,* a group of structures responsible for the manufacture, secretion, and drainage of tears (Figure 24-1). A pad of fat separates the orbital cavity from the fascia. The fatty tissue supports and protects the eye. The eyebrows, eyelids, eyelashes, and a thin, mucous membrane lining the eyelids, known as the *conjunctiva,* as well as tears provided by the lacrimal apparatus, serve to protect the eyes from invasion by foreign objects.

The ear is divided into three parts: an *external ear,* located on the lateral surface of the head; a *middle ear,* contained within the temporal bone of the cranium; and an *inner ear,* consisting of a complex network of canals in the temporal bone (Figure 24-2). The outer ear is designed to direct sound waves inward. It consists of an outer appendage known as the *pinna* or auricle, an *external auditory canal* leading to the middle

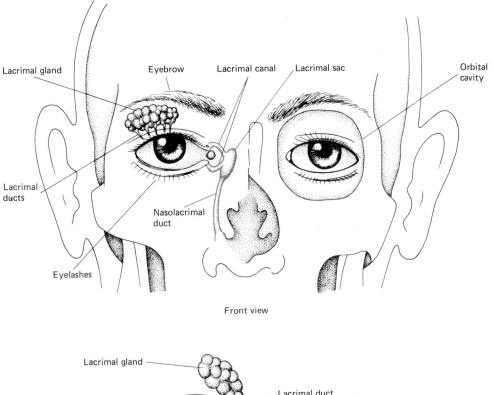

Front view

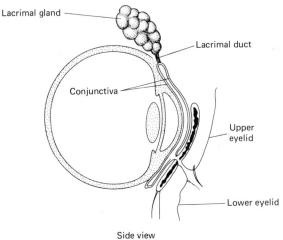

Side view

Figure 24-1 Relationship of the lacrimal apparatus to other eye parts of accessory organs as seen from the front and side.

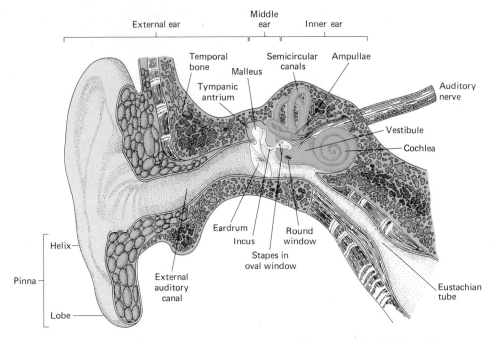

Figure 24-2   Structure of the ear showing major parts of the external, middle, and inner ear.

ear, and the *eardrum* or tympanic membrane, which separates the external auditory canal from the middle ear. The external auditory canal contains some hairs and wax-producing glands which, along with the eardrum, prevent foreign objects from entering the ear.

The middle ear is an air-filled cavity containing three small bones known as *ossicles*, two small muscles, and nerve fibers. It is separated from the internal ear by a thin, bony structure containing two small openings known as the *oval* and *round windows*. The three small bones, the *malleus, incus,* and *stapes*, articulate with each other; the malleus is attached to the eardrum; the stapes is attached to the oval window. Microorganisms from the nasopharynx can gain

entrance to the middle ear by means of the eustachian tube and sometimes invade the mastoid process of the temporal bone.

The inner ear consists of three fluid-filled canals: the *vestibule*, the *cochlea*, and the *semicircular canals*. Collectively, those structures are often called the *bony labyrinth* to distinguish them from a tubular membrane within the canals known as the *membranous labyrinth*. The two labyrinthine structures are separated by a fluid called *perilymph*. The fluid within the membrane-lined cavities is known as *endolymph*. Infections of the inner ear frequently produce disturbances in equilibrium or loss of hearing if there is an interruption in transmission of impulses.

MICROBIAL INFECTIONS OF THE EYE

The microorganisms which cause infections of the eye include bacteria, chlamydiae, viruses, protozoa, and fungi. You may recall that one filarial worm, *Loa loa*, has an affinity for ocular tissue. *Toxocara canis, T. cati,* and *Taenia solium* also invade the eye and cause marked allergic responses. Trauma to ocular tissue can provide a portal of entry for any organism. The aqueous and vitreous humors, the fluids of the anterior and posterior chambers of the eye, make excellent culture media. Some microorganisms demonstrate a particular affinity for a specific part of the eye or accessory structure. No infection of the eye should be considered lightly since manifestations of the infection may be serious enough to cause impaired vision or even loss of sight.

BLEPHARITIS

Blepharitis is an inflammation of the eyelid margins caused by an infection of the sebaceous glands. The most common causative agents are staphylococci, although other organisms can be involved. The chronic form of the disease produces thickening of lid margins and loss of lashes.

Transmission. Staphylococci in the indigenous flora of the skin and eye are readily available as potential invaders in blepharitis. Injuries so small as to go unnoticed or excessive secretion of sebum may provide conditions favorable for colonization by staphylococci. Rubbing eyes with hands may contribute to the vulnerability of the eyelids to invasion by microorganisms.

Laboratory Diagnosis. The organisms causing blepharitis are rarely present in large numbers. Swabs are therefore used for direct plating on chocolate agar and blood agar, as well as for inoculating enriched liquid broth. Gram stains of direct smears may or may not reveal the presence of bacteria. Procedures required for identification of staphylococci and streptococci were discussed in Chapter 16.

Immunity. It is doubtful that any lasting immunity to staphylococci or streptococci is produced in eye infections since they tend to remain localized and somewhat sequestered.

Prevention. Avoidance of unnecessary rubbing of eyelids and appropriate attention to ordinary eye care can, no doubt, be deterrents to blepharitis. Prompt treatment with an appropriate antimicrobial agent can prevent spread of the infection to other parts of the eye.

CONJUNCTIVITIS

Conjunctivitis, inflammation of the conjunctiva, can be caused by a variety of bacteria, herpes simplex viruses, and adenoviruses, chiefly of serotype 8. *Moraxella lacunata, Haemophilus aegyptius, Neisseria gonorrhoeae, Corynebacterium species,* staphylococci, and streptococci have been isolated from cases of conjunctivitis. *H. aegyptius* produces the very contagious infection which is sometimes called "pinkeye." The disease is characterized by a profuse catarrhal discharge. Purulent conjunctivitis in adults and the newborn (known as ophthalmia neonatorum) is generally caused by *N. gonorrhoeae*.

Transmission. Transmission of purulent conjunctivitis is usually by direct contact with the causative organism. The newborn acquires *N. gonorrhoeae* during delivery; in an adult the organism spreads to the eye from an infection of the urogenital tract. Other types of conjunctivitis may be transmitted indirectly by the use of common towels.

Laboratory Diagnosis. Gram stains of pus from purulent conjunctivitis usually reveal the presence of the typical gram-negative diplococci of *N. gonorrhoeae*. Gram stains of smears from nonpurulent conjunctivitis may reveal the gram reaction and morphology of the causative organism. However, despite the presence of oppressive symptoms, organisms are often not present in sufficient numbers to be seen on stained smears. Chocolate agar, blood agar, Loeffler's serum medium, and an enriched broth can be employed for primary isolation. Cells of *M. lacunata* die out rapidly at room temperature, but survive for several weeks in the incubator. Morphological, cultural, and biochemical characteristics of other bacterial pathogens have been described elsewhere in Unit Four.

If a viral agent is suspected, a swab, moistened with a sterile diluent, can be rubbed over the infected area, placed in a small quantity of tissue culture medium, and frozen for transfer to an appropriate laboratory. Embryonic kidney cells or continuous cultures of human neoplastic tissues support the growth of commonly isolated adenoviruses. A definitive cytopathic effect (CPE) generally occurs within a few days if adenovirus is present. Serological tests are required to type any isolated adenoviruses.

Immunity. It is unlikely that any lasting high-grade immunity occurs as a result of bacterial or viral conjunctivitis.

Prevention. Ophthalmia neonatorum can be successfully prevented by application of 1 percent silver nitrate to the eyes of the newborn (Figure 24-3). The practice is mandated by law in many

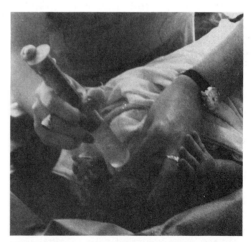

Figure 24-3 Administration of 1 percent silver nitrate in the eyes of a newborn. (Courtesy, National Society for the Prevention of Blindness, Inc., New York.)

parts of the world, including the United States. Avoiding common towels for wiping the face and hands can be an important deterrent to the spread of other types of conjunctivitis. Strict adherence to asepsis in ophthalmological procedures can prevent transmission of the disease by contaminated hands or instruments.

INCLUSION CONJUNCTIVITIS

Inclusion conjunctivitis is an acute inflammation occurring in the newborn as well as in older individuals. The etiological agent, *Chlamydia trachomatis*, can also infect the genitourinary tract. Neonatal conjunctivitis, caused by the chlamydial agent, has a longer incubation period than the gonococcal disease. A copious mucopurulent exudate occurs approximately five days after exposure. Recovery from inclusion conjunctivitis is spontaneous about ten days later.

Transmission. Inclusion conjunctivitis is transmitted to the neonate during delivery if the mother has a genitourinary tract infection. Adults can be exposed to *C. trachomatis* by sexual intercourse or by swimming in unchlorinated swimming pools which are contaminated with exudates from an infection of the eyes, urethra, or cervix.

Laboratory Diagnosis. Scrapings of epithelial cells from the conjunctiva, urethra, or cervix reveal inclusion bodies in the cytoplasm when a Giemsa stain or immunofluorescent technique is applied. *C. trachomatis* can be grown in yolk sacs of embryonated eggs where the chlamydial agent produces elementary and initial bodies. Serological tests are of limited value since some individuals do not develop measurable levels of antibody during an acute infection.

Immunity. No natural or acquired immunity to inclusion conjunctivitis has ever been demonstrated.

Prevention. Since genitourinary tract infections caused by *C. trachomatis* are often inapparent in adults, it is difficult to apply preventative measures. Unfortunately, neither 1 percent silver nitrate nor penicillin ointment affects the chlamydial agent in neonates. Prompt treatment of recognized cases of inclusion conjunctivitis and appropriate chlorination of swimming pools are important deterrents to the spread of the infection.

TRACHOMA

Trachoma is a chronic inflammation of the conjunctiva followed by papillary hyperplasia, invasion of the cornea, eyelid deformities, and progressive loss of vision (Figure 24-4). It is the major cause of preventable blindness in the world. The disease, caused by immunofluorescent types A, B, and C of *Chlamydia trachomatis*, is widespread in India, Africa, and South America. It is common among both Indians and Mexican immigrants in the southwestern part of the United States.

Transmission. Trachoma is readily transmitted by contact with exudates from infected eyes and by flies. Crowding, poor hygiene, and poverty seem to

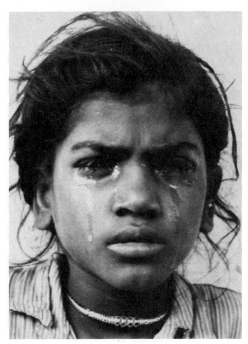

Figure 24-4 Trachoma in a young Indian girl. The suffering caused by the disease is reflected in her face. (Courtesy, World Health Organization, Geneva, Switzerland.)

be factors contributing to the spread of the disease.

Laboratory Diagnosis. Scrapings of epithelial cells from the conjunctiva reveal the presence of inclusion bodies in the cytoplasm using a Giemsa stain or an immunofluorescent technique. The trachoma organism can be cultured in yolk sacs of embryonated eggs, but recovery of the organism is not feasible as a routine laboratory procedure. Serological tests are of limited value.

Immunity. Children appear more susceptible to the trachoma agent then do adults. Recovery from an infection caused by *C. trachomatis* results only in immunity of a low order.

Prevention. Trachoma can be prevented in endemic areas by extensive treatment campaigns using topical tetracyclines. Improvement of basic hygiene for economically underprivileged individuals in developing countries could substantially reduce the number of cases of this debilitating disease. To date, no vaccine has been developed which can successfully combat the infection.

KERATITIS

Keratitis is an inflammation of the cornea. Ulcers are sometimes produced. The infection occurs in conjunction with an infection of the conjunctiva. Acute purulent keratoconjunctivitis may be caused by a variety of bacteria, fungi, and viruses. *Streptococcus pneumoniae* is the most common cause of exogenous infections; it occurs primarily in persons working in particular occupations where airborne environmental debris is unavoidable. Mycotic keratitis is a frequent complication in individuals on corticosteroids or those using eyedrops containing an antimicrobial agent. Herpetic keratitis, caused by the herpesvirus, produces a progressive and painful ulceration of the cornea. The sometimes recurrent nature of the infection is disturbing since scarring can seriously impair vision. Several large outbreaks of keratoconjunctivitis, caused by adenovirus type 8, occur each year in the United

States. That virus is believed to have been the cause of an epidemic of "pink-eye" among West Coast shipyard workers during World War II.

ORBITAL CELLULITIS

Orbital cellulitis is an inflammation of the tissues supporting the eye. It can occur as an infection secondary to sinusitis, pharyngitis, or an abscessed tooth. A variety of bacteria can be involved, including staphylococci and streptococci. Fungi belonging to the genera *Rhizopus*, *Mucor*, and *Absidia* can be opportunistic pathogens in orbital cellulitis, if patients have been compromised by immunosuppressive therapy, leukemia, or diabetic acidosis. The fungi grow within blood vessels of orbital tissue promoting *thrombosis* (for-

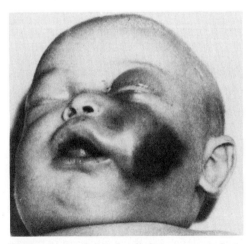

Figure 24-5 Orbital cellulitis in an infant. Occlusion of blood vessels has caused gangrene of left orbit and cheek. (From J. E. Prier and H. Friedman, eds., *Opportunistic Pathogens*, © 1974 University Park Press, Baltimore.)

mation of blood clots). The occlusion of blood vessels by thrombi cause *infarcts* (degeneration of tissue resulting from interruption in blood supply) (Figure 24-5). For this reason blindness is a frequent complication of mycotic orbital cellulitis. A diagnosis of opportunistic phycomycosis requires repeated isolation of the fungal agent from affected tissue.

ENDOPHTHALMITIS

Endophthalmitis is an inflammation of the inner eye which usually involves the vitreous humor, retina, iris, ciliary body, and choroid. Endophthalmitis, following plastic lens implantation, has been reported in several parts of the United States. If the infection spreads to the entire eye, the disease is called *panophthalmitis*. A variety of microbial agents have been implicated. Most organisms gain entrance by a penetrating wound or as a consequence of eye surgery. Strict adherence to appropriate aseptic techniques during surgery and use of protective goggles for certain hazardous occupations could reduce the number of cases of endophthalmitis and the often serious consequence of visual debility or blindness.

TOXOPLASMOSIS

Toxoplasmosis is one of the most common infections occurring in humans throughout the world. In some areas 80 percent or more of the individuals have been exposed to the protozoan causing the disease. The protozoan, *Toxoplasma gondii*, has a complex life cycle involv-

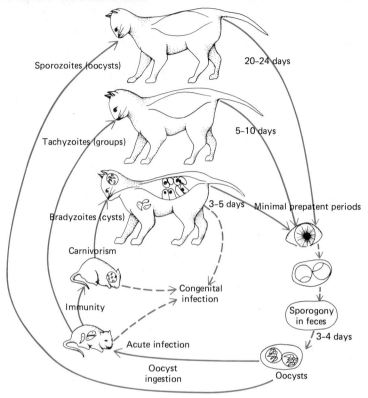

Final hosts: cats and other felines

Sporozoites (oocysts)

20-24 days

Tachyzoites (groups)

5-10 days

Bradyzoites (cysts)

3-5 days   Minimal prepatent periods

Carnivorism

Immunity

Congenital infection

Sporogony in feces

3-4 days

Acute infection

Oocyst ingestion

Oocysts

Figure 24-6 Life cycle of *Toxoplasma gondii* showing stages infective for cats and mice as well as minimal prepatent periods (days elapsing between ingestion of parasites and their appearance in feces) required for the parasites to develop in the cat. (From J. K. Frenkel, in D. M. Hammond and P. L. Long, eds., *The Coccidia,* Baltimore, University Park Press, 1973.)

ing members of the cat family as final hosts (Figure 24-6). Other warm-blooded animals serve as intermediate hosts. Cats become infected by eating mice and birds harboring the parasite. Humans are accidentally infected and very often remain asymptomatic. Toxoplasmosis is sometimes described as a common infection, but a rare disease because of the lack of demonstrable symptoms. In both the congenital and acquired forms of the infection, how-

ever, the choroid and retina can be affected. More serious consequences can occur in the congenital form of toxoplasmosis.

Transmission. In the congenital form of toxoplasmosis the protozoan is transmitted across the placenta to the fetus. The amount of damage to the fetus is related to the trimester of pregnancy in which the disease is acquired. Retinochoroiditis, hepatosplenomegaly (enlargement of the liver and spleen), hydrocephalus (accumulation of cerebrospinal fluid in the ventricles of the brain), cerebral calcification, and convulsions are possible consequences of fetal exposure. Infection may also occur during delivery. The acquired form of toxoplasmosis, occurring in adults, is believed to be transmitted by eating raw or inadequately cooked meat or poultry or by contact with cat feces.

Laboratory Diagnosis. Trophozoites or encysted forms of *T. gondii* can be observed by microscopic examination of tissues or fluids. Sputum, pleural fluid, peritoneal fluid, cerebrospinal fluid, or tissues obtained by biopsy are commonly examined for evidence of the parasite. The organism develops extracellularly as a crescent-shaped trophozoite measuring 4 to 8 μm in length and 2 to 3 μm in width (Figure 24-7). In-

tracellular forms of the parasite are smaller. Membrane-enclosed pseudocysts, measuring 20 to 100 μm in diameter, sometimes develop in the brain and eyes in chronic toxoplasmosis. Localization of the cysts in those areas is presumably caused by failure of sufficient levels of antibodies to penetrate blood-brain or blood-ocular barriers. Mice, inoculated with body fluids containing *T. gondii*, are highly susceptible to infection.

Serological tests are positive early in the acute stage of toxoplasmosis. Antibody titers against *T. gondii* tend to remain high for years following an infection.

Immunity. Although antibodies to *T. gondii* can be demonstrated in large numbers of individuals, their protective value is uncertain.

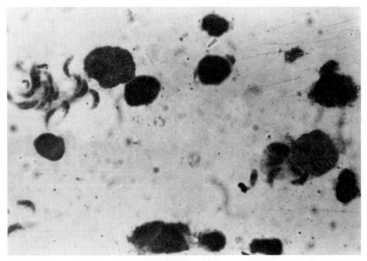

Figure 24-7 Crescent-shaped trophozoites of *Toxoplasma gondii* in pleural fluid. (Courtesy, Estelle Doheny Eye Foundation, Los Angeles.)

Prevention. Avoiding raw or inadequately cooked meat can be a significant deterrent to the spread of toxoplasmosis. In addition, pregnant women can protect themselves from exposure to the protozoan by having other members of the family clean cat-litter boxes. Periodic disinfection of litter boxes is recommended as an additional precautionary measure to avoid contact with the protozoan.

MICROBIAL DISEASES OF THE EAR

A variety of microorganisms can cause infections of the ear. Despite anatomical barriers, the organisms can enter by means of a penetrating wound, the bloodstream, or through the eustachian tube. Viral or bacterial diseases of the nose and throat predispose individuals, especially children, to otitis media and the accompanying earache. Infections of the outer ear (otitis externa) are associated with contaminated fingers, objects used in removing wax from ears, hearing aids, or swimming pool water. The protective enclosure provided by the external auditory canal provides especially favorable growth conditions.

OTITIS MEDIA

Otitis media may be an acute or a chronic infection. Fever, earache, hyperemia, and tenderness of the eardrum occur in both forms of the disease. Sufficient pus formation may cause perfo-

ration of the eardrum and scarring results in hearing impairment.

Transmission. Most cases of otitis media are caused by upward migrations of nasopharyngeal microorganisms by way of the eustachian tube. Staphylococci, streptococci, *Pseudomonas aeruginosa, Haemophilus influenzae, Proteus* species, *Aspergillus fumigatus,* and *Candida albicans* are frequent causes of acute otitis media. Anaerobes, such as *Bacteroides, Fusobacterium,* or anaerobic cocci, are often recovered from patients having chronic otitis media. Etiological agents of otitis media may remain unidentified, despite vigorous attempts to recover them.

Laboratory Diagnosis. Gram stains and cultures of nasopharyngeal secretions sometimes reveal the presence of pathogens, but the evidence is only circumstantial and not always reliable. There appears little justification for performing *tympanocentesis* (puncture of the eardrum), except if the infection does not respond to a broad-spectrum antimicrobial agent.

Immunity. The frequency of recurrent infections indicates that it is doubtful that the localized nature of middle ear infections provides any substantial immunity.

Prevention. Prompt treatment of upper respiratory tract infections and supportive care, afforded by rest, can sometimes prevent the spread of some microorganisms to the middle ear. Migrations of other infectious agents appear unavoidable. Prophylactic use of antimicrobial agents is prescribed by some pediatricians for children with recurrent otitis media.

SUMMARY

The intricate anatomical features of the eyes, ears, and their accessory organs provide effective natural barriers for infectious microorganisms under ordinary circumstances. However, the presence of underlying disease and exposure from penetrating wounds, surgical procedures, or unavoidable environmental debris constitute predisposing factors in eye and ear infections. The dependence of humans on optimal vision and hearing for creating an awareness of the environment, which permits life-saving reactions in emergencies, makes it essential that all infections of those specialized organs be diagnosed and treated promptly. Attention to local eye and ear hygiene is an important deterrent to microbial invasion and can limit ability of the organisms to spread.

QUESTIONS FOR STUDY

1. List three natural barriers which prevent microorganisms from establishing eye infections.
2. Name the common causative agents of nonpurulent and purulent conjunctivitis.
3. How can gonococcal ophthalmia neonatorum be prevented?
4. Name two natural barriers which prevent microorganisms from establishing ear infections.
5. Why do the etiological agents of otitis media often remain unidentified?

SELECTED REFERENCES

Boyd, R. F., and Hoerl, B. G. *Basic Medical Microbiology.* Boston: Little, Brown, 1977.

Davis, B. D.; Dulbecco, R.; Eisen, J. N.; Ginsberg, H. S.; and Wood, W. B., Jr. *Microbiology.* 2d ed. New York: Harper & Row, 1973.

Joklik, W. K., and Willett, H. P. *Zinsser Microbiology.* 16th ed. Englewood Cliffs, N.J.: Prentice-Hall, 1976.

Langley, L. L.: Telford, I. R.; and Christensen, J. B. *Dynamic Anatomy and Physiology.* 4th ed. New York: McGraw-Hill, 1974.

Peery, T. M., and Miller, F. N. *Pathology: A Dynamic Introduction to Medicine and Surgery.* 2d ed. Boston: Little, Brown, 1971.

Tortora, G. J., and Anagnostakos, N. P. *Principles of Anatomy and Physiology.* San Francisco: Harper & Row (Canfield Press), 1975.

U.S. Department of Health, Education, and Welfare. Eye infections after plastic lens implantation—California, Florida, Montana, Ohio. *CDC Morbidity and Mortality Weekly Report* 24:437, 1975.

U.S. Department of Health, Education, and Welfare Toxoplasmosis—Pennsylvania. *CDC Morbidity and Mortality Weekly Report* 24:285, 1975.

U.S. Department of Health, Education, and Welfare. Endophthalmitis associated with implantation of intraocular lens prothesis—United States. *CDC Morbidity and Mortality Weekly Report.* 25:369, 1976.

Wistreich, G. A., and Lechtman, M. D. *Microbology and Human Disease.* 2d ed. Beverly Hills, Calif.: Glencoe Press, 1976.

Chapter 25

Microbial Diseases of the Blood, Lymph, and Reticuloendothelial System

After you read this chapter, you should be able to:

1. Explain the role of circulating and sessile cells of the blood, lymph, and reticuloendothelial system.
2. Discuss the transmission, laboratory diagnosis, immunity, and prevention of rickettsial diseases.
3. Compare the life cycle of malarial parasites in humans and mosquito hosts.
4. Discuss the transmission, laboratory diagnosis, immunity, and prevention of malaria.
5. Compare the life cycles and geographic distribution of the causative agents of trypanosomiasis and leishmaniasis.
6. Discuss the transmission, laboratory diagnosis, immunity, and prevention of trypanosomiasis and leishmaniasis.
7. Compare the life cycles and predilection for particular tissue of the causative agents of schistosomiasis and elephantiasis.
8. Discuss the transmission, laboratory diagnosis, immunity, and prevention of schistosomiasis and elephantiasis.
9. Explain the role of rats, ticks, and lice in the transmission of febrile diseases caused by bacteria.

The blood, lymph, and reticulo-endothelial system contain a variety of circulating and sessile cells. The circulating elements include histiocytes of connective tissue, red blood cells, white blood cells, and platelets, which are fragments of cytoplasm derived from megakaryocytes found in bone marrow. The sessile cells are found in various parts of the body, including blood sinuses of bone marrow, lymph nodes, liver, spleen, adrenal cortex, alveoli, pleural membranes, peritoneum, brain, spinal cord, and subcutaneous connective tissue. The circulating or sessile cells with phagocytic activity are known as *macrophages* (Figure 25-1). The organs of the body containing large numbers of macrophages make up the *reticuloendothelial system* (RES). Unlike other systems in which organs exist in anatomic proximity to one another, the RES constitutes a diffuse system in which the organs share the common characteristic of containing noncirculating cells having phagocytic activity.

BACTERIAL INFECTIONS

In primary bacteremias causative organisms gain access directly to the bloodstream through wounds, burns, or bites of infected animals. The types of bacteria causing infections vary with geographic area, type of services rendered in health care, and level of patient care. Positive blood cultures are always significant since blood is normally sterile.

BUBONIC AND SEPTICEMIC PLAGUE

The most common form of plague in humans is a highly fatal infection called *bubonic plague*. The illness is essentially

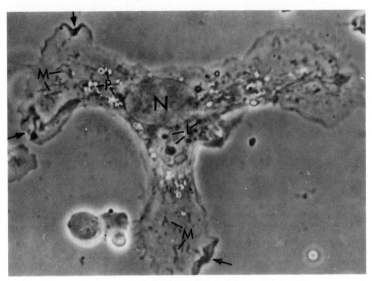

Figure 25-1 A mouse spleen macrophage two hours after removal from the animal. Structural features of the elongated cell include the oval nucleus (N), rod-shaped mitochondria (M), pinocytic vesicles (P), and lysosomes (L) of varying size. (Courtesy, R. Steinman, The Rockefeller University, New York.)

a bacteremia characterized by lymph gland involvement. Infection of the lymph glands produces swellings known as buboes (Figure 25-2). Septicemia can be present in the absence of buboes.

Transmission. The septicemic and bubonic forms of plague are transmitted by the bite of infected rat fleas (*Xenopsylla cheopis*) in other countries, but by contact with an infected animal in the United States. A pharyngeal form of primary septicemic plague can be spread by aerosols from infected individuals. The pneumonic form of the disease, which is a possible consequence of septicemic or bubonic forms, is highly communicable.

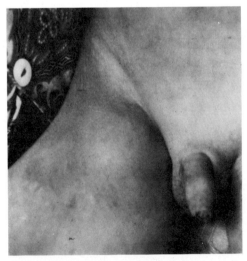

Figure 25-2 Right inguinal bubo in a 7-year-old boy with a classic case of bubonic plague. (Courtesy, Center for Disease Control, Atlanta, Georgia.)

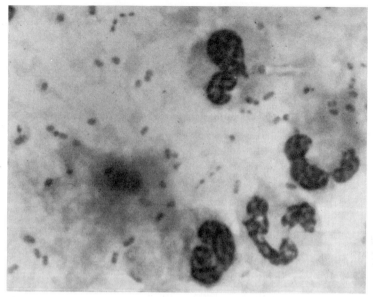

Figure 25-3 Gram stain of pus from a bubo showing *Yersinia pestis*. (Courtesy, American Society for Microbiology, Washington, D.C.)

Laboratory Diagnosis. Positive blood cultures and exudates from buboes reveal the presence of gram-negative bacilli measuring 1.0 to 2.0 μm in length and 0.5 to 1.0 μm in width (Figure 25-3). The bacilli tend to stain darker at the ends, a phenomenon called *bipolar staining.*

Immunity. Recovery from an attack of bubonic or septicemic plague confers only transient immunity to the disease.

Prevention. A vaccine containing killed cells of *Y. pestis* is available for high-risk populations. Prophylactic immunizations are recommended especially for persons traveling to countries where recent epidemics of plague have

occurred. Isolation and disinfection of materials contaminated with the infectious organisms are important deterrents to spread of the disease.

Elimination of plague would require eradication of rodent or other animal reservoirs of *Y. pestis*, as well as rat fleas. Since such massive control programs are not feasible, control measures have instead included periodic surveys in endemic and potentially epidemic areas, as well as rat-proofing of cargo vessels.

TULAREMIA

Tularemia, another bacteremia complicated by infection of lymph nodes, is caused by a gram-negative bacillus,

Franciscella tularensis, which is similar in morphology to *Y. pestis.* The febrile disease was once known as "rabbit fever" because it is most frequently transmitted to humans by handling infected rabbits. It is now known that other wild animals, such as muskrats and bobcats, can harbor the infectious organism. The disease is common throughout North America, but is especially prevalent in autumn during the rabbit hunting season. Tularemia is characterized by an abrupt rise in temperature which persists if untreated. Lymph node enlargement and headache are common and septicemia may occur in severe infections. The sequestering of the pathogens in white blood cells and sessile macrophages of the RES makes the organisms less accessible to antibodies and chemotherapeutic agents.

Transmission. Most cases of tularemia occur as a result of the direct inoculation of *F. tularensis* into the skin or conjunctival sac while handling infected animals. The disease can also be transmitted to humans by bites of ticks (*Dermacentor andersoni,* *D. variabilis,* and *Amblyomma americanum*) and flies (*Chrysops discalis*).

Laboratory Diagnosis. *F. tularensis* grows only on media enriched with cystine and glucose. The organism is highly pleomorphic. A precipitation procedure (Ascoli test) can be applied to extracts of the organism to confirm identification of isolates. Both a skin test and an agglutination test are valuable in suspected cases of tularemia when difficulty is encountered in isolating organisms.

Immunity. Despite the magnitude of the antibody response, immunity does not necessarily follow an attack of tularemia. In animal experiments immunity is conferred by activated macrophages. In persons who have had tularemia, contact with relatively avirulent strains of *F. tularensis* sometimes promotes only a localized papule. However, exposure to virulent strains is known to produce febrile disease a second time.

Prevention. Killed vaccines are of limited value. The administration of an attenuated vaccine by the intradermal multiple puncture method has reduced the incidence and severity of tularemia in laboratory workers. Preventive measures include use of rubber or plastic gloves in handling carcasses, covering exposed parts of the body to avoid bites of arthropods, and thorough cooking of wild game.

RICKETTSIAL DISEASES

The rickettsial diseases of humans can be divided into five groups: typhus fever, spotted fever, tsutsugamushi fever (scrub typhus), trench fever, and Q fever. All but Q fever are caused by rickettsiae which enter and proliferate in the endothelial lining of arterioles and capillaries (Table 25-1). The causative organism of Q fever has a predilection for lung tissue. A fever and a maculopapular rash are universal symptoms of rickettsial diseases of the blood ves-

Table 25-1 RICKETTSIAL DISEASES

GROUP	DISEASE	CAUSATIVE ORGANISM
Typhus fever	epidemic typhus	*Rickettsia prowazekii*
	Brill's disease	*Rickettsia prowazekii*
	endemic typhus	*Rickettsia mooseri*
Spotted fever	Rocky Mountain spotted fever	*Rickettsia rickettsii*
	button fever	*Rickettsia conorii*
	rickettsialpox	*Rickettsia akari*
Tsutsugamushi fever	scrub typhus	*Rickettsia tsutsugamushi*
Trench fever	trench fever	*Rochalimaea quintana*
Q fever	Query fever	*Coxiella burnetii*

sels. Fatality rates may exceed 40 percent in untreated cases.

Rickettsial diseases are worldwide in distribution, but often occur with greater frequency during spring and summer months when activity of their arthropod vectors is increased. Rocky Mountain spotted fever and Q fever are the two most common rickettsial diseases occurring in the United States. There has not been an outbreak of louse-borne typhus in the United States since 1922, but a human reservoir of the disease persists in some parts of the world because the rickettsiae may remain latent in lymph nodes or cells of the reticuloendothelial system after the patient's recovery. A recrudescent and less severe form of typhus fever, called Brill's disease, can appear ten or more years after an initial infection.

Transmission. Most rickettsial diseases are transmitted by insects, mainly fleas and lice, or arachnids, including ticks and mites (Table 25-2). The wood tick, *Dermacentor anderasoni*, is the most important vector of rickettsial disease in western United States (Figure 25-4). It transmits the agent of Rocky Mountain spotted fever. The dog tick, *D. variabilis*, is the vector of the same

Table 25-2 ARTHROPOD VECTORS AND MODES OF TRANSMISSION FOR RICKETTSIAL DISEASES

DISEASE	MODE OF TRANSMISSION	ARTHROPOD VECTOR
Epidemic typhus	feces	*Pediculus humanus corporis* (human louse)
Endemic typhus	feces	*Xenopsylla cheopis* (rat flea)
		Polyplax spinulosus (rat louse)
Rocky Mountain spotted fever	bite	*Dermacentor andersoni* (wood tick)
		Dermacentor variabilis (dog tick)
Rickettsialpox	bite	*Allodermanyssus sanguineus* (mouse mite)
Tsutsugamushi fever	bite	*Trombicula akamushi* (larval mammalian mite)
Trench fever	feces	*Pediculus humanus corporis* (human louse)

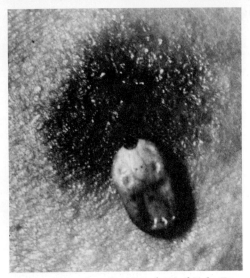

Figure 25-4 Attachment of wood tick, *Dermacentor andersoni,* to the shoulder of a victim. The tick is shown at the site of the lesion (eschar) five days after attachment. *D. andersoni* is the vector for Rocky Mountain spotted fever. (Courtesy, C. T. Taylor, Rocky Mountain Laboratory, Hamilton, Montana.)

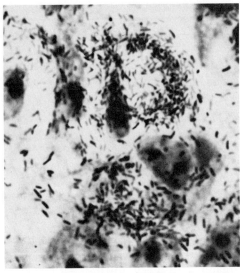

Figure 25-5 *Rickettsia rickettsii,* the causative organism of Rocky Mountain spotted fever, grown in an egg yolk sac. (Courtesy, C. T. Taylor, Rocky Mountain Laboratory, Hamilton, Montana.)

disease in eastern United States. *Allodermanyssus sanguineus,* a mouse mite, transmits rickettsial pox to humans in eastern urban areas. The mite bites humans only in the absence of its murine host. Virulent rickettsiae can, in addition, penetrate the skin or mucous membranes with no evidence of abrasion.

Laboratory Diagnosis. Rickettsiae are pleomorphic coccobacilli that range in size from 0.3 to 0.6 μm in width and 0.8 to 2.0 μm in length. The organisms can be seen in infected cells stained by the Giemsa method (Figure 25-5). Rickettsiae can be isolated from blood, but the techniques required are expensive, dangerous, and available in only a few

places in the United States. Rickettsial diseases can usually be diagnosed clinically. The severity of symptoms and fatality rates associated with the infections demand that treatment be initiated immediately in all suspected cases.

Serological tests are the most practical methods for confirming the presence of rickettsial disease. Complement-fixation (CF) and agglutination tests with rickettsial antigens are usually positive in the second or third week following onset of symptoms.

In addition, sera from individuals with typhus and the spotted fever group agglutinate some *Proteus* strains in the Weil-Felix reaction (Table 25-3). Differential diagnosis depends on the use

Table 25-3 WEIL-FELIX REACTIONS IN RICKETTSIAL DISEASES

DISEASE	OX-19	OX-2	OX-K
Epidemic typhus	4+	1+	0
Endemic typhus	4+	1+	0
Scrub typhus	0	0	3+
Spotted fever group	1+–4+	1+–4+	0
Rickettsialpox	0	0	0
Q fever	0	0	0

SOURCE: Adapted from E. H. Lennette, E. H. Spaulding, and J. P. Truant, *Manual of Clinical Microbiology*, 2d ed. (Washington, D.C.: American Society for Microbiology, 1974).

of three *Proteus* antigens, OX_{19}, OX_2, and OXK. These serological types of *Proteus* share antigens with certain rickettsial organisms so that antibodies cross react. The antigens and antisera for the *Proteus* strains are often more readily available to the small laboratory than are rickettsial antigens. Weil-Felix agglutinins may appear as early as the fifth or sixth day after onset of illness and reach their maximum early in convalescence.

Immunity. Infection with a rickettsial agent produces life-long immunity to that specific agent.

Prevention. A vaccine consisting of formaldehyde-inactivated *Rickettsia rickettsii*, grown in yolk sacs of embryonated eggs, was used in "tickbelt" states until recently. However, the vaccine not only frequently caused untoward side effects, but was subsequently shown to be of questionable value. A new vaccine consisting of killed rickettsiae, grown in monolayer cultures of cells from duck and chicken embryos, is currently being evaluated.

A vaccine prepared by growing *R. prowazekii* in yolk sacs of embryonated eggs is available for travelers to remote areas of South and Central America, Africa, and certain mountainous areas of Asia. Use of insecticides and arachnid repellents is sometimes an effective control measure.

RAT-BITE FEVER (HAVERHILL FEVER)

Rat-bite fever is an acute febrile disease contracted, as the name suggests, from the bite of a rat infected with the bacterium *Streptobacillus moniliformis*. Other bacteria have also been implicated as causative agents in some cases. Rat-bite fever is worldwide in distribution, but it is not a common disease.

Transmission. Rat-bite fever is usually transmitted by a bite, but contact with secretions of an infected animal may be responsible for some sporadic cases of the disease. Some outbreaks have occurred in rat-infested quarters without actual animal contact. One epidemic has been linked to contaminated milk.

Laboratory Diagnosis. Gram-stained smears of blood cultures or joint fluids reveal the presence of gram-negative or irregularly staining coccobacillary forms. The organisms usually measure 0.3 to 0.7 μm in width by 1 to 5 μm in length, but can occur in filaments as long as 150 μm. The microorganisms grow on serum-enriched or ascitic fluid–enriched media in an atmosphere of 5 to 10 percent CO_2. A striking feature of the organism is the spontaneous development of L-phase variants on artificial culture media. The presence of agglutinins in a titer of 1:80 against *S. moniliformis* constitutes sufficient evidence for the infective state.

Immunity. No information is available on resistance which might result from an attack of rat-bite fever.

Prevention. Control of rodent population is the most important measure in prevention.

RELAPSING FEVER

Relapsing fever is a systemic febrile disease characterized by recurrent febrile episodes occurring at intervals of 2 to 14 days. The recurrent rises in temperature are increasingly less severe and shorter in duration. The disease is caused by the spirochete *Borrelia recurrentis*, which can be found in blood during febrile periods. Transitory petechial rashes (patches of purple discoloration resulting from small hemorrhages in skin or mucous membrane) are common in some patients. Relapsing fever is worldwide in distribution, but epidemics tend to be more prevalent in overcrowded populations with poor habits of personal hygiene.

Transmission. Epidemic relapsing fever is transmitted by the lice *Pediculus humanus corporis* and *Pediculus humanus capitis*. Lice are infected by biting individuals with the disease. The arthropods remain infected for their lifetime, which ranges from five to six weeks. The *Borrelia* occupy the body cavities of their arthropod hosts and escape only when lice are injured. Consequently, one louse can infect only one person.

Endemic relapsing fever is tick-borne. The spirochetes, which can persist in coxal fluid, saliva, and feces of ticks for years, are transmitted from one generation of tick to another. In the United States soft ticks belonging to the genus *Ornithodoros* transmit relapsing fever. The ticks feed exclusively on blood. Persons are most often victimized by the ticks at night and are often unaware of bites.

Laboratory Diagnosis. Relapsing fever can be diagnosed by finding *B. recurrentis* in Giemsa-stained blood smears or in intraperitoneal fluid after inoculation of rats or mice (Figure 25-6). Animal blood should be checked daily for appearance of the spirochetes. The spirochetes are 10 to 20 μm long and 0.2 to 0.5 μm wide. *B. recurrentis* can also be stained with aniline dyes. With the Gram-stain technique the organisms appear gram-negative. Serological techniques are limited in diagnostic value since antigens of *B. recurrentis* are quite unstable.

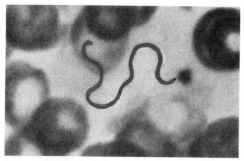

Figure 25-6 *Borrelia recurrentis* in Giemsa-stained mouse blood. (Courtesy, Center for Disease Control, Atlanta, Georgia.)

Immunity. Immunity following an attack of relapsing fever is of short duration in most individuals. When immunity is maintained over a period of years, the resistance is usually attributable to superinfection with the spirochete.

Prevention. In louse-borne relapsing fever control depends on eradication of lice. Delousing with an insecticidal powder, such as 10 percent benzenehexachloride, may be required for the individual patient and his clothing. In the tick-borne disease cleaning and spraying cabins with insecticides may be a deterrent and protective clothing may prevent exposure.

VIRAL INFECTIONS

Primary viremias (viral infections of blood which are not the result of dissemination from another part of the body), are most often the result of direct invasion of the bloodstream following the bite of an arthropod. It is still not practical for most clinical laboratories to pursue isolation of viruses, but services of regional public health laboratories are accessible without cost to the patient. It is often more practical to obtain acute and convalescent sera for serological studies then it is to attempt to obtain suitable specimens for isolation of a virus from whole blood. Demonstration of elevated titers of antibodies for a particular virus is more meaningful than isolation of a virus. Mere isolation of a virus from a clinical specimen does not necessarily implicate that virus as a cause of illness. The history of the patient, geographic area, and symptoms are important in selection of tests for particular antibodies in a suspected viremia. A number of viruses cause subclinical infections in humans, but a few viruses are highly virulent.

VIRAL HEMORRHAGIC FEVERS

The viral hemorrhagic fevers consist of a group of systemic diseases affecting humans, and sometimes animals; they include yellow fever (urban and sylvan), hemorrhagic dengue fever, Lassa fever, and at least seven other varieties of hemorrhagic diseases occurring from the Congo to the USSR. The hemorrhagic diseases are widespread geographically, but tend to be present in larger numbers in tropical and subtropical climates. None of the etiological agents occurs naturally in the United States.

The hemorrhagic fevers are extremely debilitating and some have high fatality rates. For example, average deaths of patients hospitalized with Lassa fever have been 36 percent. Hemorrhagic dengue has a fatality rate as high as 8 percent in children. Many of the diseases are transmitted by mosquitoes and ticks. The mosquito, *Aedes aegypti*, is an important vector in both yellow fever and dengue.

Only a few public health laboratories are set up to identify viral agents of the hemorrhagic fevers. The viruses stimulate production of hemagglutination-inhibiting, neutralizing, or complement-fixing antibodies.

Recovery from yellow fever confers lasting immunity. An episode of dengue fever provides immunity of long duration for the type-specific virus only and limited immunity for at least three other serological types known to cause the disease. Experience with other hemorrhagic fevers has been insufficient to determine definitive information concerning the duration of immunity following infections. There are no vaccines in general use except the attenuated tissue culture vaccine for yellow fever.

UNDIFFERENTIATED TOGAVIRUS FEVERS

A group of undifferentiated, arthropod-borne togavirus fevers occurs throughout the world. Most notable among these diseases is the classic dengue fever in the tropics, but others, such as Colorado tick fever, are found sporadically in the United States. Dengue fever is spread by *Aedes* mosquitoes, including *A. aegypti*; the arthropod host of

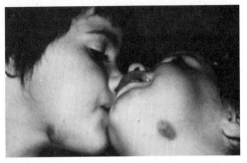

Figure 25-7 Sisters with submandibular lymphadenitis following numerous cat scratches. (Courtesy, H. G. Cramblett, Ohio State University Medical Illustrations, Columbus, Ohio.)

Colorado tick fever is the tick *Dermacentor andersoni*. Death is rare from the togavirus fevers and recovery is usually complete.

CAT-SCRATCH FEVER

Cat-scratch fever is a disease which, as the name indicates, follows the scratch of a cat. Development of a papule at the wound site is followed by lymphadenopathy (Figure 25-7). The disease is rarely serious, but the fever, chills, and swollen lymph nodes mimic other illnesses, including malignancies. The etiological agent remains unknown although chlamydiae, viruses, and bacteria are all suspected as possible causes of the febrile disease.

PROTOZOAL INFECTIONS

A few protozoa have a propensity for taking up residence within blood cells, plasma, lymph nodes, or organs of the

RES. All require an arthropod to complete their life cycle. The parasites are transmitted to humans through the bite of a protozoan-infested arthropod. The intensity of the symptoms depends on the location of the parasite within the host, the toxicogenic capacity of the protozoan, and the reaction of the host to invasion by the parasite.

MALARIA

Malaria is an acute and sometimes chronic disease which at one time was a leading cause of illness and death throughout the world. It is estimated that the disease still affects some 100 million persons each year, most in tropical and subtropical climates of Africa, Asia, Central America, South America, and the islands of the Southwest Pa-

cific. Each year over 1 million children, under the age of 14, die in tropical Africa alone from malaria. Most cases appearing in the United States are related to exposure during a tour of military duty or travel to areas in which malaria is endemic.

Human malaria is caused by four species of the protozoan *Plasmodium: P. malariae, P. vivax, P. falciparum,* and *P. ovale.* All the species are carried by the female *Anopheles* mosquito. Distribution of the species and thus the incidence of the infections they cause are related to geographic conditions (Table 25-4). The most common malarial parasite in temperate zones is *P. vivax.* Malaria can recur after many years since the plasmodia, particularly *P. vivax,* can persist in a dormant state for years in the liver. The multiplication and release

Table 25-4 CHARACTERISTICS OF INFECTIONS CAUSED BY MALARIAL PARASITES

CHARACTERISTIC	P. vivax	P. malariae	P. falciparum	P. ovale
Geographic distribution	temperate and tropical	subtropical	tropical	tropical
Exoerythrocytic period (days)	8	12	6	9
Erythrocytic period (hours)	45±	72	48	49
Average parasitemia (per mm³)	20,000	6,000	100,000–500,000	9,000
Severity	mild to severe	mild	severe	mild
Duration of infection (years)	1–3	10–30	0.5–1.5	—
Name of disease	benign tertian	quartan	malignant tertian	benign tertian
Prognosis	favorable	favorable	guarded	favorable

SOURCE: Adapted from W. H Brown, *Basic Clinical Parasitology,* 4th ed. (Englewood Cliffs, N.J.: Prentice-Hall, 1975).

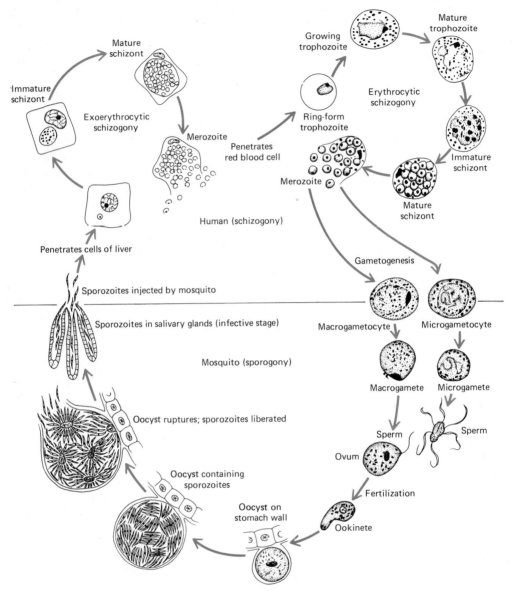

Figure 25-8   Life cycle of a malarial parasite. The sexual cycle (sporogony) takes place in the mosquito, whereas the asexual cycle (schizogony) takes place in the human.

of infective forms is often triggered by physical stress.

The life cycles of the *Plasmodium* species are complex (Figure 25-8). The human serves as the intermediate host for the phase of asexual reproduction, known as *schizogony;* the mosquito serves as the definitive host for the phase of sexual reproduction known as *sporogony.*

Life Cycle in the Human. The asexual phase of the life cycle is divided into two developmental periods: exoerythrocytic (outside red blood cells) and erythrocytic (inside red blood cells). An infected mosquito introduces infective stages of the *Plasmodium* parasite, known as *sporozoites,* into the blood when it bites a person. The exoerythrocytic period begins when the parasites are transported to the liver. Asexual progeny, known as *merozoites,* are released into the circulation in approximately 8 to 12 days, depending on the species. The merozoites penetrate red blood cells, starting the erythrocytic developmental period. The asexual phase occurring in the erythrocytes is known as *schizogony.*

Early in the erythrocytic period the parasites take the form of signet rings, but in the oxygen-rich environment of the red blood cells they soon develop into ameboid *trophozoites.* The mature trophozoites undergo mitosis and segmentation to produce *schizonts* that contain an average of 6 to 20 *merozoites,* depending on the species. When red blood cells rupture, releasing merozoites and toxins associated with metabolic processes of the organisms, the infected host experiences a fever followed by a chill.

Although in early stages of malarial infections no periodicity in fevers and chills can be recognized, symptoms occur with greater regularity as synchrony is established in developmental cycles. Intermittent paroxysms of fever occur when merozoites are released from parasitized red blood cells. The time interval required for development of *P. vivax, P. ovale,* and *P. falciparum* is 48 hours: a period of 72 hours is required for *P. malariae* (Figure 25-9). There is a progressive anemia as erythrocytes rupture upon completion of successive asexual developmental periods. The most serious illness is caused by *P. falciparum.* That organism is sometimes responsible for an acute hemolytic syndrome known as *blackwater fever.* Circulatory disturbances can also complicate infections caused by *P. falciparum* when parasites block capillaries. Obstruction of cerebral capillaries causes delirium, convulsions, coma, and ultimately death.

Some merozoites differentiate within the environment of the red blood cells to form sex cells known as *gametocytes.* The gametocytes are ingested with the blood meal by a mosquito when it bites the human host.

Life Cycle in the Mosquito. The female gametocytes (*macrogametocytes*) and male gametocytes (*microgametocytes*) undergo a short developmental period in the stomach of the *Anopheles* mosquito during which globular *macrogametes* and motile *microgametes* are formed. Fertilization occurs when

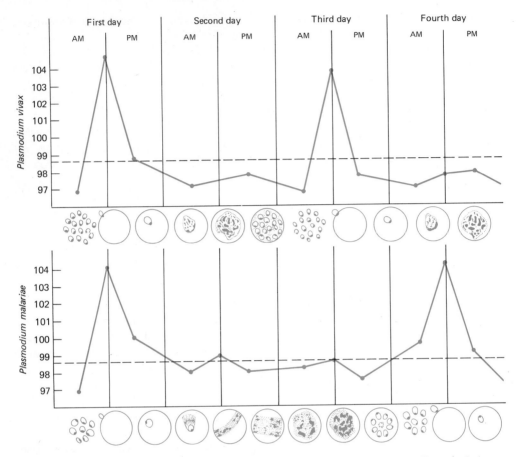

Figure 25-9 Temperature curves in benign tertian (*P. vivax*) and quartan (*P. malariae*) malaria. Temperature spikes when merozoites are released from parasitized red blood cells. (From H. W. Brown, *Basic Clinical Parasitology*, 4th ed., Englewood Cliffs, N.J.: Prentice-Hall, 1975.)

the motile microgametes enter the cytoplasm of the macrogametes to form *zygotes*. Within 12 to 24 hours the zygotes develop into *ookinetes*, elongated motile forms, which penetrate the wall of the stomach and lodge between the epithelial and muscle layers. Approximately 40 hours later *oocysts*, the encysted forms of ookinetes, are observable. A reorganization occurring within the oocysts results in the formation of thousands of sporozoites. Rupture of the sac liberates sporozoites into the body cavity of the mosquito where the actively motile forms migrate to various body parts, including the salivary glands. The sexual phase occurring in the mosquito is known as *sporogony*.

The life cycle is repeated when sporo-zoites are injected into the human host by the bite of the mosquito.

Transmission. The most common means of transmission for malaria is by the bite of an infected female *Anopheles* mosquito, but the disease can also be transmitted by blood transfusion from an infected donor. Malaria has been reported to spread among drug addicts by use of a common syringe contami-nated with the protozoa. In malaria originating from a transfusion or sy-ringe the exoerythrocytic cycle is pre-cluded, so that symptoms appear ear-lier. The plasmodia do not readily penetrate the placental barrier, but a breach in the placenta can provide a portal of entry for a congenitally ac-quired infection.

Laboratory Diagnosis. A diagnosis of malaria is made by finding the para-sites on thin or thick blood smears, after application of Giemsa stain (Figure 25-10). It is sometimes necessary to sample blood repeatedly in order to demon-strate the parasites. Blood can be taken at any stage of the infection with *P.*

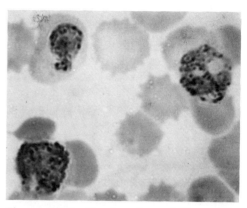

Figure 25-10 Trophozoites of *Plasmodium vivax* in a peripheral blood smear. (Cour-tesy, Carolina Biological Supply Company, Burlington, North Carolina.)

malariae, P. vivax, or *P. ovale.* If an in-fection with *P. falciparum* is suspected, peripheral blood obtained after the fever spike is more likely to contain ring forms. The appearance of more than one ring form in a single red blood cell is common in infections caused by *P. falciparum.* It takes a good deal of ex-perience and careful observation to spe-ciate malarial organisms, but a few characteristics are quite definitive (Table 25-5).

Table 25-5 DEFINITIVE CHARACTERISTICS OF THREE SPECIES OF *PLASMODIUM* AND INFECTED RED BLOOD CELLS

CHARACTERISTIC	*P. vivax*	*P. malariae*	*P. falciparum*
Size of infected cell	increased	no change	no change
Shape of infected cell	irregular	no change	no change
Parasitic forms present	all	all	rings, gametocytes
Size of trophozoites	3+	2+	1+
Inclusions	Schuffner's granules	none	Maurer's spots

Immunity. Some immunity is derived from an attack of malaria, although the amount of resistance appears quite variable. In hyperendemic areas children frequently develop an immunity for life if they are infected before the age of 3 or contract malaria several times early in life.

Prevention. Most measures for prevention of malaria have been aimed at mosquito control. The application of insecticides to breeding places can reduce the opportunity for larvae to hatch. Insect repellents, applied to the skin or clothing, and use of mosquito nets over beds are significant prophylactic measures in preventing mosquito bites. However, most mosquito-control programs are cumbersome and expensive to administrate.

Careful screening of blood donors for evidence of past infection with malarial parasites can prevent transmission of malaria by transfusions. Prophylactic use of chemotherapeutic agents, such as primaquine, chloroquine, and atabrine, has been successful in endemic areas.

Attempts to develop a suitable vaccine have been hampered until recently by the inability to culture the plasmodia outside the host. Plasmodia now can be maintained *in vitro* almost indefinitely through the use of special buffered culture media, gases, and blood free from white blood cells. However, the low immunogenicity of the malarial parasites must be overcome before a successful vaccine can be developed.

BABESIOSIS

Babesiosis is primarily a febrile disease of cattle, but it has been reported in splenectomized individuals and others in the past few years. It is caused by the tick-borne sporozoa *Babesia bovis* and *B. bigemina*. *Babesia* organisms infect red blood cells and may be confused on stained blood smears with *Plasmodium* species. The ring forms of *Babesia* are smaller than those of the malarian parasites, however. Red blood cells often contain four or five rings per cell. Recognition and control of the babesiosis in animals are important deterrents to the transmission of the disease to humans.

TRYPANOSOMIASIS

In the human host trypanosomiasis is a disease of the blood, lymph, or cerebrospinal fluid caused by the protozoan *Trypanosoma gambiense*, *T. rhodesiense*, or *T. cruzi*. *T. gambiense* and *T. rhodesiense* are limited to Africa; *T. cruzi* is confined to the Western Hemisphere. Infections caused by *T. gambiense* are generally found in West Africa; disease caused by *T. rhodesiense* is more common in East Africa. Trypanosomes spend a part of their life cycle in an invertebrate host and can affect mammals other than man.

In early stages of African trypanosomiasis lymph nodes are enlarged and fever, headache, and insomnia are present. The trypanosomes later migrate to the central nervous system causing meningoencephalitis and meningomyelitis. In terminal stages patients develop a characteristic sleeping sickness.

American trypanosomiasis (Chagas' disease) usually occurs in children. It is particularly prevalent in rural districts

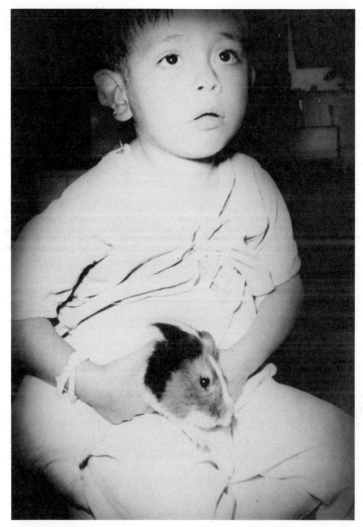

Figure 25-11   Romañas sign in a child with Chagas' disease. (From H. Zaiman, *A Pictorial Presentation of Parasites.*)

of Central and South America where the arthropod hosts of *T. cruzi* find refuge in the cracks of adobe houses. Fever, rash, lymphadenitis, conjunctivitis, and hepatosplenomegaly (enlargement of liver and spleen) are common manifestations of the disease. Edema of the eyelids (Romañas sign) often is found in acute cases (Figure 25-11). The meningoencephalitis or meningomyelitis occurring as a result of the infection can be life threatening. In chronic cases the heart or intestine may be affected.

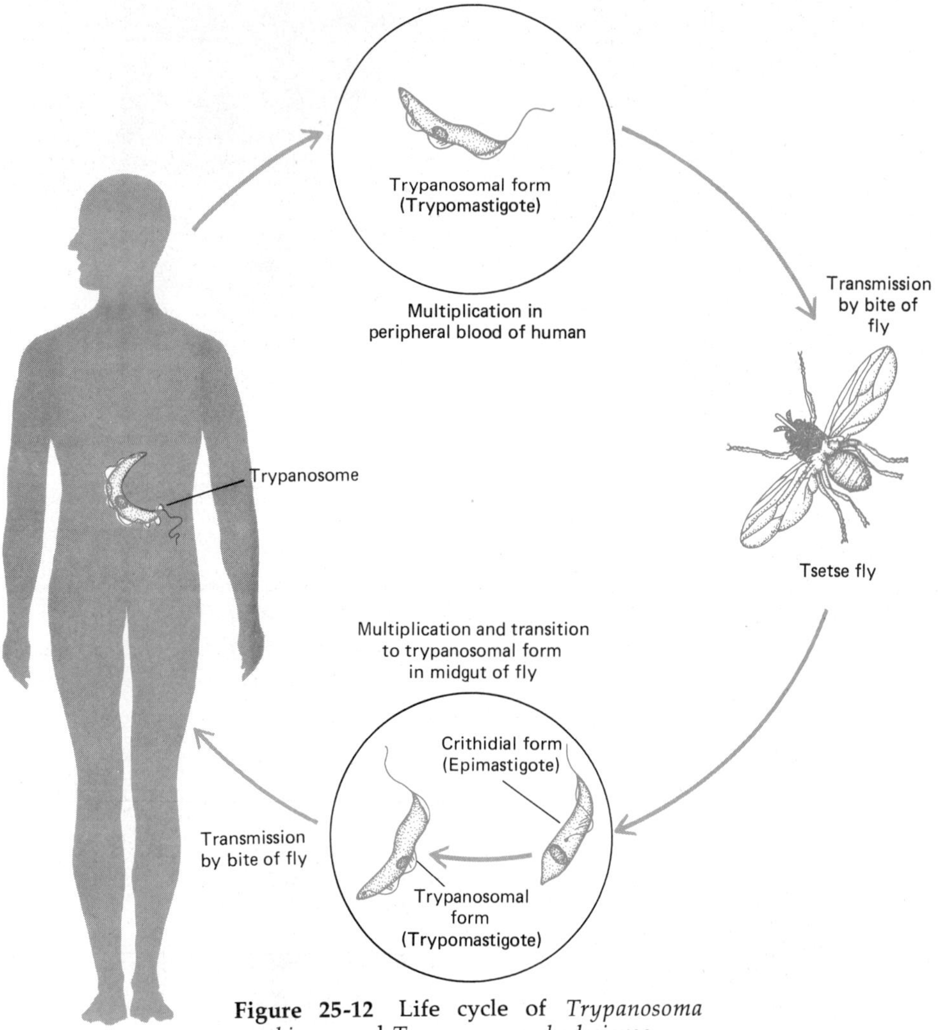

Figure 25-12 Life cycle of *Trypanosoma gambiense* and *Trypanosoma rhodesiense*.

Life Cycle. *T. gambiense* and *T. rhodesiense* spend a part of their life cycle in the *Glossina* (tsetse) flies (Figure 25-12). The crithidial form (epimastigote), occurring in the mid gut of tsetse flies, is an extracellular developmental stage in which the organism is elongated and flagellated (Figure 25-13). The extracellular trypanosomal form (trypoma-stigote) dominates in the mammalian host. It is differentiated from the crithidial form by the position of the kinetoplast, a collective term for a parabasal body and a blepharoplast. The kinetoplast is posterior to the nucleus in trypanosomal forms, and adjacent to the nucleus in crithidial forms. Completion of the life cycle is dependent on an

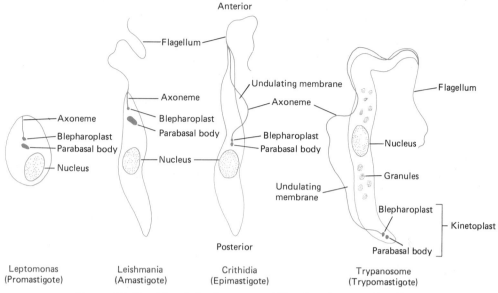

Figure 25-13   Morphologic stages of blood and tissue flagellates.

alteration between the invertebrate tsetse flies and suitable vertebrate hosts, which include pigs, goats, and cattle, as well as humans.

T. cruzi spends a part of its life cycle in the intestine of one or more species of the reduviid or kissing bug (Figure 25-14). Crithidial (epimastigote) and trypanosomal (trypomastigote) forms occur in the insects. Those forms as well

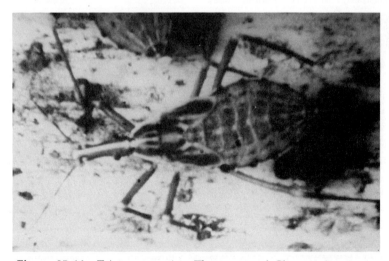

Figure 25-14   *Triatoma* species. The vector of Chagas' disease is more commonly known as the reduviid or kissing bug. (From H. Zaiman, *A Pictorial Presentation of Parasites.*)

as leptomonads (promastigote) and leishmania (amastigote) may be present in mammals, including humans (Figure 25-13). Leptomonads are elongated, slender, and flagellated forms. The kinetoplasts are located near the anterior end. Leishmanial forms are small, spherical or oval nonflagellated intracellular bodies characterized by postcentral nuclei and anterior kinetoplasts. Burrows of rodents and armadillos are often reservoirs of infected reduviid bugs.

Transmission. *T. gambiense* and *T. rhodesiense* are transmitted by the bite of tsetse flies after the parasites have undergone cyclic development in the invertebrate host. *Glossina palpalis* is the principal vector for *T. gambiense*, whereas *G. morsitans* transmits *T. rhodesiense*. Mechanical and congenital transmission can also occur, but African trypanosomiasis is not directly spread from person to person. Tsetse flies remain infected for life.

T. cruzi is transmitted by fecal material of the blood-sucking reduviid bugs. *Triatoma infestans*, *Rhodnius prolixus* and *Panstrongylus megistus* are the primary vectors, although many triatomids are infected with *T. cruzi*. The bugs defecate at the same time they bite causing contamination of the bite-wound with the infectious protozoa. Transfusion of blood containing *T. cruzi* is an alternate mode of transmission. The protozoa can also pass through the placental barrier causing congenital infection.

Laboratory Diagnosis. A definitive diagnosis of African trypanosomiasis

can be made by finding trypanosomes in blood, lymph nodes, bone marrow, or cerebrospinal fluid. *T. gambiense* is rarely found in blood except during febrile periods. The parasite has an average length of about 20 μm and is typically C- or U-shaped. Multiple examinations of thick blood smears, stained by the Giemsa technique, are desirable. Guinea pigs inoculated with blood containing either parasite demonstrate an abundance of organisms in their blood after two weeks.

T. cruzi can be detected on Giemsa-stained, thick blood smears for the first six weeks of the disease. The parasites look quite similar to the African trypanosomes, but do not multiply in blood (Figure 25-15). Organisms enter reticuloendothelial tissue, the central nervous

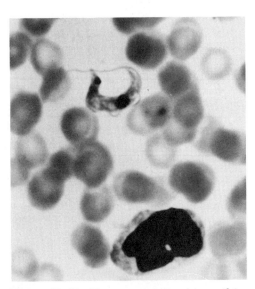

Figure 25-15 *Trypanosoma cruzi* in a thin Giemsa-stained blood smear. (Courtesy, Center for Disease Control, Atlanta, Georgia.)

system, and cardiac tissue. Within these tissues, multiplication and transition into leishmanial forms is followed by destruction of host cells. The diagnostic method of choice is *xenodiagnosis*. In xenodiagnosis trypanosome-free reduviid bugs are permitted to feed on the blood of the individual suspected of having Chagas' disease. If the person is infected, the protozoal parasites can be recovered from the bugs after approximately two weeks. Indirect hemagglutination and complement-fixation tests are available, but are reliable only in chronic cases of American trypanosomiasis.

Immunity. Susceptibility to the African or American variety of trypanosomiasis appears to be universal. Although antibodies to the trypanosomes can sometimes be demonstrated, their protective value is probably minimal.

Prevention. Prevention of trypanosomiasis is dependent on adequate control of the insect vectors. Replacement of adobe housing, where cracks provide ideal lodging places for reduviid bugs, is desirable, but not always practical. Spraying with insecticides with residual action and use of protective nets can reduce the spread of Chagas' disease. In endemic areas blood should be screened for the presence of the parasites before it is used for transfusions.

LEISHMANIASIS

Visceral leishmaniasis, or *kala azar*, is a chronic systemic disease in which the spleen, liver, bone marrow, lymph

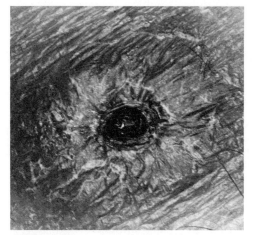

Figure 25-16 Lesion of acute cutaneous leishmaniasis, or Oriental sore. (Courtesy, R. C. Rau, Columbus, Ohio.)

nodes, intestinal mucosa, or other organs are invaded by the protozoan, *Leishmania donovani*. A more limited disease, in which parasites are restricted to intracellular invasion of white blood cells and epithelial cells of cutaneous tissues or mucous membranes, is caused by *L. tropica* or *L. braziliensis*.

A cutaneous form of leishmaniasis, caused by *L. tropica*, is endemic in some parts of Asia, North Africa, southern Europe, and both Central and South America; it is often called *Oriental sore*. Mucocutaneous leishmaniasis occurs in Mexico and much of South America. The disease is characterized by ulcers which metastasize (Figure 25-16). Ulcerative metastases constitute the primary lesions in a type of leishmaniasis known as *espundia*.

The general debility associated with both visceral and cutaneous forms of leishmaniasis makes individuals particularly susceptible to secondary bacterial infections.

Life Cycle. *Leishmania* parasites exist in different morphological forms in their vertebrate and invertebrate hosts. In humans the parasites are found only in the leishmanial form as intracellular, nonflagellated, oval bodies; the organisms in this form are called *Leishmani-Donovan* (LD) bodies. The life cycle is maintained only if leishmanial forms are ingested by sandflies belonging to the genus *Phlebotomus.* Leptomonads develop in the intestinal tract of the flies, and migrate to the buccal cavity. When the sandflies bite humans, dogs, or wild animals, leishmanial forms develop in reticuloendothelial cells of the skin, mucous membranes, or viscera.

Transmission. Both visceral and cutaneous leishmaniasis are usually transmitted by the bite of infected sandflies. Venereal transmission has been documented in one case of the visceral form of the disease, and cutaneous leishmaniasis can be transmitted by direct contact with an infected person or animal.

Laboratory Diagnosis. A diagnosis of visceral leishmaniasis depends on finding LD bodies in Giemsa-stained blood smears or aspirates of the spleen, liver, lymph nodes, or bone marrow. Splenic aspirates are the most reliable for diagnosing the disease. The LD bodies appear as blue, round or oval bodies about 2.0 to 3.0 μm in length and 1.0 to 1.5 μm in width; they typically contain two chromatin masses which stain red to purple (Figure 25-17). Fluorescent-tagged antibodies will also detect the presence of parasites on smears. Com-

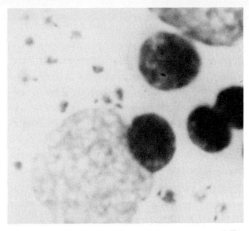

Figure 25-17 Leishman-Donovan (LD) bodies in human bone marrow smear stained with Giemsa stain. (Courtesy, R. Yaeger, New Orleans, Louisiana.)

plement-fixation tests are of limited value.

A diagnosis of cutaneous leishmaniasis can be made by observing leishmanial forms of *L. tropica* or *L. braziliensis* in scrapings from skin lesions after staining by the Giemsa technique. An intracutaneous skin test which employs antigens for *L. braziliensis* is useful as a screening procedure for detection of past or present American leishmaniasis.

Immunity. Recovery from either the visceral or cutaneous form of leishmaniasis confers lasting immunity, but there is not enough heterogenicity of antigenic components of the protozoal parasites to afford universal leishmanial resistance.

Prevention. Preventative measures include control of sandfly breeding places with insecticides and use of protective clothing and nets in endemic areas. Prompt diagnosis and treatment of infected persons is especially important in the cutaneous disease, since direct transmission of the disease is common.

HELMINTHIC INFECTIONS

A few flukes and filarial worms, upon gaining entrance through the skin, become lodged in veins or lymph nodes. The larval forms of various genera have well-developed migratory capabilities, but exhibit distinct anatomic selectivity in establishing permanent residence within a host. Accumulation of adult forms in blood vessels of particular organs or in lymph nodes predisposes affected areas to bacterial infections or malignancy. Toxic and allergic reactions may cause concomitant rashes, petechial hemorrhages, edema, and serious obstructions. External factors, such as nutrition and climate, frequently influence the severity of disease.

SCHISTOSOMIASIS (BILHARZIASIS)

Schistosomiasis is the most debilitating disease caused by helminths. Its etiological agents are three species of the blood fluke *Schistosoma: S. mansoni, S. haematobium,* and *S. japonicum.* Their geographic distribution is dependent on the habitat of their intermediate molluscan hosts. The adult worms lodge in the veins of the colon (*S. mansoni*), bladder (*S. haematobium*), or small intestine (*S. japonicum*). In urinary bilharziasis the bladder mucosa and wall as well as the blood vessels contain eggs of *S. haematobium.* The eggs may occlude blood vessels and predispose the bladder to malignancy.

Schistosomiasis occurs in Africa, South America, the Middle East, India, and the Orient (Figure 25-18). In some places more than half of the population is affected. None of the blood flukes is known to occur in North America.

Life Cycle. The mature eggs of *Schistosoma* species, excreted in urine or feces, hatch into ciliated miracidia which must find refuge in a suitable snail within approximately 32 hours (Figure 25-19). *Biomphalaria, Bulinus,* and *Physopsis* species serve as intermediate hosts for *S. haematobium; Biomphalaria* species and some species of *Tropicorbis* harbor *S. mansoni; Oncomelania* species are often infected with *S. japonicum.*

In the snail two sporocyst generations are required to produce freeswimming cercariae. The cercariae can penetrate the skin of an intermediate host or may become encysted on a leafy vegetable as metacercariae. A single miracidium may form as many as 100,000 to 200,000 cercariae.

Transmission. Schistosomiasis is transmitted by contact of the skin with fresh water contaminated with cercariae of the blood flukes. The cercariae shed their tails and enter the skin, aided by digestive enzymes of the larval forms. The cercariae can also be ingested in contaminated water.

Laboratory Diagnosis. The eggs of the schistosomes can be identified in

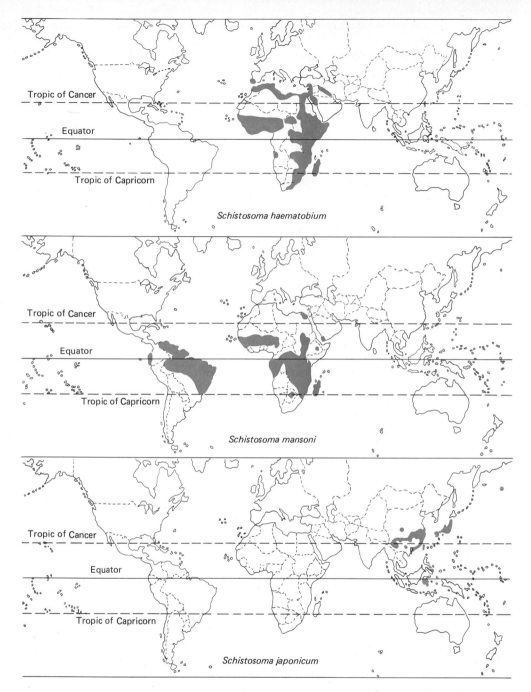

Tropic of Cancer

Equator

Tropic of Capricorn

Schistosoma haematobium

Tropic of Cancer

Equator

Tropic of Capricorn

Schistosoma mansoni

Tropic of Cancer

Equator

Tropic of Capricorn

Schistosoma japonicum

Figure 25-18   Geographic distribution of schistosomiasis by species of *Schistosoma*. (From D. L. Belding, *Textbook of Parasitology*, 3rd ed., Englewoods Cliffs, N.J., Prentice-Hall, 1965.)

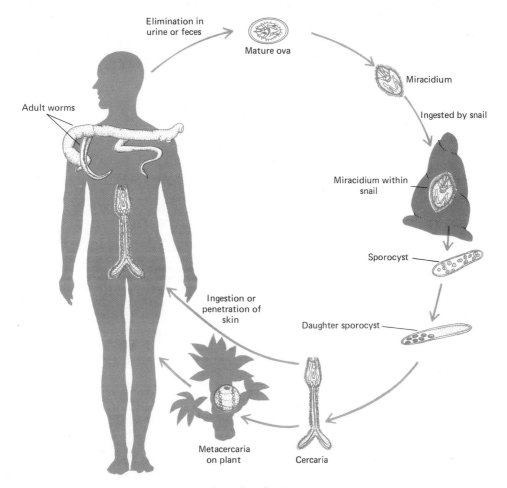

Figure 25-19 Life cycle of *Schistosoma japonicum.*

wet mounts of urine or feces. The eggs of *S. mansoni* average 150 μm in length and 60 μm in width and have a well-defined lateral spine (Figure 25-20). Eggs of *S. japonicum* are smaller and have a less conspicuous lateral spine. Eggs of *S. haematobium* are more similar in size to those of *S. mansoni,* but have a small terminal spine. Biopsies of intestinal mucosa may reveal the presence of *S. mansoni* or *S. japonicum* if stool specimens are negative. Serological tests lack specificity because cross-reactions occur with other parasitic, bacterial, and viral infections.

Immunity. Although antibodies can be demonstrated in schistosomiasis, their protective value is uncertain.

Prevention. Safe disposal of feces and urine is probably the most effective deterrent to the spread of schistosomiasis. Preventing the eggs from reaching freshwater habitats of snails interrupts the life cycle. In addition, molluscicides

571

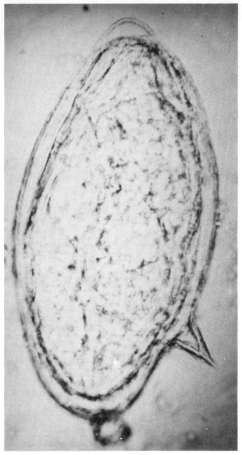

Figure 25-20 Egg of *Schistosoma mansoni* with a well-defined lateral spine. (Courtesy, Abbott Laboratories, *Atlas of Diagnostic Microbiology*, p. 67, July, 1974.)

and swamp drainage can be employed to reduce the snail population. Covering areas of the body which are exposed to contaminated water can block entrance of cercariae through the skin.

ELEPHANTIASIS

Elephantiasis is a chronic consequence of an infection caused by the filarial nematodes *Wuchereria bancrofti* and *Brugia malayi*. Mixed infections have

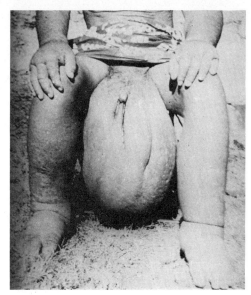

Figure 25-21 Elephantiasis of arms, legs and genitals in a resident of the Society Islands in the South Pacific. (Courtesy, J. F. Kessel, Santa Monica, California.)

been reported. In the obstructive form of the disease the scrotum, leg, or breast may be grossly enlarged because of blockage of lymphatic vessels (Figure 25-21). The parasites are worldwide in distribution, but are most common in tropical and subtropical climates. The infection was introduced in the United States with slavery, but has since disappeared. The prognosis of elephantiasis is extremely poor unless surgery can be performed to alleviate the obstruction. Superimposed bacterial infections frequently complicate the disease.

Life Cycle. Humans are the only definitive hosts for *W. bancrofti* and *B. malayi*. The adult worms live in lymph nodes where the females give birth to microfilariae. The microfilariae are transported by lymph to the bloodstream where they circulate freely. Nocturnal periodicity, that is, appearance of

572

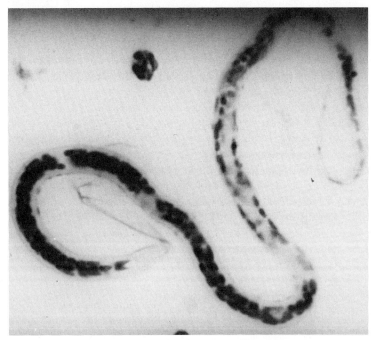

Figure 25-22 Sheathed microfilaria of *Brugia malayi* showing terminal and subterminal nuclei in tail. (From J. W. Smith, ed., et al., *Diagnostic Medical Parasitology: Blood and Tissue Parasites,* Chicago, American Society of Clinical Pathologists, © 1976. Used by permission.)

microfilariae in blood during the night, is demonstrated by some strains of *W. bancrofti.* When a blood-sucking mosquito bites an infected human, the microfilariae are transmitted to their intermediate host. In the mosquito they develop into rhabditiform larvae and ultimately into infectious filariform larvae. When an infected mosquito bites a human, the filariform larvae escape from the proboscis of the mosquito and penetrate the skin.

Transmission. Elephantiasis is transmitted by at least 48 species of mosquitoes, including many belonging to the genera *Aedes, Mansonia, Anopheles,* and *Culex.* The chief vector for wuchereriasis is *Aedes polynesiensis. Anopheles* mos-

quitoes spread Malayan elephantiasis in urban areas; *Mansonia* mosquitoes are common vectors of the disease in rural areas.

Laboratory Diagnosis. The diagnosis of elephantiasis depends on finding microfilariae in blood after application of dilute Giemsa stain. Both microfilariae of *W. bancrofti* and *B. malayi* are sheathed, but the sheath of *W. malayi* stains a bright pink color which is easily differentiated from that of *W. bancrofti* which is seldom visible. *B. malayi* is somewhat smaller, averaging only 177 to 260 μm in length; microfilariae of *W. bancrofti* are often as long as 300 μm. Nuclei extend to the tip of the tail in *B. malayi* and stain dark purple (Figure

25-22). The nuclei may overlap one another. The nuclei of *W. bancrofti* stain
blue and separation of nuclei is more
distinct.

Immunity. Data are lacking concerning immunity to infections caused by
filarial worms, including those with an
affinity for the lymph vessels. In endemic areas children exposed to the
microfilariae of *W. bancrofti* or *B. malayi*
are frequently asymptomatic.

Prevention. The chief means for preventing elephantiasis is destruction of
mosquitoes and mosquito-breeding
places with appropriate insecticides.
Protective clothing, nets, and insect repellents are recommended as additional
control measures for areas in which the
disease is endemic.

SUMMARY

Blood, lymph, and the reticuloendothelial system (RES) constitute an
entity of circulating and sessile cells.
Any infectious agent can be transported
by circulating blood and lymph, but
some microorganisms have a predilection for blood cells or endothelial cells
lining blood vessels. Some protozoa
and helminths accumulate in veins,
lymph vessels, or other tissue comprising the diffuse RES. Arthropods are important vectors for blood-transported
diseases. Diseases of the blood, lymph,
and RES are endemic in areas where
the climate and unhygienic conditions
favor growth and multiplication of
mosquitoes, fleas, flies, bugs, ticks,
mites, and lice. Effective control of the
microbial and filarial diseases spread

by these arthropods is largely dependent on effective control of the vectors
or intermediate hosts of parasites.

QUESTIONS FOR STUDY

1. Where are the circulating and ses-
   sile cells of the reticuloendothelial
   system located?
2. Name a disease transmitted by each
   vector.
   Dermacentor andersoni
   Allodermanyssus sanguineus
   Aedes polynesiensis
   Aedes aegypti
   Xenopsylla cheopis
   Pediculus humanus corporis
   Anopheles sp.
   Glossina sp.
   Triatoma sp.
   Phlebotomus sp.
   Ornithodoros sp.
   Culex sp.
3. Explain how xenodiagnosis can be
   used to detect the presence of
   Chagas' disease.
4. Why are several samples of blood
   and persistent searching for para-
   sites often required to establish a
   diagnosis of malaria?
5. Why is schistosomiasis still preva-
   lent in many parts of the world?

SELECTED REFERENCES

Brown, H. W. *Basic Clinical Parasitology*.
4th ed. Englewood Cliffs, N.J.: Prentice-Hall, 1975.
Burrows, W., Lewert, R. M.; and Rippon, J. W. *Textbook of Microbiology—*

The Pathogenic Microorganisms. 19th ed. Philadelphia: Saunders, 1968.

California State Department of Public Health. *A Manual for the Control of Communicable Diseases in California*. Berkeley: 1971.

Evans, A. S. *Viral Infections of Humans—Epidemiology and Control*. New York: Plenum, 1976.

Finegold, S. M.; Martin, W. J.; and Scott, E. G. *Bailey and Scott's Diagnostic Microbiology*. St. Louis: Mosby, 1978.

Joklik, W. K., and Willett, H. P. *Zinsser Microbiology*. 16th ed. Englewood Cliffs, N.J.: Prentice-Hall, 1976.

Lennette, E. H.; Spaulding, E. H.; and Truant, J. P. *Manual of Clinical Microbiology*. 2d ed. Washington, D.C.: American Society for Microbiology, 1974.

Maugh, T. H., II. Malaria: resurgence in research brightens prospects. *Science* 196:413, 1977.

Mims, C. A. *The Pathogenesis of Infectious Disease*. New York: Grune & Stratton, 1976.

U.S. Naval Medical School, National Naval Medical Center. *Medical Protozoology and Helminthology*. Washington, D.C.: U.S. Government Printing Office, 1965.

Wistreich, G. A., and Lechtman, M. D. *Microbiology and Human Disease*. 2d ed. Beverly Hills, Calif: Glencoe Press, 1976.

CONTROL OF MICROORGANISMS

Chapter 26

Disinfection and Sterilization

After you read this chapter, you should be able to:
1. Differentiate between disinfection and sterilization.
2. Describe the factors which influence the death of microorganisms.
3. List the physical agents commonly employed for disinfection or sterilization.
4. Contrast the efficiency of moist heat, dry heat, and steam under pressure as microbicidal agents.
5. Define thermal death time and thermal death point.
6. Discuss two methods of pasteurization.
7. Define photoreactivation, photooxidation, and photodynamic action.
8. Explain why chemical agents are unreliable for sterilization.
9. List the factors which influence the ability of physical agents to destroy microorganisms.
10. Classify the major disinfectants as protein-denaturing or membrane-altering agents.
11. Discuss the application of mechanical agents in hospital disinfection.
12. Describe two standardized methods for testing the efficiency of disinfectants.

The prevention or control of microbial growth is important in the hospital, home, and industry. The destruction of all living microorganisms is accomplished by a process called *sterilization;* the destruction of pathogenic microorganisms, exclusive of spores and viruses, is called *disinfection.* Sterilization or disinfection can be accomplished by the application of a variety of physical, chemical, and mechanical agents.

The action of an agent may be *microbiostatic* (inhibitory) or *microbicidal* (destructive) or both. A particular agent may be selective for particular organisms; a *bacteriostat* or *bactericide* controls or destroys bacteria, a *viricide* kills viruses, and a *fungicide* destroys fungi. Agents that interrrupt the life cycle of protozoa by acting upon free-living or parasitic stages are known as *protozoacides.* Those chemicals used to destroy eggs or larvae of helminths are called *anthelmintics.* In some instances successful interferences in life cycles of parasites is accomplished only by using chemical agents directed against vectors or invertebrate hosts. The World Health Organization has used the insecticides and molluscacides to control populations of certain insects and mollusks.

Although the chemical agents which inhibit or kill microorganisms are frequently called *disinfectants,* their action is not limited to pathogens. The word *germicide* more aptly describes the action of chemicals on infectious agents. The term *antiseptic* describes a chemical agent which inhibits or destroys microorganisms, but the term is usually restricted to mean a chemical agent which is applied topically. The term *sanitizer* is used to describe an agent which renders an object or environment safe by a massive reduction in total numbers of microorganisms present.

The term *asepsis* means freedom from microorganisms; techniques employed to achieve that condition are called *aseptic*. Since it is not always possible to destroy all microorganisms, asepsis is more a goal than an accomplishable feat. We can, for example significantly reduce numbers of bacteria on the hands by scrubbing vigorously with a detergent-germicide, but we cannot render our hands sterile. An object or environment containing even a single organism is *contaminated*. Aseptic techniques employed in a laboratory for the isolation of pure cultures can be successful because the conditions can be carefully controlled. The environment of a communicable disease isolation unit or an operating room presents more challenging problems.

FACTORS INFLUENCING DEATH OF MICROORGANISMS

The death of specific microbial populations is affected by physiological factors associated with the microorganisms and by forces at work in the immediate environment. Microbial death occurs when an organism, or population of organisms, is no longer capable of reproduction. The circumstances under which microorganisms die constitute the basis for the principles of disinfection and sterilization. Environmental factors may stimulate or

inhibit growth, influence synthesis of products, cause physiological variation, or completely destroy microorganisms. Combinations of more than one adverse environmental circumstance may affect death rates. An understanding of the effect of particular physical, chemical, and mechanical agents on microorganisms makes it possible to apply those agents to destroy microorganisms or keep their presence within tolerable limits.

SIZE OF THE MICROBIAL POPULATION

The ability of an agent to destroy microorganisms is dependent on the size of the initial population. When large numbers of organisms are present, some may escape a direct hit by the injurious agent. Mere density of large populations may prevent penetration of harmful agents. However, a lesser density or smaller population does not necessarily increase the number affected by the agent; the probability of a direct hit lessens with the diminishing population since the action of physical and chemical agents is random. Presumably, with enough time and killing power, one can destroy all microorganisms within a limited space, but the ubiquity of microorganisms in the atmosphere limits the ability of any method to achieve disinfection or sterilization.

TIME OF EXPOSURE

Exposure of a microbial population to a lethal agent causes a progressive reduc-

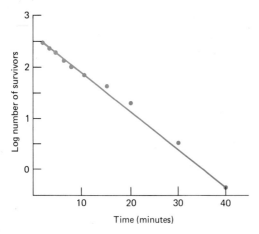

Figure 26-1 Progressive reduction of a microbial population exposed to a lethal agent. (From H. Chick, Process of disinfection by chemical agents and hot water. *J. Hyg.* 10:237, 1910, Cambridge University Press.)

tion of organisms with time. If the logarithm of the number remaining alive is plotted against time, a straight line is obtained (Figure 26-1). The microorganisms are not all killed instantaneously nor are all cells of a population equally susceptible to antimicrobial action. There is no "rule of thumb" for estimating appropriate times of exposure for particular disinfectants without identification of the contaminating organisms. The time required for complete destruction of undesirable organisms may be as little as 15 minutes or as long as 10 or more hours.

INTENSITY OR CONCENTRATION OF ANTIMICROBIAL AGENT

The intensity or concentration of an agent affects the efficiency of an-

timicrobial activity. The destructive power of most disinfectants increases exponentially with concentration up to a certain point only. For each chemical agent there is an optimal microbicidal concentration beyond which efficiency is decreased. A 70 percent concentration of isopropyl alcohol is generally more effective than absolute or 90 percent propanol. The concentration of a chemical agent required for sterilization is determined by its destructive effect on spores. Such information is available from manufacturers and is useful in the selection of appropriate dosages of physical and chemical agents.

TYPE AND AGE OF MICROORGANISMS

The various types of microorganisms vary considerably in their vulnerability to physical and chemical agents. Fungi and viruses are more resistant to both types of lethal agents than are vegetative cells of bacteria. Staphylococci and enterococci are somewhat more resistant to disinfectants than other grampositive organisms. *Serratia, Pseudomonas, Klebsiella,* and *Enterobacter* are more resistant to disinfectants than most coliforms. Tubercle bacilli are less vulnerable to the action of some aqueous chemical agents than other vegetative forms of bacteria. The resistance of mycobacteria is apparently related to the hydrophobic nature of their cell surfaces.

Vegetative cells show varying degrees of susceptibility to chemical and physical agents during growth cycles.

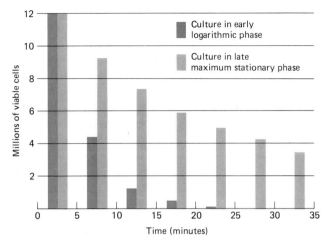

Figure 26-2 Times required to destroy cells in the logarithmic and stationary phases of growth by a lethal agent. More than one-fourth of the cells in the stationary phase remain viable after more than 30 minutes of exposure. (From M. Frobisher, R. D. Hindsdill, K. T. Crabtree, and C. R. Goodheart, *Fundamentals of Microbiology,* 9th ed., Philadelphia, Saunders, 1974.)

In general, cells in the exponential growth phase, when they are "physiologically young," are more susceptible to heat (Figure 26-2). Differences in the susceptibility of *Escherichia coli* during the growth cycle have been attributed to variations in cell-wall content.

PROPERTIES OF CONTAMINATED MATERIALS

The properties of materials to be disinfected or sterilized influence the choice of a particular physical or chemical agent. Plastic or rubber cannot withstand high temperatures; cutting edges of some surgical instruments cannot withstand moist heat or corrosive chemicals. Some fabrics are too delicate for chemical disinfection. The ability of physical and chemical agents to penetrate is dependent on the consistency of molecular constituents of contaminated materials. More viscous contaminated solutions require greater exposure times than do less dense solutions. Accumulations of extraneous organic material on the surface of microbial cells increase the penetrating force needed to destroy organisms.

ENVIRONMENTAL CONDITIONS

Conditions of the immediate environment surrounding microorganisms can influence the efficacy of antimicrobial agents. As a rule, an increase in temperature enhances the destructive ability of a disinfectant. The presence of oxygen is required for some chemicals to act upon microorganisms; an acidic environment promotes the action of other chemical agents. The synergistic effect of heat, oxygen, or an acid pH and a disinfectant often lowers the time of exposure required for disinfection or sterilization.

PHYSICAL AGENTS

An understanding of the environmental factors favoring microbial growth provides a basis for the application of physical agents in the destruction of microorganisms. Many organisms grow optimally within narrow ranges of temperature, osmotic pressure, and atmospheric conditions. Some obligate anaerobes are extremely susceptible to oxygen and do not tolerate even brief exposure to the concentration of oxygen found in the atmosphere. When a particular microbial contaminant is suspected of being present, the method for destruction is chosen on the basis of knowledge of the physiological tolerances of that particular organism. When the nature of the contamination remains speculative, as is often the case, rather stringent methods of decontamination covering a wide range of possibilities must be employed.

HEAT

Moist heat, dry heat, or steam under pressure are among the most common methods employed for destroying microorganisms, provided that the contaminated object or material can withstand the high temperatures required. Death of microbial cells subjected to dry heat is caused by an oxidation of cell substances; moist heat causes coagulation of cell proteins. Bacterial toxins vary in their susceptibility to heat, but most enzymes are heat labile. Some viruses, such as the encephalitis agents, are inactivated at room temperature. Other viruses, such as the polio and vaccina agents, are killed only when exposed to a temperature of 60°C for 30 minutes. The hepatitis viruses are destroyed by dry heat only after exposure to 180°C for an hour.

The length of time required to kill a particular microorganism at a specific temperature is called the *thermal death time*. The temperature required to kill a particular microorganism within 10 minutes is called the *thermal death point*. A knowledge of thermal death times and points is especially valuable in the canned food industry where heat processing must be adequate to destroy pathogens and spoilage bacteria.

Dry Heat. One of the most efficient methods of sterilization employs dry heat in the process of exposing objects to intense heat or direct flame. If the contaminated object, such as a dressing or animal carcass, is combustible and can be sacrificed, *incineration*, that is, the complete destruction of contaminants by burning, is recommended. If an object, like a platinum bacteriological loop, can withstand intense heat, it can be freed of microorganisms rapidly by *flaming*.

Unfortunately, all materials or objects requiring sterilization either cannot withstand direct flaming or are not expendable. Exposure to temperatures of 160° to 180°C for an hour or longer is necessary to sterilize glassware, such as Petri plates, test tubes, or pipettes. The time required for this type of dry-heat sterilization often limits it use as a method of choice, if other more rapid methods are available.

Moist Heat. A moist environment permits an article to be sterilized at lower temperatures and shorter exposure times than a dry atmosphere. *Boiling* is a readily accessible method requiring no expensive equipment. Prolonged boiling may be necessary if an object is contaminated with spores, but most vegetative cells of pathogens are killed by boiling for 20 minutes.

Flowing steam can be applied as an alternative to boiling, but prolonged exposure is necessary to destroy spores. Intermittent exposure to flowing steam or *tyndallization* employs a 30-minute period of steaming on three successive days. The process is successful in destroying bacterial sporeformers if materials are incubated at 35°C between heating periods to allow for germination of any remaining spores into the more heat-susceptible vegetative cells.

The most efficient use of moist heat employs *steam under pressure* in an instrument known as an *autoclave* (Figure 26-3). Exposure to a pressure of 15 pounds per square inch at a temperature of 121°C can accomplish sterilization. The time required to achieve sterilization at that pressure and temperature depends on the object being sterilized. For example, 15 minutes is sufficient to sterilize most bacteriological culture media. Packs of surgical dressings require exposure times of 30 minutes or longer, depending on size of packs. It is important that each pack be wrapped loosely and that sufficient space be left around the packs in the autoclave so that the steam can penetrate all the material. Most autoclaves today are equipped with electronic devices for controlling cycles and with charts for plotting temperature, thereby eliminating much of the human error inherent in the manual operation of an autoclave.

Canning Processes. A Frenchman, Nicolas Appert, has been called the "Father of Canning," for it was he who first devised a method of heating foods in sealed containers to prevent spoilage. Appert used a cork-stoppered, wide-mouthed glass jar, but most cans today are made of tin-coated steel plate. The first "tin can" was patented by Peter Durand, an Englishman, in 1810.

Canners attempt to sterilize foods, but sometimes destroy only food-spoilage organisms. The size of the can, type of food, water content, pH, and type of packing determine the temperature and time of exposure required to destroy harmful organisms. For example, spores of the pathogen *Clostridium botulinum* require 4 minutes at 120°C or 330 minutes at 100°C for inactivation.

Pasteurization. Louis Pasteur first applied heat to prevent the growth of spoilage organisms in wine, but the

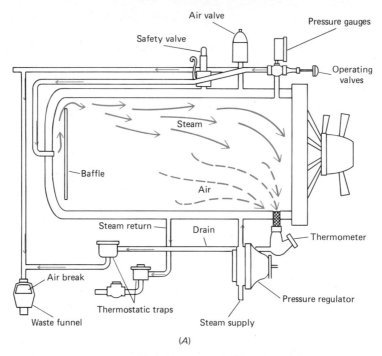

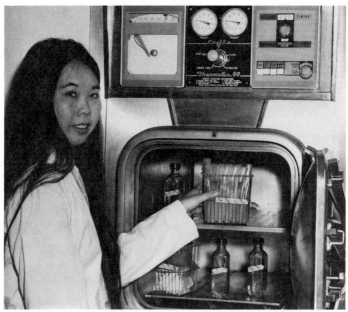

Figure 26-3 An autoclave. (*A*) Diagram of a longitudinal cross-section of an autoclave showing flow patterns for steam and air. (From S. S. Block, *Disinfection, Sterilization*, and *Preservation*, 2d ed., Philadelphia, Lea & Febiger, 1977.) (*B*) Inside of an autoclave and control panel.

greatest application of the heat treatment, or *pasteurization*, has been in the dairy industry. Pasteurization reduces the total number of microorganisms present and improves the keeping quality of milk.

A recent adaptation of the process has been used for the disinfection of respiratory therapy equipment which cannot withstand the intense heat of the autoclave. A drawback in using pasteurization for reusable equipment is that recontamination can occur during the drying period if special precautions are not taken.

The high-temperature-short-time (HTST) method of pasteurization employs a temperature of 71.7°C (160°F) for 15 seconds. The low-temperature-holding (LTH) method employs a temperature of 62.8°C (145°F) for 30 minutes. The thermal resistance of *Coxiella burnetii* and *Mycobacterium tuberculosis* is the basis for selection of the particular temperatures and times.

COLD

Low temperatures inhibit the growth of most microorganisms, but do not necessarily kill all organisms. Freezing destroys 50 to 80 percent of microbial populations if a quick freezing process is employed. A few species of bacteria and some bacterial products demonstrate unusual tolerance for cold. Cells of *C. botulinum*, type E, can elaborate toxin even at temperatures as low as 3.3°C. Endospores, spores of fungi, and cells of *Staphylococcus aureus* in the exponential phase of growth resist a temperature of −70°C even when freezing is achieved within 15 seconds.

The pH, osmotic environment, and humidity influence destruction of microorganisms at low temperatures. A high osmotic pressure is protective. A low pH contributes to bactericidal power of cold. Too much moisture favors the survival of microorganisms. In general, microbial cells can tolerate lower storage temperatures if moisture is available.

DESICCATION

Many microorganisms can survive in an environment of low moisture content, but carry on metabolic processes of such a low order that spoilage of food or textiles does not occur. Anthrax spores dried on silk threads can survive as long as 20 years.

Moisture can be removed from foods or other products in a number of ways. Sun drying is still applied to certain fruits, such as apricots, figs, prunes, and raisins. Artificial drying requires the use of heated air and carefully controlled humidity.

Rapid freezing combined with desiccation, in a procedure known as *lyophilization*, is employed rather extensively in the preservation of complement, antisera, sera, enzymes, and even bacteriological cultures. Lyophilization removes water under a vacuum and employs a quick freezing process in which the temperature is lowered to −78°C by placing product containers in a preparation of dry ice and 2-methoxyethanol.

An alternate method for maintaining stock bacteriological and tissue cultures is storage under liquid nitrogen at a temperature of −196°C (Figure 26-4).

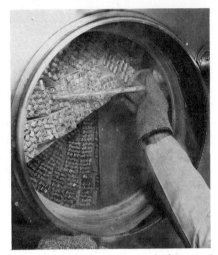

Figure 26-4 Container used for storing stock cultures under liquid nitrogen at −196°C. (Courtesy, American Type Culture Collection, Rockville, Maryland.)

Table 26-1   COMPARISON OF MINIMUM WATER ACTIVITY (a_w) FOR THREE BACTERIA AND THREE FUNGI

MICROORGANISM	MINIMUM a_w
Bacteria	
Escherichia coli	0.935–0.960
Bacillus subtilis	0.950
Staphylococcus aureus	0.900
Fungi	
Aspergillus niger	0.88
Xeromyces bisporus	0.60
Saccharomyces rouxii	0.60

SOURCE: Adapted from T. D. Brock, *Biology of Microorganisms*, 2d ed. (Englewood Cliffs, N.J.: Prentice-Hall, 1974).

The method is particularly suitable for storage of cell lines because they cannot survive the rigors of lyophilization. The lack of a cell wall makes animal cells more sensitive to severe dehydration. Some moisture is necessary to preserve the integrity of cells. In addition, during rapid desiccation hydrolytic enzymes capable of digesting cell contents may be released.

OSMOTIC PRESSURE

Most microorganisms do not tolerate an osmotic environment in which the concentration of solute exceeds by far that in the cells. A higher solute concentration in cells facilitates the movement of water molecules into cells through the cytoplasmic membranes by osmosis. Organisms which can grow in media containing excess solutes are *osmotolerant*; they include the *halophilic* (salt-loving) and *saccharophilic* (sugar-loving) species.

Osmotic tolerance is usually expressed in terms of lowest water activity (a_w) permitting growth. Water activity can be measured by determining the relative humidity of the vapor pressure over a solution. It is related to the solute concentration, the amount of dissociation, and the temperature of the environment. Most fungi show greater osmotolerance than do bacteria (Table 26-1).

SURFACE TENSION

Surface tension is the force exerted by a gas on a liquid at the interface between the liquid and the gaseous environment. At the interface of the liquid and air, less force is exerted on surface molecules than on those molecules surrounded by liquid. Molecules are most closely packed at the interface for that reason. The surface of water will support light objects which often appear to be floating on the surface. If the molecular organization of the surface is disturbed, the object will sink to the bottom.

The tension which particles suspended in a liquid exert upon the liquid is called *interfacial tension*. Surface tension can be measured on a tensiometer and is expressed in dynes per centimeter. Interfacial tension cannot be measured, but the force a microorganism exerts upon a liquid is nevertheless real.

Nutrient broth has a surface tension of approximately 50 to 65 dynes per centimeter at room temperature. Low surface tensions have a detrimental effect on most bacteria. The exact mechanism of the action of surface-tension depressants is not known, but the permeability of cell membranes appears to be altered in some manner permitting the flow of cellular constituents into the environment. The growth of streptococci is inhibited at 50 dynes per centimeter or below, but some intestinal bacteria survive lesser surface tensions without appreciable effects.

FILTRATION

Bacteria can be removed from a liquid by passing the liquid through a variety of materials which trap the microorganisms. Asbestos, sand, diatomaceous earth, porcelain, plaster of Paris, glass, or membrane filters can be used to filter microorganisms from a suspension. The membrane filters, composed of biologically inert materials and constructed so pores measure 0.01 to 10.0 μm, have largely replaced other filters in hospital and industrial laboratories for removal of bacteria.

Application of negative pressure to a flask makes filtration rapid and efficient. The process is applied to culture media which cannot withstand the heat required for autoclave-sterilization. Highly efficient particulate air (HEPA) filters are used in laminar air flow hoods or rooms in hospitals to remove airborne microorganisms from particular environments (Chapter 29).

ULTRASOUND

Ultrasonic vibrations ranging as high as 100,000 to 2,250,000 cycles per second can be produced when crystals, such as quartz, are subjected to a periodic electric field. Some phages are inactivated by exposure to sonic vibrations as low as 9,000 cycles per second; other phages and bacteria are not completely destroyed until exposed to vibrations as high as 280,000 cycles per second for a prolonged time. Some cells are literally torn apart by ultrasound; others remain intact, but are lethally damaged by the sonic vibrations. Heat is generated by ultrasonic equipment, so it is difficult to separate effects of heat and ultrasound on microorganisms. It is not practical to use ultrasonic waves on any large scale to kill microorganisms, but ultrasound can be useful in disrupting microbial cells to obtain particular intracellular fractions.

RADIATION

The propagation of energy through space as electromagnetic waves is often called *radiation*. The electromagnetic spectrum includes radio waves, hertzian waves, light, gamma rays, X rays, and cosmic rays (Figure 26-5). Wavelength of electromagnetic waves is usually expressed in Angstrom (Å) units (10^{-8} centimeter) in the near infrared, visible, and ultraviolet spectra, but the ultimate unit of wavelength is the centimeter. For convenience, other units such as nanometer may sometimes be used in expressions of wavelength.

The radio communication waves have only slight bactericidal properties, but the ultraviolet waves of light and the emissions of gamma rays, X rays, and cosmic rays are more highly bactericidal.

Ultraviolet Rays. Ultraviolet radiation (UV) ranges in wavelength from 150 to 3900 Å. Much of the shorter rays

are filtered out by materials in the atmosphere, such as ozone, so that only those rays of higher wavelengths reach the surface of the earth. UV lamps which emit wavelengths of 2600 to 2700 Å are used in surgery or inoculating hoods to reduce numbers of microorganisms.

The destruction of microorganisms by UV is caused by its action on the DNA of cells. Both purine and pyrimidine bases absorb UV radiation. The production of thymine dimers (combining of two adjacent thymine bases) is a major consequence of UV radiation on bacteria. Formation of dimers is sometimes lethal since it prevents the replication of DNA. The amount of injury inflicted is related to the duration of exposure and to the type of cell. Pigmented cells and endospores require longer periods of exposure to UV for the lethal waves to penetrate the organisms.

The amount of injury is also related to the efficiency of repair mechanisms of the organisms. Exposure to visible light, following several minutes of treatment with UV, promotes a process

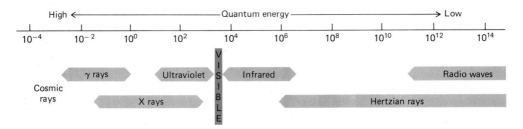

Figure 26-5 The electromagnetic spectrum showing wavelength in nm on an exponential scale. (From W. K. Joklik and H. P. Willett, *Zinsser Microbiology*, 16th ed., Englewood Cliffs, N.J., Prentice-Hall, 1976.)

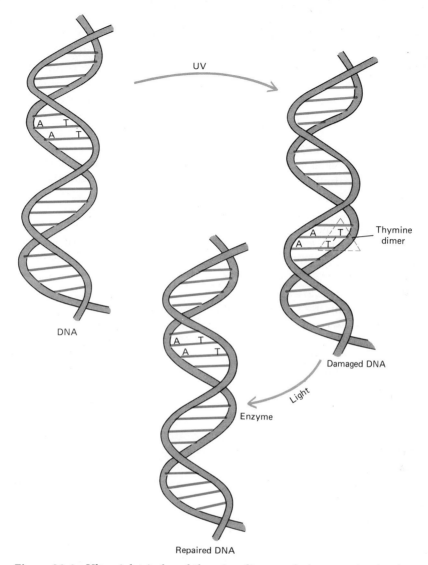

UV

A   T
A   T

DNA

Thymine
dimer

A   T
A   T

Damaged DNA

Light

A   T
A   T

Enzyme

Repaired DNA

Figure 26-6 Ultraviolet-induced thymine dimer and photoreactivation by an enzyme which splits the bond between the pair of thymines in the presence of light.

known as *photoreactivation* in which a single enzyme excises the altered region on the DNA molecule (Figure 26-6). Photoreactivation is not 100 percent efficient in populations of microorganisms damaged by UV.

Some microorganisms can promote a similar repair of the DNA in the dark through the action of a DNA-polymerase and a DNA-ligase. The ability of cells to repair UV damage has stimulated the search for repair mechanisms in cells which are believed to have become cancerous after an initial insult by exposure to radiation.

The use of UV for actual disinfection or sterilization is limited since UV is also damaging to eucaryotic cells of humans as well as to the procaryotic and eucaryotic microbial cells. No doubt the UV spectrum contributes to the lethal effect of sunlight on some microorganisms. The infrared spectrum cannot initiate chemical changes in biological systems. Any absorbed energy is lost as heat.

Visible Light. Exposure to visible light for prolonged periods can destroy microbial cells in the presence of oxygen. Death occurs as a result of *photooxidation* when light is absorbed by cytochromes and flavins of the electron transport chain. Some bacteria contain light-absorbing pigments in the cell membrane which prevent the light from reaching the vulnerable electron transport system. Most pathogens are quite susceptible to the visible spectrum since most lack protective pigments. Many airborne bacterial species are highly pigmented.

Certain dyes, when added to microbiological systems, cause a sensitization to light. Gram-positive bacteria and some viruses are somewhat more susceptible to sensitization with dyes than gram-negative species. The combined effect of dyes and light on microorganisms in the presence of oxygen is called *photodynamic action*.

Ionizing Radiation. Ionizing radiation may emanate from an X-ray machine, radioactive decay, nuclear reactors, or atomic particles from outer space. Ionizing radiation does not directly affect cells, but rather produces free radicals which injure essential macromolecules. The cosmic rays, protons, atomic nuclei, and alpha particles usually do not penetrate the atmosphere. X rays, gamma rays, and high speed electrons are the most important ionizing sources for sterilization.

Ionizing radiation affects primarily the water molecules of microbial cells. Ionization occurs when energy is transferred to the cells.

$$H_2O \longrightarrow H_2O^+ + e^-$$

Positively charged ions react with other water molecules to form additional charged molecules and hydroxyl radicals.

$$H_2O + H_2O \longrightarrow H_3O^+ + OH^-$$

The electrons (e^-) react with un-ionized water to form hydroxyl ions (OH^-) and free hydrogen radicals (H^+). Hydrogen radicals are effective reducing agents; hydroxyl radicals are potent oxidizing agents. The free radicals can react with any molecules of microbial cells, but usually cause damage to DNA. If the damage is small enough, it is repairable by dark reactivation, but not by photoreactivation.

Although effective, ionizing radiation is economically feasible in only a limited number of circumstances in the hospital. It is most suitable for sterilization of heat-sensitive sutures and disposable plastic items. The *rad* is used as the primary unit of measurement for radiation. It is equal to the absorption of

100 ergs per gram of irradiated material. The *megarad* (Mrad) is equal to 1 million rads. A dose of 2.5 Mrad destroys vegetative cells and spores. The dehydrated state of spores contributes to their resistance to ionizing radiations of lower doses.

CHEMICAL AGENTS

Chemical agents are widely used for disinfection, but are not reliable for sterilization. Spores, some viruses, and mycobacteria are especially resistant to destruction by chemical action. Some hospital equipment cannot withstand autoclaving, however, and chemical agents must be employed to render equipment as free as possible from contamination. The choice of a chemical agent for use in a hospital depends on the nature of the material to be disinfected and the type of organisms present.

PROTEIN-DENATURING AGENTS

Cells are vulnerable to any chemical agent that changes the configuration of their protein molecules. Proteins damaged by unfolding or aberrant looping of polypeptide chains are said to be *denatured.* The denaturation of cellular proteins by chemical as well as physical agents is irreversible. Acids, alkalies, and organic solvents are protein-denaturing agents. Heavy metal derivatives, oxidizing agents, dyes, and alkylating

agents alter catalytic sites on enzyme molecules by reacting with labile hydrogen atoms of specific groups on the enzymes or on phosphoric acid residues of nucleic acids.

Acids and Alkalies. The disinfectant action of acids and alkalies depends on the number of free hydrogen (H^+) or hydroxyl (OH^-) ions. The strong mineral acids, such as sulfuric and hydrochloric acids, and strong alkalies, such as potassium hydroxide, dissociate freely; organic acids, such as benzoic and tannic acids, exert a direct effect on intact molecules. The metallic action of some hydroxides appears to exert a direct toxic action on microorganisms. The cost and corrosive properties of most acids and alkalies prohibit their use in the hospital environment.

Organic Solvents. Organic solvents, such as alcohols, ethers, and acetone, alter permeability of microbial cell membranes and denature proteins. The alcohols, especially ethyl and isopropyl, are widely used in concentrations of 70 to 92 percent by weight. The alcohols are safe and quite inexpensive, but have limited action against spores and viruses. Alcoholic solutions can be applied to disinfect skin, thermometers, and anesthesia equipment. Ethers, benzene, acetone, and other ketones are highly germicidal, but are not recommended for routine use.

Heavy Metal Derivatives. Soluble salts of heavy metals destroy sulfhydryl groups ($-SH$) of cysteine residues. Derivatives of heavy metals, particularly the mercurials, have been used for years in hospitals, although most of them are not reliable germicides. The inorganic salts, such as bichloride of mercury, are toxic, irritate tissue, and corrode metal. The organic mercurials, such as Metaphen, Mercurochrome, and Merthiolate, are less offensive in their effects on tissue or metal, but are no more effective as disinfectants than the inorganic mercurials.

Silver compounds also have limited use as disinfecting agents because of their irritating and corrosive properties. Silver nitrate in a concentration of 1 percent has a selective action on the gonococcus. Its use is mandated by most states for the prevention of ophthalmia neonatorum in newborn infants.

Copper salts are fungicidal and algicidal. Their use is largely limited to spraying plants and treatment of water supplies. A concentration of 2 parts per million (ppm) copper sulfate is usually employed for control of algae.

Zinc salts, especially zinc oxide, are of value in certain superficial fungal and bacterial infections. They are constituents of powders and ointments used in the treatment of diaper rash and tinea pedis.

The arsenic derivative arsphenamine (Salvarsan), developed by Ehrlich, heralded the beginning of chemotherapy for infectious diseases. The discovery of a more selective spirocheticidal agent, namely, penicillin, has obviated the need for employing so toxic a metal as arsenic for treatment of syphilis. Arsenic compounds are still used in some protozoal infections.

Oxidizing Agents. The oxidizing agents include the halogens, hydrogen peroxide, potassium permanganate, and peracetic acid. These agents oxidize the sulfhydryl groups ($-SH$), but may also react with amino groups ($-NH_2$). Chlorine and iodine, in particular, are effective against vegetative cells, spores, fungi, and some viruses.

Iodine preparations include tincture of iodine (2 percent iodine and 2.5 percent sodium iodide in a solution of 47 percent alcohol), aqueous iodine, and iodophors (compounds containing iodine and a solubilizing agent). Iodine preparations are effective disinfectants for skin, mucous membranes, suture materials, thermometers, surgical instruments, and eating utensils.

The germicidal activity of chlorine compounds is dependent on their ability to liberate chlorine. Hypochlorite preparations are marketed as bleach for household use. Acid-fast bacilli are not killed by chlorine compounds, but chlorine products are effective disinfectants for floors, bathrooms, linens, and dishes. Dakin's solution, which is effective for cleansing of wounds, is a hypochloride containing 0.5 percent chlorine.

Hydrogen peroxide, used in a concentration of 3 percent, has limited ability to disinfect. Oxygen is released rapidly from the unstable antiseptic when it is applied to tissue.

$$2H_2O_2 \longrightarrow 2H_2O + O_2 \uparrow$$

Oxygen has a lethal effect on anaerobes of wound infections, but because the oxygen is released for a short period of time, the effectiveness of the hydrogen peroxide in killing anaerobes is sometimes minimal.

Potassium permanganate and peracetic acid are strong oxidizing agents. The potassium salt can be used as a urethral antiseptic, if diluted at least 1000 times. Peracetic acid in vapor form is an efficient method of sterilizing animal cages.

Dyes. Dyes are organic compounds derived from one or more substances found in coal tar. Most commercial dyes are distributed as salts, but those made from basic dyes are more effective bacteriostatic agents than those from acid dyes. The basic dyes have an affinity for phosphoric acid residues of nuclear material. Some aniline dyes have selective activity against gram-positive organisms. Crystal violet and brilliant green, for example, are sometimes incorporated in selective media used for culturing gram-negative bacilli because of their inhibitory effect on gram-positive organisms. Gentian violet can be successfully applied topically to lesions of tinea, candidiasis, or erysipelas to limit their spread. The acridine dyes, such as proflavine and acriflavine, can be used in the cleansing of wounds. Acriflavine, in addition, has antitrypanosomal activity.

Alkylating Agents. Formaldehyde, glutaraldehyde, and ethylene oxide inhibit enzyme activity by replacing hydrogen atoms on amino ($-NH_2$), hydroxyl ($-OH$), sulfhydryl ($-SH$), and carboxyl ($-COOH$) groups. They alter nucleic acids by replacing hydrogen atoms on $-NH_2$ and $-OH$ groups. An aqueous solution of formaldehyde is called formalin. Formalin, in concentrations of 5 to 37 percent, is active against vegetative cells and spores. It is widely used to inactivate microorganisms in vaccines, but it is irritating to tissues so care must be taken to eliminate traces of formalin in final products. Formalin can be used to disinfect instruments and as a vapor for gas sterilization of heat-sensitive materials.

Glutaraldehyde, in a concentration of 2 percent, is a potent antimicrobial agent. It is effective against acid-fast bacilli, spores, and vegetative cells. Glutaraldehyde is used extensively in the disinfection of respiratory therapy equipment.

Ethylene oxide is employed by hospitals for gas sterilization of many heat-sensitive materials.

Although new to the hospital environment, fumigation with gas has been applied for many years in the housing industry to eliminate household pests. The process, sometimes called cold sterilization, requires a special chamber in which a humidity of 25 to 50 percent and a temperature of 38° to 60°C are maintained (Figure 26-7). Other gases, such as *beta*-propiolactone or methyl bromide, can also be employed as sterilants. Installation of equipment for gas sterilization is costly, but the process can be recommended for decontamination of pillows, mattresses, shoes, artificial heart valves, and even spacecraft components.

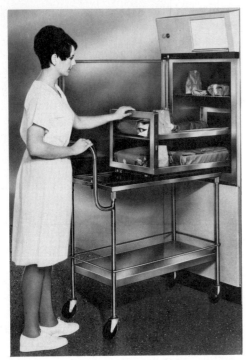

Figure 26-7 A chamber used for ethylene oxide sterilization. (Courtesy, AMSCO/ American Sterilizer Company, Erie, Pennsylvania.)

MEMBRANE-ALTERING AGENTS

The integrity of microbial membranes permits the orderly entrance and exit of soluble materials necessary for metabolic processes. Any change in membrane function through the alteration of permeability or damage may permit the loss of required metabolites or the entrance of harmful agents from the environment.

Surface-Active Agents. Chemical agents which interfere with interfacial relationships are called surface-active agents or detergents. Surface-active agents may dissociate to form negatively or positively charged ions or may be nonionic. Surface-tension depressants are not strongly bactericidal, but are often used with other disinfectants or soaps to destroy microorganisms.

Most cationic surface-active agents are quaternary ammonium salts. The "quats," as they are frequently called, are effective against gram-positive bacteria, but have only limited activity against most species of gram-negative organisms. *Pseudomonas* and *Proteus* species, both troublesome opportunistic pathogens, are remarkably resistant to the quats. Spores and mycobacteria may not be destroyed by cationic detergents. Despite these limitations, a quaternary ammonium compound, marketed under the name of Zephiran or Cepryn, is popular. The product is highly stable, nonirritating, odorless, and relatively inexpensive.

Soaps are often used with detergents for laundry, dishwashing, preoperative scrubbing, hand washing, and cleaning of walls, furniture, and floors. Soaps without disinfectant additives have no effect on microbial populations. In fact, most soaps actually support microbial growth quite well. However, the mechanical action involved in cleansing does wash bacteria away from the surface of the skin or other objects.

Phenolic Derivatives. Joseph Lister was the first to use phenol (carbolic acid) as an antiseptic spray in surgery in 1867. Phenol is a highly irritating and toxic substance which no longer has general application in hospitals. A large number of phenolic derivatives and synthetic phenolic compounds, which are less irritating and lack phenol's pungent odor, are widely used as effective antimicrobial agents, but none of the phenol homologs is reliable against spores.

Aqueous solutions of 5 percent phenol can be used to disinfect sputum, urine, feces, or contaminated glass slides. The isomeric phenols—ortho-, meta-, and paracresol—are more bactericidal than phenol. Cresols are often emulsified in soaps. The popular household disinfectant, sold under the trade name of Lysol, is an example of a cresol. Other phenolic compounds include α-phenylphenol, hexylresorcinol, and hexachlorophene. Hexachlorophene, which combines a halogen and a phenolic derivative in soap, has been used for surgical scrubs, but it is no longer recommended for infant skin care because of its carcinogenic potential.

MECHANICAL AGENTS

Mechanical agents are employed to a large degree in hospitals for cleansing before the application of or in conjunction with a chemical or physical agent. The mechanical agents alone cannot disinfect an object or area and may in fact distribute microorganisms. Their main function is to remove organic material, such as blood, secretions, or excreta, or other substances which may

interfere with the disinfecting action of physical or chemical agents or afford protection to the microorganisms. It is possible to reduce the microbial population in a hospital by substantial amounts with dry or wet agents, but none of them can be recommended exclusively for general use under all circumstances.

DRY AGENTS

Cleaning can be done by dusting, brushing, sweeping, or vacuuming. However, dry dusting, brushing, and sweeping are not recommended for hospitals. The procedures distribute microorganisms into the air and can be responsible for transmitting infectious diseases. Vacuums for hospital use require special filters which prevent dust from spreading. Microorganisms often adhere to dust particles, employing them as major vehicles for transportation.

WET AGENTS

Damp dusting, mopping, scrubbing, scouring, washing, and wet vacuuming are all mechanical means which use water or detergent-germicides. The mechanical action is, however, probably as important as the action of the disinfectants on the microorganisms. The procedures can be effective on furniture, floors, ledges, walls, shelves, and light fixtures. Disinfectants should be selected for safety, effectiveness, and economy. No one disinfectant is suitable as a universal germicide, but some

Table 26-2 RECOMMENDED CONCENTRATIONS AND APPLICATIONS OF SELECTED DISINFECTANTS

CHEMICAL AGENT	CONCENTRATION (%)	APPLICATION
Alcohols	70.0	anesthesia equipment, thermometers, skin surfaces
Chlorine compounds	0.5–1.0	toilets, lavatories, bathtubs, laundry, dishes
Ethylene oxide	25.0–50.0	heat-sensitive objects, mattresses, pillows, shoes
Formaldehyde in alcohol	20.0/70.0	surgical instruments
Formaldehyde, aqueous	16.0	surgical instruments
Glutaraldehyde, aqueous	2.0	anesthesia and respiratory therapy
Iodine in alcohol	2.0–4.5/47	suture materials, thermometers, surgical instruments, anesthesia equipment
Phenols	5.0	laboratory glassware, floors, walls, furniture
Quarternary ammonium compounds	0.1–0.13	surgical instruments, walls, floors, furniture, shelves, ledges, light fixtures, dishes, laundry

can be recommended for particular areas (Table 26-2).

EVALUATION OF DISINFECTANTS

The efficiency of germicidal activity of a disinfectant is often expressed as the *phenol coefficient*. The phenol coefficient is determined by adding a standard inoculum of *Salmonella typhi* or *Staphylococcus aureus* to various dilutions of phenol and the test disinfectant at a temperature of 20°C. Subcultures, made after 5, 10, and 15 minutes of exposure to the disinfectants, are incubated for two days and examined for evidence of growth. The bactericidal power of the test disinfectant is compared with that of phenol. The phenol coefficient is the ratio of the highest dilution of the test disinfectant killing the test bacterium in 10 minutes to the highest dilution of phenol with the same germicidal activity. A phenol coefficient of 10 would indicate that the test disinfectant had 10 times the bactericidal power of phenol; a phenol coefficient of 0.1 would mean that the test disinfectant exhibited only one-tenth as much bactericidal power as phenol against the test organisms.

A more definitive method for establishing actual dilutions of disinfectants to be used for practical purposes is recommended by the Association of Official Analytical Chemists (AOAC). The AOAC Use-Dilution Method employs three cultures obtainable from the American Type Culture Collection,

Table 26-3 CONCENTRATIONS AND TIMES OF EXPOSURE OF SELECTED DISINFECTANTS REQUIRED TO DESTROY HEPATITIS VIRUSES

DISINFECTANT	CONCENTRATION (%)	TIME OF EXPOSURE
Sodium hypochlorite	0.5–1.0	30 min
Formaldehyde in alcohol	20.0/70.0	18 hr
Formaldehyde, aqueous	16.0	18 hr
Glutaraldehyde	2.0	10 hr

SOURCE: Adapted from U.S. Department of Health, Education, and Welfare, Perspectives on the control of viral hepatitis, Type B. *CDC Morbidity and Mortality Weekly Report Supplement* 25:1, 1976.

Rockville, Maryland: *Staphylococcus aureus* (ATCC 6538), *Salmonella cholerae-suis* (ATCC 10708), and *Pseudomonas aeruginosa* (ATCC 15442). In the test procedure stainless steel cylinders are contaminated with the test organisms, dried, and transferred to specified amounts of the test disinfectant. After an incubation period of two days, the "use dilution" is calculated by examining ten cultures of each dilution of disinfectant tested. The dilution with a 95 percent level of confidence is the use dilution. The AOAC Use-Dilution Method can be applied to bacteria isolated from the environment of a particular hospital in order to establish effective disinfection procedures. Periodic monitoring of the environment, however, is necessary to insure continuing adequacy of any sterilization or disinfection procedure.

The resistance of viruses to chemical disinfection remains an enigma in many instances. The hepatitis viruses are particularly difficult to destroy. Heat sterilization is the recommended procedure, but all adherent material must be removed before heat treatment. Boiling (100°C) for 10 minutes, au-

toclaving at 15 pounds per square inch of pressure (121°C), or exposure to dry heat (180°C) for 1 hour is lethal to hepatitis viruses. In the absence of heat disinfectants can be applied (Table 26-3).

SUMMARY

A number of physical, chemical, or mechanical agents or combinations of agents can be used for disinfection or sterilization. Mechanical methods can effectively remove traces of organic material which could interfere with disinfection by chemical or physical agents. The use of heat under pressure, in a procedure known as autoclaving, is the most reliable method for sterilizing heat-resistant materials.

Factors influencing disinfection include size of the microbial population, time of exposure, intensity or concentration of the antimicrobial agent, type and age of microorganisms, properties of contaminated materials, and environmental conditions. There is no one physical or chemical agent which is universally applicable to the hospital environment. The actual procedures adopted by a hospital for disinfection or sterilization depend on the type of services offered, the design of the physical plant, and the kinds of equipment in general use. Asepsis in the hospital environment is an ongoing, largely unattainable goal, but environmental sanitation can be accomplished by prudent use of physical, chemical, and mechanical agents.

QUESTIONS FOR STUDY

1. Why is asepsis of the hospital environment usually a goal, rather than an accomplishable feat?
2. How is osmotic pressure related to water activity?
3. Compare the efficiency of heat and cold as bactericidal and bacteriostatic agents.
4. Name eight groups of disinfectants and an example of one disinfectant belonging to each group.
5. How is the phenol coefficient of a disinfectant determined?

SELECTED REFERENCES

Block, S. S. *Disinfection, Sterilization, and Preservation.* 2d ed. Philadelphia: Lea & Febiger, 1976.

Brock, T. D. *Biology of Microorganisms.* 2d ed. Englewood Cliffs, N.J.: Prentice-Hall, 1974.

California State Department of Public Health. *Cleaning, Disinfection and Sterilization. A Guide for Hospitals and Related Facilities.* Berkeley: 1965.

Carpenter, P. L. *Microbiology.* 4th ed. Philadelphia: Saunders, 1977.

Joklik, W. K. and Willett, H. P. *Zinsser Microbiology.* 16th ed. Englewood Cliffs, N.J.: Prentice-Hall, 1976.

Lennette, E. H.; Spaulding, E. H.; and Truant, J. P. *Manual of Clinical Microbiology.* 2d ed. Washington, D.C.: American Society for Microbiology, 1974.

Porter, J. R. *Bacterial Chemistry and Physiology.* New York: Wiley, 1946.

Skinner, F. A., and Hugo, W. B. *Inhibition and Inactivation of Vegetative Microbes.* New York: Academic Press, 1976.

U.S. Department of Health, Education, and Welfare. Perspectives on the control of viral hepatitis, Type B. *CDC Morbidity and Mortality Weekly Report Supplement* 25:1, 1976.

Wistreich, G. A., and Lechtman, M. D. *Microbiology and Human Disease.* 2d ed. Beverly Hills, Calif.: Glencoe Press, 1976.

Chapter 27

Antimicrobial and Chemotherapeutic Agents

After you read this chapter, you should be able to:

1. Differentiate between natural and synthetic antimicrobial agents.
2. List the target site for the major antimicrobial agents.
3. Describe problems associated with use of particular antimicrobial agents.
4. Explain the rationale for chemotherapy in cancer.
5. List several anthelminthic drugs recommended by the Center for Disease Control.
6. Describe the disc-agar method of antimicrobial susceptibility testing for typical bacteria.
7. Differentiate between the minimum inhibitory concentration (MIC) and the minimum bactericidal concentration (MCB) of an antibiotic.
8. Defend the use of generic names of antibiotics in reporting antimicrobial susceptibility tests.

Chemotherapy is the treatment of disease with chemical substances. The original sources of chemotherapeutic agents were plants. Erhlich's discovery in 1909 of the arsenical compound Salvarsan, effective against the spirochete of syphilis, was the beginning of a new dimension in the history of infectious disease. Pasteur had observed that some microorganisms produce substances which inhibit the growth of other microorganisms, but it was the discovery and purification of penicillin by Fleming, Florey, and Chain that led to the widespread use of antimicrobial agents to combat infectious diseases. The early antimicrobials were called *antibiotics* and were derived from molds or bacteria.

Most of the antibiotics of medical importance are substances not required for growth of the microorganisms. In fact, many antibiotics inhibit the growth of the very organisms that produce them. The nonessential, growth-limiting compounds are frequently referred to as *secondary metabolites* to distinguish them from primary metabolites, such as nucleic acids, proteins, or energy-rich compounds, all of which are essential for microbial metabolism.

Antibiotics derived from microbial sources are called *natural* products. Antimicrobial agents which are compounded artificially are referred to as *synthetic* products. The terms antimicrobics, antimicrobials, antibiotics, antibacterials, or chemotherapeutic agents are all used to describe drugs employed in the treatment of infectious diseases. The term chemotherapeutic agent can describe any chemical substance used for treatment in disease, but use of the term is frequently restricted to a drug used to treat a malignancy.

CLASSIFICATION OF ANTIMICROBIAL AGENTS

There are more than a hundred antimicrobial and chemotherapeutic agents in use today. We will consider the major drugs as examples of the mechanisms of drug activity. Antimicrobial agents may be classified according to the target site of their interfering activity. The understanding of antimicrobial action on target sites has paralleled the development of molecular biology.

ANTIMICROBIALS AFFECTING CELL WALLS

As bacterial cells grow, peptidoglycan is synthesized and incorporated into their walls. The enzymes responsible for promoting the synthesis and incorporation are hydrolases and synthetases. The hydrolases open up portions of the peptidoglycan; the synthetases assemble and connect new units to the polymeric network.

Normal cell growth depends on an appropriate balance of the two types of enzymes. Inhibition of synthetases leads to destruction of cell walls. Ultimately, lysis occurs when weakened cell walls can no longer withstand increases in intracellular osmotic pressure. The penicillins and cephalosporins prevent cross-linkage of amino acids between the carbohydrate moieties of the glycopeptide. Cycloserine is more specific in its action; it inhibits the formation of D-alanine from L-alanine, thereby causing depletion of an amino acid component of the peptide. Since peptidoglycan is a cell wall constituent found only in procaryotic cells, the action of the penicillins, cephalosporins, and cycloserine is selectively toxic for bacteria. Bacteria must be growing, however, for the interference in cell wall synthesis to occur.

Gram-negative organisms are usually more resistant than gram-positive organisms to the action of the penicillins because of the gram-negative organisms' constitutive ability to synthesize enzymes called penicillinases or β-lactamases. The enzymes are secreted in small amounts and remain cell bound; they destroy antibiotics coming in contact with the surface of cells before the antibiotics can affect peptidoglycan synthesis.

The resistance of some gram-positive bacteria can be explained by inducible β-lactamases secreted into the environment. The extracellular enzymes, which are produced in large quantities, degrade penicillins and cephalosporins by cleaving bonds which separate side chains (R·CH$_2$·CO) from the molecular configurations.

Penicillin

Cephalosporin

Table 27-1 PROPERTIES OF SOME NATURAL AND SEMISYNTHETIC PENICILLINS

Product	Formula	Bactericidal Activity Gram-positive	Bactericidal Activity Gram-negative	Penicillinase Resistance
Natural				
penicillin G	R= $\bigcirc$—CH$_2$C— (with =O)	+	−	−
penicillin V	R= $\bigcirc$—O—CH$_2$C— (with =O)	+	−	−
Semisynthetic				
ampicillin	R= $\bigcirc$—CH—C— (with =O, and NH$_2$)	+	+	−
cloxacillin	R= $\bigcirc$ (with Cl) —C—C—CO— (N, O, C—CH$_3$)	+	−	+
methicillin	R= $\bigcirc$ (with OCH$_2$, OCH$_3$) —C— (with =O)	+	−	+
oxacillin	R= $\bigcirc$—C—C—C— (with =O, N, O, C—CH$_3$)	+	−	+

Some strains of staphylococci are particularly resistant to the natural product of the mold *Penicillium chrysogenum.* Synthetic or semisynthetic drugs similar in structure to penicillin, but resistant to the action of penicillinases, have largely replaced the natural product in the treatment of staphylococcal infections. These drugs include methicillin, oxacillin, naficillin, and dicloxacillin. Most penicillinlike antimicrobials are bactericidal against many gram-positive and a few gram-negative bacteria. Ampicillin, a penicillin derivative, is four to eight times more effective against a variety of gram-negative organisms than other penicillins, but is destroyed by penicillinase (Table 27-1).

Some bacteria continue to survive in the presence of penicillins or cephalosporins, despite loss of all or part of their cell walls (Figure 27-1). Cell-wall–deficient bacteria have been implicated in recurrences of infections. Both protoplasts (completely wall-less forms) and spheroplasts (partially wall-deficient forms) can usually be eliminated by judicious use of a second antimicrobial agent.

Although the selective toxicity of the penicillins makes them extremely valuable therapeutic agents, some individuals are allergic to them. The penicillins are not antigenic in themselves, but can act as partial antigens, or haptens, and combine with body proteins to produce

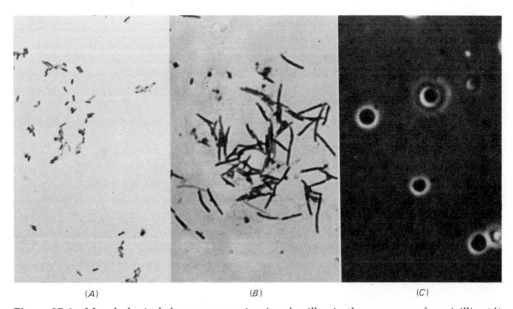

     (A)   (B)   (C)

Figure 27-1 Morphological changes occurring in a bacillus in the presence of penicillin. (A) Typical rodlike forms. (B) Conversion to filamentous protoplasts having partial cell walls. (C) Conversion to spheroplasts having no cell walls. (From H. R. Onishi, S. B. Zimmerman, and E. O. Stapley. *Annals N. Y. Acad. Sci.* 235:406, 1974.)

allergens. Fortunately, most persons who are allergic to the penicillins are not hypersensitive to cephalosporins.

Bacitracin, vancomycin, and ristocetin also inhibit peptidoglycan synthesis, but it appears that transportation of cell wall precursors is the limiting factor. Their use is usually reserved for treatment of infections caused by staphylococci or streptococci that are resistant to the penicillins or cephalosporins. Ristocetin is also active against mycobacteria. Their restricted use is due in part to possible adverse side effects. Ristocetin has a detrimental effect on bone marrow, bacitracin depresses renal tubular function, and vancomycin is associated with ototoxicity.

ANTIMICROBIALS AFFECTING CELL MEMBRANES

Cell membranes are the portals of entry and exit for large numbers of molecules essential for microbial life. The membranes aid in regulation of osmotic pressure and in bacteria contain enzymes for respiration and cell wall synthesis. Destruction of cell membranes, therefore, is lethal to cells.

The membranes of some bacteria and fungi are disrupted by polymyxins and polyenes. The subsequent release of purines, pyrimidines, and amino acids causes cell death. Unfortunately, neither polymyxins nor polyenes exhibit the degree of selective toxicity for microbial cells found in the antimicrobial agents that act upon cell walls, so many of them are limited to topical application.

The polymyxins, namely, polymyxin B and colistin, bind to phospholipids of preexisting bacterial membranes in a detergent action which causes leakage of essential cell constituents and permits penetration by environmental toxins (Figure 27-2).

The polyenes, such as amphotericin B, nystatin, and candicidin, bind selectively to the sterol component of fungal cell membranes. Since sterols are not constituents of bacterial cell membranes, except for some mycoplasmas, the drugs are of no value in the treatment of most bacterial infections. Unfortunately, polyenes do also bind with sterols of red cell membranes and can cause hemolytic anemia in patients requiring long-term therapy for systemic fungal infections. Amphotericin B is valuable in the treatment of disseminated coccidioidomycosis or systemic candidiasis. Nystatin is very effective in controlling intestinal candidiasis. Candicidin is somewhat more effective against *Candida* species than nystatin, but its use has been limited mainly to the treatment of vaginal infections.

The gramicidins, which include gramicidin and tyrothricin, a compound containing 15 to 20 percent gramicidin, interfere with respiration by uncoupling oxidative phosphorylation. Since phospholipids inhibit gramicidins, most gram-negative bacteria, all of which have abundant phospholipids in the lipopolysaccharide moiety of the cell wall, are resistant to gramicidins. The drugs are too toxic for inclusion in a regimen for treatment of systemic infectious diseases, but ointments con-

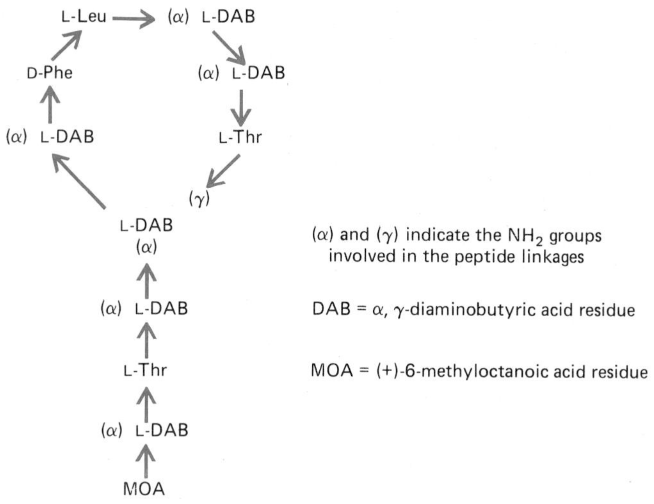
L-Leu
(α) L-DAB
D-Phe
(α) L-DAB
(α) L-DAB
L-Thr
(γ)
L-DAB
(α)
(α) L-DAB
L-Thr
(α) L-DAB
MOA
(α) and (γ) indicate the NH2 groups involved in the peptide linkages
DAB = α, γ-diaminobutyric acid residue
MOA = (+)-6-methyloctanoic acid residue

Polymyxin B

Figure 27-2 An antimicrobial that affects cell membranes. Polymyxin B binds to phospholipids permitting substances to cross membranes.

taining gramicidins can be applied to eyes, skin, nose, or throat.

ANTIMICROBIALS AFFECTING PROTEIN SYNTHESIS

Antimicrobial agents may affect one or more of the stages of protein synthesis. Chloramphenicol interferes with the attachment of mRNA to the ribosome. It is one of the most effective broad-spectrum drugs, but adverse side effects have limited its use. It has a depressive effect on bone marrow, and aplastic anemia has been known to occur after prolonged use. Chloramphenicol is not recommended for minor infections, but remains the drug of choice for typhoid fever and other salmonelloses.

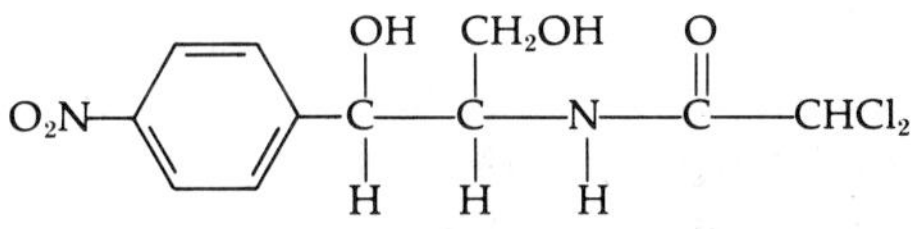
OH CH2OH O
O2N
C C N C CHCl2
H H H

Chloramphenicol

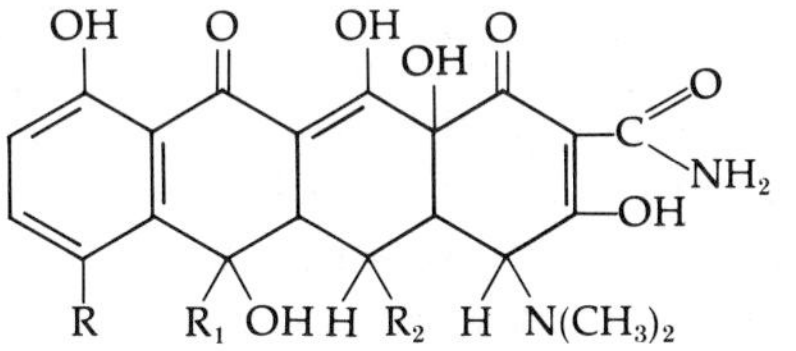
OH O OH O
OH
C O
NH2
OH
R R1 OH H R2 H N(CH3)2

Tetracycline

The tetracyclines prevent the binding of activated amino acid–tRNA complexes to the ribosome. They are broad-spectrum antibiotics reactive against a variety of gram-positive and gram-negative bacteria, mycoplasmas, rickettsiae, and chlamydia. Although allergic reactions are not common, side effects of prolonged or excessive doses of the tetracyclines include nausea, diarrhea, liver damage, anemia, photosensitivity of skin, and staining of teeth. Resistant strains of streptococci, *Escherichia, Bacteroides, Shigella,* and *Neisseria* species do occur. The mechanism of resistance in *Escherichia* and *Shigella* organisms is caused by transfer of specific resistance (R) factors by conjugation.

Erythromycin, puromycin, and cycloheximide impair elongation by inhibiting the transfer of activated amino acid–tRNA complexes. Lincomycin and clindamycin inhibit both transfer and binding of the complexes.

Erythromycin is effective against many gram-positive and some gram-negative bacteria, mycoplasmas, and atypical mycobacteria. It is particularly recommended as an alternate drug for those patients who are allergic to penicillin. No adverse effects of any consequence result from the administration of the erythromycin base, but esters of erythromycin can cause liver damage. Some staphylococci are resistant, but the mechanism of the resistance is unclear.

Puromycin is active against both eucaryotic and procaryotic cells, but the action of cycloheximide is limited to eucaryotes. Puromycin has some value as an antitumor agent, but cycloheximide is so toxic that its use is limited to an additive in culture media when selectively culturing for fungi. The range

of activity and potential for toxicity of lincomycin and clindamycin is similar to that of erythromycin, but resistance occurs less readily.

The aminoglycoside antimicrobials, including streptomycin, kanamycin, neomycin, gentamicin, and tobramycin, appear to prevent peptide elongation or to cause production of defective protein resulting from substitution of an amino acid in the peptide chain.

Streptomycin

The defective protein may be toxic *per se* or the missing protein may be a metabolite essential for a vital function.

Streptomycin, neomycin, and kanamycin are bactericidal for many staphylococci, some gram-negative bacilli, and some mycobacteria. Streptomycin and penicillin G act together effectively to exert a synergistic antibacterial activity against enterococci. All three drugs are ototoxic. Neomycin and kanamycin may cause deafness, but streptomycin's toxicity is usually limited to vertigo.

Gentamicin and tobramycin are bacteriostatic and bactericidal against many gram-negative bacilli that are often resistant to other antibiotics. In particular, most infections caused by *Proteus, Pseudomonas,* and *Serratia* species respond favorably to these drugs, although a few resistant strains of *Pseudomonas* species have been isolated. Penicillins and cephalosporins act synergistically with either gentamicin or tobramycin. Like other aminoglycosides, gentamicin and tobramycin can cause vertigo and deafness.

ANTIMICROBIALS AFFECTING SYNTHESIS OF NUCLEIC ACIDS

Many natural products inhibit the synthesis of nucleic acids. Some interfere with the replication of DNA by blocking *de novo* synthesis of purines and pyrimidines or by promoting fragmentation of DNA. Others limit the translation of information into mRNA by inhibiting the action of RNA polymerase. Several useful antimicrobial and antitumor agents are structurally similar to purines and affect the assembly of purine nucleotides.

Nalidixic acid and griseofulvin are potent inhibitors of DNA synthesis. Nalidixic acid is active against most gram-negative bacteria and has been used successfully in the treatment of urinary tract infections. Griseofulvin is most effective against dermatophytes. It may prevent the synthesis of chitin as well as DNA. Nausea, vomiting, diarrhea, and photosensitization may occur with extended use of either drug. Hypersensitivity and development of resistance do not appear to be significant problems.

Rifampin, actinomycin D, bleomycin, and mitomycin C are examples of drugs which selectively block the action of DNA or RNA polymerase.

Rifampin

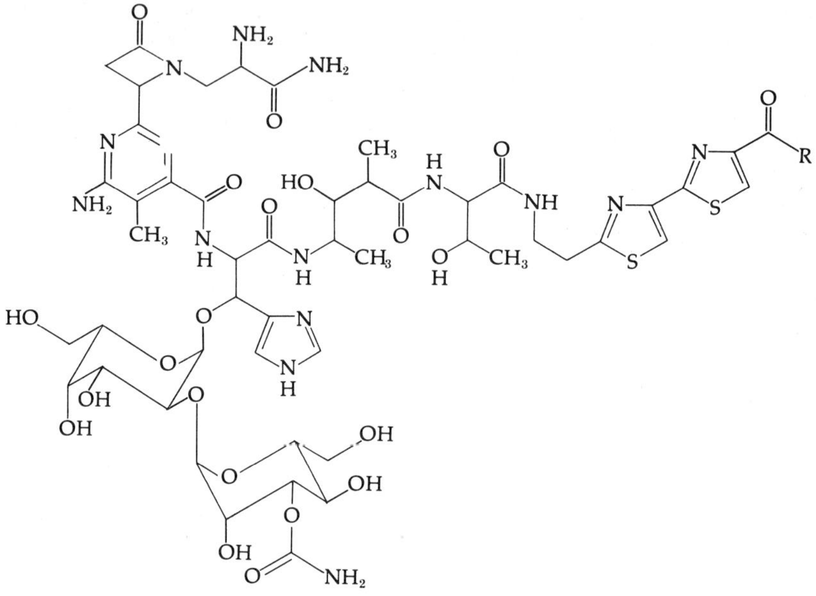

Bleomycin

Rifampin, which inhibits RNA polymerase, is active against *Mycobacterium tuberculosis* and is tolerated well by most patients. It is most frequently used in combination with other antituberculosis agents, such as isoniazid or streptomycin. Resistance is not a problem when the combinations are employed.

Actinomycin D, bleomycin, and mitomycin C, which inhibit DNA polymerase, are often included in cancer-treatment regimens in combination with an alkylating agent, that is, a chemical which limits mitosis by cross-linking with DNA. Nitrogen mustard, chlorambucil, cyclophosphamide, and the nitrosoureas are all examples of alkylating agents.

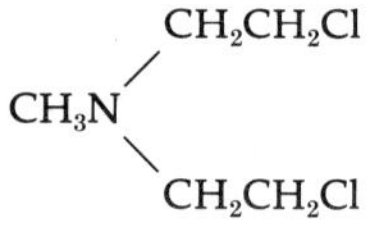

Nitrogen mustard

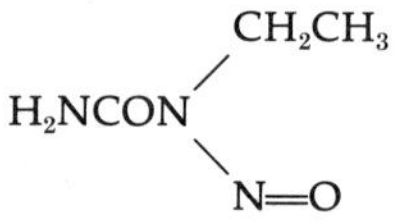

N-ethyl-*N*-nitrosourea

The proper design of combination chemotherapy for cancer is complex and may involve, additionally, a selection of steroids, antimetabolites, vinca alkaloids, and L-asparaginase. Certain types of tumors require asparagine.

Therefore, hydrolysis of blood asparagine by the exogenous enzyme inhibits growth.

The antitumor agents produce serious side effects, including depression of bone marrow activity and gastrointestinal disturbances. Another serious risk in chemotherapeutic management of cancer is the production of an increased susceptibility to other carcinogens. The rationale for chemotherapy, however, is the overall improvement in survival of cancer patients, despite toxicities of drugs.

ANTIMICROBIALS AFFECTING SYNTHESIS OF ESSENTIAL METABOLITES

Microorganisms depend on *de novo* synthesis of a number of metabolites required for growth. One essential metabolite is folic acid, which is needed by both procaryotic and eucaryotic cells for the synthesis of DNA. Folic acid cannot be transported across cell walls. Humans and other animals do not synthesize folic acid, but depend on dietary sources. Microorganisms synthesize folic acid from para-aminobenzoic acid (PABA), pteridine, and glutamate by the action of a synthetase to produce dihydrofolic acid and then a reductase to form folic acid.

The sulfonamides are structurally similar to PABA and competitively inhibit the synthetase. The synthetic antimicrobials trimethoprim, chloroguanide, and pyrimethamine limit the second step of PABA synthesis by interfering with the action of reductase.

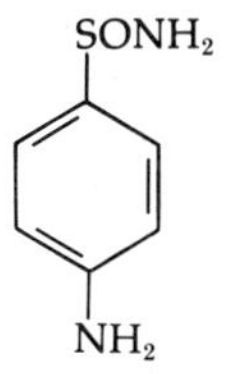

SONH₂

Sulfanilamide

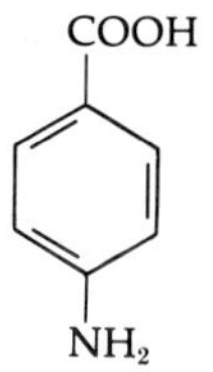

Para-aminobenzoic acid (PABA)

The combination of a sulfonamide and trimethoprim is synergistic, producing as much as a ten-fold increase in bacteriostatic activity.

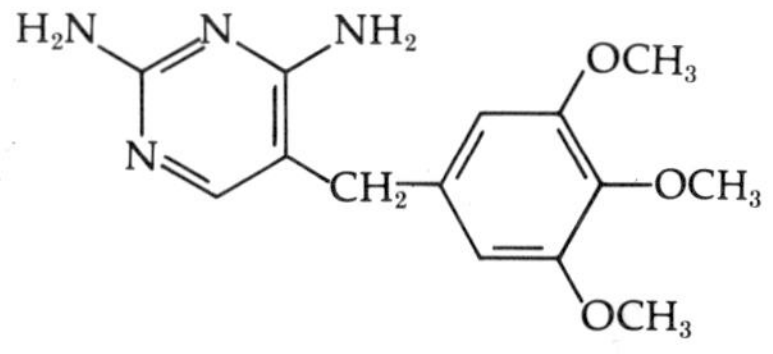

Trimethoprim

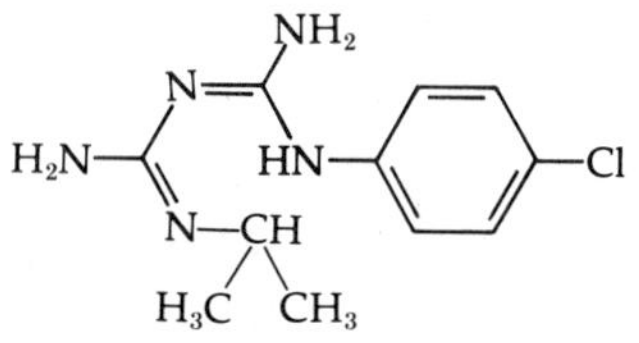

Chloroguanide

It has been shown that plasmodia synthesize folic acid in much the same manner as bacteria. Pyrimethamine inhibits the dihydrofolate reductase enzyme of plasmodia. Fortunately, the drug binds very weakly to the human enzyme. Chloroguanide is a less potent antimalarial agent than pyrimethamine. There is some evidence that chloroguanide is not active in itself, but that it is altered by the body to form a compound with antifolate activity.

The sulfonamides are especially effective in urinary tract infections caused by gram-negative bacilli. All sulfa drugs can produce serious side effects, the most important of which are bone marrow damage and renal failure in the absence of sufficient water. The kidneys and bone marrow may also be impaired as a consequence of an allergic response to the sulfa drugs. Resistance is frequently encountered in long-term sulfa-therapy regimens. Trimethoprim is better tolerated than some sulfonamides by adults, but is particularly toxic to fetuses and children and should not be used during pregnancy or for children under 12 years of age.

Idoxuridine (IDU), an analog of thymidine, is active against the herpes virus which causes a severe corneal infection. If untreated, the herpes infection can cause ulceration, scarring, and blindness. IDU is applied topically and interferes with DNA synthesis. Two other base analogs, cytosine arabinoside (ara-C) and adenine arabinoside (ara-A), as well as IDU, show promise in the treatment of systemic infections due to herpes- and cytomegaloviruses.

The antituberculosis drugs isoniazid, ethambutol, and ethionamide inhibit synthesis of essential metabolites, but the details of their action are unclear. Isoniazid is an extremely potent bactericidal agent and is generally used in combination with another antimicrobial, such as streptomycin. Resistance to isoniazid in patients who have not had previous therapy is uncommon, so isoniazid is frequently employed as the drug of choice in tuberculosis. If ineffective, combinations of other antibiotics or synthetic compounds may be substituted. Isoniazid and ethambutol may be neurotoxic; ethionamide may be hepatotoxic.

Para-aminosalicylic acid (PAS) has limited bacteriostatic activity against the tubercle bacillus and delays bacterial resistance to streptomycin and isoniazid. Gastrointestinal disturbances and mild to severe allergic reactions following PAS administration are not uncommon. Like the use of antitumor drugs in cancer, regimens for treating tuberculosis are often complex and are determined both by the severity and the site of the infection.

ANTIMICROBIALS HAVING UNKNOWN MECHANISMS OF ACTION

The exact mechanisms of action for many antiparasitic agents are unknown. Quinine, an alkaloid of cinchona bark, has been used for three centuries to treat malaria; its derivative chloroquine is popular today for treatment and prophylaxis of malaria. Emetine, another alkaloid derived from ipecacuanha roots, has been employed as an amebicide. Metronidazole is widely used for its microbicidal effect on amebas and flagellates, such as *Entamoeba histolytica* and *Trichomonas vaginalis*.

Metronidazole

The effect of alcohol is potentiated by metronidazole, so patients should be cautioned not to drink during a course of treatment.

A large number of anthelminthic drugs which exhibit selective toxicity for parasites are available. Some of these drugs are provided only on an investigational basis from the Parasitic Disease Drug Service of the Center for Disease Control in Atlanta, Georgia. Table 27-2 lists the major chemotherapeutic agents for particular protozoal and helminthic infections. Chagas' disease, clonorchiasis, and echinococcosis cannot, as yet, be treated effectively. Some trypanosomes and plasmodia have developed resistance to antiprotozoal agents, but the mechanisms of drug resistance, as well as of drug action, remain enigmas.

The analog 5-fluorocytosine was first synthesized for treatment of leukemia. It was not effective for that purpose, but it was later found to have antifungal activity. *Cryptococcus neoformans*, *Candida* species, and a rarer yeast, *Torulopsis glabrata*, are particularly susceptible to 5-fluorocytosine. Its mode of action is not entirely clear, but it appears to be converted *in vivo* to 5-fluorouracil. It is less toxic than amphotericin B and is therefore a preferred alternate drug of choice for some fungal infections.

The synthetic drugs amantadine and methisazone have antiviral activity.

Amantadine

Methisazone

The virustatic effect of amantadine is limited to the RNA viruses. It may act by interfering with penetration of virus into susceptible cells. The drug has prophylactic activity against some strains of influenza A2 viruses. Methisazone was originally known for its tuberculostatic activity, but has more recently been shown to have antiviral activity against the smallpox virus. The drug acts intracellularly, in some manner, to prevent virus maturation. Amantadine and methisazone have very limited use in the treatment of viral diseases. Both drugs demonstrate minimal to moderate toxicity.

SUPERIMPOSED INFECTIONS

Approximately 2 percent of patients treated with antimicrobial agents develop superimposed infections, often caused by indigenous bacteria or

Table 27-2 MAJOR CHEMOTHERAPEUTIC AGENTS FOR PARASITIC INFECTIONS

INFECTION	AGENT
PROTOZOA	
Amebiasis	metronidazole, tetracycline, emetine, chloroquine, diiodohydroxyquin
Giardiasis	metronidazole, quinacrine
Trichomonas vaginitis	metronidazole
Amebic meningoencephalitis	amphotericin B (?)
Pneumocystis carinii pneumonia	pentamidine isothionate
Malaria	chloroquine-primaquine, quinine, pyrimethamine, sulfonamides
Leishmaniasis	antimony sodium gluconate, pentamidine isothionate
Chagas' disease	none
African sleeping sickness	
Trypanosoma gambiense	pentamidine isothionate, suramin
T. rhodesiense	suramin, pentamidine isothionate, melarsoprol, tryparsamide
Toxoplasmosis	pyrimethamine-trisulfapyrimidines
HELMINTHS	
Tapeworms	
T. saginata, T. solium	
D. latum, H. nana	niclosamide, quinacrine
Roundworms	
E. vermicularis	pyrantel, pyrvinium, piperazine, thiabendazole
Ascariasis	pyrantel, piperazine, thiabendazole
Strongyloidiasis	thiabendazole, pyrvinium
Trichuriasis	hexylresorcinol enemas
Trichinosis	thiabendazole, steroids
Hookworms	tetrachlorethylene, bephenium, pyrantel, thiabendazole
Creeping eruption	thiabendazole
Filariasis	diethylcarbamzine
TREMATODES	
Schistosoma japonicum	tartar emetic
S. mansoni, S. haematobium	hycanthone, niridazole, antimony dimercaptosuccinate, stibophen
Clonorchis	none

SOURCE: Adapted from H. Most, Treatment of common parasitic infections of man encountered in the United States, *New Engl. J. Med.* 287:495, 1972.

yeasts. Common etiological agents in such secondary infections are resistant strains of *Proteus, Pseudomonas, Escherichia, Staphylococcus,* and *Candida* species (Figure 27-3). Individuals with impaired host defenses, such as those occurring in severe burns, organ transplantation, cancer, diabetes, collagen diseases, or neurological disorders, are especially susceptible to infectious complications following a primary infection.

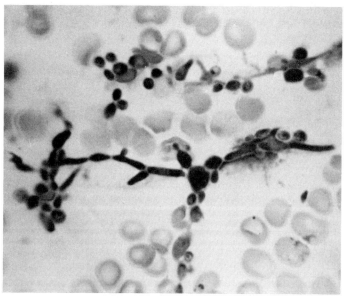

Figure 27-3 *Candida* species in a Giemsa-stained peripheral blood smear from a patient with a superimposed infection related to antimicrobial therapy. (Courtesy, M. A. Gordon and New York State Department of Health, Albany, New York.)

The judicious use of antimicrobial agents in the compromised host requires careful evaluation of multiple factors: site of the infection, toxinogenic properties of the organisms, invasive ability of the organism, and patient status. Cancer per se is usually not fatal to an individual, but the priority on nutrients is such that tumors are fed at the expense of other tissues. The resulting debilitating condition provides little defense against the invasion of microorganisms. It has been estimated that more than one-third of cancer deaths at some hospitals are caused by an infectious process. Quite clearly, the risks associated with any type of chemotherapy are real, despite its life-saving potential.

LABORATORY METHODS

The goal of drug therapy in infectious or neoplastic disease is to provide the most effective treatment with minimum risk and cost to the patient. This can be accomplished only with the aid of the laboratory in identifying the etiological agent, determining antimicrobial susceptibilities of the organism, evaluating the patient's clinical symptoms, and considering the pharmacological characteristics of available drugs. The laboratory may be needed to monitor the effectiveness of the course of therapy by assaying serum for levels of antibiotics and by taking cultures both during and after a course of therapy.

IN VITRO SUSCEPTIBILITY TESTS

In vitro antimicrobial susceptibility tests are the most reliable guides for the selection of appropriate therapy in cases in which the susceptibility of an organism is not predictable. The tests should be performed on pure cultures with antimicrobials of suitable spectra.

The Kirby-Bauer Method. The Kirby-Bauer disc-agar diffusion method is the most frequently performed test for antimicrobial susceptibility (Figure 27-4). The method employs Mueller-Hinton agar dispensed in Petri plates measuring 150 mm in diameter and 15 mm deep. The plates are somewhat larger than standard Petri plates to accommodate multiple antibiotic discs. The plates are inoculated with sterile cotton swabs from standardized suspensions of bacterial isolates. If five colonies are placed in 4.0 ml aliquots of brain-heart infusion broth, sufficient growth is obtained in two to five hours. Discs can be applied with a dispenser or forceps after allowing a few minutes for surface moisture to be absorbed. Following an overnight incubation period at 35°C, sizes of zones of inhibition are measured with calipers.

Results are reported as susceptible (S), intermediate (I), or resistant (R) after measurement of sizes of inhibition zones. Susceptibility implies that the organism should respond favorably to therapeutic doses of the drug. Resistance implies that the usual therapeutic concentrations of antimicrobials would be ineffective. Intermediate zones indicate some susceptibility to therapeutic doses and may be important in the event that a patient is hypersensitive to the drugs producing susceptibility.

MINIMUM INHIBITORY AND MINIMUM BACTERICIDAL CONCENTRATIONS

Dilution tests in broth provide a quantitative method for antimicrobial susceptibility testing. Dilution tests require serial two-fold dilutions of antibiotics in tubes or wells of plastic plates containing broth and inoculation with a standard inoculum (Figure 27-5). After overnight incubation tubes or wells are examined for turbidimetric evidence of growth. The least concentration of the antimicrobial inhibiting visible growth is reported as the *minimal inhibitory concentration* (MIC). The *minimal bactericidal concentration*

Figure 27-4 The Kirby-Bauer procedure for antimicrobial susceptibility testing. (*A*) An inoculum is collected from the tops of five colonies. (*B*) The organisms are emulsified in a test tube containing trypticase soy yeast broth and incubated for 2 to 6 hours. (*C*) The turbidity of the broth is compared with a barium sulfate standard and adjusted if necessary. (*D*) A sterile swab is dipped into the culture and excess moisture is removed by pressing swab against the side of the tube. (*E*) The swab is used to inoculate a large plate (150 mm) containing Mueller-Hinton agar. (Continued on page 618.)

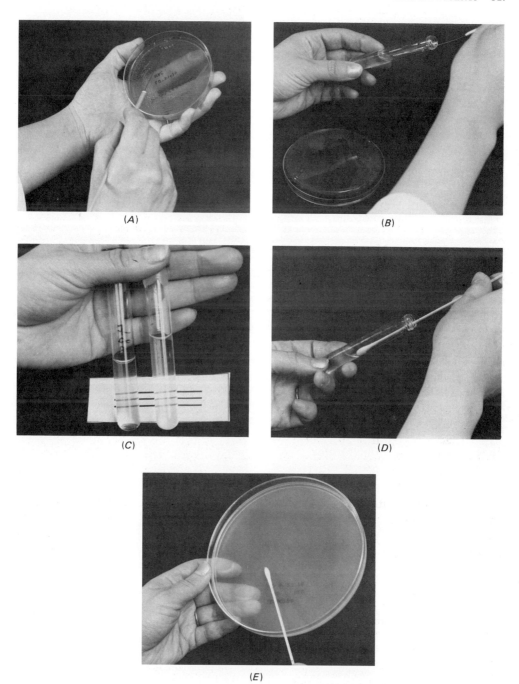

(A)

(B)

(C)

(D)

(E)

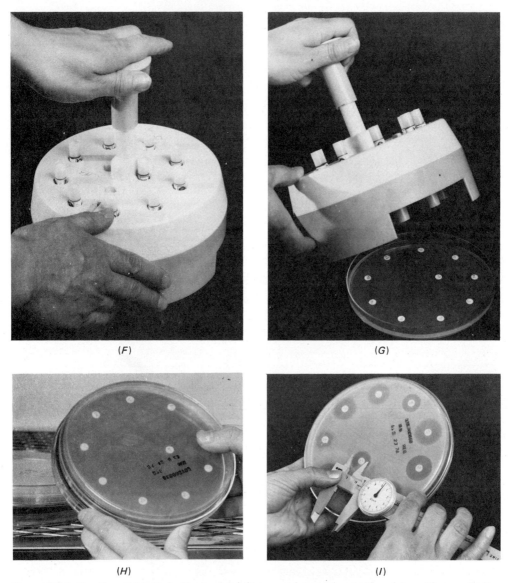

(F)

(G)

(H)

(I)

Figure 27-4 (*Continued*) (*F–G*) Antimicrobial discs are dropped onto the plate with a multidisc dispenser. (*H*) The plate is incubated overnight at 35 to 37°C. (*I*) The sizes of the zones of inhibition are measured with calipers and susceptibilities are determined by referring to a zone-size interpretive chart. (Courtesy, Saint Joseph Medical Center, Burbank, California.)

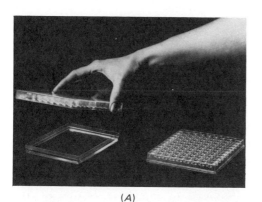
(A)

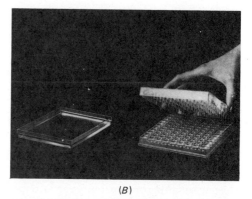
(B)

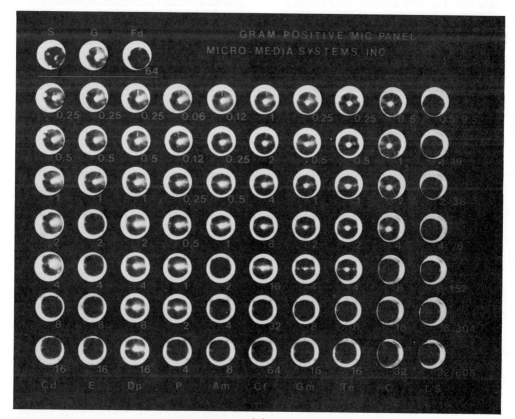
(C)

Figure 27-5 Determination of MIC. (*A*) A disposable transfer lid containing prongs is placed into a seed trough. (*B*) Plates are inoculated by lowering the prongs into the wells of antimicrobial agents which have been serially diluted two-fold. (C) The MIC test panel for gram-positive organisms. The least concentration of the antimicrobial agent inhibiting visible growth is reported as the MIC. (Courtesy, Micro-Media Systems, Inc., Potomac, Maryland.)

(MBC) can be determined by subculturing broths containing no apparent growth on an appropriate agar medium. After overnight incubation the lowest concentration of the antibiotic in the broth which fails to produce colonies on agar is the MBC. The MIC and MBC may be the same with bactericidal agents. Quantitative information is important when using particularly toxic antimicrobials and in determining synergism or antagonism between antibiotics.

ASSAY OF ANTIMICROBIALS

Assays of antimicrobials in body fluids may be useful in maintaining blood levels required for maximum therapeutic efficiency. Concentrations of antibiotics may be assayed by turbidimetric, chemical, enzymatic, radioimmunoassay, or agar diffusion techniques. Enzymatic, chemical, and radioimmunoassays are precise methods requiring meticulous attention to detail and are not suitable for most hospital laboratories.

GENERIC AND PROPRIETARY NAMES

The large number of proprietary or trade names under which antimicrobial and chemotherapeutic agents are available is astounding. Repeated attempts to require that physicians use generic names for prescription drugs have forced legislative action in some parts of the United States. There is, of course, good reason for a physician to specify a proprietary name of a particular antimicrobial if it is better tolerated or has a pharmacological characteristic consistent with the requirements of the patient. Only the antimicrobial component of chemotherapeutic agents is active *in vitro*. Generic names should be employed in reporting results of antimicrobial and susceptibility tests. A listing of some generic and proprietary names of common antimicrobial and chemotherapeutic agents may be found in the appendix.

SUMMARY

Chemotherapy has saved millions of lives, but it is not without risk to a patient. The range and degree of activities, toxic effects, and hypersensitivity potentials of the more than a hundred drugs require judicious decisions in selecting and administering therapeutic regimens. *In vitro* laboratory susceptibility testing of bacterial isolates and monitoring of serum levels of antimicrobial agents can be used as guides in the selection of appropriate drugs and dosages. The search for new antimicrobial agents and modifications of existing ones may one day yield more perfect chemotherapeutic agents, but in the meantime providing effective therapy, geared to individual needs, must be a continuing effort.

QUESTIONS FOR STUDY

1. Identify the target site for each antimicrobial agent.
   chloramphenicol
   penicillin
   streptomycin
   colistin
   nystatin
   tetracyclines
   sulfonamides
   trimethoprim
   isoniazid
   lincomycin
2. Name two drugs which have antifungal activity.
3. Name two drugs which have antiviral activity.
4. What is the basis of reporting antimicrobial susceptibility tests as susceptible (S), intermediate (I), or resistant (R)?
5. For what purpose is cycloheximide used in the microbiology laboratory?

SELECTED REFERENCES

Barker, B. M., and Prescott, F. *Antimicrobial Agents in Medicine.* Oxford: Blackwell, 1973.

Citri, N., and Pollock, M. R. The biochemistry and function of β-lactamase (penicillinase). *Advan. Enzymol.* 28:237, 1966.

Corcoran, J. W., and Hahn, F. E. *Mechanism of Action of Antimicrobial and Antitumor Agents.* Vol. 3, *Antibiotics.* New York: Springer-Verlag, 1975.

Garrod, L. P., and O'Grady, F. O. *Antibiotic and Chemotherapy.* 2d ed. London: Livingstone, 1968.

Kagan, B. M. *Antimicrobial Therapy.* 2d ed. Philadelphia: Saunders, 1974.

Kagan, B. M.; Fannin, S. L.; and Bardie, F. Spotlight on antimicrobial agents. *JAMA* 226:306, 1973.

Kucers, A., and Bennett, N. McK. *The Use of Antibiotics: A Comprehensive Review with Clinical Emphasis.* 2d ed. Philadelphia: Lippincott, 1975.

Lennette, E. H.; Spaulding, E. H.; and Truant, J. P. *Manual of Clinical Microbiology.* 2d ed. Washington, D.C.: American Society for Microbiology, 1974.

McHenry, M. C., and Gavan, T. L. Selection and use of antibacterial drugs. *Progress in Clinical Pathology.* Vol. 6. New York: Grune & Stratton, 1975.

McMahon, F. G., and Finland, M. *Drugs Useful vs. Infectious Diseases.* Mount Kisco: Futura, 1974.

Maugh, T. H., II. Cancer chemotherapy: now a promising weapon. *Science* 184:970, 1974.

Most, H. Treatment of common parasitic infections of man encountered in the United States. *New Eng. J. Med.* 287:495, 1972.

Pratt, W. B. *Chemotherapy of Infection.* New York: Oxford University Press, 1977.

Ryan, K. J.; Schoenknecht, F. D.; and Kirby, W. M. M. Disc sensitivity testing. *Hospital Practice* 5:91, 1970.

Zähner, H., and Maas, W. K. *Biology of Antibiotics.* New York: Springer-Verlag, 1972.

Chapter 28

Collection and Handling of Laboratory Specimens

After you read this chapter, you should be able to:

1. Explain how the type of specimen sent to the laboratory for microbiological examination is determined.
2. Describe the method of collecting blood for culture.
3. List five types of urine specimens which are suitable for bacteriological culturing.
4. Explain why specimens for microbiological examination should be sent to the laboratory promptly.
5. List three means of obtaining acceptable sputum specimens.
6. Explain why sputum specimens are sometimes rejected for processing by a hospital laboratory.
7. Indicate when a transport medium should be employed in collection of specimens.
8. Describe the special procedures which need to be followed if anaerobic etiology is suspected.
9. Explain why special care is required in handling specimens from individuals suspected of having syphilis and gonorrhea.
10. Describe the problems associated with surgical and postmortem samples.
11. Explain why labeling and recording the time of collection are important in processing specimens.
12. Explain when refrigeration or freezing of a specimen is indicated.

The success of the microbiology laboratory of a hospital in detecting the presence or absence of an infectious agent depends on appropriate collecting and handling of specimens. Microorganisms extremely sensitive to atmospheric oxygen or the effects of dehydration must be collected and handled with extra caution. Addition of a preservative to a specimen is sometimes required to prevent the destructive effects of an alteration in pH or overgrowth of rapidly growing organisms. Most specimens for the laboratory need to be collected under conditions of strict asepsis in sterile containers free of leakage. All specimens for microbiological examination and culture should be transported to the laboratory as rapidly as possible.

TYPES OF SPECIMENS

Some microorganisms remain confined to the site of initial entry; others extend into neighboring tissue or spread by way of the lymphatic or circulatory system to sites far removed from the portal of entry. Blood is the most effective vehicle of transportation for all microorganisms. Blood-borne microorganisms can cross the blood-brain barrier and promote infections of the central nervous system or produce foci of infection in other organs. The type of specimen collected depends on the type of infection suspected from clinical evidence or history of the patient. Multiple samples may be necessary to detect the presence of pathogens or to rule out an infectious agent as the cause of disease.

BLOOD

Blood is collected for culturing whenever there is a sudden increase in pulse rate or temperature, an onset of chills, hypotension, mild fever with a heart murmur, a history of trauma, or a rapid decline in the condition of an infant or a compromised host. Bacteremia may be intermittent so times of collection are important. Three blood cultures taken within 24 to 48 hours are usually ample. Blood taken at the first sign of fever is associated with higher recovery rates than blood obtained later in febrile disease.

Skin should be cleansed with 70 percent alcohol and treated with an iodophor, before removing blood with a syringe and needle or transfer set (Figure 28-1). Best results are obtained if blood culture bottles are inoculated at bedside. The amount of blood collected from adults should be at least 10 ml; lesser volumes can be taken from children.

Regardless of the volume obtained from a patient, a 10 percent dilution by volume of blood to liquid medium is recommended to dilute antimicrobial factors of blood. The incorporation of 0.025 percent sodium polyanetholsul-

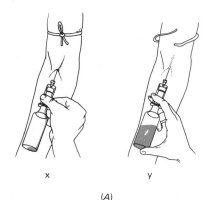

(A)

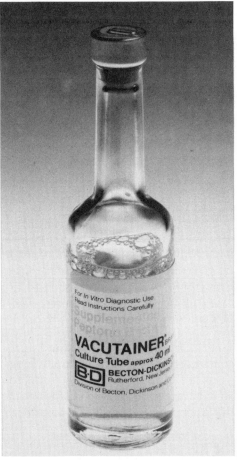

(B)

Figure 28-1 Blood culture collection. (A) Blood is collected from the antecubital vein in a Vacutainer (trademark of Becton, Dickinson and Company). (B) Actual Vacutainer containing a culture tube with a 10 ml draw tube which assures a 1:5 dilution ratio. (Courtesy, BBL Microbiology Systems, Division of Bectin, Dickinson, and Company, Cockeysville, Maryland.)

fonate (SPS) destroys both residual anticomplementary and antiphagocytic activity. Many enriched broths, such as trypticase soy or brain heart infusion, are satisfactory for recovery of aerobes, but anaerobes require prereduced media in vacuum bottles with 10 percent carbon dioxide (CO_2). Aerobic bottles need to be vented aseptically by puncturing the diaphragm with a sterile cotton-plugged needle. *Pseudomonas* species or yeast will not grow in unvented bottles. The needle should be removed, unless the bottle is to be incubated in a CO_2 incubator, to prevent excessive loss of CO_2, which may be a prerequisite for growth.

Cultures should be incubated at 35°C and inspected the same day, after an elapse of several hours, and daily for one week for evidence of turbidity, gas, hemolysis, or small colonies. Prolonged incubation may be necessary for cultures from patients already receiving antimicrobial therapy. The addition of penicillinase to blood cultures of patients receiving high doses of penicillin or cephalosporin may be necessary to obtain isolations. Examination of Gram-stained smears and subculturing are necessary to identify organisms.

URINE

Urine for routine bacteriological culture may be collected by cystoscopy, by suprapubic aspiration, from an indwelling catheter, by catheterization, or by the clean voided, midstream procedure.

Urine can be removed by cystoscopy from the bladder or ureters. To remove urine by suprapubic aspiration, a direct puncture of the bladder is made through the lower abdominal wall.

Catheterization is no longer justified for bacteriological purposes alone. If the procedure is required for diagnostic or therapeutic reasons, a sample of urine can be collected in a sterile container (Figure 28-2). Urine can be obtained from an indwelling catheter by puncturing the wall of the catheter, after

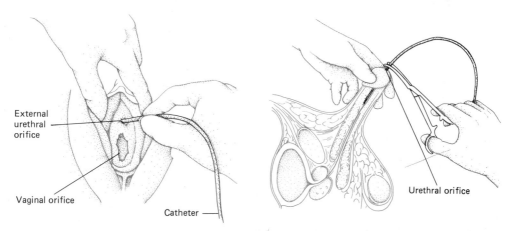

External urethral orifice

Vaginal orifice

Catheter

Urethral orifice

Figure 28-2 Technique for catheterization in female and male.

disinfection with 70 percent alcohol and an iodophor.

The reliability of a clean voided urine specimen is largely dependent on the ability of a patient to cooperate in collection of the specimen. Thorough cleaning of the vulva or glans penis with soap and water as well as adequate rinsing is required to eliminate contaminants from the genitals and perineal areas (Figure 28-3). After voiding 20 to 30 ml of urine, a midstream specimen is collected, without discontinuance of voiding, in a sterile container.

All urine specimens for bacteriological culturing, regardless of the method of collection, should be taken to the laboratory immediately for processing. If a delay is unavoidable, urine specimens should be refrigerated. Urine is a good culture medium so prolonged exposure to room temperature invalidates quantitative studies.

Quantitative studies on urine incriminate counts in excess of 10^5 as indicative of infection. Gram stains of smears prepared from uncentrifuged specimens can be of value in quantitative assessments. Usually one or more bacterial cells can be observed per oil immersion field if counts are 10^5 or greater. Quantitation by culture requires the use of a loop calibrated to deliver 0.01 or 0.001 ml of urine. Identification of any isolates is made by subculturing and biochemical testing. Although a variety of rapid methods are available for screening urines for bacteriuria, none are totally reliable. Precise identification of pathogens requires isolation and use of established procedures.

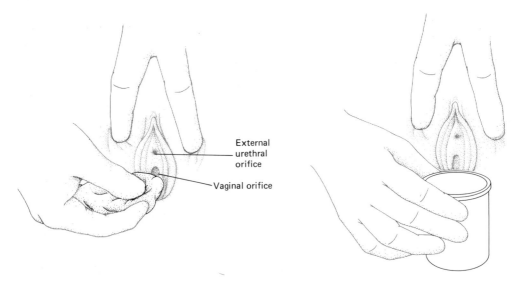

External urethral orifice

Vaginal orifice

Figure 28-3 Technique for obtaining a clean-voided specimen in the female. Gauze soaked in soap is used to cleanse urethral orifice from front to back with labia spread. Specimen is collected in a container with labia apart without allowing the body to touch the container.

Clean voided specimens are satisfactory for viral studies if 500 units of penicillin, 500 μg of streptomycin, and 200 units of nystatin per milliliter are added immediately after collection. Specimens should be frozen and maintained at $-70°C$ in a freezer until processed. Isolation of a viral agent most often requires repeated sampling.

STOOL

It is especially important that stool specimens be taken to the laboratory promptly, since many microorganisms, such as salmonellae and shigellae, do not survive a drop in temperature and subsequent alteration in pH. The use of a preservative, such as 0.033 M phosphate buffer mixed with equal volumes of glycerol, increases chances for recovery of pathogens. Either a rectal swab, obtained by rotating a swab beyond the anal sphincter, or a minute amount of stool is sufficient. Portions of stool containing blood or mucus yield especially fruitful results.

At least three stool specimens or rectal swabs should be sent to the laboratory to rule out bacterial, protozoal, or helminthic infection. Gram stains of smears from stool are usually of little or no value because of the large numbers of bacteria comprising the normal flora of the intestine. Most types of culture media selectively cultivate gram-negative bacilli, but nonselective media should be used when anaerobic or superimposed infections are suspected.

It is necessary to send larger amounts of stool and repeated specimens when looking for adult worms, proglottids, or scolices. Rectal swabs for isolation of viruses should be swirled in approximately 3.0 ml of tissue culture medium containing 500 units of penicillin and 500 μg of streptomycin per milliliter in a screw-capped vial. The specimen should be processed immediately or frozen for transport to an appropriate laboratory facility.

CEREBROSPINAL FLUID

Cerebrospinal fluid (CSF) is usually examined as an emergency procedure in patients with signs or symptoms of central nervous system disease. A fever, headache, stiff neck, or exaggerated reflexes may be present. In infants it is important to rule out meningitis in unexplained febrile disease by examination of CSF.

Specimens should be obtained by aseptic lumbar puncture, collected in sterile, screw-capped containers, and transported immediately to the laboratory (Figure 28-4). Fastidious microorganisms, such as *Neisseria meningitidis* and *Haemophilus influenzae*, do not survive very long at room temperature.

CSF must be centrifuged to concentrate any organisms present before making smears or inoculating culture media. Gram stains of smears are of value in the presumptive diagnosis of an infectious process since CSF is normally sterile. However, gram reactions of bacteria from CSF may not always be typical. The type of white blood cells present in sediments is often a clue in the differential diagnosis of meningitis. Polymorphonuclear cells are characteristic of bacterial meningitis, while mon-

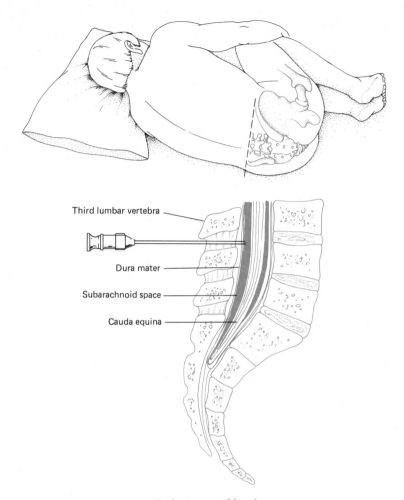

Third lumbar vertebra

Dura mater

Subarachnoid space

Cauda equina

Figure 28-4   Techniques of lumbar puncture.

onuclear cells predominate in tuberculous, viral, fungal, or protozoal infections. Glucose concentrations are decreased in bacterial and tuberculous meningitis.

If studies for viruses are requested, CSF should be frozen at −70°C as soon as possible after collection as viruses are not stable in CSF at room temperature.

SPUTUM

Specimens of sputum often yield unreliable results because of contamination with microorganisms from the nose, mouth, or pharynx. Gram stains may indicate the appropriateness of a specimen for culturing. Squamous epithelial cells in sputum are indicative of oropharyngeal contamination. In purulent infections polymorphonuclear white blood cells are present. Some hospital laboratories routinely reject specimens for processing if more than 10 squamous epithelial cells per high power field are seen. If unsatisfactory sputum specimens are not rejected by the laboratory prior to culturing, the reports on sputum cultures need to be interpreted with some caution. Bacteria which predominate in cultures, if not part of the indigenous flora, are candidates as etiological agents in infectious disease.

Specimens obtained by bronchoscopy, an induced sputum technique, or transtracheal aspiration are reliable when collected aseptically. Transtracheal aspiration or induced sputum from inhalation of an aerosol of heated hypertonic saline containing propylene glycol are particularly recommended for individuals who have difficulty in raising sputum (Figure 28-5). Cultures of 24-hour sputum specimens are fraught with error because of overgrowth of contaminants from the upper respiratory tract.

SKIN AND NAILS

Scrapings of skin or nails are sent to the laboratory if infection by a dermatophyte is suspected. Scrapings are obtained with a sterile scalpel after an area

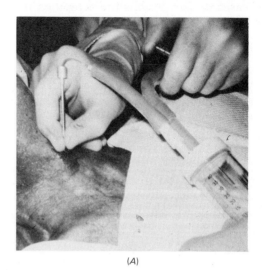

(A)

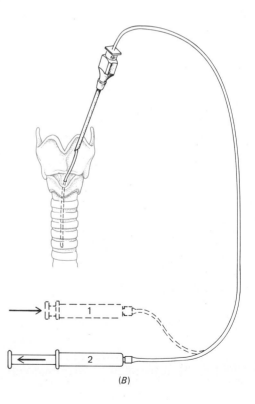

(B)

Figure 28-5 Transtracheal aspiration technique for obtaining lower respiratory tract secretions which are free from oropharyngeal contamination. (A) Photograph of aspiration in process. (Courtesy, J. G. Bartlett, Boston.) (B) Diagram showing placement of needle.

is cleansed with 70 percent alcohol. In cases of skin lesions the scrapings include tissue from active borders of lesions and some healthy tissue. For appropriate nail sampling surface scrapings are discarded and only deeper scrapings are sent to the laboratory for culture. Both skin and nail scrapings can be conveniently transported to the laboratory in sterile Petri plates.

PUS

Suppurative material from wounds, lesions, or abscesses must be collected carefully. A swab from a single lesion rarely contains enough material to establish a diagnosis, so that generous portions from several lesions or multiple specimens from large lesions are usually required. Curettage of sinus tract linings and excision of ulcers are often necessary to obtain satisfactory specimens. Parts of the walls from abscesses are excised and sent to the laboratory. Gram stains of smears from pus or fluids, if collected properly, are particularly useful. Etiological agents are usually present in sufficient amounts to be visualized with ease. Isolates require subculturing, biochemical testing, and sometimes serological tests for definitive identification. In certain fungal infections animal inoculation may be indicated.

Fluids or scrapings from bases of lesions for viral studies should be collected early after eruption of lesions, following a wash with sterile saline. Aspirated fluids or swabs can be placed in 2 ml of nutrient broth or tissue culture fluid. All specimens should be frozen at −70°C until processed.

FLUIDS OTHER THAN CSF

Specimens of peritoneal, pericardial, pleural, or synovial fluid require collection under strict aseptic conditions and immediate transfer to a transport medium since anaerobes are frequently encountered. Most body fluids are excellent culture media so contamination, with even a few microorganisms, results in prolific growth. The addition of an anticoagulant, such as heparin, is often required to prevent clotting.

Gram stains of smears prepared from centrifuged specimens may reveal the presence of invading microorganisms. Both aerobic and anaerobic conditions of incubation should be provided for isolation of infectious agents. Subculturing and biochemical testing are necessary to identify isolates.

EAR, EYE, NOSE, AND THROAT

Most physicians do not feel that tympanocentesis is justified in ear infections unless treatment with a broad-spectrum antimicrobial agent does not clear up the infection.

For reliable eye cultures conjunctival swabs are taken before application of topical anesthesia. Corneal scrapings are taken after application of an anesthetic. The paucity of available material is always a problem, and recovery of causative agents of conjunctivitis or keratitis is difficult.

The most reliable nasopharyngeal specimens for culture are obtained with

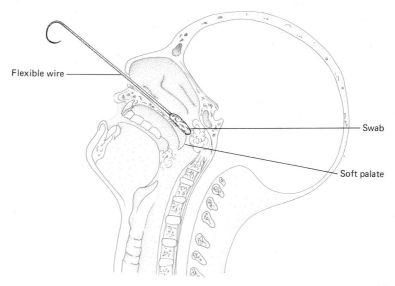

Flexible wire

Swab

Soft palate

Figure 28-6   Collection of a nasopharyngeal specimen using a dacron
swab on a flexible wire.

a dacron swab on a flexible wire (Figure 28-6). The wire can be inserted into the nasopharynx through the nose. Gram stains of smears made from swabs are of value only if a predominant organism is present. Results of cultures require careful interpretation, since large numbers of bacteria isolated may be indigenous to the nasopharynx. The nasopharyngeal route is a potential portal of entry for opportunistic pathogens causing hospital-acquired infections.

For throat cultures a dacron swab should be used to obtain material from both tonsillar areas, the posterior pharynx, and any other areas of ulceration or inflammation. A liquid or semisolid holding medium is recommended for transport to the laboratory to prevent desiccation of pathogens. Gram stains of smears prepared from swabs sometimes reveal a predominant pathogen, but the microorganisms need to be differentiated from indigenous flora using appropriate cultural, biochemical, or serological techniques.

Swabs or washings from the ear, eye, nose, or throat for viral studies, other than for respiratory syncytial virus, can be placed in 2.0 ml amounts of nutrient broth or tissue culture medium and frozen at $-70°C$ until they can be processed by the laboratory. The respiratory syncytial virus is inactivated by freezing. If shipment to a regional public health laboratory is required, it is best to check with the laboratory for exact collecting or handling procedures.

SPECIMENS REQUIRING SPECIAL HANDLING

Some specimens require special handling either because of the nature of the collection procedure, the circumstances of collection, or the characteristics of the etiological agents. Specimens may be difficult to obtain, may be impossible to duplicate, or may require expensive surgical procedures. The etiological agents may be destroyed by transfer to the *in vitro* environment unless special precautions are taken during collection, or unless special transfer or storage conditions are supplied.

PUS OR SCRAPINGS FROM SEXUALLY TRANSMITTED DISEASE (STD)

The collection and handling of specimens used for the diagnosis of STD deserve special attention. Swabs from suspected gonococcal disease are usually obtained from the urethra, cervix, pharynx, rectum, or conjunctiva. Less frequently blood, pus from abscesses, synovial fluid, or prostatic fluid yield cultures positive for gonococci.

The gonococcal organism is especially sensitive to drying and to even trace amounts of disinfectants. At least one hour should elapse after urination before collections from the urethra are made. A transport medium, prewarmed to room temperature, should be employed if the swab cannot be taken immediately to the laboratory after collection.

The presence of intracellular gram-negative diplococci, history, and symptoms constitute presumptive evidence for a diagnosis of gonorrhea, but absence of the typical gonococci does not rule out the disease. Examination of smears from men with gonorrhea is more productive than smears obtained from women with the infection. Cul-

tures should be set up on Thayer-Martin (TM) medium to confirm a presumptive diagnosis and to investigate further all instances of negative or equivocal smears.

Scrapings from chancres of syphilis require that dark-field microscopic examination be done immediately upon collection of the specimen. Treponemes are very delicate and are sensitive not only to drying, but also to temperature and other more subtle atmospheric conditions. Serum exudate must be obtained for adequate sampling of a chancre. Direct dark-field microscopic examination for detecting *Treponema pallidum* is not a common laboratory procedure. Collection and observation of specimens should be attempted only by experienced physicians and laboratory technologists.

All hospital personnel required to handle specimens from patients suspected of having syphilis must be aware that *T. pallidum* can remain viable for extended periods in some body fluids and on some types of organic matter. If hands become contaminated, immediate hand washing is necessary to avoid possible infection through small breaks in the skin. If containers are broken or leak during transport, laboratory personnel must assess the risk to all individuals who may have been exposed to the organism.

PUS OR FLUID FROM SUSPECTED ANAEROBIC INFECTIONS

If an anaerobic etiology is suspected, specimens of pus or fluid should be aspirated after thorough cleansing of skin or mucosa with 70 percent alcohol and an iodophor. Many anaerobes are destroyed by even brief exposure to atmospheric oxygen, so specimens are transported to the laboratory in the syringe after the needle is capped or transferred to transport tubes containing a reducing agent. A swab can be used to inoculate a tube of prereduced anaerobically sterilized (PRAS) medium upon receipt in the laboratory. If a delay cannot be avoided, storage in the refrigerator inhibits growth of facultative organisms. Gram stained smears of pus or fluid may provide the first evidence that an anaerobe is present. The presence of gram-positive sporeforming bacilli or gram-negative fusiform bacilli are good reasons for suspecting anaerobes as etiological agents.

SURGICAL SPECIMENS

Surgical specimens or autopsy material are obtained at some cost to the patient or relatives. Since it is usually impossible to obtain repeated specimens, tissue sent to the laboratory for examination or culturing must be handled with great care. Histopathological studies are often not definitive in establishing the diagnosis of an infectious disease. Upon receipt in the microbiology laboratory, tissue for culture is minced with sterile scissors and ground aseptically with a mortar and pestle using a 60-mesh aluminum oxide. A suspension of approximately 20 percent in nutrient broth is made for culturing on selective media. Any suspension remaining can be stored at 5°C, in case additional culturing is required after histopathological assessment has been made.

Tissue impression smears may be used for examination of tissue for some viruses, bacteria, or protozoa. Fresh lymph nodes, liver biopsy material, brain tissue, or bone marrow can be lightly impressed on a clean glass slide from a freshly cut surface. Fluorescent antibody techniques can be applied for identification of specific viruses, such as the rabies virus, or rickettsiae. Blood stains can be applied to tissue impression smears for identification of protozoa, such as *Leishmania* and *Toxoplasma*.

Cultures performed on a single postmortem sample of tissue are usually of limited value and must be interpreted with caution. Indigenous microorganisms migrate freely after death and may be abundant in tissue obtained at autopsy. Embalming of tissue diminishes chances for recovery of infectious agents.

WHOLE BLOOD FOR SEROLOGICAL STUDIES

Whole blood is obtained from patients when serological studies are necessary to establish a diagnosis. Blood is collected aseptically with a sterile needle and syringe or Vacutainer (trademark of BBL Microbiology Systems, Becton, Dickinson, and Company, Cockeysville, Maryland) after application of 70 percent alcohol to the skin. The specimen is sent to the laboratory promptly where serum can be separated from the clot aseptically after centrifugation.

For viral or rickettsial studies an acute-phase serum, obtained 5 to 7 days after onset of illness, is refrigerated until the convalescent-phase specimen can be collected, 14 to 21 days after onset. No anticoagulants or preservatives should be added.

OTHER SPECIMENS FOR VIRAL OR RICKETTSIAL STUDIES

The isolation of viruses and rickettsiae from clinical specimens is not always practical or even possible. The isolation techniques require expertise which is more frequently available in regional public health or reference laboratories than in hospital laboratories.

Transport vials and guidelines for collection of specimens are available from laboratories equipped to process such specimens. The type of specimen required depends on the suspected viral agent (Table 28-1). It is important that swabs or pieces of tissue be placed in a transport medium immediately upon collection. A balanced salt solution containing small amounts of gelatin and antibiotics is frequently employed as a transport medium. Fluids, stool, or autopsy material can be placed in sterile containers with secure caps.

All specimens should be frozen upon receipt by the hospital laboratory and stored at −70°C until they can be examined. Frozen specimens to be sent to another laboratory are packed in dry ice. Because some viruses are particu-

Table 28-1   SPECIMENS REQUIRED FOR ISOLATION OF PARTICULAR VIRUSES

Virus	Throat Swab	Stool	CSF	Conjunctival Swab	Vesicle Fluid	Urine
Adenovirus	X	X		X		X
Arbovirus			X			
Coxsackievirus	X	X	X			
Cytomegalovirus	X					X
Echovirus	X	X	X			
Herpesvirus	X		rare	X	X	
Influenza virus	X					
Mumps virus	X		X			X
Parainfluenza virus	X					
Poliovirus	X	X	rare			
Reovirus	X	X				
Respiratory syncytial virus	X					
Rhinovirus	X					
Rubella virus	X					
Rubeola virus	X		X			
Vaccinia-variola viruses					X	
Varicella-zoster virus					X	

SOURCE: L. M. Clark and M. F. Sierra, Virology: preventing and treating viral diseases. *Lab World* 29:62, 1978. Reprinted from *Lab World* with permission.

larly susceptible to injury incurred in even one freeze-thaw cycle, for maximum recovery rates care must be taken to prevent intermittent freezing and thawing during storage and shipment.

BLOOD SMEARS FOR PROTOZOAL OR HELMINTHIC PARASITES

Blood smears for examination of malarial parasites, trypanosomes, and microfilariae are best obtained at bedside. Peripheral blood from a fingertip or earlobe is preferable to venous blood. The skin is cleansed with 70 percent alcohol and broken with a sterile lancet. Blood should be free flowing; squeezing the finger or earlobe dilutes any parasites with tissue fluid and thereby decreases the probability of detecting them.

Thin or thick blood films can be prepared on clean glass slides (Figure 28-7). It may require some practice to make satisfactory smears. A thin film should contain a single layer of well distributed red blood cells. Thick smears have the advantage of concentrating any parasites, but they are more difficult to read. Multiple samplings of blood on three to four successive days may be

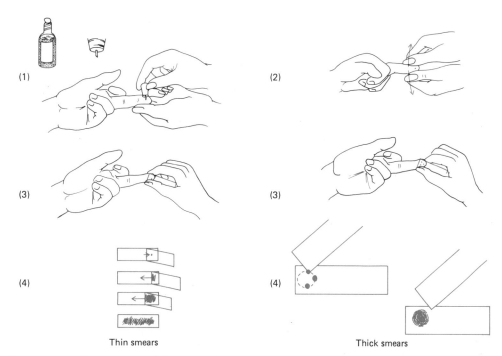

Thin smears

Thick smears

Figure 28-7   Preparation of thin and thick blood smears. (U.S. Naval Medical School, National Naval Medical Center, *Medical Protozoology and Helminthology*, Washington, D.C.: U.S. Government Printing Office, 1965.)

required to rule out protozoal or helminthic disease.

LABELING OF SPECIMENS

The individual collecting a specimen must also assume responsibility for labeling it and sending the request form to the laboratory. Writing must be legible and patients must be identified by number and name. Time of collection must be indicated for blood cultures and for other specimens in which multiple samples are required. Most laboratories record the time of arrival of specimens on the request forms so that delays in transport can be detected.

SHIPMENT OF SPECIMENS

Regulations on shipment of diagnostic specimens, including cultures of infectious agents, are contained in the Interstate Quarantine Regulations (*Federal Register*, Title 42, Chapter 1, Part 72, revised July 30, 1972). Specimens should be sent only to those laboratories entitled by permit to receive them. Packing must be sufficient to resist possible rough handling in the mails. Stoppers and covers on tubes or other containers must be secure, and double containers are required to prevent infection of a handler should breakage occur. All specimen containers must be clearly marked "ETIOLOGIC AGENT/ BIOMEDICAL MATERIAL."

SUMMARY

While only trained microbiologists can perform diagnostic tests in the laboratory, it is important for all health personnel to be familiar with the methods for collecting and handling microbiological specimens. The successful recovery of pathogens is dependent on appropriate sampling techniques, use of sterile containers, appropriate transport media, care in packing for transport, and prompt delivery to the laboratory. Multiple specimens are often required to isolate etiological agents or to rule out infectious disease. Upon arrival in the laboratory, immediate processing is necessary to avoid destruction of more fastidious organisms or to prevent overgrowth of indigenous flora. All specimens for viral or rickettsial studies need to be kept frozen until processed. If specimens are to be sent to another laboratory, they must be packaged and shipped according to governmental regulations.

QUESTIONS FOR STUDY

1. Why is the time of delivery of specimens for bacteriological studies to the laboratory so critical?
2. What is meant by a clean voided urine?
3. Why are multiple specimens sometimes required to diagnose or rule out an infectious disease?
4. What problems are associated with collection of sputum and identification of possible pathogens?

5. What special precautions must be taken when collecting or handling specimens from suspected anaerobic infections?

SELECTED REFERENCES

Barry, A. L.; Smith, P. B.; and Turck, M. Laboratory diagnosis of urinary tract infections. *Cumitech* 2:1, 1975.

Bartlett, R. C.; Ellner, P. D.; and Washington, J. A. Blood cultures. *Cumitech* 1:1, 1974.

Bodily, H. L.; Updyke, E. L.; and Mason, J. O. *Diagnostic Procedures for Bacterial, Mycotic, and Parasitic Infections*. 5th ed. New York: American Public Health Association, 1970.

Clark, L. M., and Sierra, M. F. Virology: preventing and treating viral diseases. *Lab World* 29:58, 1978.

Finegold, S. M.; Shepherd, W. E.; and Spaulding, E. H. Practical anaerobic bacteriology. *Cumitech* 5:1, 1977.

Kellogg, D. S., Jr.; Holmes, K. K.; and Hill, G. A. Laboratory diagnosis of gonorrhea. *Cumitech* 4:1, 1976.

Lennette, E. H.; Spaulding, E. H.; and Truant, J. P. *Manual of Clinical Microbiology*. 2d ed. Washington, D.C.: American Society for Microbiology, 1974.

Markell, E. K., and Voge, M. *Medical Parasitology*. 4th ed. Philadelphia: Saunders, 1976.

Sonnenwirth, A. C. *Bacteremia — Laboratory and Clinical Aspects*. Springfield, Ill.: C. C. Thomas, 1973.

Chapter 29

Control of Hospital-Acquired Infections

After you read this chapter, you should be able to:

1. List several personnel factors which contribute to hospital-acquired infections.
2. Describe a procedure for hand washing which prevents the spread of microorganisms.
3. Describe procedures for masking and unmasking.
4. Describe a procedure for gloving.
5. List the environmental factors which contribute to hospital-acquired infections.
6. Describe adequate procedures for disinfecting floors, walls, ceilings, furniture, fixtures, windows, drapes, and linen.
7. Describe an efficient washing and rinsing process for laundry.
8. Describe how to minimize infections obtained by the parenteral route.
9. Describe problems associated with the use of common equipment for patients.
10. Discuss water as a source of hospital sepsis.
11. Design a procedure for safe disposal of hospital wastes.
12. Explain how antimicrobial therapy, immunosuppressive therapy, and immobilization predispose patients to infection.
13. List the major responsibilities of the institution in preventing hospital-acquired infections.
14. Explain the criteria necessary to classify infections as nosocomial in origin.

The hospital environment represents a very special ecological niche. The types of microorganisms found in any hospital are those brought to that environment by hospital personnel, visitors, and patients. Since new patients and visitors enter the hospital daily and personnel changes are frequent, the potential for variety in a microbial population is maintained. Many microorganisms which under usual circumstances do not cause disease become invasive because of hospital-associated alterations in normal defense mechanisms. Infections that develop in a patient after admission to a hospital are called hospital-acquired or *nosocomial* infections. Such infections must be differentiated from those acquired in the community.

Careful surveillance of hospitals has revealed that predisposing factors for nosocomial infections may be associated with personnel, the environment, and patients.

PERSONNEL FACTORS

Hospital personnel may have transient pathogenic bacteria in the nasopharynx, in the gastrointestinal tract, or on the skin without evidence of disease. Personnel must, therefore, be considered as potential reservoirs of microorganisms capable of causing disease in patients. It is particularly important that food-handlers be free of those organisms causing shigellosis or salmonellosis. Even in the absence of known infectious disease, certain precautions must be taken to prevent hospital-acquired infections.

HAND WASHING

Careful hand washing is probably the most important factor in the prevention

639

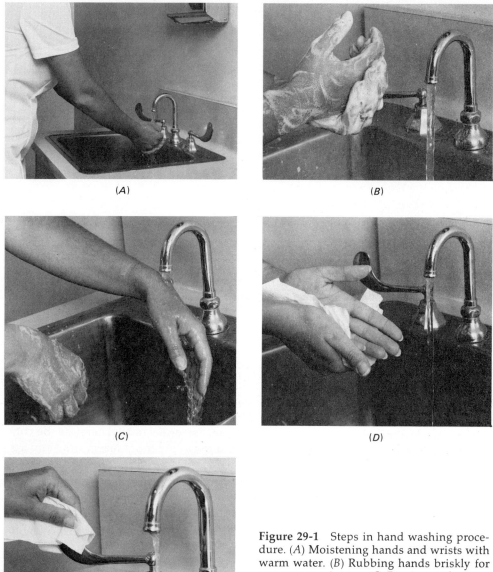

Figure 29-1 Steps in hand washing procedure. (A) Moistening hands and wrists with warm water. (B) Rubbing hands briskly for one or two minutes. (C) Rinsing with warm water flowing from wrists to fingertips. (D) Drying hands with paper towel. (E) Turning the faucet off with a clean, dry towel. (Courtesy, Saint Joseph Medical Center, Burbank, California.)

Procedure for Hand Washing

1. Moisten hands and wrists with warm water.
2. Apply a heavy lather of disinfectant-containing soap well beyond areas of possible contamination.
3. Rub hands briskly with special attention to fingers and nails for one to two minutes.
4. Rinse hands in warm water by allowing water to flow downward from wrists to finger tips.
5. Repeat hand washing procedure.
6. Dry hands thoroughly with a clean paper towel.
7. Turn the faucet off with a clean, dry paper towel.

of hospital-associated infections. Although hand washing is a simple task requiring no special skills, it is the procedure most frequently violated in patient care. Hands should be washed thoroughly: (1) between patients, (2) after handling objects such as bed pans, dressings, or specimen containers, (3) after visits to the bathroom, (4) before eating snacks or meals, and (5) before and after the end of a shift (Figure 29-1).

MASKING

Masks are worn to prevent the spread of infection by aerosols. Masks should be worn in surgery, the delivery room, isolation units, and during collection of any specimen when aerosols from nasal, tracheal, or pharyngeal sources could be transferred to hospital personnel (Figure 29-2). In some instances the patient as well as the attendant should wear a mask. It must be remembered that masks do not prevent transmission of microorganisms from person to person, but merely reduce the transmission of potential invaders.

GOWNING

Gowns are worn to prevent the clothing of hospital personnel from becoming contaminated and to eliminate the possibility of cross-infections. Gowns should be worn in surgery, the delivery room, nurseries, isolation units, and during collection of nasal, tracheal, or pharyngeal specimens (Figure 29-3).

GLOVING

Scrubbing hands and forearms before gloving for a procedure in surgery or patient care removes many microorganisms from the skin, but may bring other microorganisms from deeper skin layers to the surface. Gloves serve both in preventing the transmission of surfaced organisms to patients and in protecting the hands of personnel from contamination. Gloves must be worn in surgery, in the delivery room, for particular types of examinations, for patient care in some isolation units, for changing dressings, and for handling specimens obtained from persons with infectious diseases (Figure 29-4).

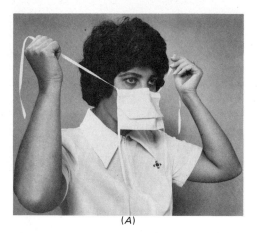 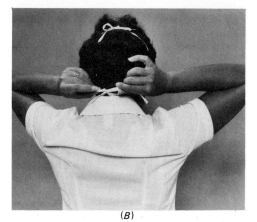

(A)   (B)

Figure 29-2 Steps in masking procedure. (A) Positioning mask while holding it by the strings. (B) Tying upper and lower strings behind the head. (Courtesy, Saint Joseph Medical Center, Burbank, California.)

Procedure for Masking

1. Wash hands thoroughly.
2. Pick up mask by strings.
3. Shake to unroll mask.
4. Position mask by pulling upper strings over ears and tying behind head.
5. Tie lower strings behind the head.

Procedure for Unmasking

1. Untie bottom strings.
2. Untie top strings.
3. Remove mask by gripping top strings.
4. Discard immediately in container for contaminated masks.
5. Wash hands thoroughly.

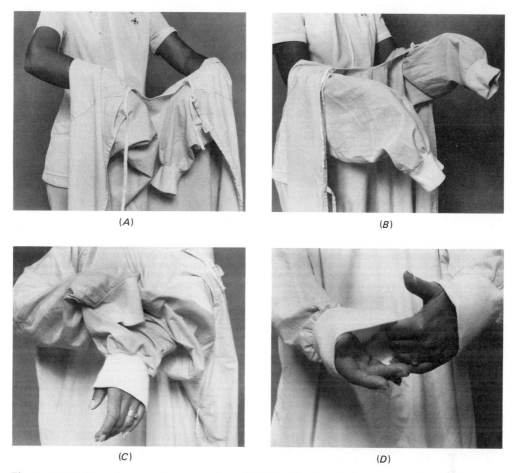

Figure 29-3 Steps in gowning procedure. (*A*) Slipping hands into gown sleeves at shoulders. (*B*) Placing arms through sleeves. (*C*) Pulling up on shoulders. (*D*) Adjusting wrist bands. (Courtesy, Saint Joseph Medical Center, Burbank, California.)

Procedure for Gowning

1. Wash hands thoroughly.
2. Slip hands into sleeves at shoulders.
3. Place arms through sleeves and pull up on shoulders touching only inside of gown.
4. Adjust wrist bands.
5. Tie neck and waist strings.

Procedure for Ungowning

1. Untie waist strings.
2. Wash hands thoroughly.
3. Untie neck strings.
4. Roll shoulders and arms forward to slip out of gown.
5. Discard immediately in container for contaminated gowns.
6. Wash hands thoroughly.

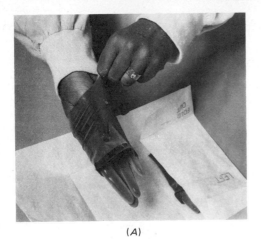

(A)

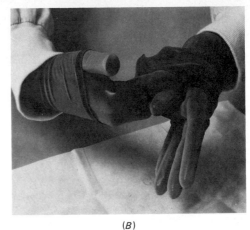

(B)

(C)

Figure 29-4 Steps in gloving procedure. (A) Pulling inside of one cuff firmly until fingers are in place. (B) Placing second glove in position. (C) Pulling glove cuffs over gowned wrists. (Courtesy, Saint Joseph Medical Center, Burbank, California.)

Procedure for Gloving

1. Grasp the inside cuff of one glove.
2. Insert the hand and pull firmly until fingers are in place.
3. Grasp the inside cuff of the second glove.
4. Insert the hand and pull firmly until fingers are in place.
5. Pull glove cuffs over the gowned wrists.

ENVIRONMENTAL FACTORS

The ubiquitous nature of microorganisms provides most environments with a plethora of potential infectious agents. The hospital environment is associated with special risks for the patient, however, and special care must be exercised to maintain low microbial populations.

Some equipment must of necessity be shared by patients requiring diagnostic procedures, surgery, or supportive therapy. Many specialized procedures employed in patient care represent potential hazards in the spread of disease. The risk may be minimized by special attention to aseptic technique, such as careful management of closed drainage systems, adequate perineal care, appropriate skin preparation before injection or surgery, removal of inner dressings with sterile forceps, prompt disposal of contaminated dressings, and capping of stopcocks.

It is not within the scope of this text to provide details for such procedures and for other activities involved in the control of microbial populations, but the informed health professional will recognize not only the ubiquity of microorganisms, but also will be aware of host factors which may predispose hospital populations to infectious disease. There is no substitute for an alert staff member in preventing invasion of frank pathogens or opportunistic microorganisms by providing good patient care. The awareness of potential sources of contamination in the environment needs to be created and maintained in all hospital personnel.

FLOORS

There is no substantial evidence correlating the incidence of specific infections to floor, table top, wall, or ceiling contamination. It is outside the realm of possibility to have floors remain decontaminated for any period of time. Not only do dust particles settle to the floor, but the flow of traffic is responsible for the dissemination of large numbers of microorganisms.

A wet method of mopping or vacuuming is necessary to remove dried contaminated material (Figure 29-5). A

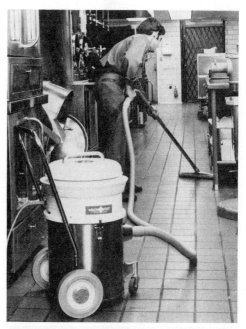

Figure 29-5 Vacuuming equipment designed for wet or dry use. (Courtesy, The Kent Company, Elkhart, Indiana.)

detergent and a germicide, such as chlorine or a quaternary ammonium compound, can be added to water. Operating room, delivery room, and nursery floors require special attention to maintain low bacterial populations. Carpeting does not increase infection hazards and may actually reduce the number of airborne organisms by entrapping them, but special steam cleaning may be required if rooms or corridors are carpeted.

WALLS AND CEILINGS

It is not necessary to clean walls and ceilings as often as floors, but grease does adhere to walls and can attract dust particles as well as microorganisms. A regular schedule for wall and ceiling washing should be followed. In addition, any room that has been occupied by a person with a communicable disease should be thoroughly cleaned and disinfected immediately after use. The choice of an appropriate detergent and disinfectant may depend on the wall finish. Whatever cleaning agent is used, rinsing should be thorough.

FURNITURE, FIXTURES, AND WINDOWS

Furniture and light fixtures should be cleaned every day. Damp dusting with a detergent-germicide is preferable to dry dusting because it produces less dissemination of microorganisms. Plumbing fixtures, such as sinks and toilets, should be cleaned twice daily with a detergent-germicide. Tubs and showers should be scrubbed immediately after each patient's use. It is usually adequate to clean windows once a month.

DRAPERIES AND CURTAINS

Cubicle curtains may be a reservoir of staphylococcal organisms. One study found that curtains around the bed of an infected patient became colonized within 24 hours. A check on cubicle curtains in other parts of the same hospital revealed that 54 percent of the curtains contained viable staphylococcal organisms. Curtains in isolation rooms should always be changed after the discharge of the patient.

LINENS, MATTRESSES, AND PILLOWS

Hospital bedding can be a significant reservoir for pathogenic bacteria. It may soon be possible to supply hospitals with linens treated with a chemical which will provide long lasting antimicrobial activity.

It is not always possible or practical to launder all blankets between patients in nonisolation units, but it is important to adhere to a schedule so that blankets are washed at regular intervals. Cotton blankets may be washed with sheets and pillow cases, but woolen blankets may require special care. Woolen blankets from isolation units must be autoclaved or subjected to gas sterilization.

A minimum amount of shaking should be done in gathering linens for

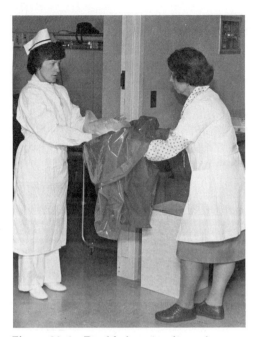

Figure 29-6 Double bagging linen from an isolation area. The use of a red outer bag clearly identifies laundry from an isolation unit. (Courtesy, A. S. Jacobs and Wilmington Medical Center Photography Department, Wilmington, Delaware.)

laundering. A linen hamper may be brought to the room or soiled linen can be bagged and placed in a laundry chute. Linen from isolation areas should be double bagged and clearly marked (Figure 29-6). Some hospitals make a practice of using different colored laundry bags for linen from isolation areas. Such linens are usually handled separately by the laundry.

Hampers or carts distinctly labeled "soiled" or "clean" can do much to avoid mixing soiled and clean linens. Carts, hampers, and chutes should be disinfected daily. A disinfectant spray

can be most effectively employed for laundry chutes.

It should be possible to empty laundry bags into washers without sorting, but if this is not possible, the sorting area should be removed from the rest of the laundry. Laundry personnel should handle the laundry as little as possible and should wear gowns, masks, and gloves for maximum protection. Conditions of washing and rinsing may vary from hospital to hospital, but minimum standards of water temperature, cleaning agents, and procedure should be met.

Linens for patients who may be particularly susceptible to infections (transplant patients, burn cases, or patients compromised in other ways) and linens for obstetrical and operating rooms should be autoclaved.

Mattresses and pillows are often protected by reusable covers or disposable bags made of impenetrable plastic materials. Coverings should be cleaned with a detergent-germicide and bags should be changed between patients.

An Efficient Washing and Rinsing Procedure

1. Use water at a temperature above 71°C (160°F).
2. Use a suitable detergent or soap.
3. Add bleach or laundry sour.
4. Wash for a minimum of 25 minutes.
5. Rinse several times in water above 71°C (160°F).

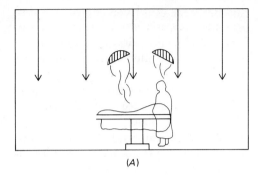

(A)

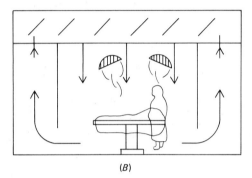

(B)

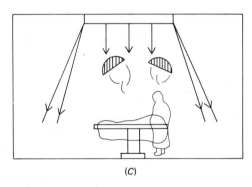

(C)

Figure 29-7 Vertical air flow in an operating room. (A) Whole room with small lamps to minimize turbulence. (B) Recirculating system with plastic curtains defining work area. (C) Downflow confined within a set of higher velocity air jets. (Reprinted with permission from *Proceedings of the International Conference on Nosocomial Infections*, published by the American Hospital Association.)

VENTILATION SYSTEMS

The quality of air and the direction of air currents are important factors in the spread of infections, but the best way to achieve a high quality of air free from pathogenic organisms, dust, and odors remains conjectural. Special needs for clean air exist in operating rooms, isolation units, and laboratories. The rate of air circulation currently required in operating rooms by federal or local regulations is 8 changes per hour, but many have ventilation rates of 15 or more changes per hour. Frequent exchanges of air can be supplied by a directed-flow ventilation system with minimal air turbulence. Such systems, called laminar flow systems, operate with low, but uniform velocities of filtered air (Figure 29-7). Installation of unidirectional flow ventilation is costly, however, and the effectiveness of such systems in operating rooms has not been proved.

NEEDLES, SYRINGES, AND PARENTERAL SOLUTIONS

The use of plastic, disposable sterile needles and syringes has greatly reduced the number of infections originating from contamination of reusable needles and syringes. Packages containing those items should not be opened until immediately before use. If the needle touches any surface or object, it must be assumed to be contaminated and should be discarded. If a filled syringe is not to be used at once, the plastic needle protector should be applied. Sterile gauze pads may be substituted if protectors are not available.

Microorganisms, such as strepto-cocci, staphylococci, or diphtheroids, may be inadvertently introduced into a host by inadequate disinfection of a patient's skin before use of a hypodermic needle. It is important that a fresh supply of disinfectant be maintained and that it be applied to cotton or gauze pads immediately before use.

If injections are to be given intravenously or if blood is to be removed from a vein or artery, it is sometimes necessary to palpate the blood vessel. In such cases the finger of the physician, technologist, or nurse should also be decontaminated by application of the same disinfectant applied to the skin of the patient.

One nationwide epidemic of hospital-acquired sepsis from contaminated bottle closures of intravenous fluids focused attention on the parenteral route of infection. Any type of injectable material can be involved in accidental parenteral infection (Figure 29-8). The increased use of total parenteral

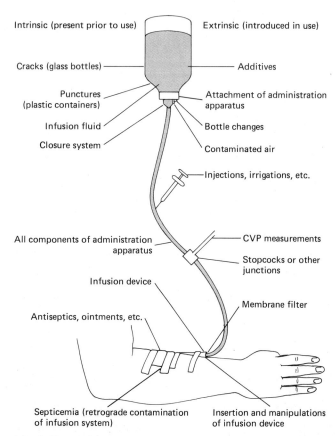

Figure 29-8 Potential intrinsic and extrinsic sources of contamination of intravenous infusion systems.

nutrition (TPN) in severely ill adults and children has substantially increased the risk of infections transmitted by that route.

Legal requirements for blood to be used for transfusion make it mandatory that blood donors have no active infections or histories of specific diseases, such as syphilis, hepatitis, or malaria. Routine serological tests for detection of antibodies against syphilis and the surface antigen (HB$_s$AG) of the hepatitis B virus are performed. Since other microorganisms may be present in donors having latent infections, it is not realistic to hope that the presence of all microorganisms will be detected. In addition, the amount or method of handling may increase the risk of contamination of whole blood fractions. Visual inspection of blood or injectable materials is of limited value in revealing contamination since materials may not normally be clear. The use of single-dose vials for medications and storage of multiple-dose vials under refrigeration, however, can substantially reduce the risk of parenterally introduced infections.

THERMOMETERS

It has long been recognized that thermometers are ideal vehicles for transmitting many microorganisms, including viruses. Unless disposable thermometers are available, the safest procedure is to provide a thermometer which can be kept bedside for each patient. Thermometers can be stored safely in 70 percent ethyl or isopropyl alcohol containing 0.2 percent iodine.

The disinfectant should be changed at least every three days. For terminal disinfection between patients, thermometers are usually sent to central supply for sterilization by ethylene oxide after mechanical cleansing with a detergent. Pressure applied with a brush accomplishes no more than wiping and eventually may destroy markings on thermometers.

RESPIRATORY THERAPY EQUIPMENT

Equipment used to assist respiration mechanically may be the source of contaminated aerosols. When such aerosols are inhaled by a patient, droplet nuclei pass directly into the distal portions of the bronchial capillaries. Epidemics caused by gram-negative bacilli, such as *Pseudomonas, Klebsiella,* and *Serratia* species, have been clearly traced to respiratory therapy equipment.

Some nebulizers and tubing are difficult to clean and cannot be autoclaved. If disposable nebulizers are not available, such equipment can be washed with a detergent and subjected to ethylene oxide sterilization. If materials permit, autoclaving is the most efficient and economical sterilizing procedure. Pasteurization at temperatures below 100°C in a water bath can destroy contaminating microorganisms, but equipment so processed is wet following treatment and recontamination can occur during the drying period, unless drying is done in an ultrafiltered drying oven.

Cold sterilants, such as glutaraldehyde, have been used effectively, but thorough rinsing with sterile distilled water is required since residues of the chemical may act as irritants. Decontamination with 0.25 percent acetic acid was at one time recommended, but is probably the least satisfactory method. Nebulizers need to be replaced every 24 hours for patients receiving multiple daily treatments.

HEMODIALYSIS EQUIPMENT

The so-called artificial kidney provides the means for detoxifying blood of patients with acute renal failure and an increasing number of patients with irreversible renal insufficiency. In the procedure arterial blood is pumped through a dialyzing membrane that allows metabolic wastes to accumulate in a surrounding bath and is returned to the venous system.

Bacterial infections are common in patients on regular hemodialysis. Staphylococcal infections and bacteremias are frequently encountered, and osteomyelitis has been reported as a sequela of such infections. Certain gram-negative bacilli, *Pseudomonas, Xanthomonas, Aeromonas,* and *Flavobacterium,* grow especially well in dialysates containing metabolic products from patients' blood. Both endotoxins and exotoxins may pass through intact membranes and cause pyrogenic reactions.

The factors influencing microbial contamination in hemodialysis systems are multiple. They include the water supply, the distribution system, and the actual dialysis machines. Most of them are associated with an indwelling cannula (small tube) which connects a vein and an artery in the forearm or leg. The contamination of renal dialysis units with viruses of hepatitis presents more difficult problems than does bacterial contamination. However, certain control measures, if applied diligently, can keep levels of bacteria and viruses to a minimum (Table 29-1).

The specific recommendations for water treatment should be made by the physician in charge of a dialysis unit. Standards developed by the ASAIO (American Society for Artificial Internal

Table 29-1 CONTROL MEASURES IN HEMODIALYSIS SYSTEMS

FACTOR INFLUENCING CONTAMINATION	RECOMMENDED CONTROL MEASURE
Water supply	treatment by reverse osmosis; weekly disinfection of reverse osmosis unit with 1.5–2.0 percent aqueous formaldehyde
Water and dialysate distribution system	disinfection with 0.5–1.0 percent sodium hypochlorite immediately before use of the system
Dialysis machines	overnight disinfection with 1.5–2.0 percent aqueous formaldehyde; design to allow outlet taps at equal elevation and at highest point of system

SOURCE: Adapted from M. S. Favero, N. J. Petersen, L. A. Carson, W. W. Bond, and S. H. Hindman, Gram-negative water bacteria in hemodialysis systems, *Health Laboratory Science* 12:321, 1975.

Organs) state that water used to prepare dialysis fluids should not contain more than 100 bacteria per milliliter. Dialysis fluids should not contain more than 1000 bacteria per milliliter. Contamination in excess of 1000 organisms per milliliter in dialysates is associated with a risk of a pyrogenic reaction or a septicemia for the patient. For monitoring purposes samples of water and dialysate should be collected and sent to the laboratory at monthly intervals.

ANESTHESIA EQUIPMENT

The breathing bags and hoses which are a part of anesthesia equipment provide sufficient moisture to support the growth of a variety of bacteria. Whereas a majority of patients can probably withstand the microorganisms encountered in anesthesia equipment, general anesthetics do interfere with some normal defense mechanisms of the body. In particular, mucous membranes of the upper respiratory tract may be traumatized so as to prevent ciliary action. Endotracheal catheters and pharyngeal airways may be disinfected with heat, glutaraldehyde, or ethylene oxide, depending upon materials of which they are made. Rubber and plastic components may be sanitized by placing in glutaraldehyde for 10 minutes. The use of glutaraldehyde should always be accompanied by thorough rinsing in sterile distilled water.

WATER AND MOPS

Water is used for drinking, diluting, and irrigating as well as cleaning. It is a common source of hospital-acquired infections. There are few nutrients in water, so only organisms like the pseudomonads survive for any length of time. However, pseudomonads can act as opportunistic pathogens and may cause infections that resist treatment.

For some uses, water should be sterilized to minimize the risk of infection. Only sterile distilled water should be placed in nebulizers. Containers of sterile distilled water should be carefully capped and bottles replaced with a fresh supply of water every 24 hours.

It is not uncommon to find microorganisms from saliva contaminating water in bedside carafes, if the lid of the carafe also serves as a drinking cup. Thorough washing and disinfection of carafes once a day insures a safe supply of drinking water for patients.

Mopheads should be used for a single day in general areas and only once in operating rooms, delivery rooms, or isolation units before washing. Under no circumstances should mops be allowed to stand overnight in water. Ideally, mopheads should be autoclaved, but washing at 71°C and tumbling until dry does reduce bacterial counts.

DISPOSAL OF WASTES

The appropriate and safe disposal of wastes can be a complex problem in a hospital because of the variety and amount of waste products resulting from patient care. Methods for the safe disposal of such products depend on the type of community sewage system. For example, although most body wastes may be disposed of by flushing down a toilet or hopper, excreta from patients with communicable diseases may need treatment with a chemical agent, such as 5.0 percent phenol, before being emptied into a toilet or hopper. Local sanitation officers can be helpful in recommending adequate procedures.

Wet garbage may be placed in an automatic waste disposal or into a can for collection by a local agency. Cans should be covered and disinfected after emptying. Dry garbage can be emptied into a large common container with little handling. Disposable, plastic inner liners for baskets often facilitate safe handling of articles such as paper, discarded flowers, or other trash.

Infectious material, such as surgical specimens, dressings, autopsy materials, sputum, stool containers, culture plates, and contaminated swabs, should be incinerated, if permitted by local health authorities, or taken to a land-fill operation where appropriate waste treatment can be applied.

PATIENT FACTORS

Most patients admitted to hospitals have either an infectious disease or an underlying disease which makes them more susceptible to infections. In addition, prolonged anesthesia, manipulative procedures, major surgery, and even supportive therapy increase the risk of infection. Identification of high risk patients may be helpful so that special precautions can be taken and more aggresive approaches can be used to detect colonization in patients.

PREDISPOSING DISEASES

Malnutrition has long been thought to influence the incidence and course of infectious diseases. For example, bacterial infections are not only frequent, but often fatal in patients suffering from severe protein deficiency.

The patient with diabetes has long been known to have both frequent and severe infections. Increased concentrations of glucose provide sufficient nutritional enrichment permitting rapid growth of microorganisms. Concomitant vascular problems in diabetics prevent phagocytic cells from responding maximally to localized infection.

Persons who have had extensive skin damage caused by burns appear to be especially susceptible to infections caused by *Pseudomonas* species. Appropriate isolation procedures can minimize exposure of those patients to *Pseudomonas* organisms and other opportunistic pathogens in the hospital environment. Although it seems a stringent precaution, flowers are sometimes not allowed in rooms of burn patients, since the water in vases is often a reservoir for pseudomonads.

Neoplastic disease severely interferes with normal defense mechanisms. A large number of patients with terminal neoplasms die of infectious diseases. The patients often become infected with microorganisms of endogenous origin, but microorganisms of the hospital environment may also be involved in infectious complications.

ANTIMICROBIAL THERAPY

The institution of life-saving antimicrobial therapy against a specific infectious agent may predispose the patient to another infectious disease. The reasons for this may vary, but one underlying factor is alteration in indigenous microorganisms which substantially reduces competition for essential growth factors. Only the most hardy microorganisms survive, and without competition from the primary invader and more susceptible indigenous organisms, they proliferate rapidly and become invasive.

IMMUNOSUPPRESSIVE THERAPY

Drugs which produce a suppression of both cellular and humoral immune responses have been widely used for patients receiving organ transplants and for those having malignancies. As a result of such therapy a new spectrum of etiological agents and new patterns of disease are emerging. In particular, the altered host appears to be more susceptible to some common fungi, protozoa, and viruses. Phycomycosis, candidiasis, aspergillosis, or herpes simplex infections are frequent complications in immunosuppressed patients.

IMMOBILIZATION

The stasis imposed by severe illness or recovery from surgery predisposes a patient to respiratory infections. Most common among these infections is viral pneumonia. Pneumonias are most likely to occur in the elderly or in infants. The practice of requiring postsurgical patients to be ambulatory as soon as possible after surgery has done much to prevent hospital-acquired pneumonias.

MISCELLANEOUS PREDISPOSING FACTORS

There are a number of additional circumstances related to the patient which predispose an individual to hospital-acquired infection. The length of time that hospitalization is required can be an important factor. Illnesses requiring long periods of confinement increase the time of exposure to microbiota of the hospital environment. The need for repetitive procedures requiring instrumentation, such as catheterizations, suctionings, cystoscopies, or intravenous feedings, also increases the risk for the patient. Any wound incurred as a result of surgery is associated with some risk, since a major portal of entry has been provided. Obese patients are at least twice as susceptible as non-obese patients to postsurgical wound infections. Furthermore, emergency operations are apt to be associated with higher infection rates than elective surgical procedures.

Alcoholics and patients who have had splenectomies appear to be extremely susceptible to pneumococcal infections. The infections often fulminate and lead to death within a few hours. The cause for this dramatic susceptibility to the pneumococcal organisms is not well understood.

INSTITUTIONAL CONTROL MEASURES

Certain responsibilities for control of hospital-acquired infections need to be assumed by the institution. Some hospitals publish a handbook, containing rules governing procedures and practices, which is given to every employee. Most hospitals and medical centers are assuming a larger role in providing educational programs for hospital personnel as well as for patients. Regular communication between the staff of the microbiology laboratory, administrative personnel, and health care personnel can often avert potential hazards for patients.

ISOLATION

When clinical or laboratory evidence confirms the presence of a communicable disease or when immunosuppressive therapy must be maintained for long periods of time, it becomes necessary to place a patient in isolation. The extent of precautions necessary to prevent the spread of disease depends on the degree of communicability of the specific infection and the degree of susceptibility of the individual. Whereas private rooms are sometimes necessary, persons with infections caused by non-airborne microorganisms may be placed in two- or four-bed rooms. Premature infants are quite susceptible to airborne infections and for that reason may be placed in special units called isolets.

Many hospitals have adopted separate procedures for respiratory, enteric, wound and skin infections as well as procedures for protective and strict isolation (Table 29-2). Notices of isolation and requirements for personnel or visitors may conveniently be posted on doors of patients' rooms. The reasons for protective measures should be carefully explained to both patients and visitors. It is usually safer to be overly cautious, but hospitals may make adjustments as dictated by physical facilities or psychological needs of patients.

Table 29-2 DISEASES REQUIRING PROTECTIVE PRECAUTIONS AND ISOLATION

DISEASES REQUIRING WOUND AND SKIN PRECAUTIONS
1. Burns, extensive, not infected with *Staphylococcus aureus* or group A streptococcus
2. Gas gangrene
3. Impetigo
4. Staphylococcal skin and wound infections
5. Streptococcal skin infection
6. Wound infection, extensive

DISEASES REQUIRING RESPIRATORY ISOLATION
1. Chickenpox
2. Herpes zoster
3. Measles (rubeola)
4. Meningococcal meningitis
5. Meningococcemia
6. Mumps
7. Pertussis (whooping cough)
8. Rubella (German measles)
9. Tuberculosis, pulmonary—sputum-positive (or suspect)
10. Venezuelan equine encephalomyelitis

Table 29-2 (*Continued*)

DISEASES REQUIRING ENTERIC PRECAUTIONS
1. Cholera
2. Enteropathogenic *E. coli* gastroenteritis
3. Hepatitis, viral (infectious or serum)
4. Salmonellosis (including typhoid fever)
5. Shigellosis

CONDITIONS REQUIRING PROTECTIVE ISOLATION
1. Agranulocytosis
2. Severe and extensive, noninfected vesicular, bullous, or eczematous dermatitis
3. Certain patients receiving immunosuppressive therapy
4. Certain patients with lymphomas and leukemia

DISEASES REQUIRING STRICT ISOLATION
1. Anthrax, inhalation
2. Burns, extensive, infected with *Staphylococcus aureus* or group A streptococcus
3. Diphtheria
4. Eczema vaccinatum
5. Melioidosis, pulmonary, or extrapulmonary with draining sinus(es)
6. Neonatal vesicular disease (herpes simplex)
7. Plague
8. Rabies
9. Rubella (German measles) and congenital rubella syndrome
10. Smallpox
11. Staphylococcal enterocolitis
12. Staphylococcal pneumonia
13. Streptococcal pneumonia
14. Vaccinia, generalized and progressive

NOTE: Lists are based on guidelines in U.S. Department of Health, Education, and Welfare, *Isolation Techniques for Use in Hospitals*, HEW Publication No. (HSM) 71-8042 (Washington, D.C.: U.S. Government Printing Office, 1973). The publication gives details of precautionary measures and recommended duration of isolation.

MONITORING THE ENVIRONMENT

An effective monitoring system should include routine culturing of autoclaves, infant formulas, irrigation fluids, and instruments having direct contact with deep tissues of the body. The Joint Commission on the Accreditation of Hospitals requires that all steam and hot air sterilizers be checked weekly, and that every load from ethylene oxide sterilizers containing equipment or fluids for use in deep tissues be checked. Gas sterilizers are much less reliable because of difficulties in maintaining standard amounts of humidification.

Commercially available strips of spore-impregnated filter paper and ampules containing a thermal-sensitive indicator and spore suspensions are used for monitoring the efficiency of sterilization procedures. Spore strips or ampules should be placed in the center of the largest items to be sterilized.

A daily record of temperature achieved by a sterilizer should be kept. Paper or tape treated with a chemical which turns from white to black upon reaching the sterilizating temperature is also used to minitor sterilization cycles. Such chemical indicators are not reliable indicators of adequate sterilization, but may be useful to show at a glance if packs or other items have undergone a sterilization process (Figure 29-9).

Dry spore strips are acceptable for testing the efficiency of steam, gas, or dry heat sterilization procedures. Spores of *Bacillus stearothermophilus* are

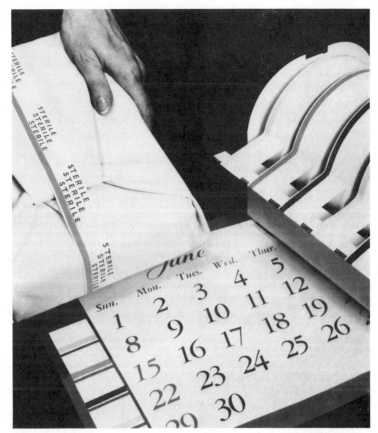

Figure 29-9 A test pack after completion of a sterilization cycle. The appearance of the word *sterile* on the test tape indicates that an acceptable temperature was reached. Tapes are color coded according to week of the month in which pack was processed. (Courtesy, Professional Tape Company, Inc., Hinsdale, Illinois.)

preferred for steam sterilizers, whereas spores of *B. subtilis* are more efficient biological indicators for dry heat or ethylene oxide sterilization. Ampules containing both a chemical and a biological indicator are required for use in washer-sterilizers or in sterilization procedures for solutions (Figure 29-10).

A chemical indicator in the inner glass tube of a 5.0 ml ampule melts and turns red when the sterilizing temperature is reached. Maintenance of the red hue for seven days of incubation at 55° to 60°C verifies effectiveness of the sterilizing procedure. The occurence of a yellow color and turbidity in ampules after incubation for seven days constitutes evidence for growth of the spores of the indicator organism (*B. stearothermophilus*).

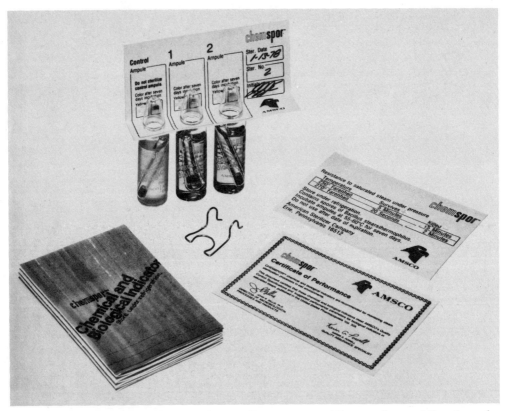

Figure 29-10   A sterility testing system containing spores of *B. stearothermophilus*. Ampules containing chemical and biological indicators can be used to verify sterility in wet environments after incubation for seven days at 55 to 60°C. (Courtesy, American Sterilizer Company, Erie, Pennsylvania.)

Spore strips of *B. subtilis* or *B. stearothermophilus* must be sent to the laboratory for transfer to trypticase soy broth. Evidence of turbidity after a seven-day incubation period at 35° to 37°C or 55° to 60°C, respectively, constitutes evidence of growth and, therefore, inadequate performance by the sterilizer.

Nonsterilized control strips or ampules are always sent to the laboratory at the same time as test strips or am-

pules to assure viability of spores. Records sent to the laboratory with control and test strips or ampules should include date, contents of load, sterilizer identification, and load number.

No materials or equipment should be released for use until laboratory reports of no growth are obtained for spore strips or ampules for the load in which they were subjected to the sterilization procedure. If reports indicate that a sterilizer is not performing satisfactorily, tests should be repeated before notifying the maintenance department or service repairman.

Some public health departments require monitoring of infant formulas in hospitals. Samples are sent to the laboratory for culturing on a weekly or biweekly basis. Recognized standards are less than 25 colonies per milliliter with no pathogens. Milk, unlike water, is a good culture medium. The presence of even a few microorganisms may result in gross contamination if milk is left at room temperature for any length of time. The use of commercially prepared sterile infant formulas has eliminated the need for monitoring infant formulas in many hospitals.

The lack of uniformly accepted standards for control of hospital equipment make it difficult to assess results of cultures taken from hospital equipment. A set of guidelines prepared by the Wilmington Medical Center in Wilmington, Delaware, derived from several sources as well as from their own experience, appears to contain achievable environmental standards (Table 29-3). The most reliable results are obtained when broth can be passed through equipment, collected under aseptic conditions, and sent to the laboratory promptly.

Table 29-3 GUIDELINES FOR ENVIRONMENTAL MICROBIAL STANDARDS

ITEM	FREQUENCY	STANDARD
Autoclaves*	weekly	no growth after 7 days
Ethylene oxide sterilizers†	each cycle	no growth after 7 days
Infant formulas	weekly	25 SPC and 1 coliform per ml
Water and ice	monthly	100 SPC and 2.2 coliforms per 100 ml
Dishes, utensils	monthly	25 SPC by swab rinse method
Liquids, soaps, lotions	monthly	10 SPC
Floor of operating room or delivery room proper	monthly	12 on Rodac plate
Floor of operating room and labor room	monthly	25 on Rodac plate
Operating room, walls, shelves, patient tables, light instrument tables, anesthesia masks, airways, endotracheal tubes	monthly	5 on Rodac plate; 7 by swab rinse method
Anesthesia and respiratory therapy equipment	monthly	15 by swab rinse method
Scrub room sinks (clean)	monthly	15 by swab rinse method
Sterile instruments, packs, etc.	every 2 or 3 months	no growth after 7 days

*Biological indicator containing 10^5 spores of *Bacillus stearothermophilus*.
†Biological indicator containing 10^6 spores of *Bacillus subtilis*.
SOURCE: Adapted from Committee on Continuing Education, *Infection Control in the Hospital Environment*, Washington, D.C.: American Society for Microbiology, 1976; V. Lorian, *Significance of Medical Microbiology in the Care of Patients*, Baltimore: Williams & Wilkins, 1977.

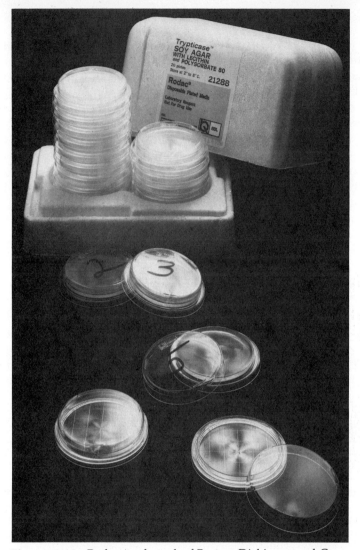

Figure 29-11 Rodac (trademark of Becton, Dickinson and Company) containing trypticase soy agar. (Courtesy, BBL Microbiology Systems, Division of Becton, Dickinson, and Company.)

Some hospitals routinely culture surfaces and air from surgery, delivery rooms, nurseries, intensive care units, and coronary care units. The Rodac plate (a product of BBL Microbiology Systems, Becton, Dickinson, and Company, Cockeysville, Maryland) can be used for sampling surfaces or air. The plates are exposed to air for 10 minutes or their agar surfaces are applied to flat areas of furniture (Figure 29-11). It is recommended that sampling of floors and overbed tables in patients' rooms be done one-half hour after cleaning. A count of less than 25 colonies indicates low-level contamination. Counts between 25 and 100 suggest doubtful disinfection practices. Counts over 100 mean that sanitation procedures are inadequate.

The American Association of Blood Banks has recommended culturing of random units of blood periodically. The number of bottles selected and the times are left to individual laboratories and depend on the volume of blood used. If contamination is suspected, however, the complete administration unit should be sent to the laboratory for culturing. In addition, blood cultures must be obtained from the patient. All blood used in transfusions should, of course, be sterile.

Drinking water or ice cannot be expected to be sterile and may contain relatively large numbers of bacteria. However, not more than 2.2 of 100 organisms found in such samples should be coliforms. Regular culturing of ice and water samples may reveal reservoirs of other organisms, such as *Pseudomonas* species, which can be troublesome as opportunistic pathogens.

Most microbiologists warn against the overmonitoring of hospital environments as expensive and unwarranted. Low air or surface bacterial counts may serve to allay fears of some physicians, but work loads resulting from monitoring procedures should not be allowed to detract from the major services of the microbiology laboratory in the diagnosis of infectious disease.

MONITORING PERSONNEL

Routine culturing of specimens obtained from hospital personnel, with the possible exception of dietary service employees, cannot be justified. Many hospitals require that at least three stool specimens from applicants for jobs involving food handling be evaluated for ova, parasites, or bacterial pathogens. Some hospitals require annual stool examinations on all dietary service employees. A few hospitals require applicants for jobs in nurseries to have nasopharyngeal cultures to detect possible carriers of *S. aureus*. Most hospitals give tuberculin skin tests and make chest X rays as part of the routine physical examination on new employees. X rays should be mandatory for all potential employees with positive tuberculin skin tests.

SURVEILLANCE

Whereas surveillance is the job of everyone on the medical care team, the responsibility for infection control is that of the hospital administrator. The hospital is necessarily concerned with both community-acquired and hospital-acquired infections. The hospital administrator must, of course, delegate some of the responsibility to supervisors of various departments and work closely with laboratory personnel and public health agencies. Some hospitals employ nurse-epidemiologists to perform surveys and accumulate data on community and hospital-acquired infections.

REPORTING COMMUNICABLE DISEASES

The list of notifiable diseases, that is, those which are to be reported to public health agencies, varies in different jurisdictions, but most agencies are guided by the U.S. Department of Health and Welfare's Public Health Service with headquarters in the Center for Disease Control in Atlanta, Georgia. Most frequently, the system of reporting functions at several levels, with communicable diseases first being reported to a local public health agency. The local agency may be a city, county, or district department of public health. Data are next collected by the state

health departments and, ultimately, forwarded to the Center for Disease Control in weekly communications.

Diseases reportable to the Center for Disease Control include some bacterial, viral, rickettsial, chlamydial, protozoal, and helminthic diseases (Table 29-4). Numbers of cases of illness and death are reported weekly in the *Morbidity and Mortality Weekly Report.* In addition, weekly reports also contain accounts of outbreaks of particular diseases, environmental hazards, or unusual cases of infectious disease.

Summaries from state health departments are published annually. The annual publication shows trends of communicable diseases, including emerging patterns of disease, which may be associated with travel or spe-

Table 29-4 DISEASES REPORTABLE TO THE CENTER FOR DISEASE CONTROL

Anthrax	Mumps
Aseptic meningitis	Poliomyelitis, total, paralytic, nonparalytic, unspecified
Botulism	Psittacosis-ornithosis
Brucellosis	Rabies in man
Chickenpox	Rabies in animals
Diphtheria	Rubella (German measles)
Encephalitis, primary infectious	Rubella congenital syndrome
Encephalitis, postinfectious with pre- or coexisting illness specified	Tetanus
Hepatitis, serum	Trichinosis
Hepatitis, acute infectious including unspecified cases	Tuberculosis, new active
Legionnaires' disease	Tularemia
Leprosy	Typhoid fever
Leptospirosis	Typhus, flea-borne, murine
Malaria	Typhus, tick-borne, Rocky Mountain spotted fever
Measles (rubeola)	Venereal diseases: syphilis, primary and secondary; gonorrhea
Meningococcal infections, total military, civilian	

cific geographic areas. National health authorities cooperate with the World Health Organization by reporting certain communicable diseases so that worldwide patterns may be available for further study and action. Reports of the World Health Organization may be found in the *Weekly Epidemiological Record*.

The responsibility for reporting communicable diseases present in a hospital usually falls to a nurse-epidemiologist or a member of the laboratory staff. Many states require that anyone working in a public or private school report at once to the local health officer the suspected presence of a communicable disease. Some jurisdictions require that any person having knowledge of a reportable disease contact the local public health agency.

MONITORING HOSPITAL-ACQUIRED INFECTIONS

Definitions for nosocomial infections must be rigidly adhered to in establishing infections as hospital associated. The following definitions are recommended by the American Hospital Association.

Definitions of Nosocomial Infections[1]

A. Urinary Tract Infection
   1. Asymptomatic Bacteriuria — colony counts in urine of >100,000 organisms per ml without pre-

[1] Reprinted with permission from *Proceedings of the International Conference on Nosocomial Infections,* published by the American Hospital Association.

vious or current manifestations of infection; classified as nosocomial if an earlier culture when the patient was not on antibiotics was negative. If patient is admitted with a urinary tract infection and a subsequent culture (>100,000 organisms per ml) is of a different pathogen, the new infection is regarded as nosocomial.

2. Other Urinary Tract Infection — onset of clinical signs or symptoms of urinary tract infection (fever, dysuria, costovertebral-angle tenderness, suprapubic tenderness) in a hospitalized patient plus one or both of the following factors developing after admission is classified nosocomial:
   a. Colony counts of >100,000 pathogens per ml of urine (carefully collected midstream specimen) or visible organisms on a gram stain of unspun fresh urine.
   b. Pyuria of >10 WBC per high-power field in an uncentrifuged specimen, with urinalysis negative for pyuria on admission.

   If a patient had prior negative urinalysis and/or culture (not repeated) and develops clinical symptoms of UTI while hospitalized, classify UTI as nosocomial. Also, if infected patients have new organisms cultured or clinical continuation of deterioration, classify as a new nosocomial UTI.

B. Respiratory Infections
   1. Upper Respiratory Infections
      (URI) — clinically manifest infec-
      tions of the nose, throat, or ear
      (singly or in combination). Signs
      and symptoms vary widely by
      site. Coryzal syndromes, strepto-
      coccal pharyngitis, otitis media,
      and mastoiditis are all included;
      the specific diagnosis should be
      entered on the line-listing form
      to allow for separate analysis.
      Majority are viral or of uncertain
      etiology. Attention must be paid
      to incubation period to differen-
      tiate community-acquired infec-
      tions that develop after admis-
      sion, and nosocomial infections.
   2. Lower Respiratory Infections
      (LRI) — clinical signs and symp-
      toms (cough, pleuritic chest pain,
      fever, and particularly purulence)
      developing after admission are
      regarded as evidence of LRI,
      even without sputum cultures or
      chest x-rays.
         When there is evidence of con-
      current upper and lower respira-
      tory infections enter both on the
      line-listing form.
         Other conditions (congestive
      heart failure, post-operative ate-
      lectasis, pulmonary embolism,
      etc.) with similar signs or symp-
      toms can be differentiated by
      clinical course. Classify as LRI if
      one or more of the following is
      present: purulent sputum (with
      or without recognized pathogen
      on sputum culture) or suggestive
      chest x-ray. An existing respira-
      tory infection may be superin-
      fected; classify as nosocomial in-
      fection when a new pathogen is
      cultured from sputum, and clini-
      cal or radiologic evidence in-
      dicates that the new organism is
      associated with deterioration of
      the patient's condition. Care
      must be used to distinguish su-
      percolonization from superinfec-
      tion.
C. Gastroenteritis
      Clinical gastroenteritis with
   onset after admission and with
   cultures of a known pathogen is
   regarded as nosocomial. However, if the incubation period for
   the pathogen is known (e.g., salmonella, shigella) the interval between admission and onset of
   symptoms must be greater than
   the incubation period. Alternately, classify as nosocomial if a
   prior stool culture or cultures,
   obtained on or after admission
   from a patient with gastroenteritis, was negative for the pathogen in question. Diagnosis of
   nosocomial gastroenteritis of
   viral etiology rests on epidemio-
   logic data indicating likelihood
   of cross-infection.
D. Skin and Subcutaneous Infections
   1. Burn Infections — colonization of
      burn surfaces with bacteria is
      nearly universal, and isolation of
      pathogenic organisms is not suf-
      ficient diagnosis of infection.
      Purulent drainage from the burn
      site and/or clinical evidence of
      bacteremia in a patient hospital-
      ized for treatment of a burn sig-
      nifies burn infections. Such in-

fections are often caused by organisms carried by the patient on admission; nonetheless, regard as nosocomial if the clinical onset occurs after admission. Regard superinfection of burns as a new nosocomial infection.

2. Surgical Wound Infections (SWI) — purulent drainage from any surgical wound signifies nosocomial infection, regardless of source (endogenous or exogenous) of organisms.

3. Other Cutaneous Infections — any purulent material in skin or subcutaneous tissue developing after admission signifies nosocomial infection. Category includes nonsurgical wounds, dermatitis, and decubitus ulcers. In patients admitted with skin or subcutaneous infections, a change in pathogens cultured from the infected site signifies nosocomial infection if continuing purulent drainage can be attributed to a new pathogen. Bacterial cellulitis usually has no purulent drainage; diagnosis depends on clinical judgment perhaps confirmed by culturing tissue fluid.

E. Intra-Abdominal Infections

1. Appendicitis, cholecystitis, and diverticulitis are not classified as infections. Secondary infectious complications (e.g., abscess, peritonitis, cellulitis) are generally classified as community-acquired infections.

2. Wound infection following surgery for uncomplicated appendicitis, cholecystitis, or diver-

ticulitis should be classified as nosocomial. SWI following surgery involving any infectious complication of the above can be classified as nosocomial only if there is clear anatomical and/or temporal separation of the infectious processes.

F. Other Sites of Infection

1. Any culture-documented bacteremia in a hospitalized patient admitted with no evidence of bacteremia is regarded as nosocomial infection, unless the organism is a contaminant. Nosocomial bacteremias can occur without underlying infection, or originate from a nosocomial infection or from manipulation of a site infected on admission (e.g., catheter, drain, incision, and drainage).

2. Intravenous Catheters and Needles — purulent drainage from the site of an intravenous catheter or needle signifies nosocomial infection. Inflammation without pus or strong clinical evidence of cellulitis is not regarded as infection unless a positive culture is obtained from aspirates of tissue fluid.

3. Endometritis — purulent cervical discharge accompanied by either a positive culture for pathogens or systemic manifestations of infection signifies nosocomial endometritis if onset occurs after admission.

4. Other sites must sometimes be considered. Application of the principles outlined above will

make classification possible. CLINICAL IMPRESSIONS/DIAGNOSIS (if available) always supersede laboratory or radiological data.

The Joint Commission on Accreditation of Hospitals requires that every hospital establish an infections committee. The main function of the committee is to reduce the number of hospital-acquired infections. This may be done by maintaining an infection surveillance system, by providing infection control educational programs, and by periodic review of hospital practices which relate to infection control. Regular meetings should be held in which reports on infections among patients, environmental or personnel monitoring, and antimicrobial susceptibility patterns are reviewed. Emphasis on productive personnel relationships can do much to correct any deficiencies which represent potential hazards in patient care.

SUMMARY

It is not possible to set up guidelines for infection control which would be applicable to all hospitals, since not only will hospital populations change, but predisposing factors will differ with time. The hospital environment is a dynamic reservoir for microorganisms. Surveillance and educational programs are costly in terms of dollars, energy, and time, but so are lawsuits for infections acquired through negligence. Policies for infection control must be developed after a careful assessment of needs and available resources in the hospital environment. There is a universal need for greater emphasis on frequent and careful hand washing to reduce the risk of hospital-acquired infections.

QUESTIONS FOR STUDY

1. What is the most important factor in the prevention of hospital-acquired infections?
2. What are the sources of microorganisms causing nosocomial infections?
3. What factors predispose hospitalized patients to infections?
4. Name the potential sources of microorganisms in contamination of intravenous infusion systems.
5. What are the responsibilities of an infections committee in a hospital?

SELECTED REFERENCES

American Hospital Association. *Infection Control in the Hospital.* Chicago: American Hospital Association, 1974.

Block, S. S. *Disinfection, Sterilization and Preservation.* Philadelphia: Lea & Febiger, 1977.

Brachman, P. S., and Eikohoff, T. C. *Proceedings of the International Conferences on Nosocomial Infections.* Chicago: American Hospital Association, 1970.

California State Department of Public Health. *A Manual for the Control of Communicable Diseases in California.* 6th ed. Berkeley: California Office of State Printing, 1971.

Committee on Continuing Education. *Infection Control in the Hospital Environment*. Washington, D.C.: American Society for Microbiology, 1976.

Dubay, E. C., and Grubb, R. D. *Infection Prevention and Control*. St. Louis: Mosby, 1973.

Lennette, E. H.; Spaulding, E. H.; and Truant, J. P. *Manual of Clinical Microbiology*. 2d ed. Washington, D.C.: American Society for Microbiology, 1974.

Lorian, V. *Significance of Medical Microbiology in the Care of Patients*. Baltimore: Williams & Wilkins, 1977.

Maki, D. G.; Goldman, D. A.; and Rhame, F. S. Infection control in intravenous therapy. *Annal. Intern. Med.* 79:867, 1973.

Rogers, D. E.; Des Prez, R. M.; Heller, P.; Reeves, T. J.; Greenberger, N. J.; Bondy, P. K.; and Epstein, F. H. *The Year Book of Medicine*. Chicago: Year Book Medical Publishers, 1972.

Rogers, D. E.; Des Prez, R. M.; Heller, P.; Braunwald, E.; Greenberger, N. J.; Bondy, P. K.; and Epstein, F. H. *The Year Book of Medicine*. Chicago: Year Book Medical Publishers, 1974.

Stefanini, M. *Progress in Clinical Pathology*. Vol. 4. New York: Grune & Stratton, 1972.

U.S. Department of Health, Education, and Welfare. *Isolation Techniques for Use in Hospitals*. DHEW Publication No. (HSM) 71-8042. Washington, D.C.: U.S. Government Printing Office, 1973.

U.S. Department of Health, Education, and Welfare. *Manual of Procedures for National Morbidity Reporting and Surveillance of Communicable Diseases*. DHEW Publication No. (HSM) 72-8113. Atlanta: Center for Disease Control, 1972.

Wood, L. A. *Nursing Skills for Allied Health Services*. Vols. 1, 2. Philadelphia: Saunders, 1972.

APPENDIXES

Appendix A

Classification of Medically Important Groups or Classes of Microorganisms and Helminths

CLASSIFICATION OF BACTERIA

Group	Predominant Habitats	Major Genera of Human Pathogens
1. Phototrophic bacteria	mud and stagnant water	none known
2. Gliding bacteria	soil, decaying vegetation	none known
3. Sheathed bacteria	slowly running fresh water	none known
4. Budding and/or appendaged bacteria	soil	none known
5. Spirochetes	fresh water, marine environments, sewage, polluted water, mollusks, ticks, lice, animals, birds, humans	*Treponema* *Borrelia* *Leptospira*
6. Spiral and curved bacteria	fresh water, stagnant water, marine environments, animals, birds, humans	*Spirillum* *Campylobacter*
7. Gram-negative aerobic rods and cocci	soil, fresh water, marine environments, hot springs, plants, animals, humans	*Pseudomonas* *Brucella* *Francisella* *Bordetella*
8. Gram-negative facultatively anaerobic rods	fresh water, marine environments, polluted water, plants, animals, birds, humans	*Escherichia* *Edwardsiella* *Salmonella* *Shigella* *Klebsiella* *Enterobacter* *Serratia*

(Continued)

671

CLASSIFICATION OF BACTERIA (*Continued*)

GROUP	PREDOMINANT HABITATS	MAJOR GENERA OF HUMAN PATHOGENS
		Proteus
		Yersinia
		Flavobacterium
		Haemophilus
		Pasteurella
		Acinobacillus
		Streptobacillus
		Calymmatobacterium
		Aeromonas
		Vibrio
9. Gram-negative anaerobic bacteria	animals, humans	*Bacterioides*
		Fusobacterium
10. Gram-negative cocci and coccobacilli	animals, humans	*Neisseria*
		Moraxella
		Acinetobacter
11. Gram-negative anaerobic cocci	animals, humans	*Veillonella*
12. Gram-negative chemolithotropic bacteria	mud, soil, fresh water, marine environments	none known
13. Methane-producing bacteria	sediments of natural waters, soil, anaerobic sewage digestors, animals	none known
14. Gram-positive cocci	soil, water, animals, humans	*Micrococcus*
		Staphylococcus
		Streptococcus
		Peptococcus
		Peptostreptococcus
15. Endospore-forming rods and cocci	soil, decaying vegetation, animals, humans	*Bacillus*
		Clostridium
16. Gram-positive asporogenous rod-shaped bacteria	fermenting plants and animal products, animals, humans	*Listeria*
17. Actinomycetes and related organisms	plants, animals, humans	*Corynebacterium*
		Actinomyces
		Mycobacterium
		Nocardia
		Eubacterium
		Propionibacterium
18. Rickettsias	arthropods, animals, humans	*Rickettsia*
		Rochalimaea
		Coxiella
		Bartonella
		Chlamydia
19. Mycoplasmas	birds, animals, humans, citrus plants, hot springs	*Mycoplasma*

SOURCE: Classification of bacteria is from *Bergey's Manual of Determinative Bacteriology*, 8th ed., edited by R. E. Buchanan and N. E. Gibbons (Baltimore: Williams & Wilkins, 1974).

CLASSIFICATION OF FUNGI

CLASS	SEXUAL SPORES	ASEXUAL SPORES	PREDOMINANT HABITAT
Phycomycetes	zygospores oospores	sporangiospores	water, soil, bread
Ascomycetes	ascospores	conidia chlamydospores arthrospores blastospores	fruit, soil
Basidiomycetes	basidiospores	usually absent	soil, grains
Deuteromycetes* (Fungi Imperfecti)	none observed	conidia chlamydospores arthrospores blastospores	soil

*Most human pathogens belong to the *Deuteromycetes*.

MAJOR *DEUTEROMYCETES* OF MEDICAL IMPORTANCE

ORGANISM	SOME IDENTIFYING CHARACTERISTICS
Candida albicans	pseudohyphae, chlamydospores
Cryptococcus neoformans	capsules, blastospores
Sporothrix schenckii	petal-like arrangement of conidia
Blastomyces dermatdiitis	single blastospores with broad bases
Blastomyces brasiliensis	multiple blastospores with narrow bases
Coccidioides immitis	arthrospores on media, spherules in tissue
Histoplasma capsulatum	tuberculate macroconidia
Epidermophyton floccosum	oval to club-shaped macroconidia, no microconidia
Microsporum species	numerous macroconidia, fusiform to obovate, thin- to thick-walled, few microconidia
Trichophyton species	numerous microconidia; macroconidia, if produced, elongated, thin- and smooth-walled

CLASSIFICATION OF PROTOZOA
MEDICAL IMPORTANCE

CLASS	COMMON NAME	MAJOR GENERA OF HUMAN PATHOGENS
Sarcodina	amebas	Entamoeba
Mastigophora	flagellates	Naegleria* Leishmania Trypanosoma Giardia Trichomonas
Ciliata	ciliates	Balantidium
Sporozoa	sporozoa	Toxoplasma Pneumocystis Plasmodium

Naegleria is more often included with the amebas although it is strictly speaking a flagellate.

CLASSIFICATION OF VIRUSES OF MEDICAL IMPORTANCE

Group	Shape	Major Viruses Causing Human Disease
DNA Viruses		
1. Parvovirus	cubical	none known
2. Papovavirus	cubical	papilloma virus
3. Adenovirus	cubical	serotypes 1–8
4. Herpesvirus	pleomorphic	varicella-zoster virus
		cytomegalovirus
		EB virus
		herpes simplex viruses
5. Poxvirus	brick-shaped	smallpox virus
		molluscum contagiosum virus
RNA Viruses		
6. Reovirus	cubical	serotypes 1–3
7. Picornavirus	cubical	polioviruses
		coxsackieviruses
		echoviruses
		rhinoviruses
8. Togavirus	cubical	arboviruses
		rubella virus
9. Orthomyxovirus	roughly spherical	influenza viruses
10. Paramyxovirus	pleomorphic	respiratory syncytial virus
		mumps virus
		rubeola virus
11. Rhabdovirus	bullet-shaped	rabies virus
12. Retrovirus	roughly spherical	none known
13. Arenavirus	oval or pleomorphic	lymphocytic choriomeningitis virus (LCV)
		Lassa fever virus
14. Coronavirus	roughly spherical	serotypes B814, 229E, OC43
15. Bunyavirus	oval	California encephalitis virus
		Bunyamwera virus

CLASSIFICATION OF HELMINTHS OF MEDICAL IMPORTANCE

Class	Common Name	Major Genera of Human Pathogens	Class	Common Name	Major Genera of Human Pathogens
Nematoda	roundworms	*Ancylostoma*	*Cestoda*	tapeworms	*Diphyllobothrium*
		Ascaris			*Dipylidium*
		Brugia			*Echinococcus*
		Dracunculus			*Hymenolepis*
		Enterobius			*Spirometra*
		Loa			*Taenia*
		Necator	*Trematoda*	flukes	*Clonorchis*
		Onchocerca			*Fasciola*
		Strongyloides			*Fasciolopsis*
		Trichuris			*Paragonimus*
		Trichinella			*Schistosoma*
		Wuchereria			

Appendix B

Proprietary and Generic Names of Selected Antimicrobial and Chemotherapeutic Agents

PROPRIETARY AND GENERIC NAMES OF SELECTED ANTIMICROBIAL AND CHEMOTHERAPEUTIC AGENTS

GENERIC NAME	PROPRIETARY NAME
Acedapsone	Hansolar (Parke-Davis)
Amantadine	Symmetrel (Endo)
Amithiozone	Teebazone (Consolidated Midland)
Amoxicillin	Amoxil (Beecham); Larotid (Roche); Polymox (Bristol)
Amphotericin B	Fungizone (Squibb)
Ampicillin*	Polycillin (Bristol); others
Capreomycin	Capastat (Lilly)
Carbenicillin	Pyopen (Beecham); Geopen; Geocillin (Roerig)
Cefazolin	Ancef (SmithKline); Kefzol (Lilly)
Cephalexin	Keflex (Lilly)
Cephaloridine	Loridine (Lilly)
Cephalothin	Keflin (Lilly)
Cephapirin	Cefadyl (Bristol)
Chloramphenicol*	Chloromycetin (Parke-Davis); others
Clindamycin	Cleocin (Upjohn)
Clofazimine	(B663; Ciba)
Clotrimazole	Lotrimin (Delbay)
Cloxacillin	Tegopen (Bristol)
Cycloserine	Seromycin (Lilly)
Dapsone	Avlosulfon (Ayerst)
Dicloxacillin	Veracillin (Ayerst); Dynapen (Bristol); Pathocil (Wyeth)
Doxycycline	Vibramycin (Pfizer); Doxychel (Rachelle); Doxycycline Hyclate (Spencer-Mead); Doxy-II (USV)

(Continued)

PROPRIETARY AND GENERIC NAMES OF SELECTED ANTIMICROBIAL AND CHEMOTHERAPEUTIC AGENTS *(Continued)*

Generic Name	Proprietary Name
Erythromycin*	Erythrocin (Abbott); others
Ethambutol	Myambutol (Lederle)
Ethionamide	Trecator (Ives)
Flucytosine	Ancobon (Roche)
Gentamicin	Garamycin (Schering)
Griseofulvin*	Fulvicin-U/F (Schering); others
Hydroxystilbamidine	Hydroxystilbamidine isethionate (Merrell)
Idoxuridine	Dendrid (Alcon); Herplex (Allergan); Stoxil (SmithKline)
Kanamycin	Kantrex (Bristol)
Methenamine hippurate	Hiprex (Merrell); Urex (Riker)
Methenamine mandelate*	Mandelamine (Warner-Chilcott); others
Methicillin	Celbenin (Beecham), Staphcillin (Bristol)
Methisazone	Marboran (Burroughs Wellcome)
Miconazole	MicaTin (Johnson & Johnson); Monistat (Ortho)
Minocycline	Minocin (Lederle); Vectrin (Parke-Davis)
Nafcillin	Unipen (Wyeth)
Nalidixic acid	NegGram (Winthrop)
Nitrofurantoin*	Furadantin (Eaton); others
Nystatin	Mycostatin (Squibb); Nilstat (Lederle)
Oxacillin	Bactocil (Beecham); Prostaphlin (Bristol)
Penicillin G (benzathine)	Bicillin (Wyeth)
Penicillin G* (potassium)	many manufacturers
Penicillin V*	Compocillin-V (Ross); others
Phenethicillin	Syncillin (Bristol); Maxipen (Pfizer)
Polymyxin B	Aerosporin (Burroughs Wellcome); Polymixin B (Pfizer)
Rifampin	Rifadin (Dow); Rimactane (Ciba)
Spectinomycin	Trobicin (Upjohn)
Sulfisoxazole*	Gantrisin (Roche); others
Tetracycline hydrochloride*	Achromycin (Lederle); others
Tobramycin	Nebcin (Lilly)
Trimethoprim-sulfamethoxazole	Bactrim (Roche); Septra (Burroughs Wellcome)
Vancomycin	Vancocin (Lilly)
Viomycin	Viomycin (Parke-Davis); Viocin (Pfizer)

* Also available generically.
Source: *The Medical Letter* 18:16, 1976.

Appendix C

Immunizing Agents for Some Major Diseases

RECOMMENDED IMMUNIZATION FOR SOME MAJOR DISEASES

DISEASE	TYPE OF PREPARATION	PRIMARY DOSES	BOOSTERS	COMMENTS*
Poliomyelitis	trivalent oral attenuated viruses (TOPV)	3	1	recommended for children at 2, 4, and 18 months and between 4 and 6 years
Diphtheria Pertussis Tetanus	diphtheria and tetanus toxoids with a killed suspension of *B. pertussis* (DPT)	3	2	recommended for children 2, 4, and 18 months and between 4 and 6 years
	tetanus and diphtheria toxoids, adult type (TD)	3	every 10 years	recommended for schoolchildren and adults
Rubella	attenuated rubella viruses	1	0	recommended for children at 15 months
Mumps	attenuated mumps viruses	1	0	recommended for children at 15 months
Rubeola	attenuated rubeola viruses	1	0	recommended for children at 15 months

(Continued)

RECOMMENDED IMMUNIZATION FOR SOME MAJOR DISEASES *(Continued)*

Disease	Type of Preparation	Primary Doses	Boosters	Comments*
Typhoid fever	killed suspension of *S. typhi*	2	every 3 years	recommended for travelers to endemic areas or laboratory personnel
Cholera	killed suspension of *V. cholerae*	2	every 6 months	recommended for travelers to endemic areas or laboratory personnel
Yellow fever	attenuated yellow fever viruses	1	every 10 years	recommended for travelers to endemic areas or laboratory personnel
Plague	killed suspension of *Y. pestis*	3	every 1–2 years	recommended for persons involved in field operations in plague-enzootic areas and laboratory personnel
Influenza	inactivated prevalent antigenic types of influenza viruses	1	annually	recommended for high-risk individuals

*Ages for immunization of children are those recommended by the Committee on Infectious Diseases of the American Academy of Pediatrics.

Glossary

A

abortive transduction Failure of a fragment of donor DNA from a phage to multiply within a host cell.

abscess A lesion characterized by the presence of pus.

acid-fast A property of some bacteria permitting them to retain the primary stain (carbol fuchsin) in the Ziehl-Neelsen staining technique.

acquired immunity Resistance to infectious agents obtained after birth.

acrotheca Type of fungal sporulation in which conidia are borne on short protuberances on club-shaped conidiophores.

active immunity Resistance to infectious agents derived from host response.

acute Having limited duration and a sudden onset, and usually relatively severe.

adenine A nitrogenous base of nucleic acid molecules.

adenosine triphosphate Energy-storage compound of cells.

adherence The property permitting a microorganism to stick to a surface.

adjuvant A substance which enhances antibody production.

aerobe A microorganism that requires oxygen for growth.

aerosol An airborne solid or liquid particle.

affinity Attraction between a single antigenic determinant and its antibody.

aflatoxin A carcinogen produced by some strains of *Aspergillus flavus*.

agar A polysaccharide derived from seaweed used to solidify media.

agglutination An antigen-antibody reaction between a particulate antigen and specific antibody resulting in visible clumping.

allantois A fetal membranous sac arising from the posterior part of the alimentary canal.

allele An equivalent gene on a paired chromosome in a diploid cell of a eucaryote.

allergen An antigen that causes a state of hypersensitivity.

allergy An altered immune response triggered by exposure to an antigen.

allogenic Having a different genetic constitution.

allograft A transplant in which donor and recipient are of the same species, but are allogenic.

allosteric Having a binding site other than a catalytic site on an enzyme.

alpha fetoprotein (AFP) Antigen associated with tumors of the liver and fetal tissue.

alpha hemolysis Partial dissolution of red blood cells by a bacterial colony resulting in a green zone on blood agar.

amastigote Intracellular form of a blood or tissue flagellate.

amino acid Basic subunit of proteins.

amnion Fetal membrane enclosing amniotic fluid and embryo.

amphitrichous Describing a type of bacterial flagellation having a single flagellum at each pole.

anaerobe A microorganism that grows only in the absence of oxygen.

anamnestic response A sharp response in antibody production following a second or subsequent exposure to an antigen.

anaphylaxis A form of systemic shock caused by hypersensitivity to parenteral introduction of an antigen.

anergic Lacking ability to respond to antigenic stimulation.

anesthesia Partial or complete loss of sensation and sometimes consciousness induced by the administration of drugs or gases.

Angstrom (Å) A unit measurement equal to 10^{-9} of a millimeter.

anthelminthic Having a destructive effect on helminths.

anthropophilic Referring to fungi having an affinity for humans rather than other animals.

antibiotic A microbiostatic or microbicidal agent derived from a microorganism.

antibody A protein produced by a vertebrate host in response to the presence of an antigen.

anticodon A sequence of three nucleotides on RNA complementary to those on messenger RNA.

antigen A substance capable of stimulating antibody production in a vertebrate host.

antigenicity The ability of a substance to promote antibody production in a vertebrate host.

antimicrobial agent A chemical substance capable of inhibiting or killing microorganisms.

antiseptic A chemical agent which can be applied topically to inhibit or kill microorganisms.

antitoxin An antibody against a toxin.

AOAC Use-Dilution Method Method devised by the Association of Official Analytical Chemists for determining dilutions of germicidal agents recommended for general disinfection of surfaces.

apoenzyme   Protein component of an enzyme.

Arthus reaction   A localized response to repeated injections of a soluble antigen.

artifact   An artificially produced aberration in microscopic appearance.

ascitic fluid   Serous fluid which is derived from the peritoneal cavity.

Ascoli test   Precipitin test used to detect antigens of the anthrax organism.

ascus   Saclike cell bearing spores of some fungi.

aseptic   Without infection or microbial contamination.

asynchronous   Not occurring at the same time.

ataxia   Lack of muscle coordination.

atom   Smallest particle of an element that can exist either alone or in combination.

atopic   Having a seemingly hereditary basis.

attenuation   Process of modifying an infective agent to a less virulent form.

autoclave   An instrument employing steam under pressure for sterilization.

autogenous   Originating with self.

autograft   A transplant from one site of the body to another site in the same individual.

autoimmunity   A state of hypersensitivity resulting from production of antibodies against a component of the host's own body.

autotroph   A microorganism capable of synthesizing cellular require-

ments from carbon dioxide and inorganic nitrogen.

auxotroph   A nutritional mutant of a bacterium requiring one or more growth factors not needed by the parental strain.

avidity   Strength of binding between antigens and antibodies.

avirulent   Without significant pathogenicity.

B

bacteremia   Presence of bacteria in the blood.

bacteriolysis   Rupture of bacterial cells.

bacteriophage   A virus which infects bacteria.

bacteriuria   Presence of bacteria in the urine.

balanitis   Inflammation of the penis.

basement membrane   Layer of solid material beneath epithelium of mucous surfaces.

basidium   Club-shaped structure which bears spores of some fungi.

basophil   A polymorphonuclear white blood cell formed in red bone marrow.

B-cell   Lymphocyte derived from the bursa of Fabricius or its equivalent which synthesizes immunoglobulins.

BCG (Bacille Calmette-Guérin)   A vaccine for tuberculosis containing an attenuated bovine strain of the tubercle bacillus.

beta hemolysis   Complete dissolution of red blood cells by a bacterial colony resulting in a clear zone on blood agar.

binary fission Process of asexual reproduction whereby two daughter cells are produced by development of a transverse cell wall.

biodegradable Having the ability to be broken down by some form of life.

biological mimicry A phenomenon in which a microorganism and its host share antigens.

blepharitis Inflammation of the edges of the eyelids involving hair follicles and glands.

blocking antibody An antibody which coats or binds to antigens interfering with activity of complete antibody.

boil A pus-producing lesion of a hair follicle; also called a furuncle.

Brownian movement Random movement of molecules.

bubo An inflammed, swollen, or enlarged lymph node.

budding A process of asexual reproduction in which daughter cells emerge from parent cells as small buds.

buffer A chemical substance that resists changes in pH.

bursa of Fabricius Lymphoid organ in chickens necessary for development and maturation of B-cell lymphocytes.

C

capneic Requiring more carbon dioxide than in the atmosphere.

capsid Protein coat of a virus.

capsomers Subunits of protein comprising a viral capsid.

capsule A visible slime layer characteristic of some bacteria.

carbuncle A pus-producing lesion of multicentric origin.

carcinoembryonic antigen (CEA) Antigen occurring in abundance in tumors of the gastrointestinal tract and fetal tissue.

carcinogen A cancer-causing agent.

caseous Resembling cheese.

catarrh Inflammation of mucous membrane of the respiratory tract.

catheterization Insertion of a tube for removal of fluid.

cell boundary Membrane or membrane and wall that enclose cytoplasm of a cell.

cellular immunity Resistance to infectious agents mediated by sensitized lymphocytes or their products.

Celsius (Centigrade) Scale ranging from 0° to 100° used to measure temperature.

centromere The junction of chromatids.

cercaria A free-swimming stage of a digenetic fluke.

chancre Primary lesion of syphilis.

chemoautotroph An organism capable of synthesizing organic compounds using chemical energy.

chemostat A device used to maintain a continuous culture of microorganisms.

chemosynthesis Process of synthesizing organic compounds using particular chemical compounds as energy sources.

chemotaxis Attraction or repulsion that is caused by a chemical stimulus.

chemotherapy Treatment of disease with chemical substances.

chloroplast Chlorophyll-containing organelle.

chromatid Structure resulting from longitudinal splitting of a chromosome.

chromosome Elongated structure conspicuous during mitosis containing genetic material.

chronic Of long duration.

cilia short, hairlike appendages of some protozoa responsible for motility.

citric acid cycle A series of aerobic, energy-liberating reactions occurring in cells.

cladosporium Type of fungal sporulation in which chains of conidia are borne on elongated, branching conidiophores.

clone A group of cells derived from a single parent cell.

coagulase An enzyme produced by *Staphylococcus aureus* which causes normal plasma to clot.

codon Subunit of the mRNA molecule containing three nitrogenous bases.

coenocytic Having an aseptate hypha with multiple nuclei.

coenzyme A carrier molecule for an enzyme.

colicin A bactericidal agent produced by a strain of *Escherichia coli*.

colloid A solute particle ranging in size from 1 to 100 nm.

colonization Accumulation of microorganisms on the surface of an object or host or within the body of a host.

colony An association of microorganisms.

colony-forming units (CFU) A quantitative expression of numbers of colonies per milliliter growing on a particular medium under standard conditions.

communicable Transmittable directly or indirectly from one individual to another.

complement Nonspecific resistance factor which takes part in some antigen-antibody reactions.

complementarity Pairing of nitrogenous bases on molecules of DNA or RNA.

complement fixation An antigen-antibody reaction which inactivates complement.

congenital Present at birth.

conidiophore A specialized hypha which bears conidia.

conjugation Transfer of genetic material from one bacterium to another during a mating process.

conjunctiva Mucous membrane which lines the eyelids.

consolidation Solidification of pulmonary tissue by fibrinogen-containing exudates.

constitutive enzyme An enzyme synthesized in the absence of a specific substrate.

contamination Presence of microorganisms.

continuous cell line A cell line which can be consistently maintained under laboratory conditions.

continuous culture A population of microbial cells maintained in the logarithmic growth phase.

convalescence Period of recovery following illness.

core Innermost portion of an endospore.

cortex Layer enclosing protoplast of an endospore.

creeping eruption Cutaneous infection caused by migration of nematode larvae; also called cutaneous larva migrans.

cristae Inner membranes of mitochondria.

crithidia Extracellular form of a blood or tissue flagellate.

cutaneous larva migrans Infections of the skin caused by migration of nematode larvae; also called creeping eruptions.

cyanophage A virus which infects cyanobacteria.

cyst A membranous sac containing fluid; resistant encysted stage of certain protozoa and bacteria.

cysticercoid Caudate solid larva of *Taenia solium*.

cysticercus Fluid-containing bladder larva of *Taenia solium*.

cystitis Inflammation of the urinary bladder.

cystoscopy Examination of the bladder with an instrument permitting internal visualization.

cytokinesis Division of cytoplasm occurring during mitosis.

cytomegaly Increase in cell size.

cytopathic effect (CPE) Morphological change in virus-infected cells.

cytoplasm Colloidal mixture of compounds within a cell.

cytoplasmic membrane Layer of lipid and protein that encloses cytoplasm of a cell.

cytoplasmic streaming A phenomenon occurring in eucaryotic cells in which cytoplasm is in constant motion.

cytosine A nitrogenous base of nucleic acid molecules.

cytotoxic Having the ability to attack cells.

D

dalton A unit of weight equal to the weight of one hydrogen atom.

death phase Phase of bacterial growth in which the number of cells decreases with time.

decubitus Ulcer caused by pressure point obstructing capillary blood flow.

definitive host A host which supports the growth of mature parasites.

degeneracy The phenomenon whereby more than one codon contains genetic information for the same amino acid.

delayed hypersensitivity An altered immune response mediated by cells in the absence of antibodies.

denaturation Destruction of the functional ability of a molecule by physical or chemical action.

dental plaque An accumulation of bacteria adhering to the surface of a tooth and contiguous epithelium.

dermatophyte A fungus which infects skin, hair, or nails.

desiccation Process of removing moisture.

dialysis Process by which a solute passes through a membrane.

diarrhea Frequent evacuation of stool which is often a fluid.

Dick test Susceptibility test for scarlet fever employing erythrogenic toxin.

differential medium A culture medium which permits organisms to be distinguished from one another.

digenetic Having an alternation of generations between a vertebrate and a mollusk host.

dimer A two-molecule particle.

dioecious Having separate sexes.

diploid cell A cell containing two chromosomes of each type.

disinfectant A chemical agent which inhibits or kills microorganisms.

disinfection The process of destroying pathogens exclusive of spores and viruses.

disseminated Widespread.

diverticulitis Inflammation of a diverticulum of the colon.

diverticulum A sac or pouch in the walls of a canal or organ.

dysentery Inflammation of intestinal mucous membranes characterized by passage of blood and mucus.

E

ecosystem Interdependent organisms and environmental factors of a particular habitat.

ectoparasite An organism living on the external surfaces or cavities of a host.

ectothrix A type of fungal infection having growth outside the hair as well as within the shaft.

efficiency of plating (EOP) A quantitative expression of the infectivity of a viral population based on a comparison of the infectious titer with the electron microscope count.

electrolyte A substance capable of conducting an electric current in solution.

electrophoresis The movement of charged particles through a medium caused by differences in electrical potential.

electrostatic bond Bond between substances due to attraction of oppositely charged particles.

ELISA Enzyme-linked immunosorbent assay technique.

emiocytosis Cellular process for elimination of undigested debris.

encephalitis Inflammation of the brain.

endemic Occurring more or less continuously in a particular area.

endogenous Originating or produced from within.

endometritis Inflammation of the endometrium, or lining of the uterus.

endoparasite An organism living within a host.

endophthalmitis Inflammation of the inner portion of the eye.

endoplasmic reticulum System of membrane-enclosed channels in a eucaryotic cell.

endospore Resistant stage occurring in the life cycle of some bacilli and cocci.

endothrix A fungal infection within the hair shaft.

endotoxin A microbial poison released upon disintegration of organisms.

enhancement Stimulation of tumor growth by tumor-associated antibodies.

enrichment medium A culture medium containing growth supplements.

enterococci Cocci of enteric origin.

enterotoxin An exotoxin produced by

some bacteria that affects the gastrointestinal tract.

enzyme A simple or conjugated protein that catalyzes chemical reactions.

eosinophil A polymorphonuclear white blood cell formed in bone marrow.

epidemic Outbreak of multiple cases of a disease within a particular area.

epidemiology The study of the natural history of a disease in terms of factors controlling its presence and its incidence and distribution.

epimastigote Extracellular form of a blood or tissue flagellate.

episome A fragment of DNA which can exist as a chromosomal or cytoplasmic factor.

erythroblast Nucleated, immature red blood cell.

erythrocyte Red blood cell.

erythrogenic toxin Rash-producing toxin of scarlet fever.

eucaryotic cell A cell having a nuclear membrane and organelles with specialized functions.

exogenous Originating from without.

exosporium Outermost layer of an endospore.

exotoxin A microbial poison excreted into the environment.

exponential growth phase Phase of bacterial growth in which cell multiplication is proportional to time.

exudate Viscous fluid containing blood cells and debris which is released from a site of inflammation.

F

Fab fragment Antigen-binding portion of an immunoglobulin after treatment with papain.

F(ab')$_2$ fragment Antigen-binding portion of an immunoglobulin after treatment with pepsin.

facultative Having the ability to live under varying environmental conditions.

fauna Animal or animal-like life of a geographic or anatomic site.

favus A chronic and highly communicable fungal infection of the scalp.

F$^+$ cell Bacterial cell containing the fertility factor as an extrachromosomal particle with the ability to donate the factor and, less frequently, other chromosomal material to an F$^-$ cell.

F$^-$ cell Bacterial cell lacking the fertility factor with the potential for receiving the fertility factor, genetic material, or both from an F$^+$ cell.

Fc fragment Crystallizable portion of an immunoglobulin after treatment with papain which has no antibody activity.

F factor Extrachromosomal or chromosomal fertility factor occurring in some bacteria.

febrile Fever-producing.

feedback inhibition A control mechanism for enzyme reactions operating at the level of the end product.

fibrinolysin Enzyme produced by some streptococci which dissolves human fibrin.

fibroblast A connective tissue cell having a supportive function.

filarial Having an association with filariae (threadlike roundworms).

filariform   Nonfeeding, infective larval stage.

filtration   Process of removing microorganisms from a liquid by passing it through a semipermeable material.

flagella   Filamentous appendages of some microorganisms which are responsible for motility.

flagellin   Protein associated with flagella.

flame cell   A ciliated cell of the excretory system in helminths.

flaming   Application of a direct flame to kill microorganisms.

flocculation   An antigen-antibody reaction involving precipitation and occurring in the presence of relatively large amounts of antigen.

flora   Plant or plantlike life of a geographic or anatomic site.

fluidity   Characteristic of the cytoplasmic membrane permitting passage of molecules by solvent action.

fluorescence   Luminescence in the presence of short-wave radiation, usually ultraviolet.

fluorone   A fluorescent dye.

fomite   Inanimate object responsible for transmission of infectious agents.

forespore   Double-membraned structure in early stage of sporulation.

fragmentation   Process of asexual reproduction in which small portions of a filament separate from the parent organism.

frameshift mutation   A mutation involving a deletion from or addition to the genome of a small number of base pairs.

fungicide   An agent which destroys fungi.

furuncle   Pus-producing lesion of a hair follicle; also called a boil.

G

gamete   A sex cell.

gamma globulin   Fraction of immunoglobulin containing a majority of antibodies.

gamma hemolysis   Absence of dissolution of red blood cells by a bacterial colony resulting in no detectable color change on blood agar.

gastroenteritis   Inflammation of the stomach and intestines.

gene   Part of the DNA molecule constituting a unit of heredity.

generalized transduction   Transfer of any small region of donor DNA by phage.

generation time   Time required for doubling of a microbial population.

genome   Full complement of genes of an organism.

genotype   Genetic constitution of an organism, as distinguished from the physical appearance, or phenotype.

genus   Name assigned to a group of related organisms.

germicide   A chemical agent which kills infectious agents.

germination   The process which changes an endospore of a bacterium to the vegetative state.

glabrous   smooth.

glomerulitis   Inflammation of the glomeruli of the kidney.

glycolysis   Degradation of glucose to an organic acid with concomitant release of energy.

Golgi body   An organelle of a eucaryotic cell which secretes enzymes.

grana   A multilayered membranous unit of a chloroplast.

granule   An accumulation of solid material within cytoplasm.

guanine   A nitrogenous base of nucleic acid molecules.

gumma   Tertiary lesion of syphilis.

H

hair follicle   A pocket in cutaneous epithelium containing a hair.

halophile   An organism that requires or tolerates high concentrations of salt in the environment.

haploid cell   A cell containing one chromosome of each type.

hapten   An incomplete antigen capable of invoking an antibody response only when bound to a carrier molecule.

helix   A configuration in which subunits of a macromolecule are coiled around one another.

hemagglutination   An antigen-antibody reaction in which the reacting antigen is attached to the surface of a red blood cell; clumping of red blood cells.

hemolysin   An exotoxin causing dissolution of red blood cells.

hemolysis   Dissolution of red blood cells in the presence of specific antibody and complement.

hermaphroditic   Possessing reproductive organs of both sexes.

heterofermentative   Producing a mix of end products by fermentation.

heterologous   Shared by two or more species.

heterophil   An antibody reacting with other than a specific antigen.

Hfr cell   A bacterial cell containing the fertility factor integrated into the chromosome and capable of donating other genetic material with an increased frequency.

histamine   A potent vasodilator released by mast cells and basophils.

histiocytes   Macrophages of connective tissues.

histocompatibility   Immunologic ability of cells or tissues to coexist.

histones   Proteins associated with DNA in eucaryotic cells.

homocytotropism   Affinity of antibodies for reacting with surfaces of cells of the same species in which the antibodies were synthesized.

homofermentative   Producing one primary end product by the process of fermentation.

homologous   Derived from the same species.

hormone   A chemical substance produced by an endocrine gland.

humoral immunity   Resistance to infectious agents mediated by substances in body fluids.

hyaluronidase   An enzyme secreted by some gram-positive bacteria enabling organisms to break down hyaluronic acid of the connective tissue matrix.

hydatid sand   Granular deposits of capsules and scolices of larvae of *Echinococcus granulosus*.

hygroscopic   Having the capacity to absorb moisture.

hyperbaric   Having greater than normal atmospheric pressure.

hyperemia   Excessive amount of blood in a body part.

hyperplasia   Increase in the number or size of cells.

hypertrophy   Enlargement of a gland or organ.

hyphae   Individual filaments making up the vegetative portion of a mycelium.

I

icteric   Referring to yellowness of skin, whites of eyes, mucous membranes, and body fluids caused by presence of bile pigments.

immediate hypersensitivity   An altered immune response characterized by complexing of allergen with antibody.

immunity   Resistance to infectious agents.

immunocompetence   Ability to combat infectious agents by immune mechanisms.

immunodiffusion   Migration of antigens and antibodies in a semisolid medium to form a visible band of precipitation.

immunoelectrophoresis   Movement of charged molecules of antigens and antibodies through an agar medium to form a visible band of precipitation.

immunofluorescence   Luminescence occurring when an antigen reacts with an antibody conjugated with a fluorescent dye.

immunogen   An antigen used under controlled conditions to elicit an antibody response.

immunoglobulin (Ig)   A protein having antibody activity or a similar antigenic specificity.

immunoprophylaxis   Prevention of disease by administration of antibodies, antigens, or modified antigens.

immunosuppression   Inhibition of the immune response.

incineration   Destruction by burning.

inclusion body   Definitive mass occurring in the nucleus or cytoplasm of cells infected with viruses.

indigenous   Occurring naturally in a particular environment.

individual immunity   Resistance to infectious agents exhibited by one person.

inducible enzyme   An enzyme synthesized in the presence of a particular substrate.

induction   Activation of a gene in the presence of a particular substance.

inflammation   A localized reaction of tissue caused by the presence of an irritant.

integument   A covering or enclosure, such as skin or a membrane.

intercalary   Located between cells of hyphae.

interfacial tension   Force exerted at the boundary between molecules of liquids and solid particles.

interferon   A nonspecific resistance factor produced by virus-infected cells.

intermediate host   A host which supports the growth of immature stages of parasites.

intertriginous   Occurring between two folds of skin.

in utero   Within the uterus.

invasive   Having the ability to enter and disseminate in tissue.

in vitro   Outside the body or in an artificial environment.

in vivo Within the living body of an organism.

isoagglutination An antigen-antibody reaction between red blood cell antigens and antibodies of incompatible sera.

isoenzyme A different form of the same enzyme.

J

jaundice Condition characterized by yellowness of skin, whites of eyes, mucous membranes, and body fluids caused by presence of bile pigments.

K

keratin A protein made by epidermal cells of the skin.

Koplik's spots Small, red spots with blue-white centers on oral mucosa occurring before the rash of rubeola.

Kupffer cell Macrophage of the liver.

L

labile Unstable.

lacrimal Pertaining to tears.

lag phase Phase of bacterial growth in which there is no increase in cell number.

lamella Inner membrane of chloroplasts.

larva Developmental stage of helminths.

laryngotracheitis Inflammation of the larynx and trachea.

lassitude Loss of energy.

latent Inactive or concealed.

legume A plant, such as peas, beans, and clover, which is associated with symbiotic nitrogen-fixing bacteria.

leishmania Intracellular form of a blood or tissue flagellate.

lepromin Heat-treated product of *Mycobacterium leprae* used in skin testing.

leptomonas Extracellular form of a blood or tissue parasite found in an intermediate host.

leukocidin An exotoxin which destroys white blood cells.

leukocyte White blood cell.

leukopenia Decrease in white blood cells.

lipophilic Having an affinity for lipids.

lymphadenopathy Disease of the lymph nodes.

lymphocyte The smaller of the mononuclear white blood cells formed in lymphatic tissue.

lymphokine A substance released by sensitized lymphocytes associated with cellular immunity.

lyophilization Process of rapidly freezing a substance at a low temperature and removing water under vacuum.

lysis Dissolution of cells in the presence of specific antibody and complement.

lysogeny A state exhibited by a virus-infected bacterium in which the phage genome coexists with the bacterial genome.

lysosome An organelle of eucaryotic cells containing hydrolytic enzymes.

lysozyme An enzyme in biological fluids having antimicrobial activity.

lytic Producing lysis in cells; specifically, relating to a virus that replicates within a host cell causing lysis.

M

macrogametocyte A sexually differentiated cell of a malarial parasite capable of producing a female gamete.

macroglobulin Large globulin molecule.

macromolecule Large molecule made up of subunits connected by bonds.

macrophage Large, sessile or wandering phagocytic cell.

macroscopic Visible with the naked eye.

malaise A vague symptom of illness.

mammillated Having protuberances like a nipple.

mast cells Round or ovoid cells of connective tissue containing coarse cytoplasmic granules.

matrix Intercellular substance of a tissue.

megakaryocyte A giant cell in bone marrow from which platelets are derived.

meiosis Process of cell division occurring in gametes whereby the numbers of chromosomes are reduced by one-half.

meningitis Inflammation of the meninges.

merozoite A cell located within the schizont of a malarial parasite.

mesophile A microorganism which grows at temperatues ranging from 20° to 45°C.

mesosome A saclike invagination of the cytoplasmic membrane of some bacteria.

metacercaria An encysted form of a cercaria of a digenetic fluke.

microaerophilic Requiring less oxygen than in the atmosphere.

microbicidal Having a destructive effect on microorganisms.

microbiostatic Having an inhibitory effect on microorganisms.

microbiota Microscopic forms of life.

microcosm An area containing microscopic forms of life.

microfilaria Prelarval developmental stage of one group of roundworms.

microgametocyte A sexually differentiated cell of a malarial parasite capable of producing a male gamete.

microglial cell Macrophage of nerve tissue.

micrometer (μm) A unit of measurement equal to 10^{-3} of a millimeter.

microsome Fragment of endoplasmic reticulum with ribosomes attached.

microtubule A filamentous organelle particularly prominent as spindle fibers during mitosis.

miliary Characterized by disseminated nodules.

minimal bactericidal concentration (MBC) The lowest concentration of an antimicrobial agent which kills bacteria under standard conditions.

minimal inhibitory concentration (MIC) The lowest concentration of an antimicrobial agent which inhibits visible growth under standard conditions.

miracidium A ciliated larva of a digenetic fluke.

mitochondria   Organelles of eucaryotic cells which are sites of respiration.

mitosis   Process of cell division in which chromosomes are duplicated and equally distributed to daughter cells.

molecule   Two or more atoms chemically combined; smallest particle of a compound that can exist.

monocyte   The larger of the mononuclear white blood cells formed in lymphatic tissue.

monoecious   Having both sexes in a single organism.

monolayer   A single layer of cells growing *in vitro*.

monomer   Repetitive molecular subunit making up a polymer.

mordant   A substance which fixes a stain.

most probable number (MPN)   A cultural technique for estimating numbers of coliforms in milk or water samples.

M-protein   A protein occurring in the cell wall of certain streptococci.

multifocal   Having many sites.

mutagen   Any agent that irreversibly alters DNA.

mutant   An organism differing from the parent cell by at least one inheritable characteristic.

mutation   A sudden inheritable change in the composition of a genome.

mutation frequency   The number of mutants occurring in a particular population.

mutation rate   The probability that a particular mutation will occur, expressed as the average number of mutations per cell per generation.

mycelium   Filamentous vegetative structure of a fungus.

mycetoma   A cutaneous lesion extending into deeper tissues frequently occurring on the hands or feet.

N

nanometer (nm)   A unit of measurement equal to 10^{-6} of a millimeter.

natural immunity   Resistance to infectious agents without previous contact.

necrosis   Death of tissue.

neoplasm   Mass of new tissue forming a tumor.

nephritis   Inflammation of the renal tubules.

neuralgia   Inflammation of a nerve.

neuroglia   Supporting framework of the central nervous system.

neutralization   An antigen-antibody reaction involving deactivation of a toxin in the presence of specific antitoxin.

neutrophil   A polymorphonuclear white blood cell formed in red bone marrow.

nitrogen fixation   Process of converting atmospheric nitrogen into nitrogenous compounds.

nonpathogen   A microorganism which does not cause disease under ordinary circumstances.

nonsense codon   Three nitrogen bases on mRNA which do not specify any amino acid and are responsible for terminating polypeptide synthesis.

nosocomial   Hospital-acquired

nucleocapsid   Virion and capsid of a virus.

nucleolus   RNA-rich portion of a nucleus.

nucleoside A subunit of nucleic acids containing a purine or pyrimidine and a sugar.

nucleotide A subunit of nucleic acids containing a purine or pyrimidine, sugar, and phosphoric acid.

nucleus DNA-rich portion of a cell occurring as a central membrane-enclosed body in eucaryotic cells.

O

obligate Necessary or required.

oncogenic Having the ability to induce tumors.

onychia Inflammation of the nail bed.

oocyst Encysted form of an ookinete.

ookinete Wormlike zygote of malarial parasites.

oophoritis Inflammation of the ovary.

operculum Polar cap of an ovum.

operon Cluster of genes containing a regulatory gene and structural genes.

ophthalmia neonatorum Purulent conjunctivitis in a newborn.

opportunist A normally nonpathogenic microorganism which produces disease under special circumstances.

opsonin A substance which promotes adherence of microorganisms to the surface of phagocytes.

optical density A unit of measurement for the amount of light excluded by a turbid or colored solution.

optochin The chemical ethyl hydrocuprein, used to differentiate *Streptococcus pneumoniae* (sensitive) from other alpha *Streptococcus* species (resistant).

orchitis Inflammation of the testes.

organelle A structure of a cell having a particular function.

osmotolerance Ability to tolerate variation in osmotic pressure.

osteoclast A macrophage of bone tissue.

OT (old tuberculin) A product of *Mycobacterium tuberculosis.*

otitis media Inflammation of the middle ear.

ovum Female reproductive cell; egg.

oxidation Addition of oxygen or removal of hydrogen from a molecule.

P

palliative Serving to relieve rather than to cure.

pandemic Occurring at the same time in widespread parts of the world.

pannus A covering of vascular tissue.

panophthalmitis Inflammation of the entire eye.

parasite An organism dependent on another organism for resources to support life.

parenteral Pertaining to any route of entry into the body other than through the alimentary canal.

paresis Partial paralysis.

paronychia Inflammation of tissue surrounding the nail.

paroxysm Sudden attack of coughing.

passive agglutination An antigen-antibody reaction in which a soluble antigen adsorbed to particles reacts with specific antibody causing clumping of particles.

passive immunity Resistance to infectious agents acquired *in utero* or by administration of products of lymphocytes.

passive transport Movement of molecules from an area of greater concentration to an area of lesser concentration using energy created by random collisions of molecules.

pasteurization Process of heating substances at a particular temperature for a specified length of time to kill nonspore-forming pathogens and reduce the total number of microorganisms.

pathogen A disease-producing microorganism.

pathognomonic Pertaining to signs or symptoms of illness.

peplos Envelope surrounding a virus.

peptidoglycan A polymer composed of amino acids and carbohydrate derivatives making up the walls of procaryotic cells.

perforation Process of making a hole.

perineum Region comprising skin, muscles, and fasciae between the vulva or scrotum and the anus.

periplasm Space between the cytoplasmic membrane and cell wall.

peritoneum Membrane lining abdominal cavity and covering abdominal organs.

permease An enzyme facilitating active transport of molecules across a cytoplasmic membrane.

phage conversion Process of rendering a bacterium into a toxigenic strain by phage-mediated genes.

phagocyte A cell having the ability to engulf solid particles.

phenol coefficient Ratio between the greatest dilution of a disinfectant killing a test organism in 10 minutes, but not in 5 minutes, to the greatest dilution of phenol producing the same result.

phenotype Observable characteristics of an organism; produced by the genotype in cooperation with environmental factors.

phialophora A fungal sporulation in which conidia are borne by a budding process from flask-shaped conidiophores.

photoautotroph An organism capable of synthesizing organic compounds using light energy.

photodynamic action Combined effect of light and certain dyes on microorganisms.

photooxidation Chemical reaction by which absorption of light by cell substances causes death of microorganisms.

photoreactivation Process whereby visible light repairs DNA molecules following injury by ultraviolet radiation.

photosynthesis Process of making carbohydrates from carbon dioxide and water in the presence of photopigments and light.

phytohemagglutinin (PHA) A substance derived from plants which promotes mitosis in artificially cultured lymphocytes.

pili Filamentous appendages of some bacteria responsible for adherence.

plaque (dental) A mass of bacteria adhering to the surface of a tooth.

plaque (viral) A clear area on a lawn of bacterial growth or on a monolayer of cells caused by lysis of virus-infected cells.

plaque-forming unit (PFU) A quantitative expression of the number of infectious phages per milliliter.

plasma cell Progeny of a B-cell lymphocyte.

plasmid   A fragment of DNA within the cytoplasm.

pleomorphic   Having many shapes.

plerocercoid   A sparganum larva of tapeworms.

plexus   A network of nerves, blood vessels, or lymphatics.

point mutation   A mutation which usually affects only a single nucleotide of the genome.

polymer   A covalently bonded group of molecular subunits of the same type (monomers).

polyploid   Having increased numbers of chromosomes.

postabortal   Following abortion.

postpartum   Following delivery.

PPD (purified protein derivative)   A purified product of *Mycobacterium tuberculosis.*

precipitation   An antigen-antibody reaction taking place between soluble antigen and specific antibody.

precursor   A substance which precedes another in a specific pathway.

primary cell line   A cell line which can be maintained under laboratory conditions for a limited time.

procaryotic cell   A cell having no nuclear membrane or membrane-bound organelles.

procercoid   Spindle-shaped larval form of tapeworms.

prodromal   Stage of disease between the earliest symptoms and the appearance of a rash or fever.

progeny   Offspring.

proglottid   A segment of a tapeworm.

promastigote   Extracellular form of a blood or tissue flagellate found in an intermediate host.

properdin   A nonspecific resistance factor active against some viruses and gram-negative bacteria.

prophage   Nucleic acid of a temperate phage when integrated into the genome of a host cell.

prophylaxis   Prevention.

proprietary   Pertaining to the trade name of a drug.

prosthetic group   Nonprotein component of an enzyme.

protoplasm   Living material of cells.

prototroph   An organism that can synthesize nutritional growth factors.

protozoacide   An agent which destroys protozoa.

prozone   Absence of agglutination in the region of excess antibody; absence of precipitation in the region of excess antigen.

pseudohyphae   Chains of elongated yeast cells resembling hyphae.

pseudomembranous colitis   Inflammation of the colon associated with antimicrobial therapy.

pseudopodia   Projections of cytoplasm appearing during movement of some protozoa.

psychrophile   A microorganism tolerating temperatures of $-5°$ to $20°C$.

ptomaine   A nitrogenous product derived from putrefactive action of bacteria.

purine   A nine-membered cyclic nitrogen base found in nucleic acids (adenine and guanine).

purpura   Bleeding.

purulent   Pus-containing.

pyelitis   Inflammation of the pelvis portion of the kidney.

pyoderma   Infection of the skin characterized by a prolific amount of pus.

pyrimidine A six-membered cyclic nitrogen base found in nucleic acids (cytosine, thymine, and uracil).
pyrogenic Fever-producing.

Q

quellung reaction A precipitin reaction which causes capsules to swell in the presence of specific antibody.

R

racial immunity Resistance to infectious agents occurring within a particular race.
radial immunodiffusion A method for quantitating antigen in an antibody-containing agar gel which measures the area of precipitate formed around an antigen well.
radiation Energy traveling through space as electromagnetic waves.
radioimmunoassay A method for quantitating antigen or antibody which employs radiolabeled components.
reagin An antibody associated with atopic hypersensitivity; the nonprotective antibody of syphilis.
redia A saclike structure comprising a developmental stage of a digenetic fluke.
reduction Addition of hydrogen or removal of oxygen from a molecule.
replica plating A technique used for separating mutants from parent cells in a mixed population.
repression Process by which the function of a gene is inhibited in the presence of a particular substrate.
respiration Energy-liberating process of cells.

reverse transcription Process of transferring genetic information from RNA to DNA.
rhabditiform Noninfective, feeding larval stage.
rhinitis Inflammation of the nasal mucosa.
ribosome An organelle of cells responsible for protein synthesis.
rod Receptor cell for black and white on the retina.
rostellum Hook-bearing protrusion on anterior end of scolex of a tapeworm.

S

saccharophile An organism that tolerates high concentrations of sugar in the environment.
salpingitis Inflammation of the fallopian tube or eustachian tube.
sanitizer A chemical agent which renders an object or environment safe by reducing the number of microorganisms.
saprophyte A microorganism capable of living on dead organic material.
saprobe An organism which requires organic material as an energy source.
schizogony Asexual cycle of malarial parasites.
schizont Asexual dividing form of a malarial parasite.
Schultz-Charlton phenomenon Blanching of scarlet fever rash in the presence of specific antitoxin.
Schwann cells Cells comprising the membranous sheath surrounding a nerve fiber.

sclerosis Hardening or induration of tissue or an organ.

scolex Head of a tapeworm.

sedimentation constant (S) A quantitative expression of the relative sedimentation rate of molecules exposed to a gravitational field expressed in Svedberg units.

selective medium A culture medium which is inhibitory for particular organisms thereby permitting other organisms to grow.

septum A partition.

sequela Complication following an initial infection.

serology Study of the nature and reactions of humoral antibodies.

serous Serum-containing.

serum sickness An immunologic injury caused by the administration of heterologous serum.

sheath Visible slime layer of cyanobacteria.

Shwartzman reaction Localized hemorrhagic necrosis caused by injection of endotoxin.

smegma Thick secretion associated with genitalia.

somatic Pertaining to nonreproductive cells (genetics) or cell envelope (immunology).

specialized transduction Transfer of a restricted region of donor DNA by phage.

species immunity Resistance to infectious agents occurring within a particular species.

spike Surface projection on the envelope of some viruses.

sporangium Spherical, spore-bearing structure of fungi.

spore coat Layer between outer fore-spore membrane and exosporium of an endospore.

sporocyst Nonciliated, saclike structure comprising a developmental stage of a digenetic fluke.

sporogony Sexual cycle of malarial parasites.

sporozoite Infective stage of malarial parasite passed from mosquito to the human.

standard plate count (SPC) A cultural method for enumeration of bacteria.

stationary growth phase Phase of bacterial growth in which the number of viable cells is constant.

sterilization Process of destroying all microorganisms.

streptolysin Hemolysin produced by streptococci.

stye An abscess in a hair follicle of the eyelids.

subacute Having characteristics of less severity than an acute infection or disease.

substrate A substance acted upon by an enzyme.

suppurative Associated with pus formation.

surface tension Force exerted by a gas on a liquid at the interface.

symbiosis A mutually beneficial association between two organisms.

synapsis Lining up of homologous chromosomes in meiosis.

synchronous Occurring at the same time.

syncytia A network of fused cells.

syndrome A collection of symptoms.

synergism Process by which two microorganisms promote a reaction which neither can perform singly;

process by which total effect of combined substances is greater than the sum of the effects of the substances acting alone.

syngraft A transplant in which the donor and recipient are genetically identical.

T

T-antigen An antigen associated with a tumor cell.

T-cell Lymphocyte derived from the thymus responsible for cell-mediated immunity.

temperate phage A phage which can be integrated into the genome of a bacterium or replicate outside the chromosome and promote lysis.

template A single strand of DNA which acts as a pattern for synthesis of DNA or RNA.

thermal death point Temperature required to kill a particular microorganism after 10 minutes exposure.

thermal death time Length of time required to kill a particular microorganism at a specific temperature.

thermophile A microorganism which grows at temperatures of 45°C or above.

thylacoid Chlorophyll-containing membrane of cyanobacteria.

thymine A nitrogenous base of the DNA molecule.

thymus A gland in the thoracic cavity necessary for development and maturation of T-cell lymphocytes.

tinea A superficial infection of the skin caused by fungi; ringworm.

Tine test Tuberculin skin test which employs OT dried on needle points.

titer A quantitative expression of antibody concentration expressed as the reciprocal of the highest dilution of serum producing a visible antigen-antibody reaction.

toxigenic Having the ability to produce toxins.

toxin A poison produced by microorganisms.

toxoid An attenuated toxin.

transcription Process of transferring genetic information from DNA to mRNA.

transduction Process of transferring genetic material from one bacterium to another by a virus.

transfer factor An extract of human blood lymphocytes.

transfer RNA Type of RNA which transports amino acids to ribosomes.

transformation Process of transferring genetic material as soluble DNA from one bacterium to another of the same species; conversion of a cell to an altered state.

transition Replacement of a purine by another purine or of a pyrimidine by another pyrimidine on the DNA molecule.

translation Process of specifying amino acid content of a protein by mRNA.

transovarial Transferred by means of the ovary (or egg).

transtracheal Across or through the trachea.

transversion Replacement of a purine by a pyrimidine or a pyrimidine by a purine on the DNA molecule.

trauma Injury.

trophozoite Vegetative cell of a protozoan.

trypanosome Extracellular form of a blood or tissue flagellate found in intermediate and definitive hosts.

trypomastigote Extracellular form of a blood or tissue flagellate found in intermediate and definitive hosts.

tubercle A cheeselike lesion of tuberculosis.

tuberculin A protein fraction of *Mycobacterium tuberculosis*.

tubulin A protein associated with microtubules.

tumor-associated antigen An antigen produced by a neoplastic cell.

tympanocentesis Puncture of the eardrum (tympanic membrane).

tyndallization Process used to kill spore-forming bacteria by employing intermittent exposure to flowing steam.

U

ultracentrifuge A high-velocity centrifuge used to separate colloidal or submicroscopic particles.

ultrasound Vibration frequencies above 20,000 cycles per second.

ultraviolet Invisible rays emitted by the sun having wavelengths of 150 to 3900 Å.

uracil A nitrogenous base of the RNA molecule.

V

vaccination Inoculation of living, dead, or attenuated microorganisms or microbial products.

vacuole An accumulation of liquid or gaseous material within cytoplasm.

valence Degree of combining power of an element or radical.

vector An animate carrier of infectious agents.

vegetative Referring to the growing, reproducing form of a microorganism.

venereal Sex-associated.

venom Poison derived from certain animals or insects.

ventricle A small cavity.

vernacular Common.

V factor A coenzyme required for growth of some *Haemophilus* species.

Vi antigen Capsular antigen of virulent strains of *Salmonella typhi*.

viremia Presence of viruses in the blood.

viricide An agent which destroys viruses.

virion Intact infective core particle of a virus.

viropexis Process by which a virus enters a cell.

virulence Ability to produce disease; pathogenicity.

virulent phage A phage that replicates within a bacterium producing cell lysis which releases new infective particles.

virus A submicroscopic biological entity exhibiting characteristics of life in host cells.

visceral larva migrans Infections of internal organs caused by migration of nematode larvae.

W

wavelength Distance between corresponding points on any two consecutive waves.

Weil-Felix reaction Agglutination of certain *Proteus* antigens by rickettsial antibodies.

Widal test An agglutination procedure used for the detection of antibodies to typhoid and paratyphoid fevers.

X

xenodiagnosis A procedure employing laboratory-grown reduviid bugs for the diagnosis of Chagas' disease.

xenograft A transplant in which donor and recipient are of dissimilar species.

X factor Heme portion of the hemoglobin required for growth by some *Haemophilus* species.

Z

Ziehl-Neelsen stain An acid-fast staining procedure employing heat.

zoophilic Referring to fungi having a primary affinity for animals, but which can also infect humans.

zygote A cell formed by the union of a male and a female gamete.

zygotic induction Process whereby a prophage is triggered to multiply vegetatively in a host cell following conjugation or transduction.

Index

81 82 83 84 9 8 7 6 5 4 3 2 1